WinkingSkull.com

Your study aid for must-know anatomy

T0257207

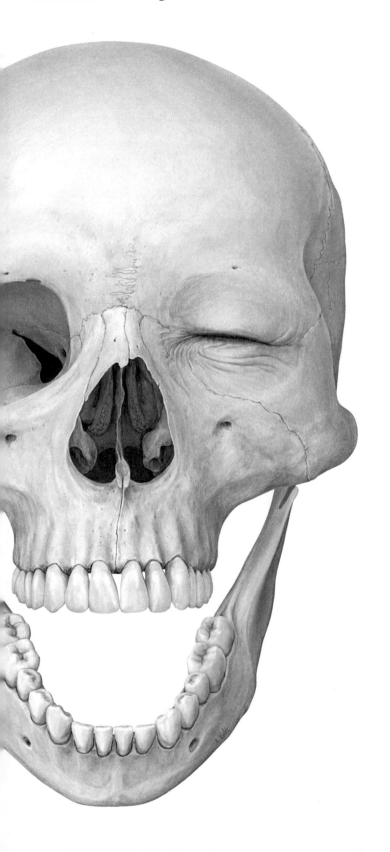

Register for WinkingSkull.com *PLUS* – master human anatomy with this unique interactive online learning tool.

Use the access code below to register for **WinkingSkull.com** *PLUS* and view over 1,200 full-color illustrations and radiographs from *Anatomy for Dental Medicine*. After studying this invaluable image bank, you can quiz yourself on key body structures and get your score instantly to check your progress or to compare with other users' results.

WinkingSkull.com *PLUS* has everything you need for course study and exam prep:

- More than 1,200 full-color anatomy illustrations
- Intuitive design that simplifies navigation
- "Labels-on, labels-off" function that makes studying easy and fun
- Timed self-tests–with instant results

Simply visit WinkingSkull.com and follow these instructions to get started today.

If you do not already have a free WinkingSkull.com account, visit www.winkingskull.com, click on "Register" and complete the registration form. Enter the scratch-off code below.

If you already have a WinkingSkull.com account, go to the "Manage Account" page and click on the "Register a Code" link. Enter the scratch-off code below.

This product cannot be returned if the access code panel is scratched off.

Some functionalities on WinkingSkull.com require support for advanced web technologies. A major browser (IE, Chrome, Firefox, Safari) within the last three major versions is suggested for use on the site.

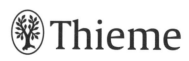

Laryngeal Function and Voice Disorders

Basic Science to Clinical Practice

Christopher R. Watts, PhD
Professor and Director
Davies School of Communication Sciences and Disorders
Texas Christian University
Fort Worth, Texas, USA

Shaheen N. Awan, PhD
Professor and Chair
Department of Communication Sciences & Disorders
Bloomsburg University of Pennsylvania
Bloomsburg, Pennsylvania, USA

179 illustrations

Thieme
New York • Stuttgart • Delhi • Rio de Janeiro

Executive Editor: Delia DeTurris
Managing Editor: Elizabeth Palumbo
Director, Editorial Services: Mary Jo Casey
Production Editor: Torsten Scheihagen
International Production Director: Andreas Schabert
Editorial Director: Sue Hodgson
International Marketing Director: Fiona Henderson
International Sales Director: Louisa Turrell
Director of Institutional Sales: Adam Bernacki
Senior Vice President and Chief Operating Officer: Sarah Vanderbilt
President: Brian D. Scanlan
Printer: King Printing
Illustrator: Alyssa Minatel

Library of Congress Cataloging-in-Publication Data

Names: Watts, Christopher R., author. | Awan, Shaheen N., author.
Title: Laryngeal function and voice disorders : basic science to clinical practice / Christopher R. Watts, Shaheen N. Awan.
Description: New York : Thieme, [2019] | Includes bibliographical references.
Identifiers: LCCN 2018001577| ISBN 9781626233904 (hardcover) | ISBN 9781626233911 (ebook)
Subjects: | MESH: Larynx--physiology | Phonation--physiology | Voice Disorders | Laryngeal Neoplasms–rehabilitation
Classification: LCC QP306 | NLM WV 500 | DDC 612.2/33--dc23 LC record available at https://lccn.loc.gov/2018001577

Thieme Publishers New York
333 Seventh Avenue, New York, NY 10001 USA
+1 800 782 3488, customerservice@thieme.com

Thieme Publishers Stuttgart
Rüdigerstrasse 14, 70469 Stuttgart, Germany
+49 [0]711 8931 421, customerservice@thieme.de

Thieme Publishers Delhi
A-12, Second Floor, Sector-2, Noida-201301
Uttar Pradesh, India
+91 120 45 566 00, customerservice@thieme.in

Thieme Publishers Rio de Janeiro, Thieme Publicações Ltda.
Edifício Rodolpho de Paoli, 25º andar
Av. Nilo Peçanha, 50 – Sala 2508,
Rio de Janeiro 20020-906 Brasil
+55 21 3172-2297 / +55 21 3172-1896
www.thiemerevinter.com.br

Cover design: Thieme Publishing Group
Typesetting by DiTech Process Solutions

Printed in the United States by King Printing   5 4 3 2 1

ISBN 978-1-62623-390-4

Also available as an e-book:
eISBN 978-1-62623-391-1

Important note: Medicine is an ever-changing science undergoing continual development. Research and clinical experience are continually expanding our knowledge, in particular our knowledge of proper treatment and drug therapy. Insofar as this book mentions any dosage or application, readers may rest assured that the authors, editors, and publishers have made every effort to ensure that such references are in accordance with **the state of knowledge at the time of production of the book**.

Nevertheless, this does not involve, imply, or express any guarantee or responsibility on the part of the publishers in respect to any dosage instructions and forms of applications stated in the book. **Every user is requested to examine carefully** the manufacturers' leaflets accompanying each drug and to check, if necessary in consultation with a physician or specialist, whether the dosage schedules mentioned therein or the contraindications stated by the manufacturers differ from the statements made in the present book. Such examination is particularly important with drugs that are either rarely used or have been newly released on the market. Every dosage schedule or every form of application used is entirely at the user's own risk and responsibility. The authors and publishers request every user to report to the publishers any discrepancies or inaccuracies noticed. If errors in this work are found after publication, errata will be posted at www.thieme.com on the product description page.

Some of the product names, patents, and registered designs referred to in this book are in fact registered trademarks or proprietary names even though specific reference to this fact is not always made in the text. Therefore, the appearance of a name without designation as proprietary is not to be construed as a representation by the publisher that it is in the public domain.

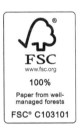

To my students: Your questions, thoughts, and insights continue to inspire me and constantly reaffirm that no person on earth has a better job than I.

To Curtis and Susan Marsh: My second parents—your support is a large reason that I have been able to pursue my professional and personal dreams.

To my parents, Michael and Glynis Watts: Mom and pop, you were, are, and will continue to be the greatest parents on earth and the most important influence on my achievements and outlook on life. I love you.

To my children, Lindsey and Emily: You are the meaning to my life. I could not love anything more than I love the two of you.

To my wife, Debbie: You ground me, center me, and give me the foundation to be a great person, father, and professional. I will always love, want, and need you. Always and forever.

—Christopher R. Watts

To my mother Samina Awan; to my brothers Paul and Martyn and their families; and, of course, to my wife Karen, my daughter Rachel and son in-law Josh, and my son Jordan. Love and thanks to all! To my father Nazir A. Awan (1930-2018)—"In God's Loving Care."

—Shaheen N. Awan

Contents

Foreword vii

Preface ix

Acknowledgments x

Media Content xi

1. Anatomy and Physiology of Phonation 1

2. Survey of Voice Disorders 28

3. The Voice Diagnostic: Initial Considerations, Case History, and Perceptual Evaluation 69

4. Acoustic Analysis of Voice 95

5. Aerodynamic Analyses of Vocal Function 161

6. Laryngeal Endoscopy and Stroboscopy 186

7. Medical Treatment of Voice Disorders 211

8. Voice Treatment: Orientations, Framework, and Interventions 225

9. Voice Rehabilitation after Laryngeal Cancer 260

    Index 285

Foreword

Laryngeal Function and Voice Disorders: Basic Science to Clinical Practice, by Christopher Watts and Shaheen Awan, is an outstanding addition to our literature. It combines the acumen of some of our field's most distinguished scholars with a wealth of experience in teaching, research, and expert practical experience. Drs. Watts and Awan have created a textbook that expertly details laryngeal function and voice disorders and will prove to be an invaluable resource for students and voice-care professionals.

Each of the nine chapters are succinctly organized into the following format: a summary, learning objectives, introduction, body of chapter, clinical case vignette, test question with detailed answers, references and suggested future readings. The abundance of carefully selected references enables readers to pursue further detail as desired.

Although the prose of a textbook is paramount, the design can take a textbook to a new level. Both prose and design are exceptional in this textbook. From high-resolution images of vocal pathologies and surgeries to clear and concise tables and graphs, the illustrations complement the prose wonderfully well. The systematic use of headings, bolded print for importance and high-definition rich color of the illustrations create a beautiful textbook for the mind as well as for the senses.

The organization of each chapter not only relates information well; for the new student, it also organizes the information for active learning. The test questions near the end of each chapter are thoughtful, but it is the detailed answers of each that continue to translate what they have *learned* into *learning*. Drs. Watts and Awan take it one step further by *applying* what has been read to clinical cases. This is how material "comes alive" for a student. Bravo.

Not only are each of the chapters clearly organized but the through-line of the entire book takes the reader through what is needed to help a patient. Said differently, the text has been organized in a practical, logical sequence for patient care. The reader learns what are the "normal" processes of laryngeal function before proceeding to the study of the abnormal processes. Next, a survey of typical voice disorders is concisely described—again, with incredibly complete tables for ease of learning. Four chapters are devoted to how to assess a patient with a voice disorder from taking a clinical history, capturing voice lab measures, and visualizing the larynx. The chapters of the book conclude with how to help patients by outlining a plethora of treatment options.

The tables, diagrams, and graphs deserve special recognition as, quite frankly, they are fantastic. The active professional wanting to find references and information quickly will find it in this book. Furthermore, the new clinician wanting to set up a voice lab (acoustics, aerodynamics, audio-perceptual) will have to look no further than this book. The reader will be impressed with the clarity of the presentations of different acoustic, aerodynamic, and audio-perceptual assessments, as well as examples of patient reported outcome measures.

Christopher Watts and Shaheen Awan in *Laryngeal Function and Voice Disorders* have written a comprehensive, beautifully designed textbook which will significantly contribute to the professional growth of speech-language pathology and laryngology, and, ultimately, care of patients. It is an invaluable addition to the literature and should be in the library of every voice-care professional.

Jackie Gartner-Schmidt, PhD, CCC-SLP, ASHA Fellow
Professor
Co-Director of the University of Pittsburgh Voice Center
Director of Speech Pathology-Voice Division
University of Pittsburgh Medical Center
School of Medicine-Department of Otolaryngology
Pittsburgh, Pennsylvania, USA

Preface

As the discipline of communication sciences and disorders enters the third decade of the 21st century, it is remarkable to consider how specialized the profession of speech–language pathology has become. Already our national credentialing organization (the American Speech-Language-Hearing Association or ASHA) recognizes four clinical specialty certifications: child language and language disorders, fluency and fluency disorders, swallowing and swallowing disorders, and intraoperative monitoring. In addition to these current specialty recognitions, a growing number of academic and community-based speech–language pathologists are focusing their research and clinical practice on voice science and populations with voice disorders. Though now over 20 years old, the term "vocologist" (Titze 1994) is being more widely used as a reference to those professionals who possess expert knowledge and skill in voice and airway disorders. In fact, in recognition of the unique knowledge and skills necessary to evaluate and treat populations experiencing voice and airway impairments, at the time of this writing, a working group of professionals associated with ASHA's Special Interest Group 3: Voice and Voice Disorders are submitting a proposal to develop a clinical specialty certification in this domain of clinical practice.

It is these developments which have motivated the authors to develop this new text, *Laryngeal Function and Voice Disorders: Basic Science to Clinical Practice*. While this book initially started as an update to a previous text entitled *The Voice Diagnostic Protocol: A Practical Guide to the Diagnosis of Voice Disorders* (Awan 2001), further discussion between the authors and feedback from a group of initial reviewers resulted in a new goal of developing a highly comprehensive learning resource for graduate students and certified clinicians which merges historical facts and experiential understanding with recent advances in scientific knowledge and evidence-based clinical diagnostic and treatment practice patterns. We chose a deliberate title to reflect the content of this text: *"Laryngeal Function"* represents a focus on laryngeal behavior across multidimensional behaviors, including laryngeal physiology in breathing, voice, and cough; *"Voice Disorders"* represents a detailed focus on the varied impairments which can lead to voice and airway disorders; *"Basic Science"* reflects inclusion of a strong foundation in the anatomical, physiological, acoustic, aerodynamic, and imaging science that informs our understanding of function in normal and disordered states; and *"Clinical Practice"* reflects a comprehensive focus on processes and options available to the speech–language pathologist for the evaluation, diagnosis, and treatment of voice and airway impairments.

In developing this text, we were motivated to merge our combined 50-plus years of knowledge and experience of laryngeal and voice science with detailed descriptions of this scientific understanding to ensure that the information provided herein can be translated into clinical practice. Our efforts to ensure this translation include (1) detailed explanations for evaluation and treatment rationale, (2) step-by-step instructions for instrumental assessments used during the process of voice evaluation, (3) frameworks to guide the clinical application of different voice treatments, (4) explanations for the roles of medical collaborators with an emphasis on otolaryngology, and (5) accompanying multimedia as a resource to facilitate learning. It is our hope and expectation that the readers of this text will find a comprehensive, detailed, yet easy-to-read resource that will aid them as they strive to improve their skills in vocology and capability to provide highly effective diagnostic and treatment services for their patients with voice disorders.

Acknowledgments

The professional accomplishments I have realized, including this textbook, would not have been possible without a solid foundation in the discipline of communication sciences and disorders, which was provided to me by the faculty of the Department of Speech Pathology and Audiology at the University of South Alabama. Much of the content within this book is an extension of knowledge created and disseminated by the legends of voice science. In compiling the data-driven information supporting many of the chapters in this book, I am indebted to the many students—my lab rats—who have worked to the point of exhaustion in compiling sources of evidence to further validate the information we have put down in pages.

—*Christopher R. Watts*

Thanks to the many esteemed colleagues in the field of voice science and disorders whom I have had the opportunity to know and work with over the years. Many of these colleagues are recognized as some of the best voice scientists in the world and their knowledge and experience has helped me benefit and develop in my own work. Of course, thanks also to my many students who have worked closely with me over the years both in the classroom and in research contexts—their desire to learn more about voice has encouraged me to do my best to provide them with the knowledge and explanations that they need to progress as highly competent clinicians and future researchers in their own right.

— *Shaheen N. Awan*

Media Content

4 Acoustic Analysis of Voice
Sample 4.1–Sample 4.25

6 Laryngeal Endoscopy and Stroboscopy
Video 6.1 Vocal fold paralysis. (From Kendall K, Leonard R. Laryngeal Evaluation, 1st ed. New York: Thieme Publishers, 2010.)
Video 6.2 Vocal tremor. (From Kendall K, Leonard R. Laryngeal Evaluation, 1st ed. New York: Thieme Publishers, 2010.)
Video 6.3 Medial compression of false vocal folds. (From Kendall K, Leonard R. Laryngeal Evaluation, 1st ed. New York: Thieme Publishers, 2010.)
Video 6.4 Normal vibratory parameters.
Video 6.5 Phase asymmetry. (From Kendall K, Leonard R. Laryngeal Evaluation, 1st ed. New York: Thieme Publishers, 2010.)
Video 6.6 Reduced amplitude of vibration. (From Kendall K, Leonard R. Laryngeal Evaluation, 1st ed. New York: Thieme Publishers, 2010.)
Video 6.7 Vibration irregularity. (From Kendall K, Leonard R. Laryngeal Evaluation, 1st edition. New York: Thieme Publishers, 2010.)

Video 6.8 Reduced mucosal wave. (From Kendall K, Leonard R. Laryngeal Evaluation, 1st ed. New York: Thieme Publishers, 2010.)

8 Voice Treatment: Orientations, Framework, and Interventions
Video 8.1 Resonant voice therapy. (From Aronson A, Bless D. Clinical Voice Disorders. 4th ed. New York: Thieme Publishers; 2009.)
Video 8.2 Vocal function exercises. (From Aronson A, Bless D. Clinical Voice Disorders. 4th ed. New York: Thieme Publishers; 2009.)
Video 8.3 The manual laryngeal muscle tension reduction technique. (From Aronson A, Bless D. Clinical Voice Disorders. 4th ed. New York: Thieme Publishers; 2009.)
Video 8.4 Lee Silverman voice treatment. (From Aronson A, Bless D. Clinical Voice Disorders. 4th ed. New York: Thieme Publishers; 2009.)
Video 8.5 Vocal cord dysfunction. (From Aronson A, Bless D. Clinical Voice Disorders. 4th ed. New York: Thieme Publishers; 2009.)
Video 8.6 Singing. (From Aronson A, Bless D. Clinical Voice Disorders. 4th ed. New York: Thieme Publishers; 2009.)

1 Anatomy and Physiology of Phonation

Summary

This chapter describes the anatomy and physiology of key laryngeal structures involved in *phonation* (i.e., vocal fold vibration). A description of the cartilaginous framework, connective tissues, intrinsic and extrinsic laryngeal muscles, and details of neural innervation are provided and physiological principles underlying vocal fold oscillation are explained. Because the process of phonation is a combination of respiratory and laryngeal function, a basic description of inspiratory and expiratory activity and control will also be provided. Finally, the relationship between normal anatomy and physiology to disordered conditions is presented.

Keywords: larynx, phonation, respiration, voice, dysphonia

1.1 Learning Objectives

At the end of this chapter, learners will be able to
- Identify the cartilaginous, soft tissue, and neurological substrates of the larynx.
- Compare and contrast the roles of intrinsic and extrinsic laryngeal muscles.
- Discuss the aerodynamic and muscular forces underlying vocal fold vibration during phonation.
- Compare and contrast muscular and neurological control during adjustments of vocal fundamental frequency and intensity.
- Identify key musculature involved in inspiration and expiration and describe the necessary coordination between respiratory and laryngeal function to produce phonation.
- Describe the key characteristics of the sound wave produced at the vocal fold level and how supraglottal function affects and transforms this sound.

1.2 Introduction

Phonation is primarily the result of aerodynamic forces acting on the inherently elastic tissue of the vocal folds, setting them into vibration and creating acoustic energy which we call "**voice.**" The characteristics of this vibration (e.g., the frequency of vibration) may be modified by muscular forces which influence the effective mass and tension of the vibrating folds. We are constantly modifying the aerodynamic and muscular forces underlying voice production to result in the wide variations of pitch and loudness produced in typical speech or in other aspects of voice function such as singing.

When laryngeal structure or physiology is impaired, the result may be a negative impact on laryngeal function, the efficiency of phonation, communication effectiveness, and subsequent perceptual characteristics of voice quality. The negative impacts on phonation and voice quality are perceptually labeled as **dysphonia**, which many speech–language pathologists will encounter during clinical practice. The purpose of this chapter is to provide an overview of the anatomy and physiology underlying normal, healthy phonation as a foundation to facilitate advanced understanding of impairments that result in dysphonia and their assessment, diagnosis, and treatment, which subsequent chapters will cover.

1.3 Evolution and Biological Roles of the Larynx

Voice production is considered an "overlaid" or nonbiological function of the larynx, taking a backseat to respiration, airway protection, and the generation of lung pressure to fixate the thorax during physical activity. According to Hirose, the larynx evolved as a simple muscular sphincter atop the primitive lung that would protect against entry of water or food.[1] This sphincter evolved into a more complicated valve capable of abduction (separation) or adduction (combination) at various levels within the larynx. Eventually, in mammals this protective structure also became used as a type of flutter valve that would vibrate during the controlled expiration.

During passive and active respiration, the **glottis** (the space between the two vocal folds) acts as an air valve. At rest, the two vocal folds lie in an **abducted** (away from midline) position creating an open glottis and a continuous passageway from the lungs to the oral cavity. During inspiratory cycles, the glottis will widen and then return to a resting open position during expiration. Deep, forceful inhalations will be accompanied by an even wider glottis. The vocal folds can be adjusted to an **adducted** (toward midline) position, so that the glottis will close forcefully to allow for the buildup of subglottal air pressure, which is required for coughing and clearing material that inadvertently falls into or irritates the larynx, trachea, or lungs. By closing the glottis in this manner, an individual can also fixate the thorax to direct muscular effort to the limbs for lifting and exercise. In a similar manner, glottal closure allows for the generation of abdominal pressures for bodily functions such as defecation.

Phonation for speech is an intentional (voluntary) behavior, but a number of involuntary reflexes mediated by the nervous system can override phonation, interrupting ongoing voice production (e.g., causing a voice break) or preventing a speaker from initiating phonation (e.g., think about food/liquid "going down the wrong pipe" when swallowing—you will experience strong laryngeal closure and/or cough, but not be able to produce voice until the stimulus is cleared). Peripheral sensory receptors located throughout the laryngeal surfaces can elicit adductor responses and cough subsequent to noxious stimuli. Central nervous system (CNS) pattern generators also mediate tonic and phasic activity in the 10th cranial nerve, called the **vagus nerve**, during respiration and swallowing.

The **laryngeal adductor reflex** is a response triggered by activation of the sensory division of the vagus nerve, which elicits activity within a brainstem nucleus called the **solitary tract nucleus** (STN—a.k.a., nucleus tractus solitaries; ▶ Fig. 1.1) in the medulla. The STN forms a reflex loop with the motor nucleus of the vagus nerve, the **nucleus ambiguus** (NA). Upon activation, the STN relays excitatory signals to the NA which then stimulates activity in the laryngeal adductor muscles via firing of **alpha motor neurons**.

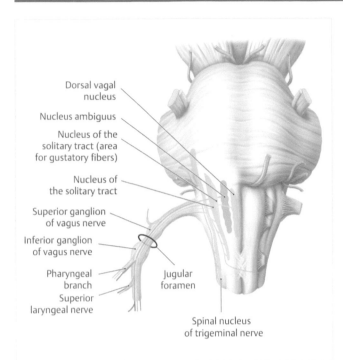

Fig. 1.1 Locations of sensory and motor nuclei of the vagus nerve in the brainstem. (From LaPointe L. Atlas of Neuroanatomy for Communication Science and Disorders, 1st ed. New York: Thieme Publishers; 2011.)

This reflex serves to forcefully close the glottis to protect the lower airway. At its most extreme, the laryngeal adductor reflex can present as **laryngospasm**, which is a prolonged tonic contraction of the laryngeal adductor muscles.

The production of **cough** can be under voluntary or involuntary control by the nervous system. Involuntary cough is triggered by stimulation of the laryngeal sensory receptors and typically serves to eliminate foreign particles or adverse sensations throughout the larynx or in the subglottic spaces.[2] The physiology of cough can be grouped into three phases: an *inspiratory phase* involving recruitment of the inspiratory muscles (diaphragm and intercostals), a *compressive phase* involving recruitment of the expiratory muscles along with strong medial compression at the glottis via recruitment of the laryngeal adductors (and subsequent buildup of subglottal pressure), and an *expulsive phase* via recruitment of additional activity in the abdominal muscles resulting in high pressure air pulses being sent through the glottis.[2] The pressure pulses flowing through the glottis help to clear the airway but also result in phonation, producing the familiar perception of a cough sound. Conscious suppression of cough is possible through cortical mechanisms; however, the neural circuitry which allows for this voluntary override of the cough reflex is not well understood.[3] Voice therapy focusing on conscious control and patterning of the respiratory muscles along with semiocclusion (narrowing) in the oral cavity during exhalation are used as a behavioral voice therapy modality to treat conditions of chronic cough.[4]

It is clear that the basic biological functions of the larynx generally have precedence over the overlaid development of behavioral voice function. In fact, the body's need to breathe or protect the trachea and lungs can interrupt phonation, which many readers of this book will have experienced when trying to speak while swallowing or after an exhausting physical exercise.

1.4 Respiratory Function

Phonation is built upon a foundation of respiration. Respiratory drive provides the power source for phonation. Speakers breathe during speech using a combination of diaphragmatic and thoracic muscular activity. Primary use of the **diaphragm** (▶ Fig. 1.2) for speech breathing is considered the most efficient method as its contraction is not resisted by bone, whereas the thoracic muscles must expand the rib cage to influence lung volume. During passive rest breathing, brainstem pattern generators control respiratory cycles at an unconscious level. However, for speech, **pyramidal (voluntary) pathways** in the CNS engage the lower motor neurons (LMN) of specific spinal nerves that form the **phrenic nerve** (nerves C3, C4, and C5) which innervates the diaphragm. Spinal intercostal **nerves** also leave the spinal cord at the thoracic level to innervate the **internal** and **external intercostal muscles** (▶ Fig. 1.3). Diaphragmatic contraction moves the lungs inferiorly, while contraction of the external intercostal muscles moves the lungs horizontally and superiorly. This has the effect of increasing lung volume and lowering air pressure within the lungs, causing air to flow in for inspiration.

Exhalation during passive breathing is accomplished by rapid relaxation of the diaphragm and/or intercostal muscles. For speech, the air must be efficiently controlled. This is accomplished through two muscular checking actions: (1) relaxation of the diaphragm and external intercostals in concert with (2) increasing activation in the abdominal and internal intercostal muscles. The abdominal muscles are antagonistic to the diaphragm, while the internal intercostals are antagonistic to the external intercostals. These checking actions help control the outflow of air from the lungs to support speech production. Exhalation is also controlled at the level of the vocal folds, which act to valve the upward flowing air. Fully adducted vocal folds will completely seal the glottis, which will cause an increase in subglottal air pressure as exhalation from the lower lungs continues.

1.4.1 Nervous System Regulation of Respiration

The primary purpose of respiration is life sustenance, with respiratory support for speech being a secondary overlaid function. Nervous system pathways and regions that modulate the activity in respiratory muscles will vary depending on whether respiration is being controlled volitionally (e.g., during speech, holding breath, and blowing) or at an unconscious involuntary level (e.g., quiet breathing while reading, watching television, and sleeping). Control from involuntary pathways will override conscious voluntary control whenever the body detects an urgent need for different blood chemical levels (e.g., oxygen).

Conscious control of the respiratory cycle (inhalation/exhalation) involves cortical motor regions which include the bilateral pyramidal pathways. Pyramidal neurons, the majority of which originate in the primary motor cortex (precentral gyrus) of the frontal lobe, are responsible for executing motor programs for volitional, planned movement including respiratory activity

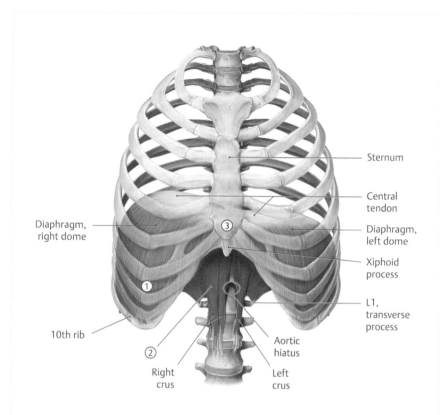

Fig. 1.2 The diaphragm. (From Baker E. Anatomy for Dental Medicine, 2nd ed. New York: Thieme Medical Publishers; 2016.)

Sternum

Central tendon

Diaphragm, left dome

Xiphoid process

L1, transverse process

Diaphragm, right dome

10th rib

Right crus

② ①

③

Aortic hiatus

Left crus

during speech production. These neurons will travel a direct route to synapse on LMNs in the brainstem and spinal cord. Target LMNs in the spinal cord include those of the intercostal and phrenic nerve, which travel into the periphery to innervate the diaphragm, intercostal, and abdominal muscles.

The brainstem **reticular formation** contains neurons which control the involuntary patterns of respiration (▸ Fig. 1.4). Located throughout the pons and medulla, the regions of reticular formation related to involuntary respiratory patterns can be organized into four areas, two in the pons (**pneumotaxic** and **apneustic** centers) and two in the medulla (**ventral respiratory group [VRG]** and **dorsal respiratory group [DRG]**). The medullary DRG acts as the pacemaker for involuntary/passive respiration. These neurons also drive activity in the VRG. The DRG needs stimulation to modulate respiratory activity—this stimulation arrives in the form of sensory information provided by peripheral sensory nerves via input from the lungs and cardiovascular system (mechanoreceptors and chemoreceptors). This peripheral stimulation also influences the **apneustic center**. When neurons of the DRG depolarize and fire, they send excitatory signals to the phrenic and intercostal nerves which innervate the diaphragm and external intercostal muscles, respectively. When ventilation demands are high, such as during physical exercise, the DRG will facilitate activity in neurons of the VRG, which then recruit additional motor neuron pools to further activate the muscles of inspiration and expiration.

The pontine pneumotaxic and apneustic centers can be thought of as "fine-tuning" the activity of the DRG. The apneustic center provides stimulation to the DRG to facilitate and prolong inspiration (e.g., when out of breath and needing to take deep, prolonged inhalations). The **pneumotaxic center** acts as an "off-switch" for inspiration. Neuronal activity in the pneumotaxic center causes termination of inspiration by inhibiting activity of the DRG. This in turn causes higher respiratory frequency (e.g., breathing faster) and reduced tidal volumes.

Activity of the brainstem respiratory pattern generator results in a resting respiratory rate of **12 to 16 breaths per minute**. Inspiration usually lasts approximately 2 seconds, and expiration lasts about 3 seconds. The normal inspiratory rate and rhythm is called **eupnea**, and difficult respiration is termed **dyspnea**. Respiratory rate and patterns can be modified when respiration is brought to a conscious level by voluntary acts (e.g., speech) and during complex involuntary reflexes such as sneezing, coughing, and vomiting. In addition, respiratory activity can be affected by conditions such as emotional state via input from the limbic system, or temperature via the hypothalamus.

The vagus nerve is also influenced by brainstem respiratory pattern generators and voluntary cortical pathways, and is active during voluntary and involuntary cycles of respiration. Laryngeal muscles controlled by the vagus are activated by brainstem respiratory centers during inspiration. The abduction–relaxation phasic action of the glottis resulting from this muscular activity is visible on laryngeal endoscopy when a patient is breathing at rest. During expiration, laryngeal muscles are also activated. Voluntary cortical control of laryngeal muscles during inspiration is present for such tasks as respiratory support for speech and deep inhalations, both of which require increased activity in laryngeal muscles via the vagus nerve to widen the glottis.

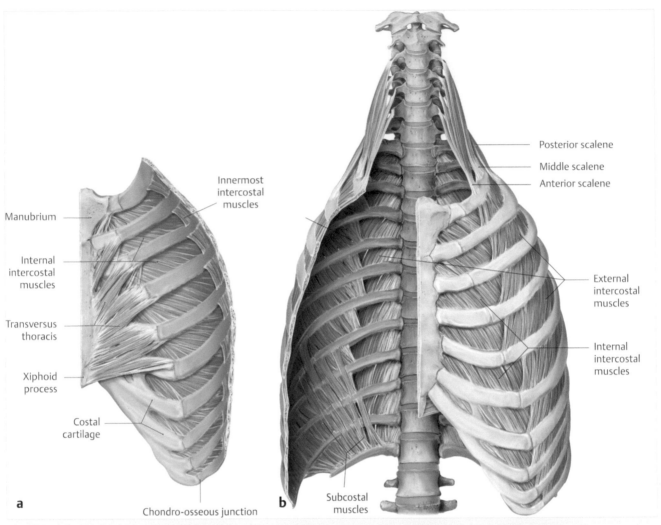

Manubrium

Internal intercostal muscles

Transversus thoracis

Xiphoid process

Costal cartilage

Innermost intercostal muscles

Posterior scalene

Middle scalene

Anterior scalene

External intercostal muscles

Internal intercostal muscles

Subcostal muscles

a

b

Chondro-osseous junction

Fig. 1.3 The intercostal muscles. (From Baker E. Anatomy for Dental Medicine, 2nd ed. New York: Thieme Medical Publishers; 2016.)

1.5 Laryngeal Framework

The larynx is located in the midline of the anterior neck (▶ Fig. 1.5), suspended from the hyoid bone above and attached to the trachea below via connective tissue (membranes, ligaments, and muscles). Removal of the connective tissue within the larynx would reveal a framework of six named cartilages (some are paired and some are unpaired). Five of these cartilages articulate with at least one other laryngeal cartilage, while the remaining one is suspended in connective tissue. Although technically not part of the laryngeal framework, the influence of the hyoid bone on laryngeal position must be emphasized. It is generally accepted that vertical hyoid position, which is determined by the degree of activation in muscles which attach to it, can have significant influence on the physiology of phonation.

1.5.1 Hyoid Bone

The hyoid is a horseshoe-shaped bone in the anterior midline of the neck positioned at the level of the third cervical vertebra. The broad central portion of the hyoid is referred to as the body, to which are fused two lateral (left and right) and superior bony projections called the "greater horns" (or cornu, which is Latin

for "horn") and "lesser horns" of the hyoid, respectively (▶ Fig. 1.6). The body, greater horns, and lesser horns serve as points of attachment for muscles and other connective tissue. The hyoid serves as an origin or insertion point for muscles that move the jaw, tongue, and larynx. Laryngeal muscles that connect to the hyoid can have the effect of elevating the hyoid bone in a superior and anterior direction, bringing the hyoid bone in closer approximation to the laryngeal framework, or depressing the larynx in an inferior direction.

1.5.2 Thyroid Cartilage

The singular (unpaired) thyroid cartilage is located in the anterior midline of the neck and forms a large portion of the anterior laryngeal border. The thyroid cartilage is shaped like a shield (▶ Fig. 1.6), formed by two broad plates (laminae) of hyaline cartilage which fuse at the midline. Numerous muscles attach to the thyroid lamina, influencing its vertical position. Superior and inferior thyroid horns (cornua) project from the posterior borders of the thyroid lamina and serve as point of attachment for connective tissue. At the apex of the thyroid midline, the fusion is incomplete creating the **thyroid notch**, which can be located by digital palpation in most adults. Immediately inferior to the notch

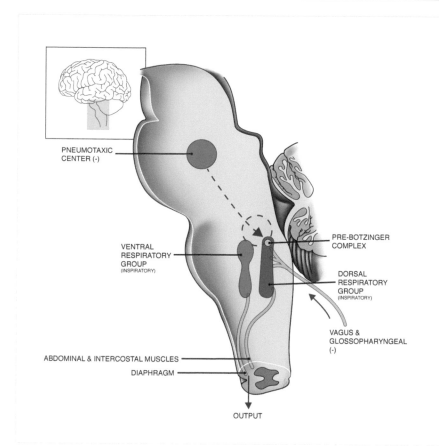

Fig. 1.4 Brainstem respiratory centers responsible for involuntary respiratory patterns. (From LaPointe L. Atlas of Neuroanatomy for Communication Science and Disorders, 1st ed. New York: Thieme Publishers; 2011.)

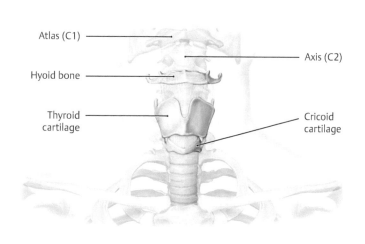

Fig. 1.5 Anterior view. The larynx is located in the midline of the anterior neck. Laryngeal structures at rest are positioned at characteristic vertebral levels in adult males: hyoid bone: C3; thyroid cartilage (superior border): C4; cricotracheal membrane: C6–C7. These structures are a half vertebra higher in females and children. (From Baker E. Anatomy for Dental Medicine, 2nd ed. New York: Thieme Medical Publishers; 2016.)

is a raised portion of cartilage known as the **thyroid prominence** (a.k.a. "Adam's Apple"), which can be very prominent in males. The vocal fold tissue is attached to the thyroid cartilage on the internal surface of the thyroid lamina just below the thyroid notch at a point called the **anterior commissure**. The superior borders of the thyroid are connected to the hyoid bone via a sheet of fibrous tissue called the **thyrohyoid membrane**. The middle and lateral margins of this membrane are thickened and referred to as the **median and lateral thyrohyoid ligaments**, respectively.

1.5.3 Cricoid Cartilage

The singular cricoid cartilage (▶ Fig. 1.6; ▶ Fig. 1.7) forms the inferior rim of the larynx. It is attached to the trachea inferiorly via the **cricotracheal ligament**. The cricoid is shaped like a ring with a thin anterior rim of hyaline cartilage which arches posterolateral (backward and to the side) to form a broad posterior lamina. A raised smooth surface is located on each lateral arch (left and right) forming **articular facets** where the cricoid communicates

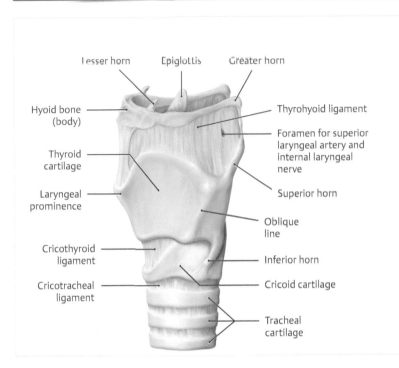

Fig. 1.6 Laryngeal framework. Oblique left anterolateral view. (From Baker E. Anatomy for Dental Medicine, 2nd ed. New York: Thieme Medical Publishers; 2016.)

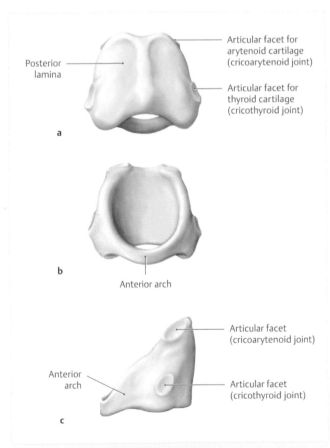

Fig. 1.7 Cricoid cartilage. **(a)** Posterior view. **(b)** Anterior view. **(c)** Left lateral view. (From Baker E. Anatomy for Dental Medicine, 2nd ed. New York: Thieme Medical Publishers; 2016.)

with the inferior horns of the thyroid, forming the **cricothyroid (CT) joint**. Additional articular facets are located on the superior surface of the posterior lamina where the cricoid communicates with the arytenoid cartilages, forming the **cricoarytenoid joint**.

1.5.4 Arytenoid Cartilages

The paired arytenoids (▶ Fig. 1.8**a**) are pyramid-shaped hyaline cartilages situated atop the cricoid at the cricoarytenoid joint. At the arytenoid base are two projections, one posterolateral and one anterior, called the **muscular process** and **vocal process**, respectively. The muscular process serves as a point of attachment for muscles which will move the arytenoid to adjust the position of the vocal folds. The vocal process serves as the posterior attachment for the vocal fold tissues. The body and apex of the arytenoids serve as attachment points for laryngeal muscles and connective tissue. Muscular contraction can move the arytenoids such that during adduction, they rotate medially to approximate each other with a slightly inferior tilt, while also sliding horizontally along the cricoarytenoid joint.

1.5.5 Epiglottis

The epiglottis is a leaf-shaped elastic cartilage attached to the inner medial surface of the thyroid just below the thyroid notch via the **thyroepiglottic ligament**. At its midpoint, the epiglottis is also attached to the hyoid bone via the **hyoepiglottic ligament**. The epiglottis (▶ Fig. 1.6; ▶ Fig. 1.9) may have a role in phonation by generating pressures above the vocal folds and also influencing resonance of sound generated during phonation. It plays a critical role in swallowing, during which inversion of the epiglottis occurs to cover the larynx to protect the lower airway.

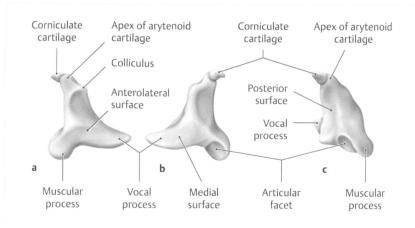

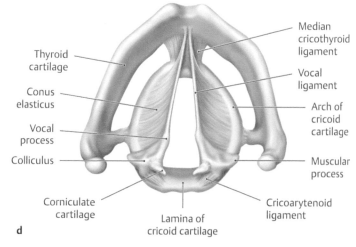

Fig. 1.8 Arytenoid and corniculate cartilages. **(a)** Right lateral view. **(b)** Left lateral (medial) view. **(c)** Posterior view. **(d)** Superior view. **(e)** Corniculate and cuneiform cartilages. Endoscopic view of the larynx showing the pyramid-shaped arytenoids capped by the pointed corniculate cartilages, with the cuneiform tubercles (the two rounded eminences) visible on the superior surface of the aryepiglottic folds. Corniculate (*left arrow*) and cuneiform (*right arrow*) cartilages. (a–d from Baker E. Anatomy for Dental Medicine, 2nd ed. New York: Thieme Medical Publishers; 2016.)

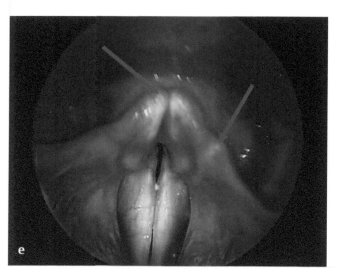

1.5.6 Corniculate and Cuneiform Cartilages

The corniculate and cuneiform cartilages provide structural integrity for the larynx but have debated influence on phonation. The paired corniculate cartilages (▶ Fig. 1.8a; ▶ Fig. 1.8b) are small horn-shaped structures situated atop the apex of the arytenoids. The paired cuneiform cartilages are embedded in a thickened rim of connective tissue called the **aryepiglottic folds**. Both cartilages

are considered "vestigial," meaning they have no known function other than possible structural support (▶ Table 1.1).

1.6 Connective Tissues

Additional membranes and ligaments line and connect the framework of the larynx and, with exception of the vocal folds, they are lined by a cellular layer of **pseudostratified, ciliated, columnar epithelium** ("respiratory epithelium"). Respiratory epithelium contains microscopic cilia which move to create a superior flow of secretions that help lubricate the larynx and remove debris (e.g., dust, and dead cells). Below the level of the vocal folds, a dense band of collagenous tissue called the **conus elasticus** connects the cricoid, thyroid, and arytenoid cartilages with each other (▶ Fig. 1.10; ▶ Fig. 1.11). The medial and lateral portions of this membrane are thickened and known as the **median and lateral cricothyroid ligaments,** respectively (▶ Fig. 1.10). Above the level of the vocal folds, another dense band of connective tissue called the **quadrangular membrane** (▶ Fig. 1.10; ▶ Fig. 1.11) connects the arytenoids, epiglottis, and thyroid cartilages. The superior rim of this membrane is thickened and called the **aryepiglottic folds**, forming the rim of the entry into the larynx known as the **laryngeal vestibule**. The most inferior portion of the quadrangular membrane is also thickened on each side (left and right), coursing horizontally where it connects the posterior arytenoids to the anterior thyroid cartilage, forming the **ventricular ligaments**. These

ligaments along with the surface epithelium and underlying musculature are known as the **ventricular folds, vestibular folds,** or **false vocal folds** (all three names are synonymous; ▶ Fig. 1.10; ▶ Fig. 1.11). A deep recess exists in the space between the ventricular folds and (true) vocal folds, called the **laryngeal ventricle** (▶ Fig. 1.11), which contains mucous glands that secrete fluids and lubricate the vocal fold tissue.

The paired vocal folds act as a dividing line, such that the laryngeal framework below the vocal folds is lined by the conus elasticus, while the framework above the vocal folds is lined by the quadrangular membrane. The space between the two vocal folds is known as the **glottis** (▶ Fig. 1.11), which can be open (abducted) or closed (adducted) depending on vocal fold position. As stated earlier, the vocal folds are attached posteriorly to the vocal process of the arytenoids and attach anteriorly at the anterior commissure of the thyroid. The vocal folds are another form of connective tissue consisting of a layered structure stratified by varying degrees of proteomic concentrations.

1.7 Vocal Fold Histology

The outermost (superficial) layer of the vocal folds is composed of **nonkeratinized stratified squamous epithelium** (▶ Fig. 1.12). The vocal fold surface is hydrated by transepithelial water fluxes moving to the surface from within, and mucus secretions from glands within the vocal folds and laryngeal ventricles.[5] Immediately below the epithelium is a **basement membrane zone** containing numerous collagen fibers which connect the epithelium to the layer immediately below the **superficial layer of the lamina propria** (SLLP). The SLLP, also known as **Reinke's space**, is composed mainly of amorphous interstitial (between the cells) proteins along with small concentrations of elastin and collagen. The SLLP is highly viscous and characterized by a consistency likened to soft gelatin. Together the vocal fold epithelium and the SLLP move as a functional unit called the **vocal fold cover**.

Deep to the SLLP, the concentration of elastin protein becomes greater, forming the **intermediate layer of the lamina propria** (ILLP). Deep to the ILLP, the ratio of collagen protein concentration becomes greatest, forming the **deep layer of the lamina propria** (DLLP). Together the ILLP and the DLLP form the

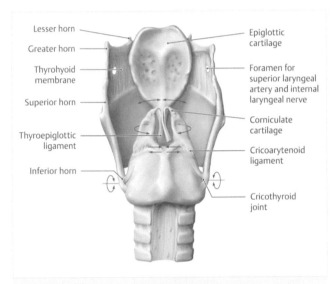

Lesser horn
Greater horn
Thyrohyoid membrane
Superior horn
Thyroepiglottic ligament
Inferior horn

Epiglottic cartilage
Foramen for superior laryngeal artery and internal laryngeal nerve
Corniculate cartilage
Cricoarytenoid ligament
Cricothyroid joint

Fig. 1.9 Posterior view of laryngeal cartilages and ligaments. *Arrows* indicate movement in the various joints. (From Baker E. Anatomy for Dental Medicine, 2nd ed. New York: Thieme Medical Publishers; 2016.)

Table 1.1 Cartilages of the larynx

Cartilage	Paired/Unpaired	Shape	Functions
Thyroid	Unpaired	Plow/Shield	a) Anterior attachment for vocal folds b) Pivots anteriorly and inferiorly to stretch vocal folds c) Attachment for laryngeal muscles
Cricoid	Unpaired	Ring	a) Connects larynx to trachea b) Attachment for laryngeal muscles c) Foundation for laryngeal joints
Arytenoid	Paired	Pyramid	a) Posterior attachment for vocal folds b) Pivots medially (adducts) and laterally (abducts) to move vocal folds c) Attachment for laryngeal muscles
Epiglottis	Unpaired	Leaf	a) Protects the laryngeal vestibule during swallowing b) Influences sound resonance
Corniculate	Paired	Cone	a) Structural support for laryngeal tissue
Cuneiform	Paired	Wedge	a) Structural support for laryngeal tissue

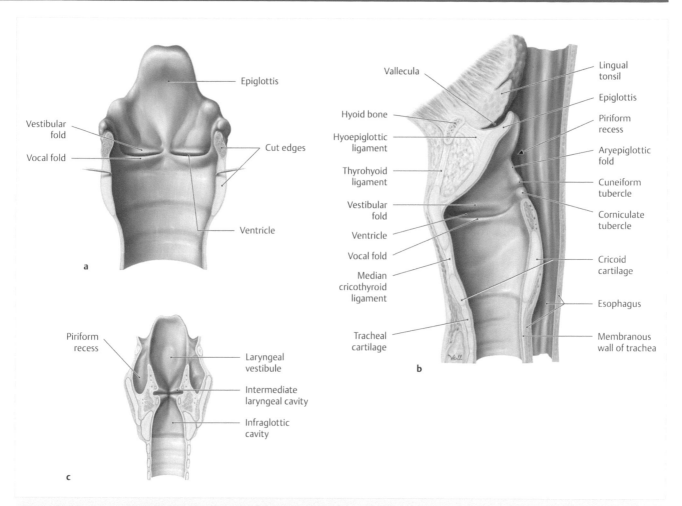

a

b

c

Fig. 1.10 Laryngeal connective tissue and spaces. **(a)** Posterior view with pharynx and esophagus cut along the midline and spread open. **(b)** Left lateral view of the midsagittal section. **(c)** Posterior view with the laryngeal levels. Regions shaded in pink are connected by the conus elasticus; regions covered in purple are covered by the quadrangular membrane. (From Baker E. Anatomy for Dental Medicine, 2nd ed. New York: Thieme Medical Publishers; 2016.)

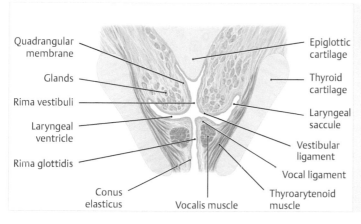

Fig. 1.11 Vocal folds, glottis, and ventricular (vestibular or false) folds. (From Baker E. Anatomy for Dental Medicine, 2nd ed. New York: Thieme Medical Publishers; 2016.)

vocal ligament, which connects the arytenoid cartilages to the thyroid and supports vibrational stresses during phonation. Deep to the DLLP is the **vocalis muscle** (see section "Laryngeal Muscles," below), which is considered the body of the vocal fold. The transition from the most superficial layer to the deepest layer of the vocal folds is characterized by an increasing stiffness gradient, with the lax and mobile cover being able to oscillate over a stiff body, with the cover connected to the body by the vocal ligament. The health of the epithelial cells of the vocal fold cover, the proteomic concentrations in the different layers of the lamina propria, and the contractile properties of the vocalis muscle influence the physiology of vocal fold vibration. An abnormality in any of these layers

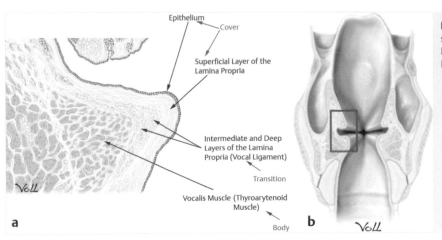

Epithelium
Cover
Superficial Layer of the Lamina Propria
Intermediate and Deep Layers of the Lamina Propria (Vocal Ligament)
Transition
Vocalis Muscle (Thyroarytenoid Muscle)
Body
a
b

Fig. 1.12 Vocal fold histologic section showing structural layers. (From Kendall K, Leonard R. Laryngeal Evaluation, 1st ed. New York: Thieme Publishers; 2010.)

Table 1.2 Membranes and ligaments of the larynx

Name	Attachments/Functions
Cricotracheal ligament	Inferior rim of cricoid to first tracheal ring; connects inferior larynx to trachea
Cricothyroid ligament (a.k.a. conus elasticus)	Connects laryngeal structures below vocal folds
Median cricothyroid ligament	Thickened medial division connecting cricoid arch to middle thyroid lamina at inferior border
Lateral cricothyroid ligament	Thinner lateral division connecting cricoid to lateral thyroid lamina at inferior border
Vocal ligament	From anterior commissure of thyroid to vocal process of arytenoid. Links vocal fold cover to vocal fold body
Cricoarytenoid ligament	Midline of posterior cricoid lamina to base of arytenoid. Stabilizes the cricoarytenoid joint
Quadrangular membrane	Broad sheet of membrane coursing upward from arytenoids to epiglottis. Covers and connects laryngeal structures above the level of vocal folds
Ventricular ligament (a.k.a. vestibular ligament)	From thyroid cartilage above the anterior commissure to anterior surface of arytenoid cartilage above the vocal process. Adducts via muscle contraction to prevent food/liquid from entering lower airway during swallowing
Aryepiglottic folds	Thickened superior borders of the quadrangular membrane. Forms the laryngeal vestibule and houses the cuneiform cartilages
Thyrohyoid membrane	From superior borders of thyroid to inferior border of hyoid bone. Connects larynx to the hyoid bone—the larynx is considered to be suspended from the hyoid via this membrane
Median thyrohyoid ligament	Thickened medial division connecting thyroid lamina to body and cornu of hyoid bone
Lateral thyrohyoid ligament	Thickened lateral division connecting superior thyroid cornu to greater cornu of hyoid bone
Thyroepiglottic ligament	From thyroid just below the notch to the petiolus of epiglottis. Connects epiglottis to thyroid cartilage.
Hyoepiglottic Ligament	From hyoid bone body to middle portion of epiglottis. Connects epiglottis to hyoid bone—when hyoid bone elevates during swallowing, the connection via this ligament results in epiglottic inversion, which covers the laryngeal vestibule

can impair phonation and disturb the resulting acoustic sound energy, resulting in the perception of dysphonia (▶ Table 1.2).

1.8 Laryngeal Muscles

1.8.1 Extrinsic Laryngeal Muscles

Extrinsic laryngeal muscles are characterized by an origin external to the larynx with an insertion on a laryngeal cartilage or on the hyoid bone. Some of these muscles originate inferior to the larynx and some superior, and their contraction will either depress the larynx or elevate the larynx, respectively. Collectively, the extrinsic muscles are referred to as the laryngeal **strap muscles**, as they act to "strap" the larynx in place within the vertical plane. As such, the extrinsic laryngeal muscles position the larynx in the vertical plane along the midline of the neck. Greater activation in the laryngeal depressors will lower the larynx, while greater activation in the laryngeal elevators will raise the larynx (▶ Fig. 1.13). While these muscles do not have a primary effect on the vibratory characteristics of the vocal folds, inefficient/ineffective use of the extrinsic musculature may "leak over" to result in inefficient use of the intrinsic musculature.

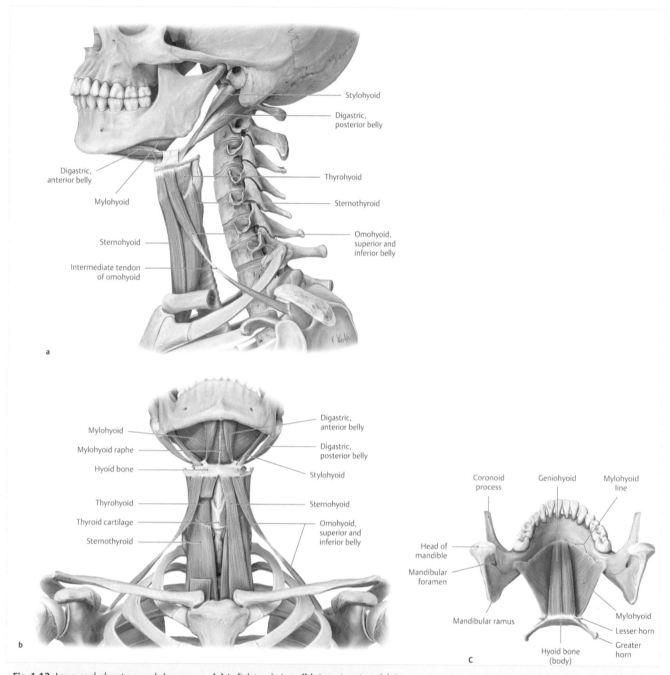

Fig. 1.13 Laryngeal elevators and depressors. **(a)** Left lateral view. **(b)** Anterior view. **(c)** Posterosuperior view. Due to their point of origin, laryngeal elevators are also referred to as the suprahyoid muscles, while the laryngeal depressors are also referred to as the infrahyoid muscles. (From Baker E. Anatomy for Dental Medicine, 2nd ed. New York: Thieme Medical Publishers; 2016.)

The laryngeal depressors include the **sternohyoid, sternothyroid, omohyoid,** and **thyrohyoid**. The thyrohyoid muscle can act as both a depressor and elevator depending on the position of the hyoid bone (e.g., fixation of the hyoid bone in an elevated position due to contraction of other laryngeal elevators, combined with contraction of the thyrohyoid, will result in laryngeal elevation). The laryngeal elevators include the **mylohyoid, geniohyoid, digastric** (anterior and posterior bellies), and the **stylohyoid**. Excessive tension in these muscles can influence the vertical position of the larynx and the relationship between the thyroid cartilage and hyoid bone. This excessive

tension is thought to be a causative factor for some voice disorders due to associated hyperfunctional influences on activation levels of the intrinsic laryngeal muscles.

1.8.2 Intrinsic Laryngeal Muscles

Intrinsic laryngeal muscles have both point of origin and insertion within the larynx, originating on one cartilage and inserting onto another such that they are named based on the two cartilages they connect. While extrinsic laryngeal muscles serve to adjust laryngeal position in the vertical midline of the neck,

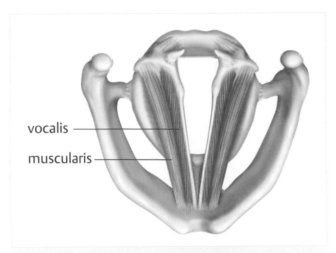

Fig. 1.14 Thyroarytenoid muscle showing vocalis and muscularis subdivisions. (From Rousseau and Branski, Anatomy and Physiology of Speech and Hearing, 1st ed. New York: Thieme Publishers; 2017.)

the intrinsic laryngeal muscles serve to adjust the position, length, and tension of the vocal folds. They adjust position by adducting the two vocal folds toward midline or abducting the vocal folds away from the midline. Adduction and abduction are possible because the arytenoid cartilages can swivel inward and outward within the cricoarytenoid joint.

The paired **thyroarytenoid** (TA; ▸ Fig. 1.14) muscle originates at the anterior commissure of the thyroid cartilage and terminates at the base of the arytenoid cartilage. This muscle has two subdivisions on each side, the medial **vocalis** and the lateral **muscularis**. The vocalis division has already been mentioned as the body of the vocal fold. It terminates on the vocal process of the arytenoid, and contraction of the vocalis influences vocal fold tension. In coordination with other muscles, the vocalis can increase tension in the cover of the vocal folds or, when contracting without opposition from antagonistic muscles (specifically, the CT muscle), can shorten the vocal folds and "relax" or decrease tension in the vocal fold cover. By adjusting vocal fold tension, the vocalis has the effect of increasing or decreasing the frequency of vocal fold vibration. The muscularis division terminates on the muscular process of the arytenoid. Due to the angle of insertion and the posterolateral position of the muscular process, contraction of the muscularis slightly adducts the vocal folds to narrow the glottis. Due to its two divisions, the TA is able to adduct, tense, or relax the vocal folds.

The **ventricular** (a.k.a., thyroventricularis) muscle is a superior extension of the TA, originating on the anterolateral margins of the thyroid cartilage below the notch and coursing posteriorly along the superior margins of the ventricle beneath the soft tissue of the ventricular folds (the false vocal folds), to insert at the lateral margins of the arytenoid cartilage. The ventricular muscle might be responsible for medial compression of the false vocal folds during "pressed" or "strained" phonation, and it is believed that contraction of this muscle stimulates glands within the ventricle to release mucous.

The paired cricothyroid (CT) (▸ Fig. 1.15) muscle originates on the anterolateral arch of the cricoid and inserts on the inner anterior surface of the thyroid lamina. Like the TA, this muscle has two subdivisions, the more vertically oriented **pars recta** and transversely oriented **pars oblique**. These two subdivisions work in concert with each other, having the effect of moving the thyroid cartilage anteriorly and inferiorly (forward and down) such that the space between the thyroid and cricoid is narrowed. The result is an increase in the distance between the arytenoids and the inner surface of the thyroid, and therefore an increase in vocal fold length. The thyroid cartilage can pivot around the cricoid due its situation within the CT joint. The anterior and inferior displacement of the thyroid elongates the vocal folds, influencing the length and tension of the vocal fold tissue. As such, the CT is a tensor of the vocal folds, it influences vibration frequency, and may also contribute to the adduction of the vocal folds by maintaining longitudinal tension.

The paired **lateral cricoarytenoid** (LCA; ▸ Fig. 1.15) muscle originates on the lateral arch of the cricoid and inserts on the muscular process of the arytenoid. Due to its angle of insertion, contraction of the LCA will adduct the vocal folds to narrow down or close the glottis. The **interarytenoid** (IA; sometimes also referred to as the "arytenoid") muscle has a paired subdivision—the **oblique**—and a singular subdivision— the **transverse**. The oblique IA originates along the base of one arytenoid and courses superiorly in an oblique line to insert near the apex of the opposite arytenoid. The transverse IA originates along the vertical length of one arytenoid and courses horizontally to insert along the vertical length of the opposite arytenoid. The divisions of the IA work in concert with each other when contracting, which has the effect of approximating the arytenoid cartilages and adducting the vocal folds to narrow or close the glottis. The **aryepiglottic** muscle (▸ Fig. 1.15) is an extension of the oblique IA. It originates on the apex of the arytenoid cartilages and terminates near the aryepiglottic folds. This muscle may be primarily responsible for the strong sphincteric closure of the larynx at multiple levels during swallowing and gagging. How the aryepiglottic muscle can contract independently of the oblique IA has yet to be established or defined.

The paired **posterior cricoarytenoid** (PCA; ▸ Fig. 1.15) muscle originates on the broad posterior lamina of the cricoid and inserts onto the muscular process of the arytenoid. Due to its angle of insertion, this muscle abducts the vocal folds and widens the glottis when contracting. It is the only active abductor muscle of the vocal folds. While the vocal folds are open at rest, during speech production they need to be rapidly abducted by the PCA for respiratory support and motor speech execution of different phonemes. Additionally, the PCA is active during periods of high ventilation demands (e.g., during physical activity), when contraction of the PCA will widen the glottis to lessen the resistance to larger volumes of air entering the trachea and lungs.

The paired **thyroepiglottic** muscle (▸ Fig. 1.15) originates at the anterior commissure of the thyroid cartilage, coursing obliquely to terminate on the lateral margins of the arytenoid cartilages, epiglottis, and aryepiglottic folds. The thyroepiglottic muscle does not influence vocal fold position, length, or tension, but instead will influence the diameter of the laryngeal vestibule (the opening to the larynx) when it contracts (▸ Table 1.3).

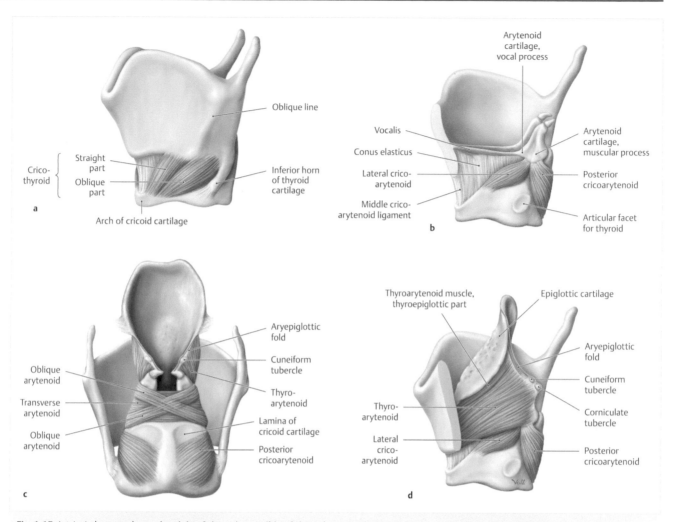

Fig. 1.15 Intrinsic laryngeal muscles. **(a)** Left lateral view. **(b)** Left lateral view with thyroid lamina, muscularis, and thyroepiglottic muscles removed. **(c)** Posterior view. **(d)** Left lateral view with thyroid lamina removed. (From Baker E. Anatomy for Dental Medicine, 2nd ed. New York: Thieme Medical Publishers; 2016.)

Table 1.3 Origin, insertion, and action of intrinsic laryngeal muscles

Intrinsic muscles of the larynx			
Muscle	Origin	Insertion	Function
Vocalis (Thyrovocalis)	Anterior commissure of thyroid	Vocal process of arytenoid	Tensor or relaxer
Muscularis (Thyromuscularis)	Anterior commissure of thyroid	Muscular process of arytenoid	Adductor
Lateral cricoarytenoid	Anterolateral arch of cricoid	Thyroid lamina	Primary adductor
Interarytenoid	Arytenoid	Contralateral arytenoid	Adductor
Cricothyroid	Lateral arch of cricoid	Muscular process of arytenoid	Tensor
Posterior cricoarytenoid	Posterior lamina of cricoid	Muscular process of arytenoid	Abductor
Thyroepiglottic	Anterior commissure of thyroid	Aryepiglottic folds	Widens laryngeal vestibule
Aryepiglottic	Apex of arytenoid	Aryepiglottic folds	Pulls epiglottis posteriorly
Ventricular	Thyroid	Arytenoid	Adducts ventricular folds

1.9 Neurology of Phonation

1.9.1 Central Nervous System

Vocalization in humans occurs due to involuntary (e.g., cry, cough, emotional vocalizations) and voluntary purposes (e.g., nonspeech vocalizations, speech). The activation of laryngeal muscles is controlled by LMN of the peripheral nervous system (PNS), but the activity of those LMN is heavily influenced by **upper motor neurons** of the CNS pathways. For emotional vo-calizations and some involuntary vocalizations such as cough and other laryngeal reflexes, pathways emanating from midbrain (periaqueductal gray area), perisylvian regions (areas of cortex surrounding the Sylvian fissure), and brainstem nuclei can drive LMN without voluntary intent of the speaker.[6] For intentional speech purposes, LMN are driven by voluntary tracts of the **pyramidal pathway** while muscle tone is adjusted during speech via contributions from the **extrapyramidal pathway**.

As illustrated in ▶ Fig. 1.16, the pyramidal pathway consists of **corticobulbar** (a.k.a. corticonuclear) and **corticospinal tracts**. LMN which go on to innervate muscles of the head and neck are controlled by UMN of the corticobulbar tract. The majority of these neurons originate in the ventrolateral (lower) region of the left and right primary motor cortex (precentral gyrus) of the frontal lobe, known as the facial area. Their axons travel inferiorly through the subcortical regions to directly communicate with LMN **cranial nerves** in the brainstem (hence another name for the pyramidal pathway—the "direct activation pathway"). The cranial nerves responsible for speech production (including pho-nation) are mostly **bilaterally innervated** by the corticobulbar tract, because approximately 50% of the corticobulbar neurons originating in the left and right cortical hemispheres cross over (decussate) near their respective LMN targets in the brainstem. This bilateral innervation of cranial nerves serves a protective purpose, as a lesion to left or right descending corticobulbar tracts will not result in complete cessation of stimulation to a cranial nerve, which can also be stimulated by corticobulbar neu-rons crossing over from the unaffected opposite side. LMN that control *lower facial muscles* and *tongue muscles* are more **unilat-erally innervated**, such that a unilateral corticobulbar tract le-sion can result in more significant effects in those muscles.

Neurons of the corticospinal tract continue through the brainstem to the level of the inferior medulla, where approxi-mately 90% of the neurons will decussate. These continue into the spinal cord as the lateral corticospinal tract, travelling as far as their respective LMN spinal nerve targets. The remainder of corticospinal neurons continue into the spinal cord as the ante-rior corticospinal tract. The majority of these neurons will also decussate, but they do this closer to their spinal nerve targets. Due to the decussation in both divisions of the corticospinal tract, the LMN spinal nerves are unilaterally innervated, such that a unilateral lesion in the corticospinal tract can have signif-icant influences on one side of the body.

During speech production, cortical and subcortical regions of the CNS prepare **motor plans** (broad spatial and temporal targets for muscles) which will be refined into **motor programs** (modi-fied motor plans with specification of muscle range, rate, tone, and force required for the intended movement) and sent to the

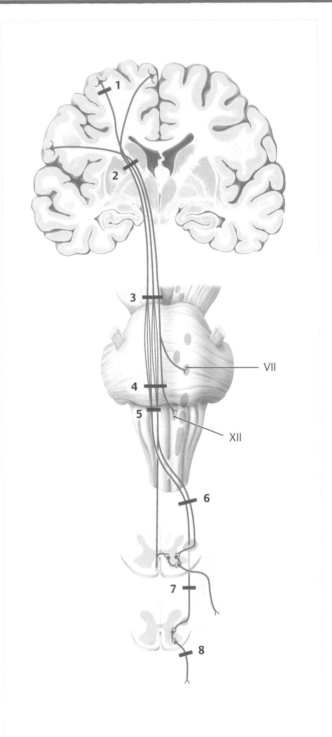

Fig. 1.16 Course of the pyramidal pathway (showing neurons in the right hemisphere only). The majority of corticospinal neurons decussate at the inferior medulla. 50% of the corticobulbar neurons decussate near their LMN targets in the brainstem, with exception to those innervating the 12th cranial nerve (hypoglossal) and neurons of the 7th cranial nerve (facial) that will innervate lower facial muscles. (From LaPointe L. Atlas of Neuroanatomy for Communication Science and Disorders, 1st ed. New York: Thieme Publishers; 2011.)

primary motor cortex to activate the pyramidal pathway. **Voicing** is a characteristic in a majority of speech sounds in many languages, and cortical planning of phonation during speech occurs along with planning for other articulators such as the tongue, lips, and jaw. The process of motor planning and motor programming involves activation of neural networks in the premotor cortex (including supplementary motor area and Broca's area) of the frontal lobe, subcortical regions, and auditory cortical regions (in temporal lobe, including Wernicke's area), with bilateral cortical activity (▶ Fig. 1.17). Once formed, motor programs are communicated to the primary motor cortex in the precentral gyrus, where most neurons which make up the pyramidal pathway originate. Extrapyramidal pathways which will affect muscle tone also send signals down to the brainstem at the same time, such that respiratory, laryngeal, and articulatory function during speech production is a product of both voluntary (pyramidal pathway) and involuntary (extrapyramidal pathway) CNS influences. Additional evidence suggests that the auditory side channel (feedback) influences ongoing voice production.[7]

1.10 Peripheral Nervous System

Pyramidal and extrapyramidal pathways converge on the LMN motor cell bodies of the cranial nerves in the brainstem (▶ Fig. 1.18). The axons of cranial nerves leave the brainstem and enter peripheral structures of the head and neck. There are 12 pairs (left and right) of cranial nerves. All *intrinsic laryngeal muscles* affecting vocal fold posture (TA, LCA, IA, CT, PCA) are innervated by only one of these, the **X cranial nerve** or **vagus nerve**. The vagus nerve is complex and consists of motor, sensory, and autonomic neurons which travel throughout the head, neck, and thorax to innervate skeletal muscles, smooth muscles, organs, and glands. Motor and sensory nuclei of the vagus reside in the brainstem medulla, and the motor cell bodies of the vagus nerve are located in the **NA**. Of its many branches, three are most important for speech and voice production. The **pharyngeal branch** of the vagus nerve splits from the main vagus trunk to provide motor innervation for the muscles of the velum (soft palate) and pharyngeal muscles, along with sensory innervation to the oropharynx and pharynx (▶ Fig. 1.19). The **superior laryngeal nerve** (SLN) branch of the vagus splits from the main vagus trunk below the pharyngeal branch. The SLN has two subdivisions, the **external branch** (eSLN) and **internal branch** (iSLN). The eSLN will provide motor supply to the CT muscle and pharyngeal constrictor muscles. The iSLN will distribute axons across the mucous membranes and other connective tissue to serve as the primary sensory nerve for the larynx. When individuals feel a sensation in their throat which makes them clear, cough, or interrupt voicing, it is due to sensory signals sent into the brainstem via the iSLN.

The **recurrent laryngeal nerve** (RLN) branches from the main trunk of the vagus below the SLN. The paired RLN is asymmetrical, being longer on the left than on the right. The left RLN travels inferiorly where it loops around the aortic arch before turning back superiorly toward the larynx. This course makes the left RLN prone to injury during thoracic surgery, especially cardiac procedures. The RLN provides motor supply to all intrinsic laryngeal muscles with exception to the CT. This translates to all adductor muscles (TA: muscularis, LCA, IA) and the abductor muscle (PCA) of the vocal folds being innervated by

the RLN. Injury to this nerve can result in significant impairment manifested by difficulty closing the glottis for voice, swallowing, and cough due to vocal fold paralysis.

Motor innervation to the extrinsic laryngeal muscles is provided by other cranial nerves including the **V trigeminal**, **VII facial**, and **XII hypoglossal** nerves. The laryngeal elevators are supplied by the trigeminal (anterior digastric and mylohyoid muscles), facial (posterior digastric and stylohyoid muscles), and hypoglossal (geniohyoid muscle) nerves. Motor innervation to the laryngeal depressors (thyrohyoid, sternohyoid, sternothyroid, and omohyoid muscles) is provided by the hypoglossal nerve via the ansa cervicalis (▶ Table 1.4).

1.11 Physiology of Phonation

The physiological processes underlying vocal fold vibration include respiratory, laryngeal, and upper aerodynamic tract (supraglottal, pharyngeal, oral, and nasal) contributions. One strategy to help conceptualize the physiology of phonation is the use of a simplified model shown in ▶ Fig. 1.20. In this three-mass model, the upper edge (m_1) and lower edge (m_2) of the vocal folds represent the cover and are able to move independently but are connected to the body (m) via the vocal ligament and surrounding tissue (the coiled springs). This model is representative of the **cover-body theory** of phonation, which proposes that a viscous and elastic cover (epithelium and SLLP) oscillates over a stiff body (vocalis) during voice production.[8]

After inhalation, a speaker will engage the muscles of exhalation (see above) creating a superior flow of air through the trachea. As this occurs, laryngeal adductor muscles (TA: muscularis, LCA, IA) will contract to create a specific degree of glottal closure and **medial compression** force, depending on the intent and/or needs of the speaker. At the same time, muscles that adjust vocal fold tension (CT and TA—vocalis) will contract to set the appropriate stiffness. As the glottis narrows, it creates a constriction to the subglottic flow of air, increasing air pressure below the glottis. As the vocal folds adduct completely along their horizontal length, subglottic pressure will continue to rise as long as the speaker continues to exhale.

The buildup of subglottic pressure will eventually overcome the degree of tension and medial compression force between the two adducted vocal folds and set them into vibration. Air will then begin to flow through the glottis (called **transglottal airflow**) by separating the bottom vocal fold edges (m_2). As air flows superiorly, it will eventually separate the top vocal fold edges (m_1). Notice in ▶ Fig. 1.21 that the bottom and top vocal fold edges do not open and close at the same time—there is a **vertical phase difference** between m_1 and m_2 during phonation. As air flows through the glottis to separate the top edge, the bottom edge will begin to close. As another vibratory cycle begins, the bottom edge will be opening while the top edge will be closing. The characteristics of airflow at the top vocal fold edge can thus be converging (called a **convergent glottis**) or diverging (called a **divergent glottis**), dependent on the point in the vibratory cycle.

The vertical phase difference during vibration causes an **intraglottal pressure gradient**, such that pressure is greater at the top vocal fold edge in a convergent glottis but greater at the bottom vocal fold edge in a divergent glottis. Sustained phonation results in continuously varying intraglottal pressure gradients between

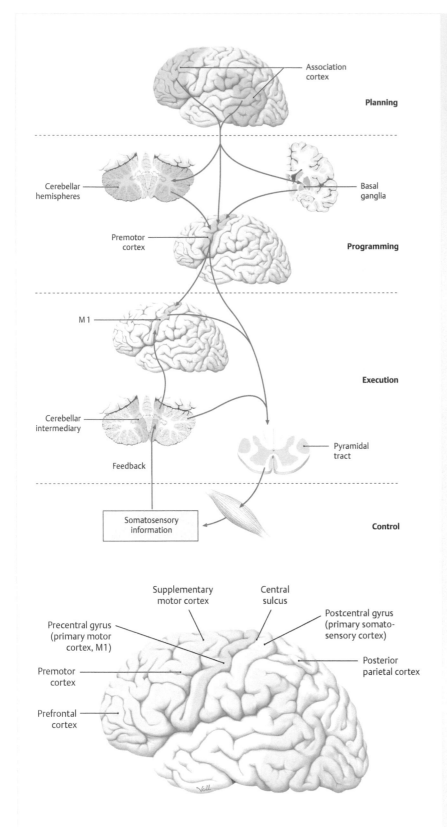

Fig. 1.17 During the planning and programming stages, cortical motor areas connect to subcortical and brainstem regions via the extrapyramidal pathway. Completed motor programs are sent to the pyramidal neurons, the majority of which reside in the primary motor cortex of the frontal lobe. The axons of pyramidal neurons descend into the brainstem/spinal cord to innervate their LMN targets, which then cause skeletal muscles to contract. (From LaPointe L. Atlas of Neuroanatomy for Communication Science and Disorders, 1st ed. New York: Thieme Publishers; 2011.)

those two regions, which creates forces that help sustain vibration. Vibration is also sustained by other aerodynamic forces. In a divergent glottis, airflow is separated along the walls of the vocal folds, on left and right sides. This separation creates small regions of turbulent airflow with extreme negative pressures, known as **flow vortices**. The negative pressure created by these vortices assists in bringing the top vocal fold edges back together.[9] The tissue of the vocal folds is also elastic. This property of elasticity

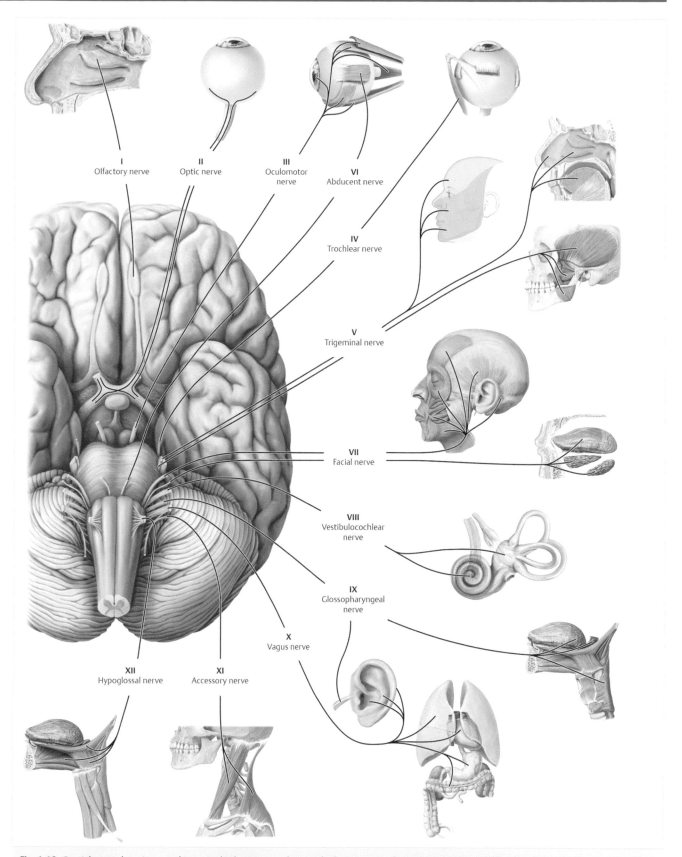

Fig. 1.18 Cranial nerve locations as they exit the brainstem, along with their targets of termination. (From LaPointe L. Atlas of Neuroanatomy for Communication Science and Disorders, 1st ed. New York: Thieme Publishers; 2011.)

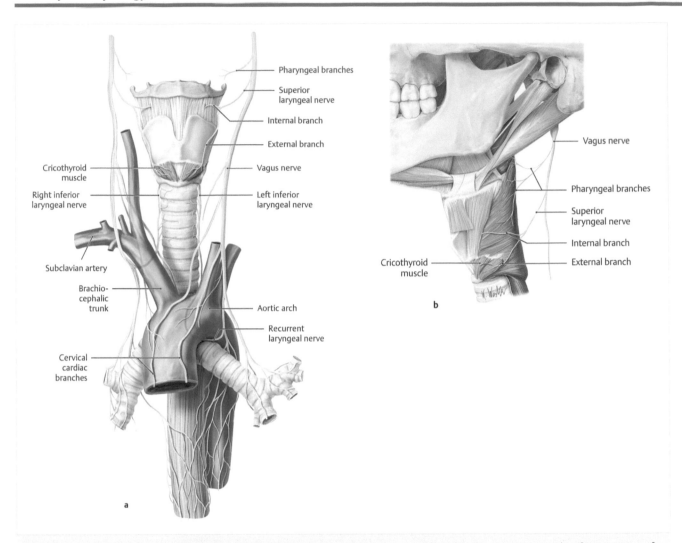

Fig. 1.19 Course of the vagus nerve showing the pharyngeal, superior laryngeal, and recurrent branches. (From LaPointe L. Atlas of Neuroanatomy for Communication Science and Disorders, 1st ed. New York: Thieme Publishers; 2011.)

Table 1.4 Peripheral innervation of the intrinsic and extrinsic laryngeal muscles

Muscle	Innervation	Influence on larynx
Intrinsic laryngeal muscles		
Vocalis	X cranial nerve, RLN	VF tensor/relaxer
Muscularis	X cranial nerve, RLN	VF adductor
Cricothyroid	X cranial nerve, eSLN	VF tensor
Lateral cricoarytenoid	X cranial nerve, RLN	VF adductor
Interarytenoid	X cranial nerve, RLN	VF adductor
Posterior cricoarytenoid	X cranial nerve, RLN	VF abductor
Thyroepiglottis	X cranial nerve, RLN	Widens vestibule
Aryepiglottis	X cranial nerve, RLN	Epiglottic inversion
Vestibular	X cranial nerve, RLN	Adducts false VF
Extrinsic laryngeal muscles		
Elevators (suprahyoid)		

Table 1.4 continued

Muscle	Innervation	Influence on larynx
Geniohyoid	XII cranial nerve	Elevates larynx
Mylohyoid	V cranial nerve	Elevates larynx
Anterior digastric	V cranial nerve	Elevates larynx
Posterior digastric	VII cranial nerve	Elevates larynx
Stylohyoid	VII cranial nerve	Elevates larynx
Depressors (infrahyoid)		
Omohyoid	XII cranial nerve	Depresses larynx
Sternohyoid	XII cranial nerve	Depresses larynx
Sternothyroid	XII cranial nerve	Depresses larynx
Thyrohyoid	XII cranial nerve	Depresses/Raises larynx

Abbreviations: RLN, recurrent laryngeal nerve; eSLN, external branch of superior laryngeal nerve; VF, vocal fold.

allows the vocal folds to separate from the midline, but will also provide a **recoil force** that helps close them. Thus, at least four forces help open and close the vocal folds during vibration: (1) subglottal pressure, (2) intraglottal pressure gradients, (3) flow vortices, and (4) elastic recoil. This influence of aerodynamic forces and tissue elasticity on vocal fold vibratory behavior has traditionally been termed the **myoelastic-aerodynamic theory of phonation.**[10]

Another force influencing phonation and traditionally included as part of the myoelastic-aerodynamic theory is the **Bernoulli effect**. This physical phenomenon occurs when air pressure lowers immediately behind and perpendicular to a flow of molecules in regions of increased flow velocity. During phonation, negative pressures are created immediately behind the transglottal flow of air. This negative pressure assists in bringing the vocal fold edges back together, just as a shower curtain might behave (it moves inward) perpendicular to the flow of water molecules. Supraglottal forces also influence vocal fold vibration. By manipulating the shape of the supraglottic larynx, pharyngeal, and oral cavities, a speaker can produce varying degrees of **inertive reactance**. Inertive reactance creates a "back pressure" on the top edges of the vocal

folds, which in theory facilitates oscillation and lowers the medial compression force needed to sustain vibration at different frequencies and vocal intensities.[11]

During sustained phonation, such as prolonging a vowel, the adductor muscles continue contracting to maintain vocal fold adduction. It is aerodynamic forces which oscillate the vocal folds once they are brought together to create the different phases of vibration (opening, open, closing, and closed). Muscular forces act to keep the vocal fold tissue approximated in this context. During connected speech, the adductor muscles and abductor muscle (PCA) contract and relax dynamically with each other to create the voiced and unvoiced sounds of speech. However, vocal fold oscillation (voicing) will only occur when the adductor muscles close the glottis to allow the aerodynamic forces to act on the vocal fold tissue. During sustained phonation or connected speech, vocal fold vibration *does not* occur by repeated contraction–relaxation (adduction–abduction) of the adductor muscles —instead, the adductor muscles sustain contraction, allowing the aerodynamic forces and elastic properties of the vocal fold tissue to facilitate the different phase of vibration.

1.11.1 Control of Fundamental Frequency

Control of fundamental frequency (F_0), perceived as vocal pitch, is controlled via a combination of respiratory drive and a dynamic interplay between the vocalis and CT muscles (► Fig. 1.22). During ongoing speech or singing, the vocalis and CT muscles are coordinated with other laryngeal and respiratory muscles to control F_0 dynamically. Both vocalis and CT are always active during sound production, although the relationship of their contraction levels differs depending on what part of a speaker's physiological frequency range is being produced.

At lower F_0 the vocalis is engaged more than the CT, which has the effect of shortening the vocal folds and "relaxing" the vocal fold cover. This results in reduced vocal fold tension and greater mass per unit length along the vocal fold, which translates to a slower period of vibration and lower F_0. To produce frequencies in the upper part of the physiological frequency range requires increased engagement (contraction) of the CT. This will elongate the vocal folds and add tension to the vocal

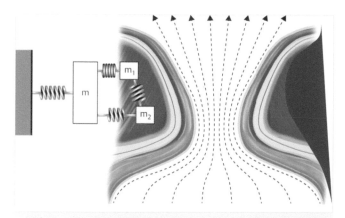

Fig. 1.20 Vocal fold three-mass model showing upper edge (m_1), lower edge (m_2), and body (m) of vocal fold. (From Rousseau and Branski. Anatomy and Physiology of Speech and Hearing, 1st ed. New York: Thieme Publishers; 2017.)

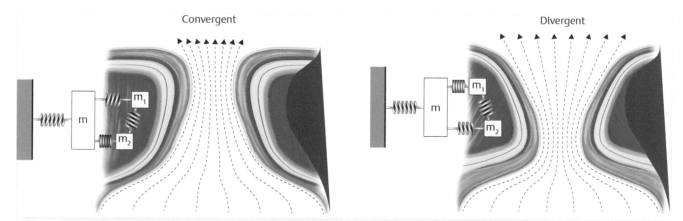

Fig. 1.21 Vocal fold oscillation showing different points of the vibratory cycle where converging and diverging glottis conditions exist. (From Rousseau and Branski. Anatomy and Physiology of Speech and Hearing, 1st ed. New York: Thieme Publishers; 2017.)

fold cover, causing the period of vibration to become faster and translating to a higher F_o. The rapid changes in F_o which occur during speech and singing result from this dynamic relationship in the degree of engagement in vocalis and CT muscles, along with the respiratory muscles that provide the airflow powering phonation.

1.11.2 Control of Vocal Intensity

Vocal intensity is the degree of acoustic sound pressure created during phonation. A number of physiological factors influence vocal intensity, including subglottal pressure, medial compression force, vocal fold tension, and glottal posture (e.g., the degree to which the vocal folds are adducted along their midline). Increases or decreases in subglottal pressure result in greater or lower vocal intensity, respectively.[12,13] Subglottal pressure is controlled by airflow rate due to respiratory muscle control along with medial compression force controlled by vocal fold adductor muscles. Vocal fold posture that results in any gap along the length of the vocal folds will create an air leak that can lower subglottal pressure. Additionally, increasing tension in the vocal folds will require greater subglottal pressure to initiate and sustain vibration, translating to greater vocal intensity.

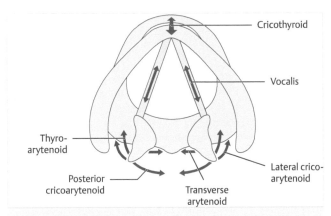

Fig. 1.22 Influence of intrinsic laryngeal muscles on arytenoids and vocal folds. (From Baker E. Anatomy for Dental Medicine, 2nd ed. New York: Thieme Medical Publishers; 2016.)

Medial compression forces and vocal fold tension influence the vibratory dynamics of the vocal folds. Among these include the duration of closed, opening, and closing phases of the vibratory cycle. When balance in the duration of these phases exists, the result is often the generation of greater vocal intensity produced with efficiency (e.g., greater output with less muscular effort). Alternatively, an imbalanced relationship in the phases of the vibratory cycle can cause the control of vocal intensity to be less efficient (▶ Table 1.5).[14]

1.11.3 Supraglottal Resonance and Voice Quality

Sound production is influenced by the physiological activation in three subsystems of voice: (1) respiratory, (2) laryngeal, and (3) articulatory, which are coupled to each other. These subsystems are coordinated such that physiological activity in one part of the system can influence physiological activity in another. An example of this is the **tracheal pull**, where the cricoid cartilage (and thus larynx) descends when inhaling due to mechanical traction of the lower airway. This movement can be palpated by placing a finger on the thyroid prominence (the "Adams Apple") and inhaling deeply—the larynx can be felt to move downward. The tracheal pull influences activity in the intrinsic laryngeal muscles during voice production, especially the CT which must adjust contraction levels to maintain F_o that is affected by the mechanical elongation of the vocal folds.[15] Similarly, it has been well established that tension in the tongue and extrinsic lingual musculature that attach to the hyoid bone can subsequently influence contraction levels of intrinsic laryngeal muscles.[16,17]

In addition to mechanical coupling of the three voice subsystems, the supraglottal vocal tract is a **resonator** of acoustic voice energy that causes specific frequencies in the spectrum of the phonatory sound wave to be amplified and accentuated. ▶ Fig. 1.23 illustrates the potential spaces which, through movement of the articulators, can be modified to resonate different frequencies in the acoustic spectrum produced by phonation. The supraglottal vocal tract also acts as a filter by dampening the energy in other frequencies. Vocal tract resonance and filtering is the product of articulation—how a speaker shapes the

Table 1.5 Influences on phonation physiology

Force/Phenomenon	Cause	Influence
Medial compression	Contraction force of VF adductor muscles	Increases subglottal pressure
Subglottal pressure	Medial compression Airflow	Separates VF in opening phase of VF vibration
Airflow	Respiratory muscle activation	Transglottal pressure gradients Flow vortices Bernoulli's effect
Transglottal pressure gradients	Differential pressures at top and bottom VF edges	Facilitates oscillation
Elastic recoil	Elasticity of VF tissues	Assists in closing phase of VF vibration
Flow vortices	Separation of VF edges	Assists in closing phase of VF vibration
Bernoulli's effect	Negative transglottal pressures	Assists in closing phase of VF vibration

Abbreviation: VF, vocal fold.

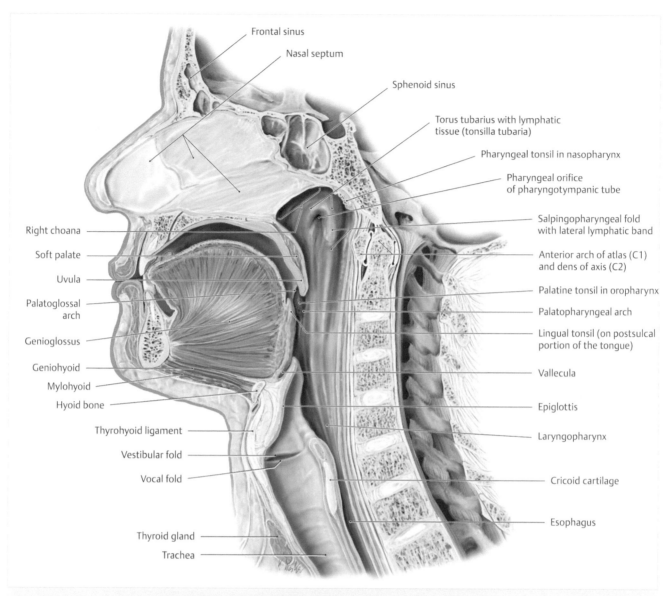

Fig. 1.23 Resonating spaces in the supraglottal vocal tract. **(a)** Laryngeal spaces immediately above the vocal folds (the "epilaryngeal" region), the pharynx, nasal cavity, and oral cavity can all be modified by the articulators to influence resonance. (From Baker E. Anatomy for Dental Medicine, 2nd ed. New York: Thieme Medical Publishers; 2016.) (*Continued*)

spaces above the glottis. This can have a significant influence on the spectrum of sound, such that at given articulatory postures, some frequencies produced by phonation will be greatly amplified while some will be attenuated to very low energy levels. You may remember this relationship from your undergraduate speech science course, where the association between the acoustic spectrum produced by vibrating folds and resonant effects on that spectrum by the supraglottal vocal tract was explained by the **source-filter theory**.

The positioning of articulators and modification of spaces in the supraglottal vocal tract can also greatly influence the physiology of vocal fold vibration. Inertive reactance—the back pressure applied to the vocal fold tissue resulting from activity in the supraglottal vocal tract—has already been discussed. Inertive reactance, which creates efficiency in vocal fold oscillation, can be increased

by semi-occlusions and elongations at the lips (e.g., via lip rounding).[18] Articulation which creates resonating spaces in the front of the oral cavity (e.g., at the lips or hard palate) or the nasal cavity (e.g., as in humming) has also been shown to influence vocal fold vibratory dynamics in a way that decreases medial compression and the force with which the vocal folds collide during oscillation, creating greater efficiency during voice production.[19] Additionally, voice production combined with wide resonating spaces in the front of the mouth is often perceived as a "resonant" or "full" sound. In contrast, constriction in the posterior supraglottal vocal tract can be accompanied by a perception of "constricted," "pressed," or "backed" sound.

The effects of inertive reactance and articulatory constrictions at different points along the supraglottal vocal tract can influence voice quality. The typical listener has auditory-perceptual

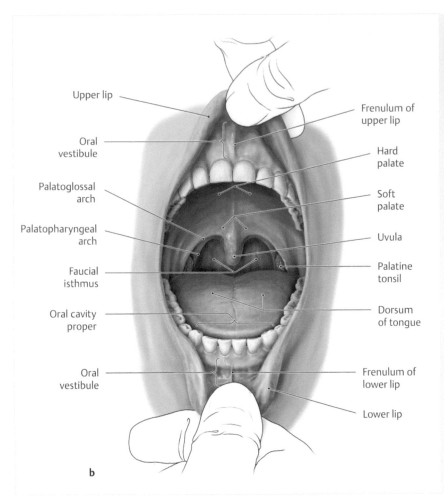

Upper lip

Oral vestibule

Palatoglossal arch

Palatopharyngeal arch

Faucial isthmus

Oral cavity proper

Oral vestibule

Frenulum of upper lip

Hard palate

Soft palate

Uvula

Palatine tonsil

Dorsum of tongue

Frenulum of lower lip

Lower lip

b

Fig. 1.23 (*Continued*) **(b)** Action of the tongue, lips, and jaw can shape the oral cavity in many different configurations to influence resonance. By protruding the lips and increasing space within the oral cavity (e.g., the "inverted megaphone" shape), a speaker can create a semi-occlusion to increase inertive reactance while creating a powerful resonating space for voice production.

awareness of acoustic features related to frequency, intensity, and spectral structure of an acoustic voice signal. When used to describe the human voice, we can think of voice quality as referring to the characteristic of a sound that distinguishes it from other sounds of similar pitch, loudness, and duration. The term "quality" is somewhat analogous to musical **timbre**. Voice quality is influenced by vocal fold vibratory dynamics that create the full spectrum of acoustic energy, in addition to the resonance of that energy by the spaces in the supraglottal vocal tract. The perception of voice quality is a psychological process unique to each listener, and is influenced by the multidimensional information embedded in the acoustic spectrum.[20,21]

1.12 Conclusion

This chapter has provided a description of the anatomy of the larynx and the nervous system control of laryngeal musculature that allows us to utilize the laryngeal mechanism for basic biological functions and for purposeful voice production. The ability of respiratory and laryngeal mechanisms to work together to produce vocal fold vibration (i.e., the physiology of phonation), along with ways in which the supraglottal

structures may affect phonatory behavior, has also be detailed. Now that the reader has a basic understanding of the structures and activities involved in the production of the voice signal, the next chapter will describe a variety of disordered states that affect respiratory-laryngeal function to result in atypical voice and dysphonia.

Clinical Case Study: Laryngomalacia

Paul is a 3-month-old male child whose parents brought him to the otolaryngologist after referral from their pediatrician. They reported that Paul exhibits abnormal vocal sounds, especially when he is breathing, which become worse when he gets upset and is crying. These sounds were not initially present at birth, but they started to notice them within a few weeks after Paul came home. They described these sounds as "like a squeaking or rustling noise." Paul's history included premature birth (31 weeks) and some "soft" neurological signs including mild hypotonicity. His parents reported some coughing during feeding, although Paul has been gaining weight appropriately. They noted that Paul often gets irritable shortly after feeding, and this behavior lasts for 30 minutes to an hour. Their biggest concern is the abnormal breathing sounds. After a general physical examination, the otolaryngologist performed a flexible fiberoptic examination of Paul's larynx using a pediatric endoscope passed through the nasal cavity. This allowed the doctor to visualize Paul's laryngeal structure, including movement of structures when breathing and crying. The following characteristics were noted by the doctor:

- Inhalatory stridor.
- Prolapsing arytenoid cartilages upon inhalation, partially obstructing the airway.
- Short aryepiglottic folds creating an omega-shaped epiglottis.
- Narrow laryngeal vestibule.

Based on the history, physical examination, and laryngeal examination, the otolaryngologist diagnosed Paul with laryngomalacia. The doctor explained the following to Paul's parents:

"Laryngomalacia is a common congenital condition. It is characterized by underdevelopment of the laryngeal cartilages, causing them to collapse into the airway during inspiration. This is the cause of the breathing sounds that you hear, called stridor, which become worse when he is upset or crying because of the increased airflow being inhaled and exhaled. Many children with laryngomalacia also experience laryngopharyngeal reflux, a condition where digestive enzymes leak up through the esophagus and into the larynx, further irritating the laryngeal tissue. Signs of reflux were noted during examination of Paul's larynx, and are likely the cause of his irritability after feeding. A majority of children with laryngomalacia, especially those with mild-to-moderate presentations such as Paul, simply resolve over time as the laryngeal structures mature. Because he is otherwise healthy, our plan will be to treat the laryngopharyngeal reflux with some behavioral feeding strategies and medicine, and then monitor Paul over the next 3 to 6 months. Most cases of laryngomalacia resolve within 12 to 18 months; so, this is a timeline that we can use to determine how Paul is progressing."

1.13 Review Questions

1. Which of the following serves as the anterior attachment for the vocal folds?
   a) Cricoid cartilage.
   b) Anterior commissure.
   c) Thyroid notch.
   d) Corniculate cartilage.
   e) All of the above.
2. Which of the following serves as the posterior attachment for the vocal folds?
   a) Vocal process.
   b) Cricoid cartilage.
   c) Anterior commissure.
   d) Epiglottis.
   e) None of the above.

3. Which of the following influences laryngeal movement in the vertical plane (up and down)?
   a) Activity of intrinsic laryngeal muscles.
   b) Activity of the lateral cricoarytenoid.
   c) Movement of the hyoid bone.
   d) Movement of the arytenoid cartilages.
   e) Both a and b.
4. What allows the arytenoid cartilages to swivel so that the vocal folds can adduct/abduct?
   a) Cricothyroid muscle.
   b) Laryngeal elevators.
   c) Cricothyroid joint.
   d) Cricoarytenoid joint.
   e) None of the above.
5. Which of the following form the vocal fold cover?
   a) Intermediate and deep lamina propria.
   b) Vocalis and superficial lamina propria.
   c) Epithelium and superficial lamina propria.
   d) True and false vocal folds.
   e) Both a and d.
6. Which of the following are forces that facilitate vocal fold oscillation during phonation?
   a) Transglottal pressure gradients and flow vortices.
   b) Medial compression and tongue pressure.
   c) Lung contraction and velar constriction.
   d) Bernoulli's effect and tracheal decoupling.
   e) All of the above.
7. How might the presence of a glottal gap influence the resulting acoustic sound spectrum?
   a) It would decrease fundamental frequency.
   b) It would elevate fundamental frequency.
   c) It would increase the amount of noise.
   d) It would decrease the amount of noise.
   e) All of the above
8. Which of the following influences fundamental frequency of phonation?
   a) Position of velum.
   b) Interplay between cricothyroid and thyroarytenoid.
   c) Position of cricoarytenoid joint and corniculate cartilages.
   d) Dynamic movement of the hyoid bone.
   e) Both a and b.
9. Which of the following plays the LEAST important role during phonation?
   a) Thyroid cartilage.
   b) Arytenoid cartilage.
   c) Cricoid cartilage.
   d) Epiglottis.
   e) None of the above.
10. Which of the following terms represents a deviation in voice quality?
    a) Loudness.
    b) Dysphagia.
    c) Dysphonia.
    d) Inertive reactance.
    e) None of the above.

11. Which of the following is the primary sensory nerve for the larynx?
    a) The pharyngeal branch of the vagus nerve.
    b) The recurrent laryngeal branch of the vagus nerve.
    c) The internal branch of the SLN (of the vagus).
    d) The external branch of the SLN (of the vagus).
    e) The glossopharyngeal nerve.

12. Which of the following are suprahyoid muscles that elevate the larynx?
    a) Omohyoid and thyrohyoid.
    b) Thyrohyoid and sternothyroid.
    c) Geniohyoid and mylohyoid.
    d) Digastric and sternothyroid.
    e) Diaphragm and external intercostals.

13. The opening into the larynx, which is the space encircled by the aryepiglottic folds, is known as the
    a) Laryngeal valve.
    b) Laryngeal vestibule.
    c) Laryngeal hole.
    d) Trachea.
    e) Diaphragm.

14. The space in-between the left and right true vocal folds is known as the
    a) Glottis.
    b) Trachea.
    c) Larynx.
    d) Vestibule.
    e) Ventricle.

15. Supraglottal pressures generated by manipulations in the vocal tract act as a force on the vocal which influences vibration. This force is called
    a) Resonance.
    b) Frequency.
    c) Pitch.
    d) Inertive reactance.
    e) None of the above.

16. Which of the following is a nonbiological role of the larynx?
    a) Impounding air to fixate the thorax.
    b) Acting as a valve for respiration.
    c) Serving as a vibratory source for voice production.
    d) Creating subglottal pressure to generate a cough.
    e) All of the above.

17. The vocal folds consist of a layered structure, functionally divided into the cover, vocal ligament, and body. Which layers make up the vocal ligament?
    a) Epithelium and superficial lamina propria.
    b) Intermediate and deep lamina propria.
    c) Deep lamina propria and vocalis muscle.
    d) Vocalis muscle and epithelium.
    e) None of the above.

18. Which of the following muscles adduct (close) the vocal folds?
    a) Posterior cricoarytenoid and interarytenoid.
    b) Lateral cricoarytenoid, interarytenoid, and thyrohyoid.
    c) Lateral cricoarytenoid, interarytenoid, and thyroarytenoid (muscularis).

d) Posterior cricoarytenoid, lateral cricoarytenoid, and interarytenoid.
e) Interarytenoid and thyrohyoid.

19. Which of the following muscles is a tensor of the vocal folds?
    a) Cricothyroid.
    b) Posterior cricoarytenoid.
    c) Lateral cricoarytenoid.
    d) Interarytenoid.
    e) None of the above.

20. The most extreme form of the laryngeal adductor reflex results in prolonged tonic contraction of the laryngeal adductor muscles, including those that adduct the ventricular folds and laryngeal vestibule. This is also known as
    a) Laryngospasm.
    b) Cough.
    c) Throat clear.
    d) Dysphonia.
    e) All of the above.

1.14 Answers and Explanations

1. Correct: Anterior commissure (**b**).
   (**b**) The vocal folds attach anteriorly to the anterior commissure of the thyroid cartilage. The two vocal folds merge as they course toward this point. (**a**) The vocal folds do not attach directly to the cricoid cartilage, although the arytenoids, to which the vocal folds do attach, sit atop the cricoid. (**c**) The thyroid notch lies above the point where the vocal folds attach to the thyroid cartilage. (**d**) The corniculate cartilages are embedded within the aryepiglottic folds and do not communicate with the vocal fold tissue.

2. Correct: Vocal process (**a**).
   (**a**) The arytenoid cartilage consists of two projections at its base: the muscular process and the vocal process. The vocal process projects toward the front and serves as the posterior attachment of the vocal folds. At rest, the two vocal processes are separated allowing for an abducted glottal configuration and allowing air to flow through the glottis for respiration. (**b**) The vocal folds do not attach directly to the cricoid cartilage, although the arytenoids, to which the vocal folds do attach, sit atop the cricoid. (**c**) The anterior commissure, which is located on the thyroid cartilage, serves as the anterior point of attachment for the vocal folds. (**d**) The epiglottis lies above the vocal fold tissue.

3. Correct: Movement of the hyoid bone (**c**).
   (**c**) The larynx is suspended, or hangs, from the hyoid bone via membranes and ligaments. As the hyoid bone moves, so moves the larynx. Hyoid movement can cause the larynx to move in a superior and anterior direction, or an inferior direction. (**a**) Intrinsic laryngeal muscles influence glottal adduction/abduction and vocal fold tension. They do not influence the position of the larynx in the vertical plane of the neck. (**b**) The lateral cricoarytenoid is an adductor of the vocal folds and an intrinsic laryngeal muscle.

(**d**) Movement of the arytenoid cartilages influences the glottal position (abducted/adducted), but not the position of the larynx in the vertical plane.

4. Correct: Cricoarytenoid joint (**d**).
   (**d**) The cricoarytenoid joint allows the arytenoid cartilages to swivel and slide along the surface of the cricoid. These movements allow the vocal processes to approximate for glottal adduction, or separate for glottal abduction. (**a**) The cricothyroid muscle influences longitudinal tension in the vocal folds by moving them anteriorly. (**b**) The laryngeal elevators pull the entire laryngeal structure superiorly and anteriorly. (**c**) The cricothyroid joint allows the larynx to move forward and down in relationship to the cricoid cartilage.

5. Correct: Epithelium and superficial lamina propria (**c**).
   (**c**) The vocal fold cover consists of the epithelium and superficial layer of the lamina propria. Together these layers are highly mobile and will oscillate quite easily during phonation when the tissue is healthy. (**a**) The intermediate and deep layers of the lamina propria are located beneath or deep to the vocal fold cover. (**b**) Together they form the vocal ligament. (**d, e**) While the superficial lamina propria is part of the vocal fold cover, the vocalis is deep to the cover and forms the body of the vocal folds.

6. Correct: Transglottal pressure gradients and flow vortices (**a**).
   (**a**) Transglottal pressure gradients and flow vortices create regions of negative pressure which influence the edges of the vocal folds to approximate each other. Along with subglottal pressure, these help sustain vocal fold oscillation. (**b**) Medial compression will influence subglottal pressure and the open–closed phase relationships during the glottal cycle, but tongue pressure will not influence vocal fold oscillation. (**c**) Lung contraction, or contraction of the respiratory muscles, is needed for airflow during phonation but velar constriction will have no influence on vocal fold oscillation. (**d**) The Bernoulli effect does influence oscillation during the closing phase of the vibratory cycle, but tracheal decoupling does not occur in normal speech production.

7. Correct: It would increase the amount of noise (**c**).
   (**c**) A glottal gap refers to an opening in the vocal folds during phonation. This results in excess air escaping through the glottis. The acoustic characteristic of this air is nonharmonic energy, also referred to as spectral noise. (**a, b**) Fundamental frequency is influenced by the temporal aspects of oscillation—specifically, the number of times the vocal folds vibrate within a given period of time. (**d**) Any glottal gap would result in obligatory spectral noise within the acoustic signal.

8. Correct: Interplay between cricothyroid and thyroarytenoid (**b**).
   (**b**) The cricothyroid muscle and thyroarytenoid muscle are antagonistic to each other. Their interplay determines the longitudinal tension of the vocal folds, which influences fundamental frequency. (**a**) The position of the velum has no influence on fundamental frequency, but rather on how sound is resonated within the nasal cavity. (**c**) The cricoarytenoid joint allows the arytenoids to rotate but does not influence

fundamental frequency—the corniculate cartilages have no known influence on fundamental frequency. (**d**) The hyoid bone influences the vertical position of the larynx but not fundamental frequency.

9. Correct: Epiglottis (**d**).
   (**d**) The epiglottis can influence the resonance properties of the vocal tract, but has minimal influence on vocal fold oscillation. (**a**) The thyroid cartilage serves as the anterior attachment for the vocal folds and moves forward and down to influence longitudinal vocal fold tension. (**b**) The arytenoid cartilages serve as the posterior attachment for the vocal fold tissue. (**c**) The cricoid cartilage houses both the cricoarytenoid and cricothyroid joints, both of which are crucial for phonation.

10. Correct: Dysphonia (**c**).
    (**c**). Negative impacts on phonation and voice quality are perceptually labeled as dysphonia. (**a**) Loudness is a perceptual feature, but when loudness is perceived as abnormal, it represents the perceptual classification of dysphonia—that is, impaired loudness is a component of dysphonia. (**b**) Dysphagia is a medical term representing an impairment in swallowing ability. (**d**) Inertive reactance is a physical force, not a perceptual attribute.

11. Correct: The external branch of the superior laryngeal nerve (of the vagus) (**c**).
    (**c**) The vagus nerve has numerous branches among which include the pharyngeal branch, recurrent laryngeal nerve, and superior laryngeal nerve. The superior laryngeal nerve itself branches into the external division and internal division. The internal branch of the superior laryngeal nerve provides the sensory receptors to the mucosa throughout the laryngeal region. (**a**) The pharyngeal branch of the vagus nerve supplies motor innervation to the region of the velum. (**b**) The recurrent laryngeal branch supplies motor innervation to all intrinsic laryngeal muscles with exception to the cricothyroid. (**d**) The external branch of the superior laryngeal nerve supplies motor innervation to the cricothyroid muscle. (**e**) The glossopharyngeal nerve forms part of the pharyngeal plexus which provides motor and sensory innervation to the oropharyngeal region.

12. Correct: Geniohyoid and mylohyoid (**c**).
    (**c**) The geniohyoid and mylohyoid originate at the inner surface of the mandible, attaching the hyoid bone inferiorly. When they contract, their muscle fibers shorten, raising the hyoid bone. As the hyoid bone elevates, it also raises the larynx, which is suspended from the hyoid bone by membranes and ligaments. (**a**) The omohyoid is an extrinsic laryngeal depressor. (**b**) The thyrohyoid muscle has its point of origin below the hyoid, but can act as a depressor or elevator depending on the action of other muscles. (**d**) The digastric muscle is a laryngeal elevator, but the sternothyroid is a laryngeal depressor. (**e**) The diaphragm and external intercostal muscles are active during inspiration and do not manipulate laryngeal position.

13. Correct: Laryngeal vestibule (**b**).
    (**b**) A vestibule is an opening to a space. The most superior region of the larynx is surrounded by the epiglottis and

aryepiglottic folds. These encircle an open space, called the laryngeal vestibule, which effectively serves as the top opening to the larynx. (**a**) The term "laryngeal valve" refers to the valving function of the larynx for respiration. (**c**) The term "laryngeal hole" is rarely, if ever, applied to the larynx. (**d**) The trachea is located inferior to the larynx. (**e**) The diaphragm is inferior to the larynx and is a muscle of respiration.

14. Correct: Glottis (**a**).

(**a**) The term "glottis" refers to the space between the vocal folds. Muscular action can serve to open the glottis or close the glottis. A patient with vocal fold paralysis that impairs his or her ability to close the vocal folds is said to have "glottal incompetency." (**b**) The trachea is located inferior to the larynx. (**c**) The larynx houses the two vocal folds. (**d**) The vestibule is the opening to the larynx. (**e**). The ventricles are located superior to the vocal folds, and lie in between the true and false vocal folds.

15. Correct: Inertive reactance (**d**).

(**d**) When the anterior vocal tract is narrowed and the regions above the vocal folds are widened, it creates a backward-directed pressure and impedance matching of intraglottal and supraglottal resistance, via a physical phenomenon known as inertive reactance. Inertive reactance serves to help separate the vocal folds during vibration and also amplify the resulting acoustic energy. (**a**) Resonance is the selective amplification and filtering of specific frequencies within the acoustic sound spectrum. (**b**) Frequency is the vibrational rate of an object, and is not a pressure or force. (**c**) Pitch is the psychological correlate of frequency.

16. Correct: Serving as a vibratory source for voice production (**c**).

(**c**) The nonbiological role of the larynx relates to voice production for communication purposes. It is considered an "overlaid" or secondary function of the larynx is not needed for survival. Although without a voice communication can be difficult, many other means of communication exists and are used on a daily basis. (**a, b, d**) Biological functions of the larynx include those related to health and physical activity. Impounding air, respiration, and cough are all biological functions needed for survival. They are needed to function during daily life activities.

17. Correct: Intermediate and deep lamina propria (**b**).

(**b**) The intermediate and deep layers of the lamina propria collectively form the vocal ligament. The vocal ligament serves to connect the vocal fold cover to the body, in addition to absorbing physical stress caused by manipulations to vocal fold length and tension. (**a, c**) The epithelium and superficial lamina propria make up the vocal fold cover. (**d**) The vocalis muscle is considered the body of the vocal fold, and is connected to the cover by the vocal ligament.

18. Correct: Lateral cricoarytenoid, interarytenoid, and thyroarytenoid (muscularis) (**c**).

(**c**) Contraction of the lateral cricoarytenoid, interarytenoid, and thyroarytenoid (muscularis) will move the vocal process medially, causing the vocal folds to adduct. The number of motor units recruited in each muscle during contraction will determine the degree of medial compression in vocal fold closure. Medial compression is one factor that can influence

subglottal pressure during phonation. (**a**) The posterior cricoarytenoid muscle is an abductor of the vocal folds. (**b**) The thyrohyoid is an extrinsic laryngeal muscle that affects vertical position, not the position of the glottis. (**d, e**) The only three muscles that actively adduct the vocal folds are the lateral cricoarytenoid, interarytenoid, and thyroarytenoid.

19. Correct: Cricothyroid (**a**).

(**a**) The cricothyroid and thyroarytenoid (vocalis) serve as vocal fold tensors. A dynamic interplay between these muscles allows a speaker or singer to adjust fundamental frequency to produce speech prosody and the various transitions between musical notes. (**b**) The posterior cricoarytenoid is an abductor of the vocal folds. (**c**) The lateral cricoarytenoid is an adductor of the vocal folds. (**d**) The interarytenoid is an adductor of the vocal folds. (**e**) Both the cricothyroid and thyroarytenoid can be considered vocal fold adductors.

20. Correct: Dysphonia (**d**).

(**d**). Dysphonia is a term that represents a perceptual change in voice quality or function. (**a**) Laryngospasm results in complete closure of the larynx, from the level of the vestibule down to the level of the false vocal folds and true vocal folds. (**b**) Cough can be reflexive or voluntary. It usually involves closure at the level of the vocal folds only. (**c**) A throat clear requires closure at the level of the vocal folds, but not necessarily levels above them.

References

[1] Hirose H. Investigating the physiology of laryngeal structures. In: Hardcastle WJ, Laver J, Gibbon FE. The Handbook of Phonetic Sciences. 2nd ed. Hoboke, NJ. Wiley-Blackwell; 2010

[2] Gestreau C, Bianchi AL, Gr, é, lot L. Differential brainstem Fos-like immunoreactivity after laryngeal-induced coughing and its reduction by codeine. J Neurosci. 1997; 17(23):9340–9352

[3] Ludlow CL. Central nervous system control of the laryngeal muscles in humans. Respir Physiol Neurobiol. 2005; 147(2–3):205–222

[4] Vertigan AE, Gibson PG. The role of speech pathology in the management of patients with chronic refractory cough. Lung. 2012; 190(1):35–40

[5] Leydon C, Sivasankar M, Falciglia DL, Atkins C, Fisher KV. Vocal fold surface hydration: a review. J Voice. 2009; 23(6):658–665

[6] Simonyan K, Saad ZS, Loucks TM, Poletto CJ, Ludlow CL. Functional neuroanatomy of human voluntary cough and sniff production. Neuroimage. 2007; 37(2):401–409

[7] Liu H, Auger J, Larson CR. Voice fundamental frequency modulates vocal response to pitch perturbations during English speech. J Acoust Soc Am. 2010; 127(1):EL1–EL5

[8] Hirano M, Kakita Y. Cover-body theory of vocal fold vibration. In: Daniloff RG, ed. Speech Science: Recent Advances. San Diego: College-Hill Press; 1985

[9] Khosla S, Murugappan S, Paniello R, Ying J, Gutmark E. Role of vortices in voice production: normal versus asymmetric tension. Laryngoscope. 2009; 119(1):216–221

[10] Van Den Berg J. Myoelastic-aerodynamic theory of voice production. J Speech Hear Res. 1958; 1(3):227–244

[11] Titze IR. The human instrument. Sci Am. 2008; 298(1):94–101

[12] Plant RL, Younger RM. The interrelationship of subglottic air pressure, fundamental frequency, and vocal intensity during speech. J Voice. 2000; 14(2):170–177

[13] Titze IR, Sundberg J. Vocal intensity in speakers and singers. J Acoust Soc Am. 1992; 91(5):2936–2946

[14] Sundberg J, Titze I, Scherer R. Phonatory control in male singing: a study of the effects of subglottal pressure, fundamental frequency, and mode of phonation on the voice source. J Voice. 1993; 7(1):15–29

[15] Leanderson R, Sundberg J, von Euler C. Role of diaphragmatic activity during singing: a study of transdiaphragmatic pressures. J Appl Physiol (1985). 1987; 62(1):259–270

[16] Brodnitz FS. Rehabilitation of the human voice. Bull N Y Acad Med. 1966; 42 (3):231–240

[17] Froschels E, Jellinek A. Practice of Voice and Speech Therapy. Boston, MA: Expression Company Publishers; 1941

[18] Titze IR. Principles of Voice Production. Upper Saddle River, NJ: Prentice Hall; 1994

[19] Verdolini K, Druker DG, Palmer PM, Samawi H. Laryngeal adduction in resonant voice. J Voice. 1998; 12(3):315–327

[20] Awan SN, Roy N. Toward the development of an objective index of dysphonia severity: a four-factor acoustic model. Clin Linguist Phon. 2006; 20(1):35–49

[21] Awan SN, Roy N, Dromey C. Estimating dysphonia severity in continuous speech: application of a multi-parameter spectral/cepstral model. Clin Linguist Phon. 2009; 23(11):825–841

Suggested Readings

[1] Titze IR. Principles of Voice Production. Englewood Cliffs, NJ: Prentice Hall; 1994

[2] Titze IR. Comments on the myoelastic - aerodynamic theory of phonation. J Speech Hear Res. 1980; 23(3):495–510

[3] Sundberg J. Science of the Singing Voice. Dekalb, IL: Northern Illinois University Press; 1989

[4] Scherer R, Titze IR. Vocal Fold Physiology: Biomechanics, Acoustics & Phonatory Control. Denver, CO: Denver Center for the Performing Arts; 1985

[5] Baken RJ, Orlikoff RF. Clinical Measurement of Speech and Voice. San Diego: Singular; 2000

2 Survey of Voice Disorders

Summary

This chapter defines and describes etiological categories of voice disorders. Descriptions, etiological and clinical characteristics, and treatment options are associated with specific voice disorder subtypes. Voice disorders are organized into functional and organic classifications. Functional voice disorders are defined as those caused by a behavior, while organic voice disorders are defined as those caused by some neurological, structural, infectious, or systemic etiology. Please note that the classifications of functional versus organic are not mutually exclusive—inefficient and ineffective behavioral voice use may result in secondary structural changes in vocal fold structures and, in turn, underlying deficits in the structure and function of the phonatory system can result in changes in the behavioral use of the voice (e.g., compensatory behaviors). The collaborative interprofessional practice recommended for management of voice disorders is also highlighted.

Keywords: Voice disorders, dysphonia, functional, organic, phonation

2.1 Learning Objectives

At the end of this chapter, learners will be able to
- Define, compare, and contrast functional and organic voice disorders.
- Describe the etiological substrates of functional and organic voice disorders.
- Describe the clinical characteristics (signs and symptoms) of functional and organic voice disorders.
- Identify and differentiate between medical and speech–language pathology options for the management of functional and organic voice disorders.

2.2 Introduction

It is apparent that most people, regardless of their degree of understanding of voice and voice disorders, are able to distinguish a typical voice from disordered voice. This statement is supported by the findings of a study by Anders et al who reported that recorded voice samples could be easily identified and ranked by trained and untrained groups alike—training did not necessarily enhance the accuracy of perceptual identification.[1] Though we may be able to perceive differences in voice, defining typical versus disordered voice is not so easy. What is it that the listener detects in the voice signal that allows for the discrimination between typical and disordered voice? It appears that there are a number of characteristics (age, gender, racial type, body size/type, etc.) that determine a range for typical voice type and quality. As we are exposed to the vast range of voice types throughout our lives, we learn that voices may be highly differentiated but still be considered within typical expectations.[2] We gain experience as to the limits of typical voice and, thereby, develop a mental scale by which typical voice is gauged. *As long as a particular voice does not deviate substantially from this internal gauge in terms of parameters such as pitch, loudness, quality, and duration, it will be considered within the typical range.*[3]

In contrast, a **voice disorder** exists when a speaker's voice quality, pitch, loudness, vocal flexibility, and/or stamina deviates from expectations related to age, sex, body type, speaking community, communication needs, and/or performance needs.[4] The clinical presentation of a voice disorder is often labeled as **dysphonia**, a word whose literal meaning can be understood as a condition ("-ia") of bad ("dys") sound ("phon"). Dysphonia is also a medical diagnosis used by healthcare professionals and the healthcare industry. The terms "voice disorder" and "dysphonia" are often used interchangeably, although one should keep in mind that a voice disorder does not require the presence of a "bad sounding" voice. For example, an individual who experiences pain and tightness when speaking may produce a perceptually normal voice and yet be diagnosed with a voice disorder due to deviations in vocal stamina and/or flexibility that limit their ability to use voice for communication or performance needs.

Voice disorders and accompanying perceived dysphonia exist along a continuum of severity, from an absence or minor degree of the observed deviant voice characteristic to an extreme amount. The lower end of this continuum may be best acknowledged as a "minimal" level, because even typical voice signals are not necessarily perfect. On the opposite end of the continuum, an extreme level of voice deviation is highly noticeable and, most probably, has a significant effect on patient and listener alike. It is important that voice therapists have parameters by which they not only designate the severity of the perceptual characteristics of the voice but also account for the impact the voice problem may have on the speaker's ability to communicate and obtain employment.[5] The following severity terminologies attempt to incorporate several of the possible diverse effects of dysphonia[3]:

- **Mild**: While the listener experienced in the perceptual characteristics of the disordered voice may consider the voice disordered, the lay listener may consider the voice to be only unusual in nature and within typical expectations. The voice characteristics are not distracting, and the ability to effectively communicate is not affected. The dysphonia does not interfere in any substantial manner with phonation.
- **Moderate**: Both trained and untrained listeners would consider the voice dysphonic. There may be intermittent periods in which the voice characteristics are highly distracting. The ability to effectively communicate is noticeably affected under certain conditions (e.g., noisy environments). The dysphonia may occasionally cause phonation to cease or become highly effortful.
- **Severe**: Both trained and untrained listeners would consider the voice extremely dysphonic. The voice characteristics are highly distracting. The ability to effectively communicate is consistently affected. The dysphonia causes phonation to be mainly absent or extremely effortful.

The voice therapist is encouraged to closely compare the perceived abnormal voice characteristic(s) to all parts of these definitions. It may be that a disordered voice does not show all the characteristics mentioned under each definition, or it may show characteristics crossing definitions. In these cases, intermediate ratings (e.g., mild-to-moderate) may be appropriate. In addition, certain dysphonia types (e.g., inappropriately high pitch) may be considered abnormal but not necessarily disrupt the ability to phonate.

Voice disorders, whether chronic or transient, mild or severe, are experienced by a large percentage of the general population across all ages of the lifespan. Lifetime prevalence rates have been estimated at approximately 30% with point prevalence rates (number of cases at a single point in time) approaching 7% in the adult population.[6,7,8] Some groups are at a greater risk for the development of voice problems. Data from treatment-seeking populations consistently demonstrate that individuals who rely on voice production for their job-related duties, the so-called **professional voice users**, experience a greater frequency of voice problems than others. Among this group include teachers, singers, actors, clergy, lawyers, and others.[9] Nonprofessional voice users also experience voice problems with great frequency, which can be explained by the range of possible causes underlying dysphonia—as you will learn in this chapter.

Underlying the onset and maintenance of voice disorders is some **impairment** or inefficiency in body function. These impairments can relate to anatomical, physiological, behavioral, and/or psychological abnormalities which disrupt the efficiency and effectiveness of voice production and the perceptual impressions of the sound produced. For example, changes in vocal fold structure, neuromuscular control, and/or behavioral regulation of vocal subsystems are impairments which can often be identified in speakers with voice disorders. When the impairment results in the inability to produce adequate voice for the needs of a speaker, it creates a **disability**. A professor who experiences vocal fatigue and progressive dysphonia during lectures could be said to have a disability if it affects the teaching process.

When a disability leads to a restriction in life activities, such as that same professor having to take time off from teaching or not being able to find a job due to his or her restricted teaching abilities, the condition is known as a **handicap**.[10] Speech–language pathologists (SLPs) and otolaryngologists seek to determine the underlying impairment(s) causing a vocal disability. The underlying impairment becomes a primary target of voice treatment through voice therapy, medical management, or a combination of those two. As an example, disabilities and handicaps related to phonation can be improved by modifying a speaker's vocal demands and/or environment. By rehabilitating or improving the anatomical, physiological, and/or behavioral impairments underlying the voice disorder, reductions in disability and handicap often naturally follow.

Any impairment has a point of origin or cause—this is known as the **etiology** of the problem. For example, a structural change in the margin(s) of the vocal fold(s) (e.g., the formation of a polyp or nodule) can be classified as an impairment, but their origin is related to excessive phonotrauma of the vocal fold tissue. The physical characteristics of the nodules, the cellular and proteomic activity leading to their development and maintenance, and the manner in which they negatively impact vocal fold oscillation are related to the **pathology**—the state, condition, or characteristics of the problem. To treat a voice disorder, it is typically necessary to identify not only the pathology but also the underlying etiology and address both as part of a treatment plan to affect a positive change in the pathological state of the voice mechanism.

2.3 Voice Disorder Classifications

Wide varieties of classification models exist which subdivide voice impairments based on one or more dimensions.[3] For the purposes of this book, we will use an etiological framework for classifying voice disorders broadly into **functional** and **organic** categories,[11,12] and a third category of **idiopathic** to account for laryngeal conditions affecting the vocal folds for which the underlying cause has yet to be definitively identified. As you will learn in later chapters of this book, the category into which a voice disorder is assigned upon diagnosis, in addition to the subtype within a category, can substantially impact the treatment options recommended to the patient.

2.3.1 Functional Voice Disorders

A functional voice disorder is caused by vocal behaviors. These behaviors are tied to neuromuscular activity under the influence of conscious and subconscious mechanisms. Vocal behaviors can be a **primary** (e.g., the first, or original) etiology of a voice problem or a **secondary** etiology. A specific criterion for the diagnosis of a primary functional voice disorder is that no structural, neurological, or other systemic condition can be identified as an existing etiology of the current impairment.[13] In some cases, a primary functional voice disorder is precipitated by an acute systemic condition such as upper respiratory infection, but at the time of clinical presentation the precipitating organic condition has resided and no other illness or impairment could otherwise explain the voice problems. A synonym for this category is "**nonorganic**," and some authorities have also used the labels "**muscle misuse**" and "**psychogenic**" voice disorders as the broad category label. The term "psychogenic" relates to the strong ties between psychological processes and voice production, and the belief by some that most subtypes of functional voice disorders are caused by emotional and psychological reactions[4] to life events. It is true that the cranial nerves controlling laryngeal muscles are intimately connected to the emotional centers of the brain,[14] and a detailed history often reveals major life events and/or stressors in the recent past of patients diagnosed with primary functional voice disorders.[15] A behavioral change in the activity of respiratory, laryngeal, and supralaryngeal muscles that are under the influence of the voluntary motor pathways is the common thread among functional voice disorders, a major reason we include these impairments within this category.

An important concept in understanding functional voice disorders is that, while structural, neurological, or systemic etiology is not necessary for diagnosis, **structural changes to the vocal folds may develop as a result of the vocal behaviors.** For example, vocal nodules are structural changes to vocal fold tissue. However, if a patient never used his or her voice, the nodules would not develop. In a majority of cases, the behavior underlying the functional voice disorder is **imbalanced or dysregulated control of laryngeal, respiratory, and/or perilaryngeal muscles** characterized by excessive muscular activation.[16] This excessive kinetic pattern of muscular contraction is sometimes referred to as **vocal hyperfunction** and voice problems resulting from these patterns are commonly labeled as **hyperfunctional voice disorders**.[4]

The neuromotor imbalance characteristic of functional voice disorders can arise from habituated muscle tension and vocal inefficiency, compensatory behaviors to some other physiological impairment, and/or psychological stress. In effect, the patient's use of the vocal mechanism has resulted in the dysphonia. **Patients can present with more than one etiology underlying their current voice difficulties.** It is not uncommon for functional voice disorders to develop in response to a primary organic etiology. **In these cases, the functional component is labeled as a secondary etiology.** One reason this can occur is that many patients attempt to compensate for a change in voice due to an organic etiology by adjusting the balance between respiration, phonation, and resonance when producing voice. This can lead to maladaptive hyperfunctional voicing patterns that cause an additional impairment. In such cases, the functional etiology would be secondary to the original organic cause.

2.3.2 Organic Voice Disorders

Organic voice disorders are caused by structural, systemic, or neurological changes to the respiratory and/or laryngeal mechanisms necessary for phonation. Organic voice disorders are *not initially* caused by vocal behaviors—conceptually, even in the absence of voice use, the organic changes would still develop. The onset of organic voice disorders can be due to **endogenous factors** (from within one's own body—e.g., inflammatory cellular activity, neurodegenerative conditions) or **exogenous factors** (from outside one's own body—e.g., surgery affecting respiratory or laryngeal structures). Organic voice disorders can also occur in conjunction with functional voice disorders. In most of those cases, the organic disorder is the primary etiology and the functional disorder is the secondary etiology, developing in response to the organic condition.

Certain structural changes to vocal fold tissue may be caused by organic and/or functional etiologies. For example, vocal process granulomas (see below) maybe due to phonotrauma via vocal behaviors (functional cause) or from reflux and/or intubation (organic causes). In these cases, it can be difficult to determine if the etiology is purely organic or if there is a functional component to the onset of the problem. Voice disorder subtypes which fall into both categories or which can be challenging to label into one specific category will be described below.

2.3.3 Idiopathic Voice Disorders

Idiopathic voice disorders have underlying etiologies which have not been conclusively identified. The impairment and disability can be understood in these conditions, and often successfully managed, but the origin of the problem has yet to be determined. This diagnosis should be used with great care and only after an exhaustive assessment has been completed.

2.4 Functional Voice Disorders

▶ Table 2.1 illustrates subtypes of commonly observed voice disorders along with associated clinical characteristics that tend to have a functional cause. It should be very obvious from this table that many clinical characteristics are similar across functional subtypes. It is also true that perceptual, acoustic, and aerodynamic characteristics can be similar when comparing functional with organic voice disorders. **These similarities indicate the vital importance of laryngeal visualization and referral to an otolaryngologist for medical evaluation prior to any final diagnosis being made and treatment being implemented.**

2.4.1 Muscle Tension Dysphonia

Description

Muscle tension dysphonia (MTD) can be of two types, primary MTD and secondary MTD. **Primary MTD** is a change in voice quality, pitch, loudness, flexibility, and/or stamina which occurs in the absence of any current structural, systemic, or neurological changes to the subsystems of voice. **Secondary MTD** results in similar voice changes but occurs in response to a primary organic etiology. MTD also goes by the broader label of **functional dysphonia**, although that term has also been used to refer to functional voice disorders primarily resulting from psychological factors.[4,13]

MTD is a common voice disorder, accounting for 8 to 45% of all diagnoses among treatment-seeking populations.[7,17,18,19] As with most functional voice disorder subtypes, MTD is diagnosed more frequently in females than in males and can occur in patients across the lifespan.[7,19] MTD presents along a continuum of perceived severity, both from the patient's perspective and the clinician's perspective. The dysphonia resulting from MTD can manifest as a wide range of changes in quality, pitch, and/or loudness. Symptoms and signs of MTD form a cluster of dimensions which can vary from patient to patient. Typical symptoms of MTD include some combination of the following:

- Tension, soreness, and/or pain in neck and/or shoulder region.
- Vocal fatigue.
- Variable or consistent changes in voice quality, pitch, or loudness (dysphonia).
- Loss of frequency range.
- Globus sensation in throat.
- Increased effort needed to produce voice.

2.4.2 Etiological Characteristics

A number of theories have attempted to explain the genesis of primary MTD, and thorough assessment will often lead the identification of one or more of the following:

- Technical misuse of the vocal mechanism, often related to heavy vocal demands or unique vocal requirements associated with a professional or social activity. The frequency and/or type of voice use can lead to musculoskeletal tension in a similar manner as one might experience in the limbs after heavy or sustained exercise. Muscular tension in the subsystems of voice can limit vocal flexibility, stamina, and phonation physiology, the third causing dysphonia. As the speaker begins to subconsciously compensate for these changes, the poor technical control can develop into a habituated (e.g., chronic) incoordination of respiratory, laryngeal, and articulatory musculature; excessive contraction of intrinsic and extrinsic laryngeal muscles; inappropriate resonant focus; and/or improper control of vocal frequency and intensity.[13,20,21]

Table 2.1 Clinical characteristics of functional voice disorder subtypes. Subtypes with * represent those with possible multifactorial etiologies in addition to functional voicing behaviors. Clinical characteristics listed are those most commonly associated with the subtypes, although there can be great variability in clinical presentation from speaker-to-speaker

Subtype	Clinical Characteristics
Muscle tension dysphonia	**Endoscopic** ○ Normal laryngeal structure (primary MTD) ○ Supraglottic compression of the false vocal folds in the medial (toward midline) dimension. ○ Supraglottic anterior-posterior compression (the petiolus of the epiglottis approximates the arytenoids). ○ Excessive medial compression at the glottis, often manifested by tight closure ("hyperadduction") at voicing onsets. ○ Posterior glottal gap ○ Vocal fold bowing during contraction **Aerodynamic** ○ Increased mean and peak subglottal pressure ○ Increased phonation threshold pressure ○ Decreased transglottal airflow **Acoustic** ○ Decreased cepstral peak prominence ○ Increased perturbation (e.g., larger measures of jitter and/or shimmer) ○ Increased spectral noise (e.g., lower measures of harmonic-to-noise ratio) ○ Increased fundamental frequency ○ Decreased physiological frequency range **Auditory-Perceptual** ○ Dysphonia often characterized by roughness associated with increased perturbation but sometimes breathiness resulting from glottal gaps secondary to the hyperfunction. ○ Strain and effort when speaking ○ Hard glottal attacks (voicing onset) **Visual & Tactile** ○ Decreased thyrohyoid space ○ Pain when palpating anterior and lateral margins of neck in the vicinity of the larynx ○ Elevated larynx ○ Bulging sternocleidomastoid muscle
Psychogenic dysphonia/ aphonia	**Endoscopic** ○ Similar to MTD **Aerodynamic** ○ Similar to MTD, unless aphonia present **Acoustic** ○ Similar to MTD, unless aphonia present **Auditory-Perceptual** ○ Dysphonia on a continuum from mild dysphonia to aphonia ○ Characteristics of dysphonia typically more variable compared to MTD **Visual & Tactile** ○ Similar to MTD
Mutational falsetto	**Endoscopic** ○ Elongated vocal folds associated with increased longitudinal tension; Otherwise normal. **Acoustic** ○ Increased fundamental frequency **Aerodynamic** ○ Possible increased phonation threshold pressure due to increased vocal fold tension **Auditory-Perceptual** ○ Abnormally high pitch **Pitch breaks** ○ Breathy voice ○ Hard glottal attacks ○ Normal sounds produced during vegetative voicing (cough, throat clear, etc.) ○ Often stimulable for lower pitch during diagnostic probes **Tactile & Visual** ○ Elevated larynx
Nodules	**Endoscopic** ○ Bilateral symmetric or quasi-symmetric exophytic masses at mid-membranous vocal folds ○ Hourglass closure pattern ○ Normal or minimally reduced mucosal wave at site of mass – will be more affected with larger/stiffer nodules ○ Normal or minimally effected vibratory amplitude, symmetry, and periodicity – will be more affected by larger/stiffer nodules ○ Compensatory hyperfunction (medial & anterior-posterior compression)

Table 2.1 continued

Subtype	Clinical Characteristics
	Aerodynamic ○ Increased subglottal pressure ○ Increased phonation threshold pressure ○ Increased transglottal airflow **Acoustic** ○ Variable effects on fundamental frequency ○ Decreased physiological frequency range ○ Increased perturbation ○ Decreased cepstral peak prominence ○ Decreased harmonics-to-noise ratio **Auditory-Perceptual** ○ Breathy or hoarse voice quality ○ Pitch breaks ○ Excessive loudness in some speakers
Polyps	**Endoscopic** ○ Unilateral exophytic mass at mid-membranous vocal fold ○ Possible contralateral reactive mass ○ Hourglass closure pattern ○ Increased vascularity – often a prominent vessel feeding into the mass ○ Reduced mucosal wave at site of mass ○ Reduced amplitude and symmetry and periodicity of vibration ○ Compensatory hyperfunction (medial & anterior-posterior compression) **Aerodynamic** ○ Increased subglottal pressure ○ Increased phonation threshold pressure ○ Increased transglottal airflow **Acoustic** ○ Variable effects on fundamental frequency ○ Decreased physiological frequency range ○ Increased perturbation ○ Decreased cepstral peak prominence ○ Decreased harmonics-to-noise ratio **Auditory-Perceptual** ○ Breathy or hoarse voice quality ○ Pitch breaks ○ Excessive loudness in some speakers
Pseudocysts*	**Endoscopic** ○ Unilateral exophytic mass at mid-membranous vocal fold, with translucent appearance ○ Reduced adduction of arytenoid on affected side may be visible. ○ Hourglass closure pattern ○ Mucosal wave, amplitude, symmetry, and periodicity may be unaffected or only minimally affected. Larger masses may exacerbate signs in this domains ○ Compensatory hyperfunction (medial & anterior-posterior compression) in more severe masses **Aerodynamic** ○ Increased subglottal pressure ○ Increased phonation threshold pressure ○ Increased transglottal airflow **Acoustic** ○ Variable effects on fundamental frequency ○ Decreased physiological frequency range ○ Increased perturbation ○ Decreased cepstral peak prominence ○ Decreased harmonics-to-noise ratio **Auditory-Perceptual** ○ Breathy or hoarse voice quality ○ Pitch breaks ○ Excessive loudness in some speakers
Cysts*	**Endoscopic** ○ Unilateral mass at mid-membranous vocal folds, often appearing as a white subepithelial capsule ○ Hourglass closure pattern ○ Reduced mucosal wave—typically to a greater extent than other mid-membranous lesions ○ Reduced amplitude, symmetry, and periodicity—will be more affected by larger/stiffer cysts ○ Compensatory hyperfunction (medial & anterior-posterior compression) **Aerodynamic**

Table 2.1 continued

Subtype	Clinical Characteristics
	◦ Increased subglottal pressure ◦ Increased phonation threshold pressure ◦ Increased transglottal airflow Acoustic ◦ Variable effects on fundamental frequency ◦ Decreased physiological frequency range ◦ Increased perturbation ◦ Decreased cepstral peak prominence ◦ Decreased harmonics-to-noise ratio Auditory-Perceptual ◦ Breathy or hoarse voice quality ◦ Pitch breaks
Granulomas*	Endoscopic ◦ Unilateral or bilateral exophytic masses at vocal process of arytenoids ◦ Possible groove in at one arytenoid caused by contralateral contact patterns. ◦ Erythema (redness) and edema in posterior larynx may accompany lesions (suggestive of reflux) ◦ Compensatory hyperfunction (medial & anterior-posterior compression) Aerodynamic ◦ May be within normal limits when no dysphonia present ◦ Increased subglottal pressure and transglottal airflow expected if granulomas interfere with glottal closure ◦ If compensatory hyperfunction is present without glottal incompetence decreased transglottal airflow could be expected Acoustic ◦ May be within normal limits when no dysphonia is present. ◦ Characteristics of MTD when compensatory hyperfunction is present Auditory-Perceptual ◦ Often within normal limits ◦ May be strain when compensatory hyperfunction is present.
Edema*	Endoscopic ◦ Unilateral or bilateral translucent or pale white puffiness in vocal fold cover ◦ In Reinke's edema, large balloon-like enlargement of vocal folds often with prominent vasculature ◦ Complete closure pattern ◦ Reduced mucosal wave, amplitude, symmetry, and periodicity Aerodynamic ◦ Increased subglottal pressure ◦ Increased phonation threshold pressure Acoustic ◦ Low fundamental frequency ◦ Decreased physiological frequency range ◦ Increased perturbation ◦ Decreased cepstral peak prominence ◦ Decreased harmonics-to-noise ratio Auditory-Perceptual ◦ Extremely low pitch ◦ Rough voice quality ◦ Strain
Vascular injury	Endoscopic ◦ Unilateral or bilateral prominent vasculature. ◦ May take form of varix, ectasia, telangiectasias, and/or hemorrhage Aerodynamic ◦ May be within normal limits ◦ With compensatory hyperfunction, may be similar to MTD Acoustic ◦ May be within normal limits ◦ With compensatory hyperfunction, may be similar to MTD Auditory-Perceptual ◦ May be within normal limits ◦ With compensatory hyperfunction, may be similar to MTD

- Musculoskeletal tension may be a learned adaptation (compensation) from an acute (transient) organic condition, such as an upper respiratory infection, allergic reaction, or laryngopharyngeal reflux (LPR). As the organic precipitator fades or heals, the speaker's muscular adaptation is so habituated that they are unable to independently restore an efficient physiological balance in the subsystems of voice.[3,20,21]

- Excessive musculoskeletal tension can be induced by psychological and/or trait characteristics of the individual. Factors such as personality, emotion, and stress have long been linked with musculoskeletal tension in the subsystems of voice.[22] Mental illness has also been associated with behavioral changes in vocal function, although we will identify this cause as a separate subtype of functional voice disorder below.[4] In the case of emotion and stress, it is believed that hyperfunctional voicing behaviors arise subsequent to disinhibition of subcortical pathways in response to environmental triggers. The subcortical emotional release may result in poor control over respiratory and phonatory subsystems. Psychological distress has also been associated with a "pressor" response that results in hyperfunctional muscular reactions in the laryngeal and respiratory muscle.[4,12,13,20]

The excessive musculoskeletal tension of secondary MTD is thought to develop as a compensatory adaption for an existing organic condition. MTD occurs in varied populations of speakers, including professional and nonprofessional voice users, singers and nonsingers, in addition to adults and children. Both primary and secondary MTDs are characterized by similar clinical signs which are detailed in ▸ Table 2.1.[23]

Clinical Characteristics

Visual inspection of the larynx with endoscopy in patients with primary or secondary MTD will often reveal signs of muscular hyperfunction. Hyperfunction can be visualized in at least three ways: (1) medial compression of the supraglottic false vocal folds (▸ Fig. 2.1), (2) anterior-posterior supraglottic squeezing which often obscures views of the anterior vocal fold regions (▸ Fig. 2.2), and (3) tightly compressed vocal folds and arytenoid cartilages at the onset of phonation. When stroboscopy is added to the endoscopic exams, it is not uncommon to observe a posterior glottal gap and shortened open phase of the vibratory cycle. Voices which are perceptually rough might include visual signs of

reduced periodicity, mucosal wave, and symmetry of vibration. In patients who manifest increased activity in the posterior cricoarytenoid, a clinical sign might include bowing either unilaterally or bilaterally while the vocal folds are adducted.

The physiological changes observed during laryngeal endoscopy and videostroboscopy influence the aerodynamic and acoustic measurements obtained during the comprehensive voice evaluation. Aerodynamic characteristics of MTD include increases in subglottal air pressure and decreases in transglottal airflow. Acoustic characteristics reflect the reduced periodicity and stability of phonation. These are manifested in elevated measures of frequency and amplitude perturbation (jitter and shimmer, respectively) and decreased cepstral peak prominence. Phonation instability can introduce additive noise in the acoustic signal, which is reflected in decreased values of harmonic-to-noise ratio. Because of the excessive muscular tension underlying MTD, reduced flexibility of laryngeal function can be measured in a compressed physiological frequency range.

Auditory-perceptual, tactile (via laryngeal palpation), and external visual signs can also inform clinical hypotheses of the presence of MTD. Voice quality is often perceived as rough and strained, although some speakers can manifest breathiness. During voicing, onsets at the initiation of a breath group might also display **hard glottal attacks**—a sharp burst of loudness during the initial sound of a word. When the larynx of patients with MTD is palpated, there is often a reduced thyrohyoid space and many patients report pain or soreness when pressure is applied centrally and laterally around the laryngeal region. In some patients, the sternocleidomastoid muscle bulges during speaking, and the larynx can be extremely elevated even at rest.

As previously mentioned the severity of MTD varies widely from patient to patient, although the reported symptoms are generally a consistent problem either throughout the day or during periods of heavy voice use. In severe cases of primary and secondary MTD, the hyperfunction of the intrinsic laryngeal

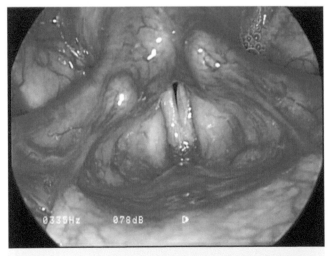

Fig. 2.1 Hyperfunctional signs in muscle tension dysphonia (MTD). Endoscopic view of larynx demonstrating medial compression of the false vocal folds in a case of primary MTD, obscuring the lateral portions of the true vocal folds. (From Bhattacharyya A. Laryngology: Otorhinolaryngology—Head and Neck Surgery Series. 1st edition. New York: Thieme Publishers, 2014.)

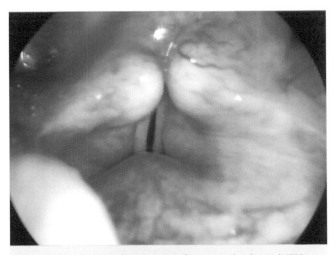

Fig. 2.2 Hyperfunctional signs in muscle tension dysphonia (MTD). Endoscopic view of larynx demonstrating anterior-posterior compression of the larynx in a case of secondary MTD subsequent to glottal insufficiency. Notice the petiolus of the epiglottis (the bump just above the most anterior part of the vocal folds) bulges posteriorly and approximates the arytenoid cartilages, obscuring the anterior vocal folds. (From Kendall K, Leonard R. Laryngeal Evaluation, 1st edition. New York: Thieme Publishers, 2010.)

muscles may be so great that the false vocal folds compress medially and closely approximate each other. This may result in vibration of the false vocal folds along with or instead of the true vocal folds, a condition known as **ventricular phonation**. The voice quality of ventricular phonation is characterized by severe roughness, low pitch, and strain.

In some cases of MTD, the hyperfunction can manifest as incomplete glottal closure, believed to occur when the vocal fold adductor muscles co-contract with the antagonistic abductor muscle, the posterior cricoarytenoid. The voice quality in these cases of MTD is characterized by breathiness, which can be subtle or extreme depending on the degree of hyperfunction. An alternative theory for breathiness associated with MTD is that glottal insufficiency results from severe fatigue in the laryngeal adductor muscles after chronic hypercontraction.[11] It is important to understand that this same voice quality can be caused by clinical psychiatric or psychological disorders, as discussed below; therefore, it is of utmost clinical importance to determine if mental illness is a possibility. If suspected, referral to a mental health professional is warranted. This referral can also be appropriate for those diagnosed with MTD where psychological processes associated with personality, emotional responses, and stress reactions are so great that the knowledge and skills of the SLP are inadequate to address them as part of a treatment plan.

Treatment

Research evidence and clinical experience support voice therapy as an effective intervention for MTD, given the presence of certain prognostic variables. Among the positive prognostic indicators include a compliant and motivated patient, recent onset as opposed to a long history of dysphonia, positive physiological health, and a lack of secondary gain associated with the voice problem. Secondary gain is an extraneous benefit that is independent of beneficial voice therapy; secondary gain may perpetuate and reinforce the disorder. Behavioral treatments targeting a physiological balance in the vocal subsystems are often effective for improving vocal outcomes within six to twelve treatments sessions, sometimes longer, when delivered by a skilled and knowledgeable clinician. As described in Chapter 8, resonant approaches, flow phonation, vocal function exercises, semioccluded vocal tract exercises, and manual circumlaryngeal massage/reposturing are some of the strategies that can be effective for treating primary or secondary MTD.[24,25,26,27,28,29]

Psychological Processes and MTD

In addition to serving as a phonemic and linguistic marker during speech production, human phonation is influenced by psychological processes in the mind of the speaker (i.e., those mental processes which include reasoning, judging, analyzing, perceiving, feeling, etc.) and causes psychological reactions in the mind of the listener. A speaker will use phonation to convey emotion, personality, and intent among other paralinguistic features. A listener will make judgments about a speaker based on their perception of voice, judgments which include decisions about a speaker's sincerity, character, motivation, sociocultural background, and also likeability.[12] Speakers are cognizant of these listener reactions, and use information from listener responses to inform subsequent use of voice. In both normal and dysphonic speakers, these psychological processes are intimately linked to and constantly influence phonation.[4]

It is logical to consider that psychological responses to life activities and the environment, including emotional and stress reactions, can influence phonation physiology in such a way that those reactions become a facilitator of dysphonia. For example, many nervous speakers have experienced acute examples of dysphonia when giving a speech to a public audience. When associated with chronic dysphonia, these psychological responses typically manifest as increased muscular tension and are linked to broader physiological impairments associated with MTD—a physiological imbalance between the subsystems of voice. The **Trait Theory** explains the development of functional voice disorders as a behavioral response to environmental stimuli which is then manifested in excessive muscle tension.[22] This can be further understood as heightened sensitivity to specific stimuli causes some speakers to respond physiologically in the form of dysregulated motor control in the subsystems of voice. According to this theory, individuals with personality dimensions of elevated neuroticism and low extraversion are most at risk for the development of functional voice disorders.[22,25,30]

It is also logical to consider that an existing dysphonia can result in subsequent psychological reactions that further influence phonation physiology. These reactions may cause dysphonia to be maintained over time or progress in severity and form. However, these are often natural, intensified psychological reactions by speakers to environmental stress and/or the sound of their own dysphonic voice. While these reactions and the stressors that trigger them can often be identified with skillful evaluation techniques, their presence does not necessarily indicate a psychological disorder. Thus, MTD in both primary and secondary forms is often associated with psychological reactions to the environment and/or a speaker's perception of their own dysphonic voice, but this should not be automatically interpreted as a speaker suffering from a mental illness.

The onset and maintenance of voice disorders have been linked to psychological factors such as reactions to interpersonal relationships, social communication, and other life-related activities.[4,31,32,33] To investigate possible psychological sources of muscular tension, it is important to utilize a screening tool as part of a comprehensive voice evaluation. An individual's personality type has also been associated with an increased risk of functional voice disorders.[25,30,34] In such cases, it can be useful to incorporate a personality profile or questions which probe more deeply into personality characteristics (e.g., introversion/extroversion). The information gained from these tools will help the clinician to better understand how a patient's psychological processing, physiological reactions to that processing, and personality relate to the voice impairment. This information can then be used to develop an effective and comprehensive treatment plan that may include counseling by the clinician and/or referral to appropriate mental health professionals.

2.4.3 Psychogenic Dysphonia

Description

It is important to realize that voice production *can* be influenced by mental illness—psychiatric or psychological disorders with specific diagnostic criteria defined by the Diagnostic and Statistical Manual of Mental Disorders.[35] In our classification model, we categorize **psychogenic dysphonia** as a subtype of functional voice disorders caused by some form of mental illness. The auditory-perceptual characteristics of psychogenic dysphonia can range from mild to severe dysphonia, and in some cases complete aphonia presenting as a whisper. Our narrow definition of psychogenic dysphonia differs from a number of previous sources; some have used this term as a categorical label for all functional voice disorders, while others have referred to psychogenic voice problems specifically as "**functional dysphonia**" or "**functional aphonia**" depending on the auditory-perceptual characteristics of the voice.[4,12,13,36]

Etiological Characteristics

Voice impairments resulting from psychogenic dysphonia have been associated with a number of psychiatric conditions, including conversion disorders, somatization disorders, and mood disorders among others.[4,35] These diagnoses are made by psychiatrists and psychologists, not the SLP, indicating the necessity for referral whenever a mental health issue is suspected. It can be difficult to differentiate MTD from psychogenic dysphonia because the clinical presentation is similar and, as noted earlier, MTD can be exacerbated by personality and reactions to life stress. It is best practice to refer patients to mental health professionals whenever psychological dysfunction is suspected.

Clinical Characteristics

Endoscopic, auditory-perceptual, and acoustic clinical signs of psychogenic aphonia can be very similar to those of MTD, making it challenging to differentiate these two voice disorder subtypes in some patients. According to Verdolini et al, features of vocal impairment associated with psychiatric or psychological voice disorders include the following[35]:

- Variable (from speaker-to-speaker) voice quality ranging from perceptually mild dysphonia to complete aphonia.
- Variable (from speaker-to-speaker) glottal adduction ranging from hyperadduction to hypoadduction.
- Odynophonia (pain during phonation—also associated with a variety of other disorders).
- Laryngeal pain (also associated with a variety of other disorders).
- In the presence of aphonia, vegetative voicing behaviors (e.g., cough, throat clear) remain intact.
- Decreased fundamental frequency (associated specifically with depression).

Treatment

A psychological screening is an important tool to consider as part of a routine voice evaluation protocol, but especially in cases where possible disordered psychological processes are suspected. Because these processes drive the physiological impairments underlying psychogenic dysphonia, referral to a mental health professional is the appropriate next step when evidence leads to the clinical hypothesis that psychogenic dysphonia is a possibility. This does not prohibit the use of clinical probes during the diagnostic process to determine if the patient is stimulable for improved voice, or even trial voice therapy to reestablish more functional voice production.

When appropriate referrals are made and the patient chooses a trial of voice therapy, the authors' collective clinical experiences have found that aphonia is easier to treat than the irregular dysphonia that is typical in patients with underlying psychological disturbances. For aphonia, an initial goal is to establish vocal fold oscillation. Vegetative voicing behaviors (cough, throat clear, vocal fry, lip trills) often succeed in eliciting phonation. Once voicing is consistently established, the goal is to shape this into sustained phonation, usually following a hierarchy of vowel prolongation to syllables to words and then **phrases**. Psychogenic dysphonia can be highly variable in its characteristics, which can differentiate it from MTD. An initial goal in these cases is to establish a more consistent phonation pattern while unloading the hyperfunctional laryngeal behaviors that are underlying the dysphonia. Similar techniques as those used with MTD can be successful, although patients with psychogenic dysphonia might require more treatment sessions than those with aphonia to establish carryover. In both psychogenic aphonia and dysphonia, our experience suggests that any secondary gain from the voice problem will make treatment prognosis less favorable.

2.4.4 Mutational Falsetto

Description

Mutational falsetto is a functional voice disorder characterized by abnormally elevated speaking fundamental frequency. It is associated with failure to naturally lower vocal pitch during puberty, which can persist through adolescence and adulthood.[37] Because of its onset around the time of puberty, it has also been called "**puberphonia.**" Mutational falsetto is most commonly seen in males, although it can also affect females.[3,37] The dysphonia of mutational falsetto occurs in the context of a normal laryngeal structure and neurological innervation.

Etiological Characteristics

The precipitating cause of mutational falsetto is not known and likely multifactorial. Various theories have been suggested, which include

- Previous experience of an embarrassing pitch break (due to natural maturation processes), resulting in the maintenance of the "childlike" pitch because the speaker believes they have greater control of this higher fundamental frequency.
- Embarrassment related to a sudden low pitch voice that is different from one's peers.
- Psychological immaturity.
- A stronger feminine self-identification in a male.
- Rewards of a higher-pitched voice related to singing.

These psychological factors are not the only possible cause of an elevated pitch in a teenage/adult male or female, reinforcing the need for a comprehensive voice evaluation and otolaryngologic evaluation prior to final diagnosis. Other causes of this voice type, which would not be mutational falsetto and not classified as a primary functional voice disorder, can include

- Endocrine disorders affecting laryngeal development.
- Hearing loss.
- Underlying weakness/dysarthria in the laryngeal muscles resulting in atrophy and/or vocal strain.

Clinical Characteristics

Clinical characteristics associated with mutational falsetto are illustrated in ▸ Table 2.1. The most common and dominant symptom reported by the patient and/or their caregivers is an abnormally high pitch. Patients might also relate negative social reactions from peers and strangers when communicating, and gender confusion by listeners when speaking on the phone. The increased vocal fold tension causing elevated fundamental frequency can be observed on endoscopy and is represented by elongated vocal folds (due to excessive cricothyroid contraction). Other features of laryngeal structure, color, and movement fall within normal limits.

Acoustic signs of mutational falsetto are typically increased fundamental frequency, which will be present during sustained vowels and connected speech. This validates the clinician's (and patient's) perception of elevated pitch. In addition, auditory-perceptual features may include pitch breaks during connected speech, mild breathiness, and hard glottal attacks. These features reflect the patient's lack of refinement in laryngeal and respiratory motor control. Interestingly, vegetative sounds such as coughing and throat clear, and sometimes humming, may be produced with normal voice quality. These behaviors can also be used during trial diagnostic probes intended to facilitate a reduction in pitch.

Treatment

The elevated fundamental frequency and subsequent high pitch in the context of a teenage or adult body is the most salient clinical characteristic of mutational falsetto. Once an accurate diagnosis is made, treatment for mutational falsetto can be efficient and highly successful. As with all voice treatments, a laryngeal exam performed by an otolaryngologist is a requirement prior to the initiation of voice therapy in order to rule in or out associated medical diagnoses. Voice therapy for mutational falsetto can often utilize a symptomatic approach focusing on the singular pitch abnormality.[31] Incorporation of circumlaryngeal massage and reposturing, shaping of low pitch vegetative voicing (e.g., grunts, growls), and humming are commonly utilized therapeutic strategies to establish a naturally lower pitch. Many patients quickly adapt their motor behaviors to accommodate the more natural pitch and are able to establish consistency in production within one treatment session. Some cases may need multiple treatment sessions, although in general cases of mutational falsetto do not require prolonged voice therapy.

2.4.5 Functional Voice Disorders Related to Phonotrauma

Phonotrauma is a physical injury that occurs to the tissue of the vocal folds secondary to vocal behaviors (phonation + trauma = phonotrauma). The vocal behaviors which lead to phonotrauma have often been labeled as **vocal abuse and misuse**. Phonotrauma can result in abnormal tissue changes to the vocal fold structure. The development of these changes can be conceptualized in this way: As the vocal folds oscillate, they continually contact each other during the closing and closed phases of vibration. These collisions create mechanical stresses on the vocal fold tissue, which include impact stress and shear stress.[38]

As a result of these stresses, the vocal folds continually experience cellular activity associated with wound healing, a normal process that maintains the health and integrity of the tissue.

Wound healing progresses in three phases: (1) inflammation, (2) proteomic deposition within the extracellular matrix (ECM) and cellular deposition in the vocal fold epithelium (epithelialization), and (3) tissue remodeling.[39] When mechanical stresses are too great or too frequent, they can overburden this wound healing process, injure the vascular supply of the vocal folds, disrupt the integrity of tissue remodeling, and lead to phonotrauma.[40] The products of this disrupted wound healing process can be a combination of edema, epithelial hyperplasia, and disorganization of the ECM leading to the development of abnormal masses in the vocal fold cover.

Certain regions of the layered vocal folds appear more susceptible to phonotrauma, including the **basement membrane zone** (BMZ), mid-membranous region of the vocal fold, and tissue in the cartilaginous glottis. As described in Chapter 1 and illustrated in ▸ Fig. 2.3, the BMZ is the region between the vocal fold epithelium and superficial layer of the lamina propria (SLLP) which bonds these two layers together. The BMZ itself is layered, consisting of a superficial **lamina lucida** and a deep **lamina densa**. The lamina lucida contains collagen and fibronectin proteins running vertically which connect this layer to the epithelium above and lamina densa below. The lamina densa also contains collagen fibers which anchor it to the SLLP below. It has been suggested that the BMZ proteomic composition and structure is crucial for maintaining tissue integrity of the vocal fold cover and its links to the vocal ligament.[41] Injury to the BMZ secondary to phonotrauma is a leading theory explaining the development of many benign masses which develop on the medial edges of the vocal folds secondary to acute or chronic phonotrauma.[39,42,43]

2.4.6 Vocal Fold Nodules

Description

Vocal fold nodules (VFN) are bilateral **exophytic** (growing outward; raised above the surface of the epithelium) masses located at the mid-membranous medial edges of the vocal folds (▸ Fig. 2.4; ▸ Fig. 2.5). Along with vocal fold polyps, cysts, and pseudocysts, they have been labeled a type of **benign mid-membranous lesion**. When a functional voicing behavior leads to phonotrauma and tissue change, the mid-membranous region is the most common area affected. Because the exophytic mass will restrict vocal fold closure on either side of the "bumps," closure pattern in mid-membranous lesions is often exemplified by an hourglass configuration, as illustrated in ▸ Fig. 2.6. VFN are symmetrical or quasi-symmetrical and can vary in size and shape depending on their stage of development and the patient's voice use patterns.

Etiological Characteristics

VFN are caused by phonotrauma and develop at the mid-membranous region (often referred to as the "nodal point") because this area absorbs the greatest impact stress from collision forces during vocal fold vibration.[38] VFN develop in stages, starting out as a soft, small edematous **excrescence** (an abnormal outgrowth)

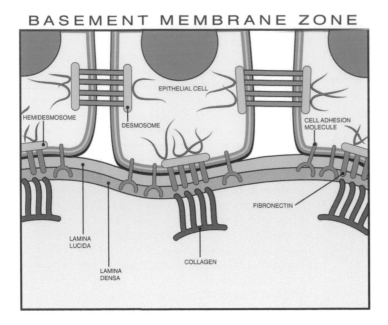

Fig. 2.3 Basement membrane zone (BMZ) of vocal folds.

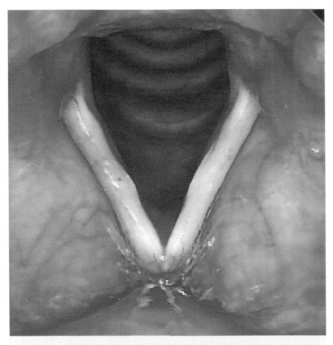

Fig. 2.4 Vocal fold nodules. Vocal fold nodules are exophytic masses at the medial edges in the middle of the membranous vocal fold (or the juncture of the anterior 1/3 and posterior 2/3 of total vocal fold tissue). They appear symmetric or quasi-symmetric calluses or bumps in the vocal fold epithelium. (From Kendall K, Leonard R. Laryngeal Evaluation, 1st edition. New York: Thieme Publishers, 2010.)

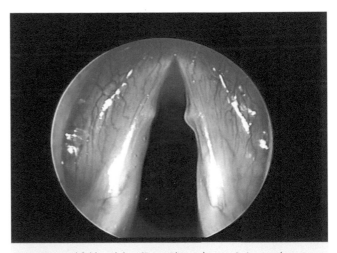

Fig. 2.5 Vocal fold nodules. (From Bhattacharyya A. Laryngology: Otorhinolaryngology—Head and Neck Surgery Series. 1st edition. New York: Thieme Publishers, 2014.)

which over time develops into a more fibrous, larger, and stiffer mass. At a microscopic level, VFN are characterized by epithelial hyperplasia (it becomes thicker), increased density of the BMZ with increased deposition of fibronectin, and possible separation from the epithelium above, along with increased levels of hyaluronic acid and disorganized elastin fibers in the SLLP.[42,43,44,45] These changes are brought on by disruptions in the normal wound healing process secondary to phonotrauma, and it is likely that some individuals are genetically more susceptible to this type of physical injury than others. For example, VFN occur with much greater frequency in adult females than in adult males, and the same degree of vocal use can induce the formation of nodules in one individual but not in another.

VFN are common in speakers or singers who habitually use their voice for long periods of time each day or who frequently push their voice to extremes (e.g., loud, forceful speaking or singing). Because VFN develop over time, it is thought that sustained phonotrauma over many weeks and

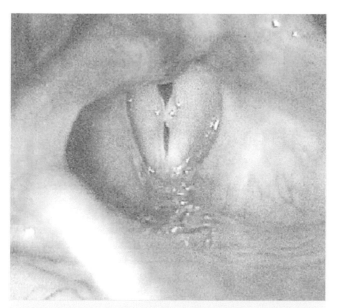

Fig. 2.6 Example of hourglass closure pattern typically seen in mid-membranous lesions. (From Fried M, Tan M. Clinical Laryngology. 1st edition. New York: Thieme Publishers, 2014.)

months promotes their development rather than an acute instance of severe phonotrauma. It is not surprising that many professional voice users experience VFN, including teachers, professional and recreational singers, actors, and clergy to name just a few. VFN are seen much more frequently in females than in males. Different theories have been proposed to explain this phenomenon including the greater frequency of collisions experienced by female vocal folds (they have a naturally higher rate of vibration) and the lower amounts of hyaluronic acid (which acts as shock absorber) in female vocal folds compared to males.[46]

Clinical Characteristics

Glottal closure pattern associated with VFN is usually an hourglass configuration with nodules in contact with each other. This glottal configuration results in aerodynamic, acoustic, and auditory-perceptual consequences. In speakers with VFN, subglottal pressure and transglottal airflow are often found to be increased. Acoustically there is increased perturbation (e.g., jitter, shimmer) and decreased cepstral peak prominence along with lower harmonic-to-noise ratio (indicating elevated noise in the acoustic signal). Perceptually the voice often has a breathy quality, or hoarse quality when a rough component (due to irregular vocal fold vibration) is also present (hoarseness is a combination of breathy and rough voice qualities). Depending on the patient's compensatory reactions to the altered tissue structure, vocal strain might also be present. Some speakers with VFN also speak with elevated vocal intensity, which can be a clinical sign of the vocal behaviors which led to the development of the nodules.

Treatment

The recommended first-line treatment for VFN is almost always voice therapy, which can directly address the etiology of the impairment (vocal behaviors). When VFN are diagnosed in their early formative stages, the prognosis for voice therapy to facilitate a return to normal tissue remodeling and improved vocal function is very good, given a skilled clinician and a motivated patient. Even with small chronic nodules that are resistant to complete resolution, voice therapy can rehabilitate vocal function by restoring an appropriate physiological balance in the vocal subsystems to produce a voice that is acceptable in quality and function for the speaker.

As nodules mature over time, the tissue changes become more resistant to complete resolution secondary to voice therapy. Some long-standing vocal nodules will require surgical excision when voice therapy does not achieve adequate improvement to serve the speaker's needs. There are some patients who undergo surgery, for various reasons, before receiving an appropriate dose of voice therapy. In such cases, voice therapy should always be recommended after surgery to facilitate restoration of a physiological balance in the subsystems of voice, promote healthier and more sustainable voice use patterns, and prevent a return of the VFN.

2.4.7 Vocal Fold Polyps

Description

The word "polyp" is a general term referring to a growth that protrudes from epithelium. Polyps can occur in many different parts of the body other than the vocal folds. Vocal fold polyps (VFP) are usually *unilateral* exophytic masses located at the mid-membranous medial edge of the vocal fold. Although VFP can occur bilaterally, a more common finding is the presence of contralateral reactionary swelling on the opposite vocal fold. These contralateral masses are often characterized by edema and are thought to form in response to repeated trauma from collisions with the stiff polyp. A period of voice rest (1–2 weeks) often reveals significant reduction in size of the contralateral swelling and illuminates the prominence of the primary exophytic polyp.

Etiological Characteristics

VFP are caused by phonotrauma and their development may be exacerbated by stimuli such as reflux, smoking, allergies, and infections.[47] One theory suggests that polyps develop secondary to phonotrauma-induced rupture of small blood vessels within the vocal folds.[47,48] On endoscopy, it is not uncommon to visualize enlarged blood vessels leading into VFP, suggesting prior injury to the vasculature. At a microscopic level, VFP are characterized by epithelial hyperplasia and sometimes atrophy, increased fibronectin clustered around abnormal vascularity along with decreased collagen deposition in the region of the BMZ, and other vascular abnormalities in the vocal fold cover.[42,43,47] It has been suggested that vocal folds experiencing the formation of VFP are characterized by reduced collagen type IV deposition in the BMZ compared to other benign mid-membranous lesions, a condition which might put a speaker at risk for polyp development over some other benign mass.[42] Although histologically they are somewhat similar, VFP appear to result in greater changes below the epithelium (submucosal), while VFN result in greater changes to the epithelium itself.[49]

VFP occur in similar clinical populations as nodules, although there is an increased frequency of polyps seen in males and VFP are uncommon in children. In addition to predominantly unilateral development, a difference between VFP and VFN is the belief that polyps can develop after an acute event, such as screaming or high intensity phonation throughout a day or multiple days. This contrasts with nodules, which develop over a longer period of time. VFP have a predilection to create stiff segments within the vocal folds which impact vibratory amplitude and mucosal wave to a greater extent than VFN.[49] This may result from VFP affecting the submucosal region to a greater extent. VFP can be characterized by a broad-based attachment at the mid-membranous region (referred to as **sessile polyps**) or be attached to this region by a thin stalk that allows the bulk of the polyp to move within the glottis during phonation (referred to as a **pedunculated polyp**).

Clinical Characteristics

Visually VFP can take on different forms including a smooth, bright red mass indicative of recent hemorrhage or dull reddish mass suggesting prior bleeding (▶ Fig. 2.7; ▶ Fig. 2.8). Some VFP take on a more fibrotic appearance as a dull opaque or dull white and smooth excrescence. The morphological qualities of polyps may depend on the age of the mass and how recent vascular injury was associated with their development. Other than specific visual characteristics, the clinical signs of VFP are very similar to those of VFN. Glottal configuration typically assumes an hourglass configuration with the polyp preventing anterior and posterior segments of the vocal folds from touching. Subglottal pressure and transglottal airflow are typically increased. Increased perturbation, decreased cepstral peak prominence, and decreased harmonic-to-noise ratio are also characteristic of VFP. The voice is often perceived as breathy or hoarse with strain present in some individuals due to functional compensation for the impairment.

Treatment

The recommended front-line treatment for VFP is often voice therapy, although prognosis for complete resolution of the mass

and return to normal tissue remodeling is not as good compared to nodules. There is also debate as to whether voice therapy or surgery is the most effective first option. Factors that might influence voice therapy prognosis include the size and age of the lesion, the vocal demands of the patient, history of past lesions, and motivation of the patient. Whether or not surgical excision comes first, it is crucial that the patient receives voice therapy to target the underlying primary etiology. This will typically require a focus on vocal hygiene to identify and reduce phonotraumatic behaviors, in addition to techniques which restore a physiological balance in the vocal subsystems during speech production.

2.4.8 Vocal Fold Pseudocysts*

Description

Vocal fold pseudocysts are exophytic polyp-like edematous masses located most commonly at the mid-membranous region of the vocal fold. This subtype is a more recent label and has been classically described as an **edematous polyp**. As with the subsequent discussion of vocal fold cysts, we qualify this diagnosis with an asterisk because, in this case, current theory suggests that pseudocysts develop secondary to phonotrauma in the context of an underlying glottal incompetence due to scar or vocal fold paresis (i.e., an associated organic etiology).[50,51,52,53]

Etiological Characteristics

Pseudocysts develop in the subepithelial space very close to the BMZ. As illustrated in ▶ Fig. 2.9, these masses are described as translucent, noncapsulated and fluid-filled, with a blister-like appearance.[53] Pseudocysts occur most frequently in young, non-smoking adult females and especially vocal professionals, and have been described as a focal type of unilateral edema in the SLLP, otherwise known as a type of unilateral localized (rather than diffuse) **Reinke's edema**.[51,52] The phonotrauma resulting in pseudocysts is thought to be a functional compensation for underlying scar or paresis that develops from viral infections, iatrogenic (e.g., surgical) injury, or idiopathic causes. It has been

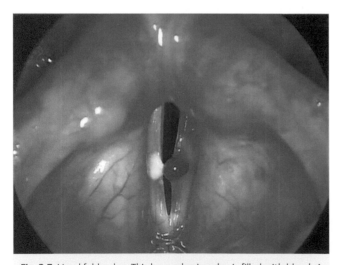

Fig. 2.7 Vocal fold polyp; This hemorrhagic polyp is filled with blood. A reactive contralateral lesion may also be present, hidden beneath the bright white mucous. (From Kendall K, Leonard R. Laryngeal Evaluation, 1st edition. New York: Thieme Publishers, 2010.)

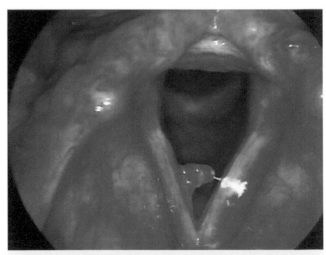

Fig. 2.8 Vocal fold polyp; This fibrous polyp has a broad base along the mid-membranous vocal fold. (From Kendall K, Leonard R. Laryngeal Evaluation, 1st edition. New York: Thieme Publishers, 2010.)

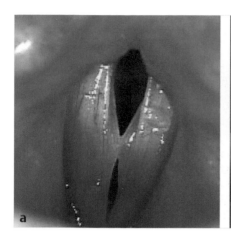 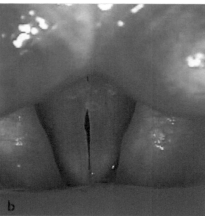

Fig. 2.9 Left vocal fold pseudocyst with reactive selling on right vocal fold; Pseudocysts appear as translucent exophytic masses that resemble a blister. These have classically been referred to as edematous polyps but recent theory suggests their development is due to phonotrauma secondary to underlying vocal fold paresis. (From Kendall K, Leonard R. Laryngeal Evaluation, 1st edition. New York: Thieme Publishers, 2010.)

suggested that unilateral paresis causes asymmetrical vocal fold closure with subsequent imbalanced sheer stress on the paretic side. In the presence of hyperfunctional effortful closure to compensate for the glottal inefficiency, the asymmetrical stress patterns cause tissue injury developing into a pseudocyst.[52]

Clinical Characteristics

The glottal configuration resulting from pseudocysts is an hourglass configuration. The glottal insufficiency subsequently affects aerodynamic, acoustic, and auditory-perceptual signs in a similar manner to other mid-membranous lesions. Perceptual signs attributed to these lesions include breathy voice quality and voice breaks with patient-reported symptoms including effortful phonation and vocal fatigue. Laryngeal endoscopy may reveal hyperfunctional characteristics similar to those seen in MTD.[52]

Treatment

Voice therapy to rebalance the vocal subsystems can "unload" laryngeal hyperfunction causing the phonotrauma, but the voice is likely to remain dysphonic unless any underlying precipitating paresis is addressed.[52] The exophytic mass will often need surgical removal, although it is understood that if the underlying paresis is not addressed there can be a high rate of recurrence.[50,53] It is also important to understand that published studies do not unanimously find 100% of patients diagnosed with pseudocysts have an underlying paresis. This suggests the likelihood that a subset of patients with pseudocyst-like exophytic lesions might present with phonotrauma as the primary and singular etiology. In such cases, a combination of trial voice therapy with subsequent medical management, if needed, would constitute an appropriate treatment approach.

2.4.9 Vocal Fold Cysts*

Description

Vocal fold cysts are unilateral or bilateral masses located most commonly at the mid-membranous region of the vocal fold. Cysts are epithelial-lined sacs that form in the SLLP. They can anchor to the BMZ or the vocal ligament, in which case they can significantly increase the stiffness of the vocal fold at the site of lesion. Cysts are a subtype of functional voice disorder that we label with an asterisk, because this lesion is also thought to

have an organic origin in a number of cases or result from a synergistic combination of functional and organic causes.

Etiological Characteristics

Vocal fold cysts can be congenital or acquired. In congenital cysts, patients will often relate that they have a long history of dysphonia. In the authors' clinical experiences and in a large number of reports, it is common that acquired cysts present in patients with heavy vocal demands or excessive voice use patterns, which along with their common mid-membranous location suggests a functional contribution to the development of cysts in many patients. There are two types of cysts that form in the vocal folds, **mucous retention cysts** and **epidermoid cysts**. Mucous retention cysts are thought to result from clogging of a mucous gland duct secondary to phonotrauma and/or some other irritant. Epidermoid cysts are thought to result from epithelial cells which become entrapped below the vocal fold surface.[35,54] Vocal fold epithelium is constantly being remodeled secondary to phonation and old cells are normally shed off into the mucociliary blanket lining supraglottal region. Theoretically, if one or more cells become trapped within the vocal fold cover, they can migrate into the subepithelial space and potentially result in the formation of an epidermoid cyst.

Clinical Characteristics

Visually, cysts can take on varied clinical appearances depending on their size and depth (▶ Fig. 2.10; ▶ Fig. 2.11). Deeper cysts may appear as a small raised surface at the medial edge of a vocal fold, while more superficial or large cysts can appear as white or translucent masses below the surface of the epithelium which protrude into the glottis. Because the epithelium covers them, very small cysts may not be visible even though their effects on vibratory dynamics observed during stroboscopy can be seen. Cysts form deeper in the vocal fold cover than do VFN and VFP and some can anchor to the vocal ligament. For these reasons, they can create stiffer vocal fold segments than VFN and VFP and their impact on vibratory amplitude, mucosal wave, and symmetry tends to be greater. Large cysts or those that form closer to the BMZ can cause an excrescence on the medial edge of the vocal fold and in some cases result in a contralateral reactionary lesion.[55] Cysts result in a similar glottal configuration (hourglass), aerodynamic,

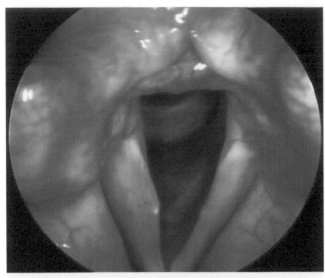

Fig. 2.10 Vocal fold cyst. A unilateral cyst on the right vocal fold. The exophytic effect at the vibrating edge will result in an hourglass or incomplete closure pattern. (From Kendall K, Leonard R. Laryngeal Evaluation, 1st edition. New York: Thieme Publishers, 2010.)

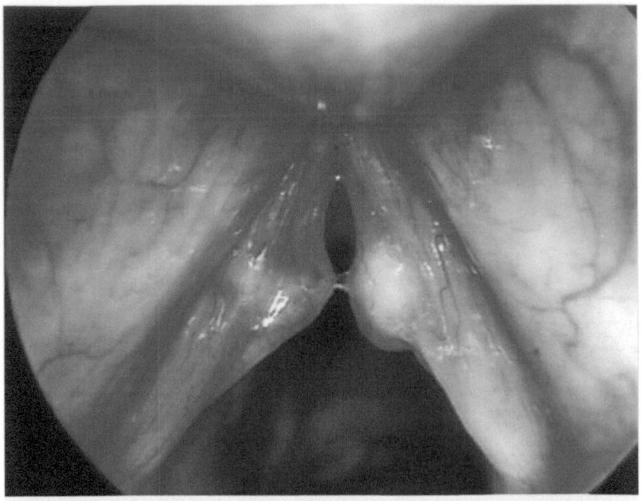

Fig. 2.11 Bilateral vocal fold cysts; Bilateral cysts occur less often than unilateral cysts. These are likely congenital as this adult patient reported a history of hoarseness since childhood. (From Fried M, Tan M. Clinical Laryngology. 1st edition. New York: Thieme Publishers, 2014.)

acoustic, and auditory perceptual features as those that occur with VFN and VFP. The severity of these clinical signs will depend on the size of the cyst, its location along the medial edge of the vocal fold, and the presence of compensatory hyperfunction by the patient.

Treatment

The prognosis for cysts to resolve secondary to voice rest or voice therapy is poor, although some advocate for a trial of voice therapy prior to surgery. In most specialty voice centers, the front-line treatment for cysts is phonosurgery. The skill of the surgeon is important for cyst removal because they can easily rupture during removal, especially when anchored to the vocal ligament, and it is believed that material left within the vocal fold can develop into another cyst during the wound healing process. Some also believe that ruptured cysts can result in the development of scar or sulcus vocalis (see sections **"Vocal Cord Scar"** and **"Vocal Fold Sulcus"** later). Because cysts are often associated with phonotrauma, postsurgical voice therapy is appropriate to restore a physiological balance to the subsystems of voice and prevent reoccurrence of benign mid-membranous lesions.

2.4.10 Vocal Process Granulomas*

Description

Vocal process granulomas are unilateral or bilateral exophytic masses located on or just above the vocal process of the arytenoid, in the region of the cartilaginous glottis. Granulomas may form secondary to ulceration of tissue at the vocal processes in response to chronic irritation, which can include phonotrauma. We also qualify this subtype with an asterisk because granulomas are known to have multiple etiologies, which can include reflux irritation and iatrogenic injury from intubation.[56]

Etiological Characteristics

Granulomas related to phonotrauma are thought to occur when the cartilaginous glottis oscillates at greater than normal amplitudes. The vocal fold tissue experiencing large amplitude oscillations and the greatest impact stress is typically at the mid-membranous region. When an individual speaks loudly, especially *forcibly loud*, they can recruit tissue oscillation in the cartilaginous glottis. Unlike anterior regions, underlying the epithelium and lamina propria at the cartilaginous glottis is hard cartilage, such that tissues at the vocal processes must oscillate over a hard surface instead of muscle. Chronic irritation subsequent to this type of phonation can cause ulceration at the vocal process and subsequent formation of granuloma tissue. At a microscopic level, granulomas are characterized by ulceration and cellular injury to the epithelium, with inflammation and edema in the vocal fold lamina propria.[57]

Clinical Characteristics

The appearance of granulomas on endoscopy can be quite varied, ranging from small and round to large and irregular shape (▶ Fig. 2.12). Color varies from pearly white to dull yellow, and mucus tends to congregate at the site of the granuloma. In some cases, a reactive lesion or additional granuloma is present on the opposite vocal process with a groove shaped by the contours of the contralateral mass. Because laryngeal sensory receptors at the level of the glottis are located in the posterior regions, some patients with these lesions may complain of pain at rest, pain during phonation, or a globus sensation in the throat. Granulomas may not cause a dysphonia or disrupt vibratory dynamics due to their posterior placement, which typically does not interfere with oscillation of the membranous vocal folds. This means that aerodynamic, acoustic, and auditory-perceptual characteristics of voice in speakers with vocal process granulomas are often within normal limits. However, a secondary MTD can develop

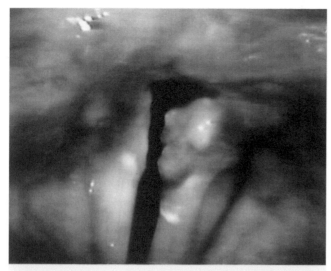

Fig. 2.12 Vocal process granuloma; Granuloma on the left vocal fold with erythema and the development of possible granulation tissue on the left vocal process. (From Kendall K, Leonard R. Laryngeal Evaluation, 1st edition. New York: Thieme Publishers, 2010.)

as a hyperfunctional response to the abnormal sensations produced by the granuloma, which would then produce clinical signs of symptoms associated with excessive muscle tension during phonation.

Treatment

The experience of otolaryngologists has found that granulomas are prone to reoccur after surgical excision. The front-line treatment for granulomas, regardless of etiology, is conservative treatment in the form of an antireflux protocol (medicine and lifestyle changes) along with voice therapy to promote an appropriate physiological balance and reduction of phonotrauma. Granulomas take time to heal, anywhere from 3 months up to a year.[56,57,58] This necessitates patience from both the speaker and the clinician, and speaker compliance with the reflux management and voicing behaviors is critical. Surgical removal may be a secondary option for granulomas which will not resolve. Surgery might also be warranted for very large granulomas which interfere with the airway. Interestingly, some professionals have noted occasional patients with a mature granuloma who reported coughing that subsequently dislodged the mass from the vocal folds.

2.4.11 Edema/Inflammation*

Description

Edema is synonymous with swelling, which is characterized by the accumulation of excess fluid within tissue. Vocal fold edema tends to accumulate in the SLLP and can be localized or distributed diffusely throughout a vocal fold. Edema can be present in symmetrical or asymmetrical volumes bilaterally. Vocal fold **inflammation** typically includes edema in addition to increased vascularity causing patches of redness (called **erythema**) throughout the vocal folds and/or laryngeal regions.

Etiological Characteristics

Vocal fold edema can be related to number of possible etiologies (hence our use of an asterisk) which include phonotrauma. Edema is part of the cycle that occurs during wound healing and it is common for vocal folds to swell immediately after prolonged or intense voice use. In the acute phase after heavy voice use, endoscopy can reveal edema in the mid-membranous region of one or both vocal folds. Voice rest or a return to typical voice habits allows the vocal fold tissue to heal appropriately in most cases. When phonotrauma is chronic, however, it can lead to persistent edema and inflammation. Laryngeal inflammation is characterized by swelling, amplified cellular activity, and increased vascular supply to the small blood vessels causing the tissue to appear reddened. These changes can cause increased pressure within laryngeal tissue and subsequently pain—when localized to the vocal folds, pain will typically be caused by inflammation in the posterior regions. Persistent edema with inflammation secondary to phonotrauma is a type of **chronic laryngitis**, a diagnosis that will show up again in the organic voice disorder category due to its multifactorial etiology.[59]

At a microscopic level, the proteomic changes that occur in edema can be like those that occur during polyp formation, with the exception that changes in polyps are focal at the site of the lesion.[42,44] Reports have indicated thickening of the BMZ with fluid-filled spaces and thickened blood vessel walls.[44] This histological similarity to polyps is perhaps one reason diffuse edema in one or both vocal folds is also referred to as **polypoid** changes (remember that "polyp" means a change within epithelium causing the surface to be raised).

Clinical Characteristics

In mild forms, edema presents endoscopically as a subtle translucent or pale white change to the vocal fold surface, giving the appearance of fullness or puffiness to the vocal fold (s) (▶ Fig. 2.13). In more severe forms, the vocal folds can become dramatically enlarged with viscous fluid and an inflamed appearance, almost as if the vocal folds are balloons filled with a thick liquid. This severe form of persistent edema is known as **Reinke's edema**, **polypoid degeneration**, or **polypoid corditis** (all are synonymous terms; ▶ Fig. 2.14). The severity of fluid accumulation and tissue changes seen in Reinke's edema is believed to result from a combination of phonotrauma and heavy smoking. The vast majority of patients with this condition, who tend to be middle-age to older females, are chronic smokers.[60]

In addition to the features noted earlier, endoscopically Reinke's edema can present with reduced mucosal wave and vibratory amplitude due to increased stiffness of the viscous subepithelial liquid. The amount of swelling in each vocal fold may not be equivalent and this can lead to asymmetry and/or irregularity of vibration, although the amount of bilateral edema typically allows for glottal closure to be complete. Perceptually the voice of Reinke's edema is characterized by a substantial low pitch and typically has a rough quality, which will be validated acoustically by a low fundamental frequency, increased perturbation, and decreased cepstral peak prominence.

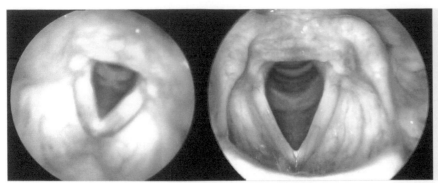

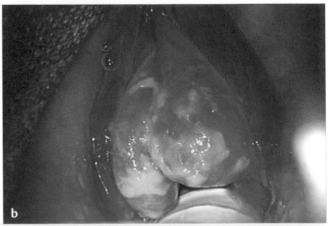

Fig. 2.13 Bilateral vocal fold edema; Healthy vocal folds appear as pearly white with minimal vasculature apparent on the surface epithelium. These vocal folds viewed through a rigid endoscope appear mildly translucent, suggestive of edema. (From Kendall K, Leonard R. Laryngeal Evaluation, 1st edition. New York: Thieme Publishers, 2010.)

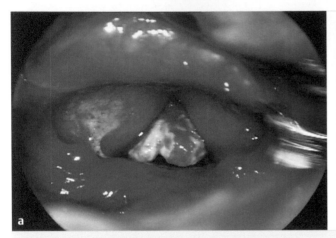

Fig. 2.14 Reinke's edema (polypoid degeneration/corditis); Reinke's edema viewed through a rigid endoscope. The SLLP if filled with thick fluid most often associated with chronic smoking. Both edema (swelling) and inflammation (increased vascularity) is evident. (From Fried M, Tan M. Clinical Laryngology. 1st edition. New York: Thieme Publishers, 2014.)

Treatment

Front-line treatment for Reinke's edema begins with recommendations for cessation of smoking. There are physicians who will not perform further management until a patient complies with this recommendation. In some cases, smoking cessation can substantially improve the edema, especially if it is not long-standing. Voice therapy to address the phonotraumatic behaviors might also be recommended in this phase. With the combination of smoking cessation and voice therapy, the management has addressed two of the primary etiologies of Reinke's edema. Edema to some degree typically remains in a large percentage of patients, but it can be reduced or eliminated completely via microlaryngoscopic surgery or office-based laser treatment.[61] Voice therapy can also be recommended postsurgery to help the patient learn appropriate physiological control of the vocal mechanism.

2.4.12 Vascular Injury

Description

The layered structure of the vocal folds contains a microvascular network of blood vessels running in parallel with the anterior-posterior dimension of the tissue. Phonotrauma can induce mechanical damage to the vessel walls in this network and cause vascular injuries which go by various labels including varices, capillary ectasias, capillary lakes, and spider telangiectasias.[54]

Varices are dilated or enlarged blood vessels appearing as prominent capillaries within the vocal fold cover (▶ Fig. 2.15). **Ectasias** are dilated pools of blood visible on the surface of the vocal fold—these are sometimes also referred to as **capillary lakes** (▶ Fig. 2.15). **Spider telangiectasias** are networks of blood vessels which run in an irregular pattern across a section of vocal fold—these appear similar to "spider veins" in legs and arms. These vascular injuries are at risk for **hemorrhage** that bleeds into the vocal fold and spreads diffusely across a large segment or length of the entire tissue (▶ Fig. 2.16). Most of these vascular injuries are visible during endoscopy on the medial vibratory edges and/or superior edges of the vocal folds.

Etiological and Characteristics

Vascular injuries can occur secondary to chronic or acute phonotrauma and are often related to performance demands of singers and actors, screaming, coughing, and throat clearing.[62] Increased vascular supply to the vocal fold tissue is a normal part of the wound healing response, but excessive phonotrauma can permanently injure the blood vessels. Chronic, enlarged vessels are a sign of prior injury.

Clinical Characteristics

Some vascular injuries can be asymptomatic, but when they affect phonation, the typical presentation is dysphonia and/or loss of frequency range. In professional voice users, vascular

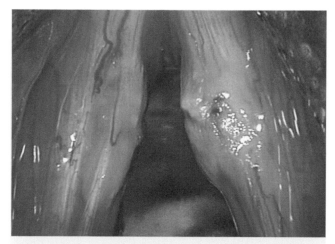

Fig. 2.15 Varices and ectasias. This 25-year old musical performer demonstrates multiple varices bilaterally and at least one ectasia on the right mid-membranous vocal fold. (From Fried M, Tan M. Clinical Laryngology. 1st edition. New York: Thieme Publishers, 2014.)

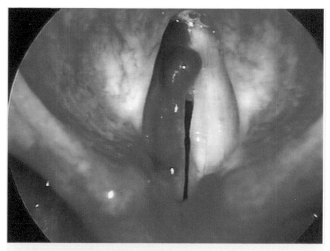

Fig. 2.16 Vocal fold hemorrhage; This figure illustrates a left vocal fold polyp with associated hemorrhage spread diffusely throughout the tissue (From Fried M, Tan M. Clinical Laryngology. 1st edition. New York: Thieme Publishers, 2014.)

injuries are a great concern due to the risk of hemorrhage and potential scar formation secondary to altered wound-healing mechanisms. Scar is irreversible (to date) and can create a permanent loss in the artistic range of a vocalist. Vascular injuries are often visible during endoscopy and can appear anywhere along the medial superior edges. Perceptually, acoustically, and aerodynamically, the effects of vascular injury will be highly variable and dependent on the specific site of lesion and its influence on vibratory dynamics.

Treatment

The typical front-line treatment for vascular injuries is strict voice rest. Surgical options include microlaryngoscopy and more recently laser treatment.[55] Voice therapy is typically warranted to reestablish an appropriate physiological balance in the subsystems of voice and prevent the phonotrauma that caused the original pathology. When working with singers, if the voice therapist is not a singing voice specialist, a referral to a singing pedagogue is recommended when the patient is not currently receiving professional voice training.

2.5 Organic Voice Disorders

Organic voice disorders are caused by structural, neurological, systemic, or infectious changes to the subsystems of voice. As illustrated in ▶ Table 2.2, the range of etiologies underlying organic voice disorders is vast, and detailed coverage of every etiology is beyond the scope of this book. We do know from published data and clinical experience that SLPs engaging in clinical practice with voice-disordered populations will encounter certain organic etiologies much more frequently than others—these will be the focus of this section.

The most commonly diagnosed etiologies of organic voice disorders in treatment-seeking populations are laryngitis and vocal fold paralysis, in that order.[7,63] The label of "laryngitis" may be overused by physicians other than otolaryngologists, evidenced by large discrepancies in the number of treatment-seeking patients receiving this diagnosis in otolaryngology

clinics compared to general practice clinics.[7] It is important for clinicians to be familiar with the range of possible organic etiologies because this knowledge will serve our interprofessional collaborative practice with otolaryngologists in addition to other health professionals, and facilitate the process of differential diagnosis. Just as a range of possible etiologies of organic disorders exists, the treatments for these disorders are varied, so accurate diagnosis is crucial.

2.5.1 Neurological Subtypes

Vocal Fold Paralysis/Paresis

Description

Vocal fold immobility (VFI) is a complete restriction or partial restriction (dysmotility) of movement in the arytenoid cartilage toward or away from the midline, or a restriction of the thyroid cartilage from moving about the cricothyroid joint. The causes of VFI include neurological etiologies, inflammation, trauma, and other organic causes many of which are listed in ▶ Table 2.3. The most common cause of VFI is paralysis or paresis, terms that refer to the inability (paralysis) or reduced ability (paresis) to adduct, abduct, or tense one or both vocal folds due to a dysfunction in the neurological pathways that influence laryngeal muscle contraction. These terms are often used interchangeably, but it is important to understand the distinction between them since *some* vocal fold movement is a better prognostic indicator than *no* movement.

All forms of vocal fold paralysis/paresis result from dysfunction in branches of the vagus nerve, specifically the recurrent laryngeal nerve (RLN) and/or external division of the superior laryngeal nerve (SLN). The dysfunction can occur unilaterally or bilaterally, though unilateral paralysis/paresis is the most common form. The vagus can be impaired itself or the central nervous system inputs that control the vagus may be the locus of injury, with the effects manifesting through the peripheral nerve. Dysfunction in the RLN can result in **adductor paralysis/paresis**

Table 2.2 Neurological, structural, and systemic or infectious conditions underlying organic voice disorders. This list is not comprehensive but represents the more common etiologies presenting in treatment-seeking individuals.

Subtype	Clinical Characteristics
Neurological	
Dysarthria	Voice effects vary based on dysarthria type. UVFP and spasmodic dysphonia are types of flaccid dysarthria and hyperkinetic dysarthria, respectively. Parkinson's disease results in hypokinetic dysarthria, characterized by glottal incompetency, bowed vocal folds, breathy voice with low volume and sometimes accelerated speech rate. Spastic dysarthria results in excess laryngeal muscle tone and restricted range of movement causing a strained and rough voice quality, reduced frequency and intensity modulation during speech (monotonicity), and a reduced speech rate.
Spasmodic Dysphonia	ADSD: Intermittent strained-strangled voice quality with roughness and perceived effort. Within-word voicing and pitch breaks occurring most often in voiced sounds. Hyperkinesia of SD disrupt the fluency of speech. ABSD: Intermittent breathiness with aphonic voicing breaks and strain occurring most often on voiceless sounds and at word onsets.
Vocal Fold Paralysis/Paresis	Adductor UVFP: Glottal incompetency due to peripheral nerve injury or dysfunction where vocal fold fails to adduct to midline. Breathy voice quality with low volume, diplophonia, reduced fundamental frequency. Compensatory hyperfunction may develop and evidenced by supraglottal laryngeal compression. Abductor UVFP: Restricted ability of vocal fold to abduct away from midline. Dysphonia may be mild due to midline position of vocal fold. Reduced vocal loudness, weak cough, and possible inspiratory stridor. Adductor/Abductor BVFP: Both are serious conditions putting health at risk. Adductor BVFP results in compromised airway protection, especially during swallowing. Abductor BVFP can obstruct airway causing breathing difficulties.
Voice Tremor	Rhythmic 4 Hz to 10 Hz modulation of voice especially noticeable during sustained vowels in moderate-to-severe cases. Patients often complain of "shaky" or "wobbly" voice. Possible aphonic voicing breaks with rushes of air. Tremor may be visible in arytenoids and other laryngeal/pharyngeal structures on endoscopy.
Structural	
Carcinoma	Laryngeal cancer is an abnormal proliferation of cells with potential of or which have realized migration to distant sites beyond their place of origin. The vast majority of laryngeal cancers are squamous cell carcinomas. Laryngeal cancers are divided into glottic, supraglottic, and subglottic sites of origin. They may occur with or without leukoplakia or erythroplakia. Severe epithelial dysplasia can be indistinguishable from carcinoma in situ. Laryngeal cancer can take on varied visual appearances and must be confirmed via histology from a biopsy specimen.
Cyst	Mucous retention and epithelial inclusion cysts may be congenital or acquired. Acquired organic etiologies are thought to be related to a blocked mucous gland duct and trapped epithelial cells. Cysts are listed also in the Functional category due to their frequent association with heavy vocal use.
Granuloma	Organic causes include intubation injury or laryngopharyngeal reflux irritating tissue at the vocal process. The epithelium at the vocal process can develop ulceration which may progress to granuloma development. Due to the posterior location of granulomas symptoms can include pain and/or globus sensation. Even with appropriate treatment granulomas can take time to resolve, and some will need phonosurgical removal.
Laryngeal web	Congenital or acquired webs form tissue bridges between left and right vocal folds, most commonly at the anterior membranous region. Acquired etiologies include intubation injury or poor wound healing from phonosurgery. Small webs may be asymptomatic. Larger webs can cause signs and symptoms including: audible inspiration, difficulty breathing, and a rough voice with high pitch.
Laryngocele	An air-filled pocket of tissue that occurs in the anterior portion of the ventricle. Larger lesions can appear endoscopically as ballooning out of the ventricular space. Laryngocele's can be congenital or acquired, with acquired etiologies related to ventricular exposure to excessive high pressures such as during coughing and playing wind instruments.
Laryngomalacia	Congenital incomplete maturation of the cartilaginous framework of the larynx. Endoscopic signs include an omega shaped epiglottis, arytenoid prolapse, and narrowed airway. Perceptual signs include inhalatory stridor or noisy breathing, and abnormal cry sound. The signs and symptoms of laryngomalacia may not appear until up to 2 weeks after birth and can worsen over the first few months. With time most cases will naturally resolve, sometime between the first and second years of life.
Papilloma	Exophytic masses appearing as wart-like lesions on the vocal fold epithelium. Caused by HPV subtypes 6 and 11, with accompanying dysplasia in a small percentage of cases. Surgical management is the mainstay of treatment, although papillomas tend to regrow and repeated surgeries are often necessary.
Presbylaryngis	Age-related laryngeal changes characterized by glottal incompetence due to vocal fold atrophy and bowing. Voice quality tends to be breathy with reduced loudness. Voice therapy can be effective for presbyphonia, but requires a patient willing to do daily exercises. Injection laryngoplasty is an effective temporary treatment for presbylaryngis.
Premalignant lesions	Leukoplakia – white patches (composed of keratin) adhering to the vocal fold cover. These are often raised from the surface of the epithelium. Erythroplakia – Red patches on the surface of the vocal folds. Erythroleukoplakia – Red patches with white "speckles" on the surface of the vocal folds.

Table 2.2 continued

Subtype	Clinical Characteristics
	All three of the above can be present with or without underlying dysplasia. Dysplasia – Abnormal epithelial cell structure and number. Dysplasia can evolve into cancer when it invades vocal fold tissues beyond the epithelium.
Laryngeal stenosis	Narrowing of the airway which can occur at supraglottic, glottic, or subglottic levels. In pediatric populations stenosis can be congenital (e.g., see Laryngomalacia and webs, above) or acquired, such as from prolonged intubation. In adults, common etiologies include inflammatory conditions such as granulomatosis, in addition to post-radiation fibrosis, prolonged intubation, and trauma.
Scar	Fibrotic epithelium developing from an abnormal wound healing responses. Most often associated with trauma from phonosurgery. Scar is best visualized using videostroboscopy, where it can appear as a mildly discolored (e.g., opaque) section of vocal fold epithelium that is extremely stiff. Scar typically causes reduced mucosal wave, reduced amplitude, and aperiodicity. There is currently no cure for scar although voice therapy and phonosurgery may be attempted to improve voice quality and function.
Sulcus	A notch or groove running horizontally along the medial edge of a vocal fold. Can be present unilaterally or bilaterally. Sulci can be of three subtypes: Type 1 – physiological sulcus Type 2 – sulcus vergeture Type 3 – sulcus vocalis These subtypes can be considered a continuum of mild to severe, with Type 1 sulci presenting as asymptomatic or mild and Type 3 sulci causing severe dysphonia. Sulci can be congenital or acquired. As with scar, voice therapy and/or phonosurgery may be used to treat the sulcus although positive clinical outcomes can be challenging.
Systemic/Infectious	
Amyloidosis	Abnormal deposits of amyloid proteins which can be present in many tissues of the body, including the larynx. These can cause exophytic masses on the laryngeal tissue with the most common symptoms including hoarseness and difficulty breathing (dyspnea). These lesions are managed primarily by surgical removal.
Arthritis	Rheumatoid arthritis is an autoimmune disease characterized by inflammation in joints. Laryngeal manifestations can affect the cricoarytenoid and cricothyroid joints, causing dysmotility or immobility of the vocal folds. Endoscopic signs can include erythema and edema especially posteriorly at the arytenoids, along with reduced adduction/abduction movements. Depending on vocal fold position stridor may also be present and reduced pitch range is possible. Pharmaceutical treatment is primary for the systemic inflammatory condition. Injection laryngoplasty or thyroplasty may be applied to correct vocal fold position.
Bacterial/fungal infections	Bacterial and fungal infections typically cause inflammation in the form of erythema and edema in tissue leading to an associated laryngitis. Fungal infections can be related to chronic use of inhaled corticosteroids and antibiotics. Fungal infections are also exemplified by white patches occurring throughout the larynx, including the vocal fold tissue. Treatment for both bacterial and fungal infections is pharmaceutical.
Laryngitis	A general term referring to inflammation in the form of edema (swelling) and erythema (increased vascularity). Multiple etiologies including viral and bacterial infections, laryngopharyngeal reflux, and abnormal responses to medications. Laryngopharyngeal reflux is thought to be a common cause in 20% or more of patients with laryngeal complaints.

Table 2.3 Etiologies of Vocal Fold Immobility resulting in paralysis, paresis, or mechanical fixation cartilage at the laryngeal joints.

Cause	Description
Iatrogenic surgical injury	Surgical injury is the most common cause of unilateral paralysis. Procedures involving the neck or left thorax risk injuring the vagus nerve. Thyroidectomy, cardiovascular, and cervical spine procedures are common surgical etiologies of vocal fold paralysis/paresis.
Neurological disease	Disease affecting the central or peripheral nervous systems can affect vagus nerve. Vocal fold paralysis/paresis is common in degenerative neurological diseases such as amyotrophic lateral sclerosis and Parkinson's disease. Stroke resulting in spastic dysarthria or lateral medullary syndrome (Wallenberg's) are also etiologies of paralysis/paresis.
Tumors	Benign or malignant tumors can restrict joint mobility or impinge upon the vagus nerve to cause paralysis/paresis. Because the RLN courses into the left superior chest tumors in that region can also cause paralysis/paresis.
Inflammatory/Infectious conditions	Osteoarthritis and rheumatoid arthritis are chronic inflammatory that can affect mobility of laryngeal joints. Allergies and immune system disorders can also result in chronic inflammation affecting voice. Sarcoidosis and Amyloidosis are conditions that can also affect the larynx and effect vocal fold movement.

Table 2.3 continued

Cause	Description
Viral	SLN or RLN paralysis/paresis can occur in the context of recent history of severe upper respiratory infection, which is thought to be a significant cause of temporary or permanent SLN injury.
Physical trauma	Immobility from intubation or blunt/penetrating trauma to the head or neck can cause paralysis or mechanical fixation. Paralysis/paresis from prolonged intubation is a common etiology in children born premature with severe health issues.
Congenital	Congenital malformations (e.g., cleft) can affect laryngeal structure and restrict vocal fold movement. Some children are born with motor impairments (e.g., cerebral palsy) causing dysarthria with a dysphonic component.
Idiopathic	Sometimes there is no explanation for the onset of vocal fold paralysis/paresis. Often these cases have an acute onset, although a minority of cases can experience gradual onset. When there is no identifiable cause to an existing paralysis/paresis it is called idiopathic.

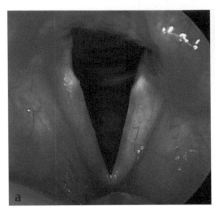
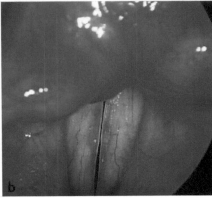

Fig. 2.17 Unilateral vocal fold paralysis. (a) Left unilateral vocal fold paralysis showing affected vocal fold near paramedian position. (b) Incomplete closure along the midline the of the glottis. (From Kendall K, Leonard R. Laryngeal Evaluation, 1st edition. New York: Thieme Publishers, 2010.)

or **abductor paralysis/paresis**, while dysfunction in the SLN can affect a speaker's ability to increase tension in the vocal folds for manipulating pitch. This form is typically called **SLN paralysis/paresis**.

Etiological Characteristics

The most common form of paralysis affecting the larynx is unilateral vocal fold paralysis (UVFP). The most frequent etiology associated with UVFP is iatrogenic injury subsequent to surgery. Of surgical populations, the most common procedure causing UVFP is **thyroidectomy**. Idiopathic paralysis/paresis and cardiovascular surgeries are other common causes. Because the SLN and RLN branch off the main stem of the vagus nerve at different levels (RLN lower than SLN), the locus of injury can affect one or both branches. When isolated SLN paralysis/paresis is present the etiology is often related to thyroid surgeries, although it is not uncommon for a patient with SLN to report a recent upper respiratory infection preceding the onset of vocal difficulties. Bilateral vocal fold paralysis (BVFP) occurs much less frequently than UVFP and can be associated with trauma to the head/neck, stroke, surgical procedures, and neurological disease.

Clinical Characteristics

Unilateral Adductor/Abductor Paralysis/Paresis

Vocal fold paralysis/paresis can range from mild paresis to complete paralysis. While endoscopy can provide visual evidence of movement disorders associated with the condition, definitive diagnosis may require laryngeal electromyography performed by the otolaryngologist. In **adductor UVFP**, important clinical signs are the position of the vocal fold relative to midline and residual movement in the affected arytenoid. Adductor UVFP causes glottal incompetency characterized by incomplete closure along the length of the vocal folds during adduction (▸ Fig. 2.17). Vocal fold position in adductor paralysis can be midline, paramedian (e.g., halfway between midline and abducted), abducted, or some range in between those positions. The closer to midline a vocal fold is, the more likely that aerodynamic forces can induce the vocal fold into vibration.

The perceptual qualities associated with adductor UVFP vary widely depending on vocal fold position and the degree of compensatory hyperfunction, but typically include breathiness, reduced loudness, diplophonia, and low pitch. The breathiness and reduced loudness are associated with the glottal incompetence, which will be more severe the farther away from midline an affected vocal fold is positioned during voicing. Over time, a paretic vocal fold can atrophy and its vertical position relative to the nonparalyzed vocal fold can change, creating a vertical level difference that can affect vibratory dynamics (▸ Fig. 2.18). This can impact the periodicity of vocal fold vibration, increasing perturbation and introducing a rough quality to the auditory-perceptual features of the voice. A vertical level difference can also occur soon after injury when the laryngeal muscles on the affected side lose tone and cause the ipsilateral arytenoid cartilage to prolapse inward toward the glottis (▸ Fig. 2.19).

The perceptual features in **abductor UVFP** can be mild when the paretic vocal fold is positioned at midline. This position allows the unaffected fold to narrow the glottis sufficiently to achieve phonation. In some cases, the voice quality may be perceptually near normal with only subtle deviation in perceptual dimensions. However, because one vocal fold lacks tone and is unable to generate strong medial compression

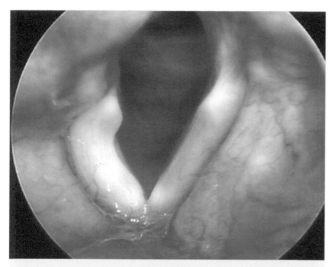

Fig. 2.18 Unilateral paralysis with atrophy. (From Kendall K, Leonard R. Laryngeal Evaluation, 1st edition. New York: Thieme Publishers, 2010.)

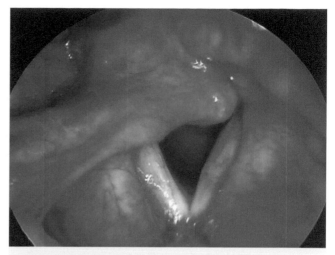

Fig. 2.19 Unilateral paralysis with arytenoid prolapse. (From Kendall K, Leonard R. Laryngeal Evaluation, 1st edition. New York: Thieme Publishers, 2010.)

forces, it is common for patients with abductor UVFP to present with a weak cough and difficulty generating elevated vocal loudness. Also, because the paretic vocal fold is stuck at midline, there may be an inspiratory stridor when breathing, especially after physical exertion.[64]

Superior Laryngeal Nerve Paralysis/Paresis

SLN injury will affect the function of the cricothyroid muscle, the main tensor of the vocal folds. Unilateral SLN injury is most common although bilateral injury can also occur. Endoscopic signs of unilateral SLN injury can include asymmetry of arytenoid adduction with the strong side rotating past midline toward the weak side, a flaccid vocal fold with increased mucosal wave during vibration, a vertical level difference between left and right vocal folds during adduction, and possible bowing.[64,65] Perceptually, the most salient feature of unilateral SLN injury is reduced pitch range. This might go unnoticed in non-singers, but vocalists will be acutely aware of the problem and often report a limited pitch range or a singing impairment. Singers and nonsingers may also complain of vocal fatigue.[65]

Bilateral Adductor/Abductor Paralysis/Paresis

BVFP is associated with etiologies including surgery (including the effects of prolonged intubation), trauma, infections, and degenerative diseases such as amyotrophic lateral sclerosis. BVFP can also be a congenital condition. Both adductor and abductor forms are much more serious conditions than UVFP. In adductor BVFP, the vocal folds are positioned away from midline without the ability to close the glottis. If the patient is able to produce voice, this results in a severely breathy quality with reduced loudness, but more importantly this condition presents the risk of laryngeal penetration and aspiration during swallowing. In abductor BVFP, the vocal folds are positioned at midline. This presents immediate breathing concerns due to obstruction of the airway, and immediate surgical solutions are typically warranted.

Treatment

Most patients with significant adductor or abductor BVFP will require surgical procedures to improve the airway by widening or narrowing the glottis. In some cases, these patients may also need voice therapy, but the primary concern for many will be breathing and/or swallowing. The majority of paralysis patients who seek management for voice problems are those with adductor UVFP. The preferred treatment will depend on many factors which include voice impairment severity, the position of the paralyzed vocal fold, the presence of compensatory hyperfunction, time post onset of the impairment, the patient's need for voice, and the treatment orientation of the voice care team (based on their knowledge, skills, and training). Many laryngologists will treat adductor UVFP first with injection laryngoplasty, as this procedure can lead to immediate voice improvement without permanent surgical alteration to the nervous system or cartilaginous structure.[66] Injection laryngoplasty is a temporary treatment (injection materials are absorbed by the tissues within 3 to 12 months), so that the patient has a more functional voice while the nervous system has time to recover spontaneously. Beliefs regarding the temporal limit of spontaneous recovery from UVFP range from 6 to 12 months, after which a patient may decide on a more permanent solution. Long-term solutions for improving glottal closure subsequent to adductor UVFP include **thyroplasty** using varied substances, arytenoid manipulation procedures, and laryngeal reinnervation (see Chapter 7).

Research and clinical experience demonstrate that voice therapy can be highly effective for improving glottal closure and overall vocal function secondary to adductor UVFP. The greatest prognosis for voice therapy occurs when it can be implemented in the acute stage post-onset, when the paretic vocal fold is somewhere between midline and paramedian positions, and when there is some residual arytenoid movement during adduction.[67,68] Voice therapy may be initiated prior to any surgical procedures or combined with injection laryngoplasty in the acute stages of impairment. As described in Chapter 8, voice therapy in cases of adductor UVFP targets the primary etiology of glottal incompetence, although, ironically, some patients can develop inappropriate hyperfunctional behaviors in an effort to compensate for the paralysis. In these cases, the clinician must consider finding the appropriate physiological balance to improve glottal closure while not overtaxing muscular effort.

Effective treatment approaches for glottal incompetence secondary to paralysis/paresis include modified vocal function exercises, increasing respiratory support, isometric contraction exercises while voicing (i.e., pushing), accent method, glottal attacks at voicing onset, and resonant focus in the context of increasing vocal loudness.[68,69,70,71,72] Voice therapy is also the front-line treatment for SLN paralysis/paresis, with rehabilitation focused on increasing vocal fold tension and dynamic flexibility for intonation and pitch control. Frameworks for selected approaches are discussed further Chapter 8.

Spasmodic Dysphonia

Description

Spasmodic dysphonia (SD) is a type of **dystonia** caused by involuntary hyperkinesia in the laryngeal muscles (it is also called **laryngeal dystonia**). SD is task specific to phonation, meaning that the dystonia does not occur at rest and is typically present only during voicing behaviors. The onset of SD is usually in middle age with average diagnosis at approximately 50 years.[4] SD can manifest in two forms: **adductor SD (ADSD** —by far the most common) and **abductor SD (ABSD)**. In some patients, an underlying vocal tremor may also be present. ADSD is characterized by adductor hyperkinesia (hyperadduction) during phonation, while ABSD is characterized by abductor hyperkinesia thought to be caused by co-contraction of the antagonistic posterior cricoarytenoid.

Etiological Characteristics

SD affects more females than males (between 1:2 and 1:3 male-to-female ratio) and approximately 10% of patients report a familial history of dystonia.[73] Classically, there existed a debate regarding the underlying etiology of SD. Contemporary theory labels SD as a subtype of neurological dystonia, although what precipitates the onset of neurological dysfunction is not well understood. Neuroimaging studies have linked abnormalities of dopaminergic neurons in the striatum of the basal ganglia to clinical characteristics of SD, including loss of motor inhibition (facilitating the dystonic episodes) and abnormal sensorimotor integration.[74,75]

Clinical Characteristics

Adductor Spasmodic Dysphonia

SD in all forms typically presents as a progressive neurological disorder whose course is variable from patient to patient. The onset is characterized by a mild hoarseness initially that progresses over the course of months to years. There is often a plateau of severity, though the time course of progression and degree of eventual severity cannot be predicted. Perceptually ADSD is characterized by roughness, strain, and effort often described as a "strained-strangled" quality, and inconsistent within-word voice and pitch breaks. ADSD interrupts

the smooth flow of connected speech and can resemble characteristics of dysfluency including tense pauses and prolonged syllables.[76,77]

Endoscopically, the adductor hyperkinesia is visible in some patients, typically those with moderate to severe impairment. When tremor accompanies SD, the rhythmic oscillation of the arytenoid cartilages can also be evident during phonation. During dystonic moments, the arytenoid cartilages can appear tightly pressed together along with medial compression of the false vocal folds and anterior-posterior laryngeal squeezing, the latter behaviors often being the result of compensatory hyperfunction. Vibratory dynamics may be impaired during hyperadduction with or without tremor but normal during nondysphonic moments.

It can be challenging to differentiate the clinical features of ADSD from moderate-to-severe MTD. The process of differential diagnosis can be informed by evidence from task-specific vocalizations. For example, speakers with ADSD tend to be perceived as less dysphonic during sustained vowels compared to connected speech, while perceptions of dysphonia in speakers with MTD tend to be more consistent across voicing tasks.[78] Speakers with ADSD also tend to be more dysphonic on stimuli loaded with voiced sounds compared to stimuli loaded with unvoiced sounds.[79] The consistency of features in MTD compared to the variable inconsistency of ADSD features is a differential characteristic of these two disorders.

Abductor Spasmodic Dysphonia

Perceptually ABSD is characterized by intermittent breathiness with aphonic voice breaks and strain. Physiologically, the dystonia of ABSD results in irregular hyperabduction causing transient glottal gaps during phonation. The hyperkinesia of ABSD can occur at the onset of words resulting in aphonic or very breathy onsets, sometimes perceived as a prolonged word initiation.[49] In contrast to ADSD, ABSD occurs more frequently on voiceless sounds. Clinical stimuli containing words and sentences with voiced and voiceless contrasts can thus be useful in distinguishing between the two forms of SD. A voice tremor can also be present and is a confirmatory sign of SD versus MTD.[4,49] Endoscopically, the abductor dystonia, if able to be visualized, can present as very brief and asymmetric vocal fold abduction movements during vibratory cycles.

Treatment

Currently, the front-line treatment for ADSD and ABSD is unilateral or bilateral injections of **botulinum toxin** (BT).[73] When injected into muscles, BT is taken into the terminal branches of motor neurons where it damages SNARE proteins ("SNARE" stands for **s**oluble **N**-ethylmaleimide-sensitive factor **a**ttachment **re**ceptor). SNARE protein functions to bind synaptic vesicles filled with neurotransmitter to the presynaptic membrane of the neuron, so that the neurotransmitter can be released into the synaptic cleft and stimulate the postsynaptic receptors of muscle cells. By damaging the SNARE proteins, BT prevents neurons from releasing normal amounts of neurotransmitter, which will cause a paresis in the target muscle. Over time, the neurons affected by BT will recover primarily through the process of **axonal sprouting**, where new axon terminals are formed. The evolution from initial paralysis/paresis to functional neuronal recovery via axonal sprouting can take between 2 and 6 months, although in some patients the effects of BT can last longer. Unfortunately, neuronal recovery in cases of SD means that those neurons can once again carry the hyperkinetic signals transmitted from the central nervous system to the laryngeal muscles, with the return of dystonia. BT injection is covered more extensively in Chapter 7.

Voice therapy as the primary treatment has not demonstrated great success in confirmed cases of SD. When combined with BT management, voice therapy has been shown to improve clinical outcomes, although there are conflicting reports in the literature and additional research is needed to better inform clinical practice.[80,81] When voice therapy is combined as an adjuvant modality, the specific treatment approaches target the compensatory hyperfunction that often accompanies both ADSD and ABSD. These techniques are similar to those used to treat MTD, as this compensatory hyperfunction can be thought of as a type of secondary MTD.

Essential Voice Tremor

Description

Tremor is an involuntary repetitive (rhythmic) oscillation in muscles. Tremor can occur in otherwise healthy individuals or from neurological injury such as degenerative neurological conditions (e.g., Parkinson's disease [PD]), and can affect most parts of the body. **Physiologic tremor** is considered normal, with tremor frequency ranging between 8 and 12 Hz. Physiologic tremor is typically not visible because the amplitude is so low. The amplitude of physiologic tremor can be increased and become more apparent in certain contexts such as anxiety, stress, pharmaceutical use, excessive caffeine consumption, and physical exhaustion among others. Pathological tremors are typically higher in amplitude and slower in frequency. The most common pathological tremor is **essential tremor**, considered a "benign" tremor that most frequently affects the hands but can also include the head, neck, larynx, tongue, legs, and trunk. Typical frequencies of essential tremor range between 4 and 10 Hz.[82] When essential tremor affects the larynx and induces dysphonia, the condition is called **essential voice tremor** (**EVT**) or **organic voice tremor**.

Etiological Characteristics

EVT is thought to be related to dysfunction in thalamic and cerebellar motor pathways.[83] Although the sex demographics of essential tremor are relatively equivalent, the EVT subtype occurs more frequently in females than males by a wide margin. Patients frequently report a familial history of tremor, thought to occur in 30% to 50% of diagnosed cases and suggesting strong genetic links in a large percentage of the treatment-seeking population.[82] EVT can be considered a disease of aging, with a majority of diagnoses occurring between the ages of 50 and 70 years.[82]

Clinical Characteristics

EVT typically has a gradual onset, is slowly progressive, and patient complaints can be variable. Upon diagnosis, patients will often ask how bad their voice will get in the future, but the rate and extent of progression is difficult to predict. In severe cases, patients may complain of a "shaky" or "wobbly" voice. In mild cases, the patients may be unaware of tremor but realize that they have a dysphonia. Other symptoms include reduced loudness (though there may be other age-related causes to that also), hoarseness, vocal instability, and difficulty breathing when speaking. These symptoms can be exacerbated during times of fatigue, anxiety, or heavy vocal demands.[82] Many patients also present with a concomitant tremor in the hand or some other part of the body, although it is important to understand that EVT can occur as an isolated tremor. Some patients also report a beneficial effect of alcohol on the severity of their tremor.

Clinical signs of EVT can be evident on endoscopic, perceptual, and acoustic analyses. Endoscopy can reveal tremulous activity not only in the arytenoids during rest breathing and phonation but also in supralaryngeal and pharyngeal structures. Tremors can be visualized in the horizontal plane at the level of the glottis, vestibular folds, and/or arytenoid cartilages, or in the vertical plane in other supraglottal laryngeal regions. Auditory-perceptual features include a quavering, unsteady voice which in severe cases may be staccato-like.[4] When EVT is suspected, it is useful to compare perceptual features during sustained vowel versus connected speech. Connected speech can mask tremor, especially in milder cases, but attempts at controlled sustained voicing such as vowel prolongation often reveal the saliency of the tremor. During vowel prolongation, the tremor can resemble a vibrato as in singing. The voice tremor can be measured acoustically from recordings of sustained vowels, which will provide the clinician and patient with an objective calculation of the tremor rate (frequency) and amplitude. Acoustic analyses may also reveal subtle aphonic voice breaks and voiceless rushes of air.[82]

Treatment

Front-line treatment for EVT is primarily pharmaceutical in the form of BT. While antitremor or anticonvulsant medicines are effective for controlling tremor in many patients with essential tremor, their effectiveness for EVT has been poor in a majority of cases.[82] BT injections into the thyroarytenoid improve vocal function in 60 to 80% of patients, with effects manifesting as reduced tremor amplitude.[82,84] Similar to treatment in SD, voice quality immediately postinjection can be extremely breathy followed by stabilization of improved function. As the clinical effect wanes over several months, patients will typically require repeated injections.

Dysarthria

Description

Dysarthria is an umbrella label for a collective group of speech disorders resulting from disturbances in muscular control over the speech mechanism secondary to paralysis, weakness, and/or incoordination.[85] It is important to understand that some etiologies of voice disorders are also dysarthrias—for example, UVFP due to peripheral nerve injury is a type of flaccid dysarthria, and SD and EVT are types of hyperkinetic dysarthrias. These three voice disorders result in focal impairment to laryngeal muscular control. A number of other dysarthrias also cause voice impairment, although the laryngeal dysfunction in many of these cases is only one element within a cluster of deviant speech dimensions.

Dysarthria Subtypes

One of the most common dysarthrias affecting vocal function for which patients routinely seek out voice therapy is the **hypokinetic dysarthria** of PD. PD is a neurodegenerative disease affecting motor and non-motor pathways in the central and peripheral nervous systems. The cardinal clinical signs of PD include resting tremor, rigidity, bradykinesia (slow movement), and postural/balance difficulties. The clinical phase of PD is associated with the onset of dysfunction in basal ganglia neural networks which utilize the neurotransmitter dopamine, although there is a long subclinical phase of neurodegeneration that progresses from the lower brainstem into higher subcortical and cortical neurons in addition to peripheral autonomic pathways.[86] When this progressive degeneration reaches the basal ganglia motor networks, a process that can take 10 or more years from initial onset, the resulting motor impairment typically causes a patient to seek evaluation from a physician, leading to diagnosis. Initial motor signs often include tremor in one hand, rigidity ("stiffness") in a hand or leg, and/or balance difficulties. The specific pathophysiology causing the neurodegeneration in PD is the presence of abnormal alpha-synuclein protein deposits in neuronal cell bodies and axonal projections, which form **Lewy bodies** and **Lewy neurites** that impair neuron function.[87]

Pharmaceutical treatment in the form of dopamine replacement and dopamine agonists is the front-line treatment for PD. In many patients, these medications can substantially improve limb motor function during the early years of treatment (unfortunately, after years of treatment, the dopamine replacement can itself cause motor disturbances in the form of dyskinesias). Surgical procedures such as deep brain stimulation have also shown positive effects on limb motor function in many patients. Interestingly, medication and surgery used to treat PD do not have similar positive effects on speech. The reasons for this are still unclear, although theories have suggested that the central connections of cranial nerves, which are in some ways different from those of spinal nerves, may be related to the differential effects of limb versus speech motor function after pharmaceutical treatment.[88]

The laryngeal manifestations of PD include glottal incompetence, which has been associated with bowing of the vocal folds. Respiratory support can also be compromised by increased muscle tone, causing rigidity in the muscles of inhalation/exhalation. Theories have associated the vocal fold bowing in PD with rigidity in the laryngeal muscles similar to that which occurs in limb muscles, although alternative theories (e.g., atrophy) have also been put forth.[89,90,91] The salient clinical presentation of this impairment includes reduced loudness and a breathy voice quality. The changes in vocal fold tone and/or glottal closure may not be the only cause of reduced loudness, however. Alternative explanations have suggested that impaired scaling of vocal effort, related to basal ganglia mediation for the sense of physical effort, may contribute to the reduced vocal loudness that is characteristic of speakers with PD.[88]

Upon voice evaluation, PD usually presents as a cluster of clinical signs which are similar from patient to patient. Endoscopically, glottal incompetence is a common finding that can confirm the perceptual impression of a breathy and low volume voice quality. Some patients may compensate for the glottal incompetence with hyperfunctional recruitment of laryngeal muscles. This recruitment can be visible on endoscopy and perceived as an added rough or harsh component to the breathy voice. Acoustically the glottal incompetence and impaired vocal fold oscillation can lead to decreased measures of CPP and HNR. It is also typical for physiological frequency range to be reduced secondary to the hypokinetic dysarthria of PD. The presence of glottal incompetence will also be detected by aerodynamic measurements, which can be characterized by increased subglottal pressure and increased transglottal airflow. In more moderate-to-severe cases, articulation can also be compromised, and clinicians must be aware that increased speech rate (unique to hypokinetic dysarthria) and articulatory imprecision can cause degrees of unintelligibility during conversational speech.

Surgical options such as injection laryngoplasty are available to treat the glottal incompetency found in PD.[92] Voice therapy does not target the cause of PD (the underlying neuropathology), but a strong science base supports the benefits of voice therapy for rehabilitating motor function in the subsystems of voice and subsequently improving vocal function and quality of life. Voice therapy for the dysarthria of PD targets the physiological impairment of glottal incompetence and some treatments also focus on cognitive awareness and motor recalibration of amplitude scaling during speech.[88,93] A robust evidence base supports the application of the **Lee Silverman Voice Treatment** (**LSVT-LOUD**) for the voice impairment of PD. This proprietary treatment approach utilizes daily exercises under clinical guidance which requires an individual to progress through a hierarchy of vocalization types while increasing activity in voluntary motor pathways (those controlling respiratory, laryngeal, and articulatory muscles), vocal loudness, and cognitive scaling of effort. LSVT-LOUD has demonstrated short- and long-term gains in vocal loudness and speech intelligibility in large cohorts of patients.[94] An associated treatment with emerging evidence is **Speak-Out!**, which is structured in a very similar manner as LSVT-LOUD, although with different clinical prompts and no lower limit restriction on the recommended number of treatment sessions.[9,95] Other treatment approaches for the glottal incompetency of PD include **vocal function exercises**, in both traditional form and modified by increasing vocal effort and perceived loudness. These approaches are discussed in more detail in Chapter 8.

Spastic dysarthria is a dysarthria subtype resulting from bilateral injury to the pyramidal and extrapyramidal motor pathways of the central nervous system. It is often associated with head injury, stroke, or degenerative neurological disease including amyotrophic lateral sclerosis (ALS). The laryngeal effects of spastic dysarthria include increased muscle tone and possible hyperadduction that can be visible through endoscopy as medial and anterior-posterior laryngeal compression.[4] This creates the perception of a rough and strained voice quality (often described as "harsh") that lacks intonation flexibility. Because hypertonicity can reduce the speed and range of movement, speakers with spastic dysarthria can also exhibit a slow speech rate with imprecise articulation. ALS, which can begin in either the central or peripheral nervous system, will exhibit these vocal characteristics when the CNS pathways to the vagus nerve

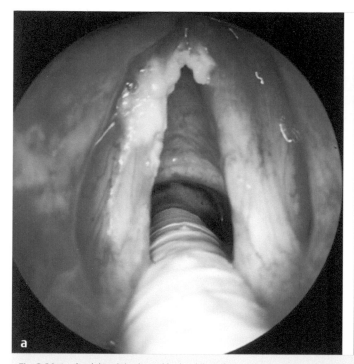

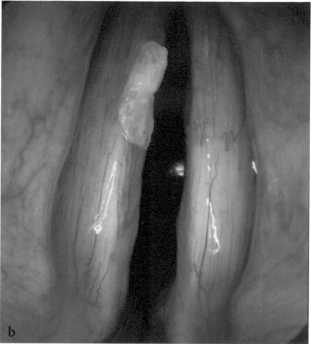

Fig. 2.20 Leukoplakia. **(a)** Bilateral leukoplakia. **(b)** Focal area of leukoplakia involving one vocal fold. (From Kendall K, Leonard R. Laryngeal Evaluation, 1st edition. New York: Thieme Publishers, 2010.)

are impaired. In the early stages of ALS disease progression, a change in voice can be the most salient feature of the disease. When ALS begins in the PNS, the laryngeal manifestation can be a **flaccid dysarthria** in the form of UVFP or BVFP. Often the voice problems are a secondary concern, whereas the articulatory disturbance causing unintelligibility and the possible swallowing impairments can be the primary concern.

2.5.2 Structural/Infection/Systemic Subtypes

Premalignant Lesions

Description and Clinical Characteristics

Vocal fold premalignant lesions are abnormal structural changes to the vocal fold which are limited to the epithelium and have not invaded surrounding layers or distant tissues. These lesions are most often associated with chronic smoking, smoking combined with moderate or heavy alcohol use, or LPR. Four types of premalignancies are most common to the vocal folds with the potential to cause dysphonia: leukoplakia, erythroplakia, erythroleukoplakia, and dysplasia. **Leukoplakia** can be translated as a "white surface," and this is exactly what the laryngoscopic characteristics of leukoplakia are—white patches on the vocal fold cover (▸ Fig. 2.20). Histologically, leukoplakia is an accumulation of keratin, which is normally not produced by the nonkeratinizing epithelium of the vocal folds. **Erythroplakia** means "red surface." The "red surface" is due to increased visibility of vasculature supplying the epithelium of the vocal folds (▸ Fig. 2.21). Some otolaryngologists will refer to these white or red lesions as a type of vocal fold **plaque** (a general term meaning "raised patch" or "focal tissue damage"). **Erythroleukoplakia** (▸ Fig. 2.22) appears as a

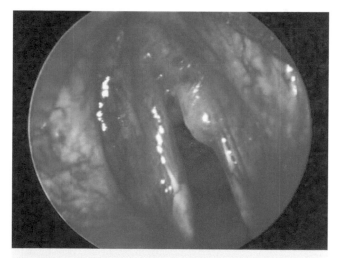

Fig. 2.21 Erythroplakia with severe dysplasia (From Bhattacharyya A. Laryngology: Otorhinolaryngology—Head and Neck Surgery Series. 1st edition. New York: Thieme Publishers, 2014.)

combination of the two, and is often described as a red lesion with white "speckles."[96]

Dysplasia refers to an abnormality in cellular structure and number, and often occurs with any of the three premalignancies noted earlier. Laryngeal dysplasia may initially be diagnosed as **leukoplakia**, **erythroplakia**, or **erythroleukoplakia** (all three are based on visual appearance), followed by histological visualization of cell abnormality which confirms dysplasia on lab testing.

These four conditions are considered premalignant lesions at risk for transformation into cancer. Leukoplakia, erythroplakia, and erythroleukoplakia can all develop dysplasia which, when

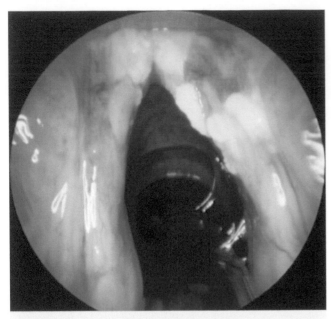

Fig. 2.22 Erythroleukoplakia showing red and white speckled appearance. (From Kendall K, Leonard R. Laryngeal Evaluation, 1st edition. New York: Thieme Publishers, 2010.)

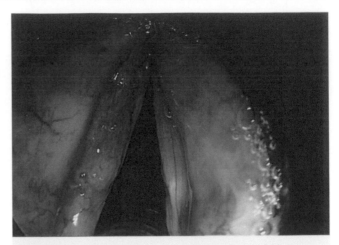

Fig. 2.23 Early invasive (T1) carcinoma of the left vocal fold. (From Bhattacharyya A. Laryngology: Otorhinolaryngology—Head and Neck Surgery Series. 1st edition. New York: Thieme Publishers, 2014.)

severe, can then evolve into a **carcinoma** (cancer that affects epithelium). Not all discolored vocal fold plaques will develop into carcinoma, but all can develop dysplasia and statistics show that 8 to 14% of laryngeal dysplasias will evolve into cancerous lesions.[97,98] As dysplasia becomes more severe, it has a greater risk for developing into cancer. The diagnosis of cancer means that the abnormal dysplastic cells have invaded into deeper levels of the vocal fold tissue. When laryngeal dysplasia is severe but still confined to the epithelium, it is sometimes called "**carcinoma in situ.**" Carcinoma in situ means "cancer in its original place." Therefore, severe forms of vocal fold dysplasia and early forms of glottic cancer are histologically very similar—both represent significant cellular abnormalities on the stratified squamous epithelium of the vocal fold cover.

Treatment

When a white or red plaque is identified on the vocal fold epithelium, it is impossible to know with endoscopy if there is an underlying dysplasia and/or carcinoma. Up to 50% of leukoplakias can develop an underlying dysplasia, which may eventually evolve into carcinoma.[99] Because of this risk, the otolaryngologist will be concerned that conservative management might allow a dysplasia time to evolve into cancer. On the other hand, surgical excision or ablation of a plaque runs the risk of permanent injury to the vocal fold tissue and chronic dysphonia. This can create a quandary for the physician, and thus it is not surprising that management decisions for premalignant lesions vary from center to center and can include observation of the lesion over time, excision via microlaryngoscopy or laser, or even radiation treatment.[97] When excised, all premalignant lesions will undergo biopsy to determine the presence of dysplasia, its severity, and/or whether the abnormal cells have proliferated to such a degree that they are cancer. In many cases, the surgeon at the time of

biopsy can excise margins of normal tissue surrounding the lesion and remove all plaque or dysplastic tissues. In some cases, this can result in a cure (i.e., the abnormal tissue may not return).

Laryngeal Cancer

Description and Clinical Characteristics

Cancer is an abnormal proliferation of cells with potential or which have realized migration to distant sites beyond their place of origin. The vast majority (95%) of laryngeal cancers are **carcinomas**, a type of cancer that affects the squamous epithelial cells lining the larynx. The greatest risk factor for laryngeal cancer is chronic smoking, and heavy alcohol use combined with smoking dramatically increases this risk. Laryngeal cancers can also be associated with the human papilloma virus (HPV). Laryngeal cancer is classified based on region of origin: glottal, supraglottal, and subglottal. Over 13,500 new cases of laryngeal cancer are diagnosed in the United States each year, with incidence much larger in males than in females.[100] The majority of laryngeal cancers originate at the glottis, representing approximately 60% of all cases. Approximately 35% and 5% originate in the supraglottal and subglottal regions, respectively.

Supraglottic and subglottic cancers may have no effect on voice—their initial symptoms are often pain or globus sensation in the throat. Some subglottal cancers can go undetected until they metastasize to distant sites. Initial signs of glottic cancer are often pain or dysphonia. Approximately 74% of all glottic cancers originate in the anterior one-third of the vocal fold, whereas 12% originate in the mid-membranous region and 4% in the posterior one-third. The remaining lesions originate at multiple sites or the exact site of origin cannot be determined.[101] Glottic cancer can evolve from leukoplakia, erythroplakia, or erythroleukoplakia and can have a highly variable appearance (▸ Fig. 2.23). Other than carcinoma in situ, the diagnosis of glottic cancer necessitates abnormal cellular invasion into the BMZ and superficial lamina propria. Unfortunately, evidence of deeper cellular invasion may be obscured by the presence of superficial plaque. However, on endoscopy, glottic cancer will often result in significant stiff segments across a broad section of the vocal fold, with erythema (redness) and edema at the site of lesion.

Treatment

Cancerous cells pose a risk to life due to their ability to metastasize. The diagnosis of laryngeal cancer is thus significant. Stage 1 and stage 2 laryngeal cancers are typically treated with surgery, radiation, or a combination of these two. Management of more advanced laryngeal cancers has evolved over the past few decades with a bias toward laryngeal preservation in the form of radiation or chemoradiation, which has replaced the traditional laryngectomy as the initial treatment approach in a majority of late-stage laryngeal cancers. Specific surgical options, tumor staging, and voice restoration second to laryngectomy are further discussed in Chapter 9.

Vocal Fold Cysts

Description and Clinical Characteristics

Cysts are included under the organic and functional categories due to their likely multifactorial etiology. As previously mentioned, these lesions occur frequently in speakers with heavy vocal demands or those who are excessive talkers. Organic etiological contributions include congenital cysts, mucous gland duct blockage, and trapped epithelial cells in the superficial lamina propria. Congenital cysts tend to be more of the epidermoid type than mucous retention type.[62] In acquired cysts, the degree to which functional behaviors and organic influences combine is unclear, although leading theory suggests these factors are synergistic for cyst development in many cases. Additional characteristics of cysts can be found in section **2.4.9, Vocal Fold Cysts**.

Vocal Process Granuloma

Description and Clinical Characteristics

Granulomas are included under both organic and functional categories due to their multifactorial etiology. Organic etiologies of vocal process granulomas include **postsurgical intubation injury** and LPR. Intubation injury occurs when the endotracheal tube used for ventilation irritates the posterior vocal fold tissue. This can result in **ulceration** and/or granuloma development in the region of the vocal process. It is thought the longer intubation occurs the more at risk the patient is for vocal fold injury, including ulcer and granuloma development in addition to a risk for vocal fold paralysis.

Chronic LPR results in digestive fluids moving in a retrograde direction through the **upper esophageal sphincter** (UES).[102] The posterior larynx lies directly above and in front of the UES putting it in the path of these fluids. Over time, the chemicals of these fluids can irritate and damage the tissue at the vocal processes and surrounding vocal fold and laryngeal tissue. This can result in ulceration and/or granuloma development at one or both vocal processes over time. As discussed in section **2.4.10, Vocal Process Granulomas**, treatment for granulomas, regardless of etiology, includes three elements: antireflux treatment, voice therapy to reduce or eliminate phonotrauma, and time. Granulomas can take quite a long time to resolve, in some cases up to a year. A minority of granulomas will not resolve and may require phonosurgery, depending on the severity of their effects on the speaker.

Presbylaryngis

Description

Presbylaryngis denotes age-related changes to the larynx and subsequent alterations in voice quality. Structural changes to the larynx are considered a natural consequence of physiological aging, though in some individuals these changes may be so great to cause voice impairment, which in the absence of additional neurological, structural, or behavioral etiologies is diagnosed as presbylaryngis. Physiological changes of aging affecting the larynx include loss of muscle bulk (atrophy), reduced density in elastic fibers, ossification of laryngeal cartilages, and changes to epithelial thickness which may be different in females and males (e.g., thickened epithelium in females vs. thinner epithelium in males).[62,103] Voice impairment because of aging is common with reported incidence approximating 30% of those older than 65 years.[104]

Clinical Characteristics

A primary physiological impairment causing dysphonia in presbylaryngis is glottal incompetence. Glottal incompetence in presbylaryngis is characterized by an **elliptical closure** pattern related to loss of vocal fold tone and **vocal fold bowing** (▶ Fig. 2.24). The suspicion of vocal fold bowing and atrophy can be supported by observing **prominent vocal processes**. This appearance emanates from the atrophy and/or concave shape of the membranous vocal fold at its attachment to the vocal process. Endoscopic signs can also include compensatory hyperfunction in the form of supraglottic laryngeal compression (▶ Fig. 2.24).

Perceptual characteristics of presbylaryngis can be similar to those of the hypokinetic dysarthria of PD, which also occurs more commonly in advanced age. The aged voice contains salient features that listeners use, quite successfully, to determine whether or not a speaker is older or younger. **Breathiness** and **reduced loudness** are the most salient perceptual characteristics of presbylaryngis and are the basis for describing this condition by its other name, **presbyphonia**. Hoarseness may be more prominent than breathiness when phonation periodicity is significantly degraded, creating a rough component on top of the breathiness. Measures of cepstral peak prominence and harmonic-to-noise ratio tend to be reduced as a result of the glottal incompetence and phonation instability. Aerodynamic measures, as with most cases of glottal incompetence, tend to be characterized by increased subglottal pressure and transglottal airflow.

Treatment

The glottal incompetence of presbylaryngis can be treated successfully with voice therapy and/or surgical options. Evidence-based approaches for glottal incompetence include vocal function exercises, phonation resistance training exercises (PhoRTE), LSVT, and vocal exercises combined with neuromuscular electrical stimulation.[105,106,107,108] Successful voice therapy for presbylaryngis will require a motivated patient who is willing to perform vocal exercises multiple times each day, as the beneficial effects of treatment will take time to manifest. Surgical treatment for the glottal incompetence has

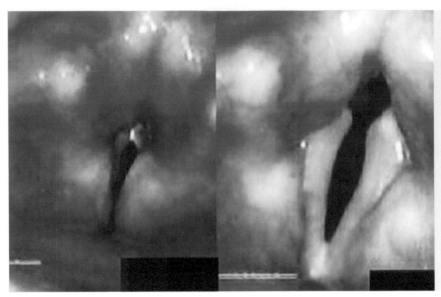

Fig. 2.24 Vocal fold bowing with incomplete elliptical closure secondary to presbylaryngis. Note the prominent arytenoids in the right panel, and signs of compensatory hyperfunction in the left panel. (From Kendall K, Leonard R. Laryngeal Evaluation, 1st edition. New York: Thieme Publishers, 2010.)

most recently included injection laryngoplasty to add bulk to the vocal folds and improve glottal closure.[109] While injections can provide an immediate benefit to vocal function, the effects will be temporary due to material reabsorption. Patients who develop a secondary MTD due to compensatory hyperfunction will likely benefit from voice therapy, whether or not they receive injections.

Laryngeal Papillomatosis

Description

Laryngeal papillomatosis is a condition caused by infection of the HPV virus, resulting in growth of epithelial lesions called **papillomas**. These develop primarily on the vocal folds but can also appear at other sites in the larynx. Papillomas cause dysphonia when they interfere with glottal closure and/or epithelial oscillation during vibration. Laryngeal papillomatosis is associated with a number of different HPV subtypes but most frequently HPV 6 and HPV 11, which are believed to be passed to a child from the mother at birth or at any other time by human-to-human contact.[110] Laryngeal papilloma is seen more commonly in children, but there are a growing number of adults being affected by the HPV virus and at risk for papilloma development.

Clinical Characteristics

Papillomas are benign exophytic masses that can develop anywhere along the length of the vocal folds. They grow out of the vocal fold epithelium and appear endoscopically as clusters of small wart-like pods that have been likened to a cauliflower or raspberry appearance when viewed up close (▶ Fig. 2.25). These lesions vary in size but can be so large that they interfere with respiration by partially obstructing the airway. There is some concern that severe cases of papillomatosis have potential to develop into malignancy as approximately 28% papillomas related to HPV 6 and 11 have been associated with underlying dysplasia.[110]

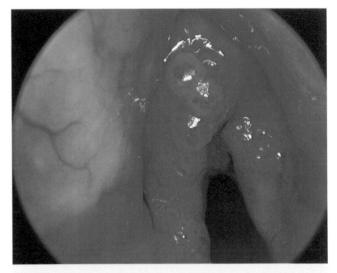

Fig. 2.25 Laryngeal papillomatosis. (From Kendall K, Leonard R. Laryngeal Evaluation, 1st edition. New York: Thieme Publishers, 2010.)

Treatment

Surgical treatment is the front-line management for papillomas, although there are considerations which must be taken into account with this disorder that are unique. Papillomas tend to reoccur and it is common for those affected to undergo repeat surgeries. Repeated incision to the vocal fold mucosa runs the risk of permanent scar. Surgical strategy is dependent on the surgeon, and has included microlaryngoscopic removal with cold steel instruments, lasers, and microdebriders.[111] Some physicians use adjuvant agents such as antiviral medications, most notably cidofovir, in an attempt to attack the underlying viral etiology of the disorder.[112] The degree of dysphonia severity will depend on the extent of the lesion, the degree to which it impedes glottal closure and disrupts vibratory dynamics, and the presence of compensatory hyperfunction. Perceptual, acoustic, and aerodynamic measurements will be influenced by those factors and should be expected to be outside of normal limits as dysphonic severity increases.

Laryngitis

Description

Laryngitis is a general term referring to inflammation of the larynx. Inflammation is characterized by edema and erythema within tissue, and this inflammatory response can be generalized throughout the larynx or localized to different regions. Laryngitis is the most common diagnosis given by primary care physicians for patients seeking treatment for throat-related ailments. This diagnosis reflects a tissue response and not an etiology, and it is not surprising that the frequency with which laryngitis is diagnosed by otolaryngologists is much less.[7]

Etiological Characteristics, Clinical Characteristics, and Treatment

Laryngeal inflammation can result from many different causes, and differential diagnosis of the underlying etiology can be very challenging. Endoscopically, the laryngeal and vocal fold mucosa appears red and swollen with increased mucous. Sometimes the mucous can be viscous, sticky, white, and pool on the vocal fold surface. The degree of dysphonia caused by laryngitis will be a function of the amount of swelling, irritation, and existence of compensatory hyperfunctional responses. In some patients, finding the cause of laryngitis can take time and involves a process of elimination based on response to different treatments. Some of the more common etiologies associated with acute and chronic laryngitis include

- Laryngopharyngeal reflux.
- Allergic responses.
- Chronic phonotrauma.
- Bacterial, viral, and fungal infections.
- Smoking.
- Radiation.
- Environmental irritants.

LPR is thought to be one of the most common causes of laryngeal inflammation in otolaryngologic clinics, with estimates of incidence in 20 to 30% of treatment-seeking patients with laryngeal complaints, although some authors put the incidence rate much higher.[102] Symptoms of LPR can be variable as illustrated in ▶ Table 2.4. In more severe cases of LPR, the posterior region of the larynx can become visibly edematous at the interarytenoid space, appearing as puffy translucent or white epithelium (some refer to this as "**pachydermia**"). Treatment typically follows three stages: (1) behavioral and lifestyle changes, (2) pharmaceutical management, and (3) surgery. Behavioral and lifestyle recommendations for inhibiting reflux include modifying diet (e.g., reducing acidic and fatty foods), modifying eating patterns (e.g., no food at least 2 hours prior to sleep), and sleeping with the head elevated. A number of different drugs and drug combinations can be prescribed or recommended by the physician, including **proton-pump inhibitors** (e.g., Omeprazole, Lansoprazole), **H2-blockers** (e.g., Ranitidine, Famotidine), and over-the-counter **antacids**.

Table 2.4 Otolaryngologic symptoms and associations with laryngopharyngeal reflux. From Fried, MP, Tan M. Clinical Laryngology. 1st edition. New York: Thieme Publishers, 2014

Symptoms	Associations
Dysphonia	Rhinosinusitis
Globus (foreign body) sensation	Otitis media
Chronic cough	Laryngospasm
Soreness or burning in throat	Granuloma
Throat clearing	Airway stenosis
Excessive mucous production	Leukoplakia
Dysphagia	Lingual tonsil hypertrophy
	Obstructive sleep apnea
	Laryngeal carcinoma

It is accepted that pharmaceutical control of LPR can take months to show effect, so patients must be compliant with medication schedules. When behavioral/lifestyle modifications combined with pharmaceutical management are not effective for controlling LPR, and the diagnosis is certain, some patients may be candidates for surgical management. Currently, the most common surgical procedure for LPR is **fundoplication**. This surgery adds tone to the lower esophageal sphincter (LES) by twisting the fundus (entry of the stomach) around the lower esophagus.

Infections are also a common cause of inflammation associated with laryngitis. **Viral** upper respiratory infections and the potential laryngeal effects of these conditions will be familiar to most individuals. Viral infections most commonly cause acute laryngitis lasting less than 2 weeks, although in some cases infection can be chronic or the patient can develop phonotraumatic behaviors as a result of the infection which leads to additional vocal impairments. Various pharmaceuticals can be prescribed to combat the physiological responses of viral infections, responses that in addition to inflammation can include increased mucous production and cough. **Bacterial** infections can also cause inflammatory laryngeal responses and should be confirmed with cultured specimens.[59] These will be treated with various antibacterial medications. **Fungal infections** causing laryngitis are most often associated with yeast infection (**candidiasis**) throughout the larynx. Candidiasis appears as white or discolored patches on the vocal fold and surrounding laryngeal tissue (▶ Fig. 2.26). Fungal infections can be caused by different etiologies including the use of inhaled steroids (e.g., by those with asthma), antibiotic medications, and immune disease, among others. Antifungal medications are typically effective for treating these infections.

A large number of **medications** are confirmed or suspected to have a negative effect on the tissue of the larynx and might have the potential to facilitate dysphonia or problematic laryngeal sensations. For this reason, a patient's current use of prescription and nonprescription medications is an important part of the history component of the voice evaluation. Many medications influence the vocal fold tissue systemically from within. Some medications are inhaled, however, and can influence the tissue at the surface.[113] One example is **inhaled corticosteroids**, the primary treatment for individuals with chronic asthma. The incidence of dysphonia in users of inhaled corticosteroids has been reported as high as 58%, with suggested mechanisms including mucosal changes at the vocal fold surface and underlying changes to the TA muscle.[113] For a review of various medications on vocal function, see the review article by Abaza et al.[114]

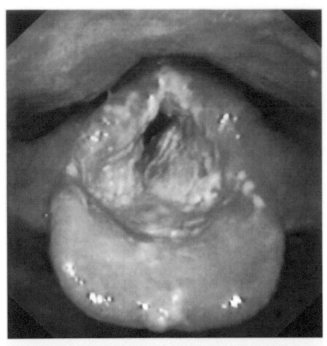

Fig. 2.26 Laryngitis caused by fungal infection. (From Bhattacharyya A. Laryngology: Otorhinolaryngology—Head and Neck Surgery Series. 1st edition. New York: Thieme Publishers, 2014.)

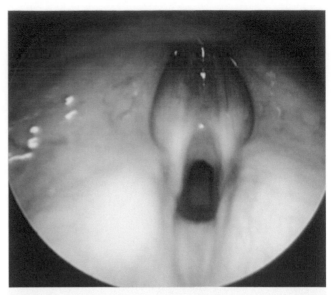

Fig. 2.27 Congenital laryngeal web at anterior glottis. (From Fried M, Tan M. Clinical Laryngology. 1st edition. New York: Thieme Publishers, 2014.)

Laryngeal Web

Description, Clinical Characteristics, and Treatment

Laryngeal webs are a form of laryngeal stenosis (narrowing) characterized by tissue bridges connecting the left and right laryngeal regions together (▶ Fig. 2.27). Laryngeal webs most often occur at the level of the glottis, causing an absence of space between the two vocal folds at the location of the web. **Congenital webs** result from separation failure of the two vocal folds during fetal development. **Acquired webs** most often result from tracheal intubation or phonosurgery which irritates the tissue. During the wound healing response, the left and right vocal fold epithelium can migrate toward each other and connect to form a bridge. Laryngeal webs occur in both pediatric and adult populations, and the vast majority form anteriorly where the two vocal folds most closely approximate each other.[115]

In pediatric populations, webs can be very serious because they can obstruct the airway and cause breathing difficulties. In cases of substantial airway obstruction, immediate surgery may be required to establish patency. The effects of congenital and acquired webs on phonation can be variable, and are dependent on the size of the web in the horizontal plane. Very small webs may be asymptomatic. Larger webs can cause **audible inspiration**, **difficulty breathing**, and a **rough voice** with **high pitch** due to the short segments of vocal fold able to oscillate.[31]

Small webs that are asymptomatic will likely be monitored over time. For more severe webs, the primary treatment is surgery. Surgical options include laser resection or other phonosurgical approaches which divide the web, freeing up the glottic space. Preventing webs from reforming can be a challenge due to the close proximity of the left and right vocal folds at the anterior region. To prevent the vocal fold edges from reconnecting, a silicone or silastic keel can be placed on the tissue at the site of resection, which can later be removed after adequate healing has taken place.

Laryngocele

Description and Clinical Characteristics

A laryngocele is an air-filled pocket of tissue that occurs in the anterior portion of the ventricle known as the **laryngeal saccule**. Some laryngoceles can fill with fluid and/or become infected. Endoscopically, these appear as dilated ventricles protruding medially, in some cases obstructing views of the ipsilateral vocal fold. This can give the appearance of a ventricle being filled with air like a balloon. Various theories exist to explain laryngocele formation including congenital malformations and exposure of the laryngeal saccule to intense intralaryngeal pressure. Such pressures might be related to singing, playing wind instruments, blowing glass, or coughing, among others.[111] It is not surprising that some patients with chronic cough develop laryngoceles secondary to the chronic high pressures delivered to the larynx. If the laryngocele is large enough, it can put pressure on the vocal folds, disturbing vibratory dynamics and causing hoarseness. Additional symptoms include cough, globus sensation, stridor, snoring, and in severe cases dysphagia.[111] The primary treatment for laryngocele is surgery which may include drainage of any fluid before excision of the lesion.

Laryngomalacia

Description and Clinical Characteristics

Laryngomalacia is a congenital condition caused by incomplete maturation of the cartilaginous framework of the larynx. It is one of the most common causes of inhalatory stridor in infants. The

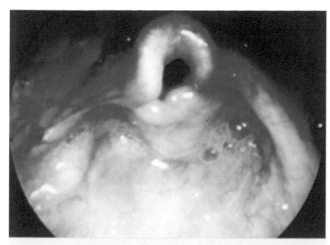

Fig. 2.28 Laryngomalacia showing omega shaped epiglottis and prolapsed arytenoids with narrowing of airway. (From Fried M, Tan M. Clinical Laryngology. 1st edition. New York: Thieme Publishers, 2014.)

condition affects the rigidity of the laryngeal cartilages, resulting in abnormal pliability and positioning of cartilages that can obstruct the airway. Endoscopic signs of laryngomalacia include an omega-shaped epiglottis, arytenoid prolapse, and narrowed airway (▶ Fig. 2.28). The condition takes on varied forms of severity and, in some cases, is so mild to be asymptomatic. In some children, the symptoms of laryngomalacia may not be present immediately at birth, but have gradual onset within the first 2 weeks. Treatment for laryngomalacia is typically observation over time. As the child grows, the laryngeal cartilages mature and symptoms typically subside within a few years. In severe cases causing airway obstruction, surgical procedures to improve airway patency can be performed.[115]

Vocal Fold Scar

Description, Etiological, and Clinical Characteristics

Vocal fold scar represents fibrotic, stiff epithelium which develops secondary to injury of the vocal fold mucosa. Scar forms when there is a breakdown in the normal wound-healing response. It is believed that scar forms early during the first week of wound healing, and is characterized by fragmented and disorganized elastin fibers, thick collagen bundles, and decreased hyaluronic acid.[40,116] Scar tissue is not pliable, so its existence will significantly impact the vibratory dynamics of a vocal fold. Scar is also currently irreversible and is a great concern to singers and the laryngologists who perform phonosurgery on that population. The prevention of scar formation is a preeminent focus of scientific investigation in laryngology, with several groups currently working on potential treatments for this debilitating pathology.

The most common cause of vocal fold scar is iatrogenic injury from phonosurgery. Any time the vocal fold tissue is excised, there is a potential for scar formation, and the otolaryngologist will spend dedicated time going over these risks with a patient. Some also consider chronic phonotrauma as an etiology, which would mean that scar could also be placed in the functional category of voice disorders. For example, some believe that scar can develop secondary to vocal fold blood vessel rupture. Scar tissue may appear as a dull discolored region, either flat or

raised, on the vocal fold cover. However, its presence can best be visualized during laryngeal videostroboscopy. It will affect most of the vibratory characteristics, including reduced amplitude, symmetry, and mucosal wave especially at the location of the scar. Scar tissue can also be so fibrotic that the shape of the vocal fold at the site of the scar is compromised, causing a notch or incomplete closure pattern. This type of scar can also attach to deeper vocal fold layers or wrap inward to appear as a longitudinal groove along the medial surface of the tissue, and has been considered as a type of a **sulcus** (see next section).

The perceptual, acoustic, and aerodynamic effects of vocal fold scar depend on the severity, which can range from mild and barely symptomatic to so severe that it ends a performer's career. The perceptual effects are generally hoarseness with reduced pitch range, most noticeably a loss in the higher pitches. These perceptual effects correspond to acoustic characteristics of increased perturbation and decreased cepstral peak prominence and harmonic-to-noise ratio. Reduced physiological frequency range will correspond to the pitch limitations. Because speakers with scar must work harder to set the vocal folds into vibration, aerodynamic profiles can be characterized by increased subglottal pressure.

Treatment

There is currently no cure for vocal fold scar. Voice therapy can improve vocal function secondary to scar by promoting the most efficient and effective physiological balance in the vocal subsystems. However, the presence of significant scar tissue will reduce vocal flexibility by limiting physiological frequency range in addition to causing permanent irregularities in vocal fold vibratory periodicity. There are a number of surgical approaches for treating scar. In general, these attempt to separate the vocal fold epithelium from the lamina propria and then fill the space underneath the epithelium with a pliable substance such as collagen-based products, fat, or hyaluronic acid. Surgery for scar can be difficult, does not completely cure the scar, and carries the risk of additional scar tissue forming during the healing process after surgery.

Vocal Fold Sulcus

Description, Etiological, and Clinical Characteristics

Vocal fold sulci appear as grooves or notches along the medial vocal fold edges and represent a continuum of scarring characterized by abnormal epithelial organization. Sulci can occur unilaterally or bilaterally. Some have distinguished vocal fold sulcus from scar as a flat or raised epithelial disturbances (scar) versus epithelial indentations (sulci).[117] Sulci have been differentiated based on their histological characteristics and functional impact. Ford et al identified three types of sulci: Type 1, **physiological sulcus**, a superficial sulcus characterized by minor atrophy in the vocal fold epithelium which is anchored to the superficial lamina propria, causing a slight inward depression or notch in the vocal fold cover. Physiological sulci may be asymptomatic or have only very mild effects; Type 2, **sulcus vergeture**, a deeper sulcus running horizontally along the vocal fold margin. Vergeture means "stretch mark" and describes the visual characteristics of this lesion. These sulci can extend into the vocal ligament and cause substantial dysphonia; Type 3, **sulcus**

vocalis, the deepest sulcus which may extend past the vocal ligament and cause the most severe degree of dysphonia.[118] Sulci running along the entire length of a vocal fold can create the visual appearance of bowing on endoscopic examination, and on videostroboscopy will reveal stiffness along the length of the sulcus with an incomplete elliptical closure pattern.[119]

The etiology of sulci is unclear and possibly multifactorial. Both congenital and acquired etiologies have been proposed. Congenital hypotheses suggest incomplete development of the vocal fold tissue at birth or early rupturing of a congenital epidermoid cyst which subsequently damages the vocal fold cover. Acquired etiologies have included phonotrauma, infection, and abnormal wound healing secondary to phonosurgery.[119] Perceptual, acoustic, and aerodynamic characteristics will be dependent on the type and severity of sulcus.

Treatment

The presence of sulcus, especially Types 2 and 3, cause dysphonia and may lead to the development of a secondary MTD. Voice therapy can be effective for rebalancing physiology to promote improved voice quality and function, although "normal" voice quality may be difficult to achieve with voice therapy alone. A number of different surgical options exist to treat sulcus including injection laryngoplasty and sulcus resection. The management choice will be a collaborative decision between the patient, otolaryngologist, and SLP.

2.5.3 Idiopathic Voice Disorders

Idiopathic voice disorders include those impairments affecting laryngeal function for which no conclusive underlying etiology can be identified. While the signs and symptoms of these conditions are discernable, including effects on breathing, cough, and phonation, it is not clear if these are primarily related to neurological impairment, systemic conditions, functional misuse, psychological abnormality, or some combination of those factors. The two idiopathic clinical conditions most often encountered are paradoxical vocal fold movement (PVFM) and chronic cough, which will be described below.

Paradoxical Vocal Fold Movement

Description and Clinical Characteristics

Paradoxical vocal fold movement, also known as **vocal cord dysfunction** (VCD), is characterized by transient but repetitive episodes of **inappropriate and involuntary adduction of the vocal folds during inspiration**. This has the effect of narrowing the airway and causing dyspnea, and can result in compensatory hyperfunction in the laryngeal and respiratory muscles that cause expiration to be labored and rushed with a negative impact on phonation. To come close to experiencing what patients go through during PVFM episodes, try to inhale at the same time you hold your breath—breathing is difficult, unpleasant, and worrisome. It is not uncommon for patients later diagnosed with PVFM to be initially diagnosed with asthma, and report a history of admission to emergency rooms due to difficulty breathing. It is also typical for these patients to report that inhaled corticosteroids prescribed for asthma do not help with PVFM episodes. The reason for this is that asthma is caused by an inflammatory airway obstruction below the larynx, while PVFM occurs at the level of the vocal folds and is not inflammatory.

In addition to asthma, PVFM is associated with a number of medical conditions, which include laryngopharyngeal reflux.[120] During the evaluation process, a guided case history can reveal one or more factors, known as "triggers," which precede the onset of a PVFM episode. While specific triggers vary across patients and can be unique to individuals, collectively reports of physical exertion during **exercise**, noxious **odors** such as smoke or inhaled chemical smells, psychological **stress**, and **throat irritation** are commonly reported as inciting factors for PVFM episodes.[120] Individuals with exercised-induced PVFM, many of whom are athletes, can have so great a difficulty breathing during episodes that they are unable to continue performance.

Unfortunately, it can be difficult to elicit a PVFM episode during the evaluation process, unless the clinician is able to expose the patient to one or more of the possible triggers. When PVFM episodes do occur during evaluation, the abnormal adductor movements can be visualized during endoscopy as substantial and sometimes near complete closure of the glottis, most often with a narrow posterior gap through which a limited amount of air can be inspired. Perceptual signs of PVFM episodes include the obvious **dyspnea** in addition to inhalatory **stridor** (and on occasion exhalatory stridor), **wheezing**, **choking**, and **hoarse voice** quality with vocal strain.

Treatment

Although the etiology of PVFM is idiopathic, behavioral voice therapy can be effective for controlling the disorder. Effective approaches employ motor learning principles to control respiratory cycles during the initial phases of PVFM onset to prevent or control full-blown episodes. Voice therapy for PVFM focuses on motor behavior during inspiration and expiration, identification and elimination, or modification of triggers and the physical and psychological perceptions which precipitate episodes. Medical treatment is employed along with voice therapy when laryngopharyngeal reflux or other systemic conditions are identified as potential precipitating factors.

Chronic Cough

Description and Clinical Characteristics

Involuntary cough is a protective reflex controlled by brainstem nuclei that are sensitive to afferent signals from laryngeal mucosa in addition to mucosa in the lower and upper airway. The physiology of cough includes activation of respiratory and laryngeal muscles to produce a powerful burst of high-pressure air which moves through the airway at a high velocity. The cough reflex includes recruitment of intrinsic laryngeal adductor muscles (LCA and TA), which are coordinated with the vocal fold abductor (PCA) to produce the laryngeal valving necessary for cough production.[121] Productive cough is purposeful, as it removes irritants (e.g., phlegm, foreign particles) from the airway or protects the lower airway from irritants above.

From a medical perspective, cough is categorized based on symptom duration: **acute cough** lasting less than 3 weeks (e. g., most typical with an upper respiratory infection/cold), **subacute cough** lasting between 3 to 8 weeks, and **chronic cough**.[122] **Chronic cough** is defined as a persistent cough present for more than 8 weeks. It can be related to multifactorial etiologies (▸ Table 2.5) and can be resistant to medical treatment (chronic refractory cough).[123] It can be present as a singular diagnosis but is also associated with a number of medical conditions including laryngopharyngeal reflux, asthma, and systemic responses causing postnasal drip.[120] Chronic cough occurs up to three times more frequently in females than in males with onset most often between the ages of 50 and 70 years.[124] Dysphonia can be a consequence of chronic cough and is related to, among other things, the repeated phonotrauma experienced by the vocal fold tissue.

Treatment

Cough can be difficult to control and medical management is often a stepwise process of exclusion. ▸ Fig. 2.29 illustrates a management algorithm for cough in adult patients and highlights the multifactorial etiological possibilities which must be investigated to arrive at the appropriate treatment.[122] Among the possible treatments to alleviate the frequency and severity of cough is voice therapy provided by SLPs. Management of chronic cough from the perspective of speech–language pathology includes four components: (1) education, (2) cough control techniques, (3) vocal hygiene training, and (4) psychoeducational counseling.[125] Outcome studies focusing on the application of these treatment components have reported significant clinical effects not only for cough symptoms but also for the frequency and severity of breathing and voice difficulties.[120]

2.6 Conclusion

This chapter has summarized the etiologies, clinical characteristics, and possible treatment options for a myriad of voice disorders that the clinician may experience in voice practice. We have seen that most cases fall into *functional* (i.e., disorders that initially develop due to the patient's use of the voice), *organic* (i.e., disorders that initially develop due to some underlying disease process), or *idiopathic* (i.e., no known cause) categories. However, we have also described cases (e.g., vocal fold cysts) in which the underlying etiology may arise from multiple categories.

As we build our foundation of knowledge regarding voice production and the disordered states that may affect it, we will

Table 2.5 Common causes of cough based on duration

Cough classification	Most common causes
Acute: < 3 weeks	• Viral upper respiratory tract infection (URTI) • Exacerbation of underlying lung disorder (chronic obstructive pulmonary disorder, asthma) • Acute environmental exposure to irritant • Acute cardiopulmonary disease (e.g., pneumonia, pulmonary embolism)
Subacute: 3–8 weeks	• Postinfectious cough (URTI < pertussis) • Non-postinfectious cough
Chronic: > 8 weeks	• Active cigarette smoking or chronic irritant use • Angiotensin-converting enzyme inhibitor use • Radiographic apparent disease process of the lung with normal chest radiograph: • Upper airway cough syndrome (chronic cough) • Asthma • Non-asthmatic eosinophilic bronchitis • Gastroesophageal / Laryngopharyngeal reflux

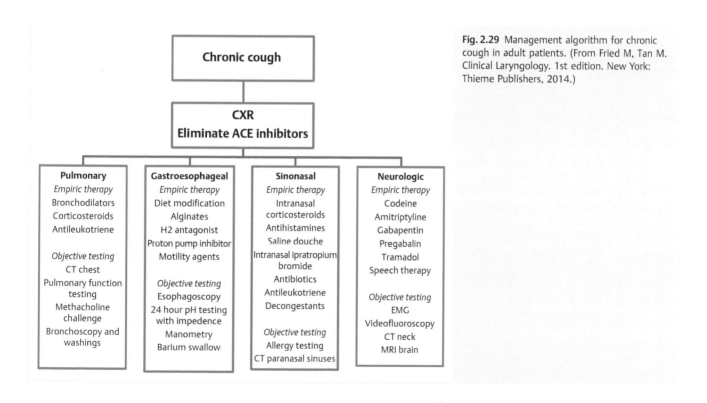

Fig. 2.29 Management algorithm for chronic cough in adult patients. (From Fried M, Tan M. Clinical Laryngology. 1st edition. New York: Thieme Publishers, 2014.)

now move on to a more detailed discussion of the diagnostic procedures that will be used to document the highly variable characteristics of the voice. In particular, our next chapter will review important concepts and terminology used to describe the type and severity of dysphonia that the patient may present with, review key elements of case history examination, and detail some of the practices and issues related to the perceptual description of the voice, whether typical or disordered.

Clinical Case Study: Unilateral Vocal Fold Paralysis

Amy is a 46-year-old female who was referred to the SLP by her otolaryngologist for symptoms of dysphonia. During the evaluation, the patient complained of the following symptoms: a "whispery" voice quality with low volume, low speaking pitch, wheezing when breathing especially after exercise, and vocal fatigue at the end of a working day. The current symptoms occurred suddenly after recent thyroidectomy surgery approximately 2 months prior to the evaluation date. Prior to that surgery, there was no history of voice problems. The following clinical signs were noted by the SLP:

- Inhalatory stridor.
- Reduced breath groups during connected speech (more frequent breaths).
- Consistent breathiness.
- Consistent low speaking intensity.
- Weak cough.
- Speaking fundamental frequency = 175 Hz.
- Cepstral peak in vowel = 5.50 dB; Cepstral peak in speech = 3.25 dB.
- Low/High spectral ratio = 28 dB.
- Physiological frequency range = 12 semitones.
- Vital capacity = 3.5 L.
- Subglottal pressure—comfortable phonation = 15 cm H_2O.
- Phonation threshold pressure = 8 cm H_2O.
- Transglottal airflow—comfortable phonation = 265 mL/s.
- Maximum phonation time = 10 seconds.
- s/z ratio = 1.8 s.

Based on the patient's history, description of the problem, and observed signs, the clinical hypothesis developed by the SLP was vocal fold paralysis or paresis. Subsequent laryngeal endoscopy with videostroboscopy revealed reduced adductory movement in the left vocal fold. This was accompanied by impaired vibratory dynamics (asymmetry, reduced amplitude on left, irregular periodicity, increased mucosal wave on left, midline glottal gap). With effort, the patient could achieve closure, although there was a consistent large posterior gap. The SLP reviewed the videostroboscopic examination with the otolaryngologist, who subsequently diagnosed the patient with UVFP.

2.7 Review Questions

1. Which of the following is a characteristic that differentiates functional from organic voice disorders?
   a) Organic voice disorders can cause exophytic lesions to develop on the vocal folds.
   b) Functional voice disorders include a behavioral hyperfunction.
   c) Functional voice disorders have no known primary etiology that is neurological, structural, or systemic.
   d) Organic voice disorders occur without behavioral hyperfunction.
   e) All of the above.

2. Which of the following is *not* an impaired characteristic of a voice disorder?
   a) Quality.
   b) Dialect.
   c) Loudness.
   d) Flexibility.
   e) None of the above.

3. Which of the following correctly describes a vocal handicap?
   a) The individual cannot adduct one vocal fold completely.
   b) The individual is unable to generate the same amount of loudness.
   c) The individual exhibits a vocal tremor when speaking.
   d) The individual must take time off from work because of voice problems.
   e) Both a and d.

4. Which of the following are etiologies of vocal process granulomas?
   a) Vocal behaviors and laryngopharyngeal reflux.
   b) Intubation and medication.
   c) Medication and vocal behaviors.
   d) Laryngopharyngeal reflux and viral infections.
   e) Both c and d.

5. Why do benign mid-membranous lesions tend to occur and where?
   a) The length of the vocal folds causes the middle to swell first.
   b) That region of the vocal folds experiences the greatest impact stress.
   c) The frequency of vibration is greatest in that region.
   d) It is by random chance.
   e) None of the above.

6. What is the key difference between primary MTD and secondary MTD?
   a) Secondary MTD can result in breathiness and roughness.
   b) Primary MTD is present without structural, neurological, or systemic causes.
   c) Primary MTD is caused by functional hypercontraction of laryngeal muscles.
   d) Secondary MTD can lead to changes in the vocal fold tissue.
   e) All of the above.

7. Why would vocal process granulomas cause pain but not vocal fold nodules?
   a) Impact stress is greater in the posterior region of the vocal folds.
   b) Granulomas can be larger than nodules.
   c) There are pain receptors in the posterior region of the glottis.
   d) Granulomas require surgery, which will result in painful swelling.
   e) All of the above.

8. Endoscopic signs of MTD might include
   a) Supraglottal constriction of the larynx.

b) Anterior laryngeal webbing.
c) Loud voice with low pitch.
d) Glottal insufficiency with one vocal fold failing to adduct.
e) None of the above.

9. Nodules and polyps are thought to develop from phonotrauma that damages what vocal fold layer?
   a) Intermediate lamina propria.
   b) Deep lamina propria.
   c) Vocalis muscle.
   d) Basement membrane zone.
   e) All of the above.

10. Which organic voice disorder is characterized by a tissue bridge at the anterior region of the glottis?
    a) Papilloma.
    b) Unilateral vocal fold paralysis.
    c) Laryngeal web.
    d) Laryngopharyngeal reflux.
    e) None of the above.

11. What theory explains the underlying etiology leading to the development of pseudocysts?
    a) There is a viral infection isolated to the larynx.
    b) There is an underlying vocal fold paresis.
    c) There is a bacterial infection throughout the body.
    d) There is an endocrine disorder causing a hormonal imbalance.
    e) Both a and c.

12. What theory explains the development of a vocal fold epidermoid cyst?
    a) There is blockage of a mucous gland duct.
    b) There is viral infection isolated to the vocal fold lamina propria.
    c) There is a trapped epithelial cell in the vocal fold lamina propria.
    d) There is arthritis in the cricoarytenoid joint.
    e) All of the above.

13. What is believed to be the cause of laryngeal papillomatosis?
    a) Human papilloma virus.
    b) Bacterial infection leading to tissue change.
    c) Vocal fold paralysis.
    d) Phonotrauma.
    e) None of the above.

14. A difference between vocal fold nodules and polyps is_____.
    a) Polyps occur at the mid-membranous region.
    b) Nodules are due to phonotrauma.
    c) Polyps occur in males and females.
    d) Nodules are typically bilateral.
    e) All of the above.

15. Symptoms of adductor spasmodic dysphonia become more severe on what type of stimuli?
    a) Unvoiced sounds.
    b) Voiced sounds.
    c) Phrases.
    d) Sentences.
    e) None of the above.

16. Which of the following correctly describes the impairment of paradoxical vocal fold motion?
    a) Involuntary vocal fold abduction during exhalation.
    b) Increased muscle tone causing rigidity at rest and during phonation.

c) Involuntary vocal fold adduction during inspiration.
d) Adduction occurs at the onset of phonation.

17. Which of the following vocal tasks often perceptually reveals a vocal tremor best?
    a) Sustained vowel.
    b) Rapid breathing cycles.
    c) Reading the rainbow passage.
    d) Reading CAPE-V sentences.
    e) All of the above.

18. Perceptual characteristics of presbylaryngis include
    a) Excessive loudness and low pitch.
    b) Rough voice quality with tremor.
    c) Voice breaks with hoarse voice.
    d) Reduced loudness and breathy voice.
    e) None of the above.

19. Incomplete maturation of the laryngeal cartilages at birth can cause a condition known as
    a) Laryngocele.
    b) Laryngomalacia.
    c) Osteoarthritis.
    d) Papillomatosis.
    e) All of the above.

20. Why is laryngopharyngeal reflux most likely to irritate the posterior larynx than the anterior larynx?
    a) The upper esophageal sphincter is located behind the posterior larynx.
    b) Reflux migrates from the anterior larynx to the posterior larynx.
    c) Tissue in the posterior larynx is different from that of the anterior larynx.
    d) There are more sensory receptors in the posterior larynx.
    e) Both b and c.

2.8 Answers and Explanations

1. Correct: Functional voice disorders have no known primary etiology that is neurological, structural, or systemic. (**c**).
   (**c**) A primary difference between functional and organic voice disorders is that functional disorders are caused by behaviors, while organic disorders are not. Organic disorders are caused by neurological, structural, or systemic conditions. (**a. b**) Both functional and organic disorders can result in exophytic lesions. (**d**) Organic voice disorders can result in compensatory functional compensation, although the primary disorder remains organic.

2. Correct: Dialect (**b**).
   (**b**) Dialect is a linguistic or articulatory attribute, not a vocal attribute. (**a**) Voice quality includes perceptual characteristics of the voice and serves as an essential characteristic of voice perception. (**c**) Vocal loudness refers to the perception of vocal intensity and is often impaired in disorders of hypofunction. (**d**) Vocal flexibility can refer to the physiological frequency range or the characteristics of vocal intonation.

3. Correct: The individual must take time off from work because of voice problems (**d**).
   (**d**) A handicap is a restriction in life activities—an individual who has to take time off work due to a voice problem would meet this definition. (**a, b, c**) The inability to adduct the vocal folds, generate vocal loudness, or the presence of a vocal tremor are physiological impairments. These may or may not

lead to a disability and resulting handicap, but by themselves do not meet the definition of a handicap.

4. Correct: Vocal behaviors and laryngopharyngeal reflux (**a**).
(**a**) Vocal process granulomas can be caused by multiple actors, including vocal behaviors, reflux, and intubation trauma. (**b, c, d**) While intubation trauma can cause the formation of granulomas, medications do not. Viral infections are not known to cause vocal process granulomas.

5. Correct: That region of the vocal folds experiences the greatest impact stress (**b**).
(**b**) During oscillation, the mid-membranous region of the vocal folds experience the greatest amount of impact stress due to the physical properties of the vocal fold tissue and physical forces influencing their oscillation. Early swelling after heavy vocal use tends to occur in this region, as do *benign lesions such as nodules, polyps, and cysts.* (**a**) Vocal fold length has no bearing on the development of mid-membranous lesions—they occur in long and short vocal folds. (**c**) The entire length of a vocal fold typically vibrates at the same frequency. (**d**) The reason why mid-membranous lesions occur where they do is because of impact stress at that location, not random chance.

6. Correct: Primary MTD is present without structural, neurological, or systemic causes (**b**).
(**b**) Primary MTD is the presence of dysphonia without an accompanying organic condition. It is due to functional behaviors that persist over time, and does not develop secondary to some other condition. (**a**) Breathiness and roughness can be a characteristic of either primary or secondary MTD. (**c**) Functional hypercontraction of the laryngeal muscles is the underlying physiological impairment of both primary and secondary MTD. (**d**) Primary and secondary MTD can both lead to a change in the vocal fold tissue —for example, vocal fold nodules.

7. Correct: There are pain receptors in the posterior region of the glottis (**c**).
(**c**) Pain receptors within the larynx at the level of the vocal folds are located primarily in the posterior glottal region, at the region of the vocal processes and interarytenoid space. The lack of pain receptors on the vocal fold tissue explains why we do not feel pain when they collide during phonation. (**a**) Impact stress is greatest at the mid-membranous portion of the vocal folds. (**b**) Granulomas can take on varied appearances, from very small to very large. They are not always larger than nodules. (**d**) Treatment for granulomas should always start conservatively, requiring surgery only after many months of voice therapy and antireflux medication.

8. Correct: Supraglottal constriction of the larynx (**a**).
(**a**) MTD is characterized by hypercontraction of laryngeal muscles. This can include the ventricular muscles, which are extensions of the thyroarytenoid. This will cause the false vocal folds (the ventricular folds) to move medially and constrict or narrow the larynx. (**b**) Laryngeal webs are organic disorders, not functional. (**c**) A loud voice with a low pitch is not necessarily a sign of muscle tension dysphonia—it can be a habitual voice pattern of a speaker. (**d**) Glottal

insufficiency secondary to MTD would be characterized by both vocal folds failing to completely adduct the glottis.

9. Correct: Basement membrane zone (**d**).
(**d**) The basement membrane zone lies immediately beneath the vocal fold epithelium, and contains fibers that connect the epithelium to the superficial layer of the lamina propria. Damage to these connections, and the repair process that follows, is thought to lead to the development of vocal nodules secondary to chronic phonotrauma. (**a**) The intermediate layer of the lamina propria is part of the vocal ligament, and is not involved in vocal fold nodules. (**b**) The deep lamina propria is part of the vocal ligament, and is not involved in vocal fold nodules. (**c**) The vocalis muscle is part of the vocal fold body, and is not involved in vocal fold nodules.

10. Correct: Laryngeal web (**c**).
(**c**) Laryngeal webs are characterized by tissue of the left and right vocal folds attached, or bridged, together. Most often this occurs at the anterior commissure and anterior regions of the vocal fold tissue. (**a**) Papilloma can occur anywhere along the length of the vocal folds, and can also occur at other locations within the airway. (**b**) Unilateral vocal fold paralysis is characterized by the inability of one vocal fold to adduct or abduct. (**d**) Laryngopharyngeal reflux influences the posterior region before affecting anterior regions.

11. Correct: There is an underlying vocal fold paresis (**b**).
(**b**) Pseudocysts appear as blister-like exophytic lesions at the mid-membranous region of the vocal folds. Contemporary theory links their formation to an underlying paresis, which results in compensatory phonotrauma leading to the appearance of an edematous cyst-like lesion. (**a**) Viral infections typically lead to different degrees of laryngitis, although they can cause coughing and throat clearing leading to vocal fold edema. (**c**) Bacterial infections most often cause forms of laryngitis. (**d**) Endocrine disorders can cause generalized edema and erythema throughout the larynx, but are not related to the formation of pseudocysts.

12. Correct: There is a trapped epithelial cell in the vocal fold lamina propria (**c**).
(**c**) Throughout the day, the vocal fold epithelium continually replaces cells. Old cells are typically shed off and swallowed or cleared via secretions and saliva. If a cell becomes trapped within the epithelium, it is thought the cellular response can lead to formation of a cyst, entrapping the old epithelial cell. (**a**) Cysts that form secondary to a mucous gland duct blockage are referred to as mucous retention cysts. (**b**) Systemic laryngeal infections typically affect the entire laryngeal region, and are not isolated to the lamina propria. (**d**) Arthritis would inhibit movement of laryngeal cartilages at the joints, but are not related to cyst formation.

13. Correct: Human papilloma virus (**a**).
(**a**) Laryngeal papillomatosis is associated with a number of different human papilloma virus (HPV) subtypes but most frequently HPV 6 and HPV 11, which are believed to be passed to a child from the mother at birth or at any other time by human-to-human contact. (**b**) Bacterial infections result in laryngeal edema and erythema but are not associated

with the formation of papillomatosis. (**c**) Vocal fold paralysis causes the inability of one or both vocal folds to abduct or adduct. (**d**) Phonotrauma can result in exophytic lesions such as nodules and polyps, but not papillomatosis.

14. Correct: Nodules are typically bilateral (**d**).

(**d**) Vocal fold nodules are symmetrical or quasi-symmetrical bilateral lesions which can vary in size and shape depending on their stage of development and the patient's voice use patterns. (**a**) Both polyps and nodules occur at the mid-membranous portion of the vocal folds. (**b**) Both nodules and polyps occur secondary to phonotrauma. (**c**) Both nodules and polyps occur in males and females.

15. Correct: Voiced sounds (**b**).

(**b**) The process of differential diagnosis for SD can be informed by evidence from task-specific vocalizations. Speakers with ADSD also tend to be more dysphonic on stimuli loaded with voiced sounds compared to stimuli loaded with unvoiced sounds. (**a**) Unlike speakers with MTD, speakers with SD tend to have less difficulty with unvoiced sounds compared to voiced sounds. (**c**) Regardless of phrase length, speakers with SD will have more dysphonic moments on voiced sounds than unvoiced sounds. (**d**) Speakers with SD will have equal difficulty on words, **phrases**, or sentences when they are loaded with voiced sounds.

16. Correct: Involuntary vocal fold adduction during inspiration (**c**).

(**c**) Paradoxical vocal fold movement (PVFM) is characterized by transient but repetitive episodes of inappropriate and involuntary adduction of the vocal folds during inspiration. This has the effect of narrowing the airway and causing dyspnea, and can result in compensatory hyperfunction in the laryngeal and respiratory muscles that cause expiration to be labored and rushed with a negative impact on phonation. (**a**) PVFM is most evident during inhalation, not exhalation. (**b**) Muscular rigidity is a feature of hypokinetic dysarthria (e.g., Parkinson's disease) rather than PVFM. (**d**) Adduction normally occurs during phonation—in PVFM, the problem is adduction during inspiration.

17. Correct: Sustained vowel (**a**).

(**a**) Vocal tremor, especially when mild, is best perceived when a patient produces a sustained vowel. Because healthy phonation is typically stable during sustaining vowels, the rhythmic nature of the tremor will stand out during these productions. (**b**) Rapid breathing, without attempts at phonation, will do little to help distinguish whether or not a speaker has vocal tremor. (**c**) The rainbow passage consists of sentences produced in connected speech. Severe tremor might be elucidated when reading this, but mild vocal tremor can be difficult to discern in connected speech. (**d**) Like the rainbow passage, vocal tremor can be difficult to discern in connected speech, such as when reading the CAPE-V sentences, especially when tremor is mild.

18. Correct: Reduced loudness and breathy voice (**d**).

(**d**) Breathiness and reduced loudness are the most salient perceptual characteristics of presbylaryngis and are the basis for describing this condition by its other name, presbyphonia. (**a**) Excessive loudness and low pitch may or may not be associated with a voice disorders, although they are not typically features of presbylaryngis. (**b**) Rough voice quality and tremor are more characteristic of vocal tremor rather than presbylaryngis. (**c**) Voice breaks are typically not a feature of presbylaryngis, although they are common in spasmodic dysphonia.

19. Correct: Laryngomalacia (**b**).

(**b**) Laryngomalacia is a congenital condition caused by incomplete maturation of the cartilaginous framework of the larynx. It is one of the most common causes of inhalatory stridor in infants. The condition affects the rigidity of the laryngeal cartilages, resulting in abnormal pliability and positioning of cartilages that can obstruct the airway. (**a**) A laryngocele is an air sac within the larynx, often visible as a protrusion in the region of the laryngeal ventricle. (**c**) Osteoarthritis will affect the laryngeal joints and typically associated with laryngeal aging. (**d**) Papillomatosis results in wart-like clusters of exophytic lesions. These are due to viral infection, not congenital malformation.

20. Correct: The upper esophageal sphincter is located behind the posterior larynx (**a**).

(**a**) Reflux consists of stomach contents which migrate upward through the esophagus. The superior opening of the esophagus is the upper esophageal sphincter, which sits immediately behind the posterior region of the larynx. (**b**) If reflux material migrates within the larynx, it would move from a posterior location to an anterior location. (**c**) Tissue in the posterior and anterior larynx is similar, although the vocal fold tissue is a different type of epithelium than that of other laryngeal regions. (**d**) There are more sensory receptors in the posterior laryngeal regions, although this does not explain why reflux irritates and damages posterior tissue more than anterior tissue.

References

[1] Anders LC, Hollien H, Hurme P, Sonninen A, Wendler J. Perception of hoarseness by several classes of listeners. Folia Phoniatr (Basel). 1988; 40 (2):91–100

[2] Fex S. Perceptual evaluation. J Voice. 1992; 6(2):155–158

[3] Awan SN. The Voice Diagnostic Protocol. Gaithersburg, MD: Aspen; 2001

[4] Aronson AE, Bless DM. Clinical Voice Disorders. New York: Thieme; 2009

[5] Higgins MB, Chait DH, Schulte L. Phonatory air flow characteristics of adductor spasmodic dysphonia and muscle tension dysphonia. J Speech Lang Hear Res. 1999; 42(1):101–111

[6] Cohen SM. Self-reported impact of dysphonia in a primary care population: an epidemiological study. Laryngoscope. 2010; 120(10):2022–2032

[7] Cohen SM, Kim J, Roy N, Asche C, Courey M. Prevalence and causes of dysphonia in a large treatment-seeking population. Laryngoscope. 2012; 122 (2):343–348

[8] Roy N, Merrill RM, Thibeault S, Gray SD, Smith EM. Voice disorders in teachers and the general population: effects on work performance, attendance, and future career choices. J Speech Lang Hear Res. 2004; 47(5):542–551

[9] Watts CR. The prevalence of voice problems in a sample of collegiate a cappella singers. J Speech Path Ther. 2016; 1:105

[10] World Health Organization. International Classification of Impairments, Disabilities, and Handicaps - A Manual of Classification Relating to the Consequences of Disease. Geneva: WHO; 1980

[11] Brodnitz FS. Rehabilitation of the human voice. Bull N Y Acad Med. 1966; 42 (3):231–240

[12] Brodnitz FS. Vocal Rehabilitation: A Manual Prepared for the Use of Graduates in Medicine. Rochester, MN: American Academy of Ophthalmology and Otolaryngology; 1971

[13] Roy N. Functional dysphonia. Curr Opin Otolaryngol Head Neck Surg. 2003; 11(3):144–148

[14] Jürgens U. The role of the periaqueductal grey in vocal behaviour. Behav Brain Res. 1994; 62(2):107–117

[15] Aronson AE. Importance of the psychosocial interview in the diagnosis and treatment of "functional" voice disorders. J Voice. 1990; 4(4):287–289

[16] Hillman RE, Holmberg EB, Perkell JS, Walsh M, Vaughan C. Objective assessment of vocal hyperfunction: an experimental framework and initial results. J Speech Hear Res. 1989; 32(2):373–392

[17] Cohen SM, Kim J, Roy N, Wilk A, Thomas S, Courey M. Change in diagnosis and treatment following specialty voice evaluation: a national database analysis. Laryngoscope. 2015; 125(7):1660–1666

[18] Coyle SM, Weinrich BD, Stemple JC. Shifts in relative prevalence of laryngeal pathology in a treatment-seeking population. J Voice. 2001; 15(3):424–440

[19] Herrington-Hall BL, Lee L, Stemple JC, Niemi KR, McHone MM. Description of laryngeal pathologies by age, sex, and occupation in a treatment-seeking sample. J Speech Hear Disord. 1988; 53(1):57–64

[20] Morrison MD, Rammage LA. Muscle misuse voice disorders: description and classification. Acta Otolaryngol. 1993; 113(3):428–434

[21] Roy N, Ford CN, Bless DM. Muscle tension dysphonia and spasmodic dysphonia: the role of manual laryngeal tension reduction in diagnosis and management. Ann Otol Rhinol Laryngol. 1996; 105(11):851–856

[22] Roy N, Bless DM. Toward a theory of the dispositional bases of functional dysphonia and vocal nodules: exploring the role of personality and emotional adjustment. In: Kent R, Ball M, eds. Handbook of Voice Quality Measurement. San Diego, CA: Singular Publishing Group; 1999

[23] Kang CH, Hentz JG, Lott DG. Muscle tension dysphagia: symptomology and theoretical framework. Otolaryngol Head Neck Surg. 2016; 155(5):837–842

[24] Kapsner-Smith MR, Hunter EJ, Kirkham K, Cox K, Titze IR. A randomized controlled trial of two semi-occluded vocal tract voice therapy protocols. J Speech Lang Hear Res. 2015; 58(3):535–549

[25] Roy N, Gray SD, Simon M, Dove H, Corbin-Lewis K, Stemple JC. An evaluation of the effects of two treatment approaches for teachers with voice disorders: a prospective randomized clinical trial. J Speech Lang Hear Res. 2001; 44(2):286–296

[26] Roy N, Weinrich B, Gray SD, Tanner K, Stemple JC, Sapienza CM. Three treatments for teachers with voice disorders: a randomized clinical trial. J Speech Lang Hear Res. 2003; 46(3):670–688

[27] Roy N. Assessment and treatment of musculoskeletal tension in hyperfunctional voice disorders. Int J Speech-Language Pathol. 2008; 10(4):195–209

[28] Watts CR, Diviney SS, Hamilton A, Toles L, Childs L, Mau T. The effect of stretch-and-flow voice therapy on measures of vocal function and handicap. J Voice. 2015; 29(2):191–199

[29] Watts CR, Hamilton A, Toles L, Childs L, Mau T. A randomized controlled trial of stretch-and-flow voice therapy for muscle tension dysphonia. Laryngoscope. 2015; 125(6):1420–1425

[30] Dietrich M, Verdolini Abbott K. Vocal function in introverts and extraverts during a psychological stress reactivity protocol. J Speech Lang Hear Res. 2012; 55(3):973–987

[31] Boone DR, McFarlane SC, Von Berg SL, Zraick RI. The Voice and Voice Therapy. 9th ed. Boston, MA: Pearson; 2014

[32] Dworkin J, Meleca R. Vocal Pathologies: Diagnosis, Treatment, and Case Studies. San Diego, CA: Singular Publishing; 1997

[33] Prater RJ, Miller J, Deem JF, Swift RW. Manual of Voice Therapy. 2nd ed. Austin, TX: Pro-Ed; 1999

[34] Dietrich M, Verdolini Abbott K, Gartner-Schmidt J, Rosen CA. The frequency of perceived stress, anxiety, and depression in patients with common pathologies affecting voice. J Voice. 2008; 22(4):472–488

[35] Verdolini K, Rosen CA, Branski RC. Classification Manual for Voice Disorders - I. Mahwah, NJ: Lawrence Erlbaum; 2006

[36] Ruotsalainen JH, Sellman J, Lehto L, Jauhiainen M, Verbeek JH. Interventions for treating functional dysphonia in adults. Cochrane Database Syst Rev. 2007(3):CD006373

[37] Dagli M, Sati I, Acar A, Stone RE, Jr, Dursun G, Eryilmaz A. Mutational falsetto: intervention outcomes in 45 patients. J Laryngol Otol. 2008; 122(3):277–281

[38] Titze IR. Mechanical stress in phonation. J Voice. 1994; 8(2):99–105

[39] Branski RC, Verdolini K, Sandulache V, Rosen CA, Hebda PA. Vocal fold wound healing: a review for clinicians. J Voice. 2006; 20(3):432–442

[40] Thibeault SL, Rousseau B, Welham NV, Hirano S, Bless DM. Hyaluronan levels in acute vocal fold scar. Laryngoscope. 2004; 114(4):760–764

[41] Gray SD, Pignatari SS, Harding P. Morphologic ultrastructure of anchoring fibers in normal vocal fold basement membrane zone. J Voice. 1994; 8(1):48–52

[42] Courey MS, Shohet JA, Scott MA, Ossoff RH. Immunohistochemical characterization of benign laryngeal lesions. Ann Otol Rhinol Laryngol. 1996; 105(7):525–531

[43] Nunes RB, Belilau M, Nunes MB, Paulino JG. Clinical diagnosis and histological analysis of vocal nodules and polyps. Rev Bras Otorrinolaringol (Engl Ed). 2013; 79(4):434–440

[44] Dikkers FG, Nikkels PG. Lamina propria of the mucosa of benign lesions of the vocal folds. Laryngoscope. 1999; 109(10):1684–1689

[45] Gray SD, Hammond E, Hanson DF. Benign pathologic responses of the larynx. Ann Otol Rhinol Laryngol. 1995; 104(1):13–18

[46] Butler JE, Hammond TH, Gray SD. Gender-related differences of hyaluronic acid distribution in the human vocal fold. Laryngoscope. 2001; 111(5):907–911

[47] Martins RH, Defaveri J, Domingues MA, de Albuquerque e Silva R. Vocal polyps: clinical, morphological, and immunohistochemical aspects. J Voice. 2011; 25(1):98–106

[48] Thomas JP. Why Is There a Frog In My Throat? Portland, OR: James P. Thomas; 2012

[49] Kendall KA, Leonard RJ. Laryngeal Evaluation: Indirect Laryngoscopy to High-Speed Digital Imaging. New York: Thieme Medical Publishers; 2010

[50] Akbulut S, Gartner-Schmidt JL, Gillespie AI, Young VN, Smith LJ, Rosen CA. Voice outcomes following treatment of benign midmembranous vocal fold lesions using a nomenclature paradigm. Laryngoscope. 2016

[51] Estes C, Sulica L. Vocal fold pseudocyst: a prospective study of surgical outcomes. Laryngoscope. 2015; 125(4):913–918

[52] Koufman JA, Belafsky PC. Unilateral or localized Reinke's edema (pseudocyst) as a manifestation of vocal fold paresis: the paresis podule. Laryngoscope. 2001; 111(4, Pt 1):576–580

[53] Rosen CA, Gartner-Schmidt J, Hathaway B, et al. A nomenclature paradigm for benign midmembranous vocal fold lesions. Laryngoscope. 2012; 122(6):1335–1341

[54] Choudhury N, Ghufoor K. Benign lesions of the larynx. In: Kirtane MV, de Souza CE, Bhattacharyya AK, Nerurkar NK, eds. Laryngology. New York: Thieme Medical Publishers; 2014

[55] Zeitels SM. Benign lesions of the vocal folds. In: Fried M, Tan M, eds. Clinical Laryngology. New York: Thieme Medical Publishers; 2015

[56] Lemos EM, Sennes LU, Imamura R, Tsuji DH. Vocal process granuloma: clinical characterization, treatment and evolution. Rev Bras Otorrinolaringol (Engl Ed). 2005; 71(4):494–498

[57] Shin T, Watanabe H, Oda M, Umezaki T, Nahm I. Contact granulomas of the larynx. Eur Arch Otorhinolaryngol. 1994; 251(2):67–71

[58] Havas TE, Priestley J, Lowinger DS. A management strategy for vocal process granulomas. Laryngoscope. 1999; 109(2, Pt 1):301–306

[59] Berzofsky C, Pitman MJ. Laryngeal inflammation. In: Fried MP, Tan M, eds. Clinical Laryngology. New York: Thieme Medical Publishers; 2015

[60] Vinson KN, Garrett GC. Microanatomy and cellular physiology. In: Kirtane MV, de Souza CE, Bhattacharyya AK, Nerurkar NK, eds. Laryngology. New York: Thieme Medical Publishers; 2014

[61] Koszewski IJ, Hoffman MR, Young WG, Lai YT, Dailey SH. Office-based photoangiolytic laser treatment of Reinke's edema: safety and voice outcomes. Otolaryngol Head Neck Surg. 2015; 152(6):1075–1081

[62] Sataloff RT. Clinical Assessment of Voice. San Diego: Plural Publishing; 2005

[63] Van Houtte E, Van Lierde K, D'Haeseleer E, Claeys S. The prevalence of laryngeal pathology in a treatment-seeking population with dysphonia. Laryngoscope. 2010; 120(2):306–312

[64] Bhattacharyya AK, Stimpson P, Purushotan S. Vocal fold paralysis. In: Kirtane MV, de Souza CE, Bhattacharyya AK, Nerurkar NK, eds. Laryngology. New York: Thieme Medical Publishers; 2014

[65] Stemple JC, Glaze L, Klaben B. The Voice and Voice Therapy. 4th ed. San Diego: Plural Publishing; 2010

[66] Vinson KN, Zraick RI, Ragland FJ. Injection versus medialization laryngoplasty for the treatment of unilateral vocal fold paralysis: follow-up at six months. Laryngoscope. 2010; 120(9):1802–1807

[67] Mattioli F, Bergamini G, Alicandri-Ciufelli M, et al. The role of early voice therapy in the incidence of motility recovery in unilateral vocal fold paralysis. Logoped Phoniatr Vocol. 2011; 36(1):40–47

[68] Mattioli F, Menichetti M, Bergamini G, et al. Results of early versus intermediate or delayed voice therapy in patients with unilateral vocal fold paralysis: our experience in 171 patients. J Voice. 2015; 29(4):455–458

[69] Busto-Crespo O, Uzcanga-Lacabe M, Abad-Marco A, et al. Longitudinal voice outcomes after voice therapy in unilateral vocal fold paralysis. J Voice. 2016; 30(6):767.e9–767.e15

[70] D'Alatri L, Galla S, Rigante M, Antonelli O, Buldrini S, Marchese MR. Role of early voice therapy in patients affected by unilateral vocal fold paralysis. J Laryngol Otol. 2008; 122(9):936–941

[71] El-Banna M, Youssef G. Early voice therapy in patients with unilateral vocal fold paralysis. Folia Phoniatr Logop. 2014; 66(6):237–243

[72] Schindler A, Bottero A, Capaccio P, Ginocchio D, Adorni F, Ottaviani F. Vocal improvement after voice therapy in unilateral vocal fold paralysis. J Voice. 2008; 22(1):113–118

[73] Blitzer A. Spasmodic dysphonia and botulinum toxin: experience from the largest treatment series. Eur J Neurol. 2010; 17 Suppl 1:28–30

[74] Simonyan K, Berman BD, Herscovitch P, Hallett M. Abnormal striatal dopaminergic neurotransmission during rest and task production in spasmodic dysphonia. J Neurosci. 2013; 33(37):14705–14714

[75] Stamelou M, Edwards MJ, Hallett M, Bhatia KP. The non-motor syndrome of primary dystonia: clinical and pathophysiological implications. Brain. 2012; 135(Pt 6):1668–1681

[76] Cannito MP, Burch AR, Watts C, Rappold PW, Hood SB, Sherrard K. Disfluency in spasmodic dysphonia: a multivariate analysis. J Speech Lang Hear Res. 1997; 40(3):627–641

[77] Cannito MP, Woodson GE, Murry T, Bender B. Perceptual analyses of spasmodic dysphonia before and after treatment. Arch Otolaryngol Head Neck Surg. 2004; 130(12):1393–1399

[78] Roy N, Gouse M, Mauszycki SC, Merrill RM, Smith ME. Task specificity in adductor spasmodic dysphonia versus muscle tension dysphonia. Laryngoscope. 2005; 115(2):311–316

[79] Roy N. Differential diagnosis of muscle tension dysphonia and spasmodic dysphonia. Curr Opin Otolaryngol Head Neck Surg. 2010; 18(3):165–170

[80] Murry T, Woodson GE. Combined-modality treatment of adductor spasmodic dysphonia with botulinum toxin and voice therapy. J Voice. 1995; 9 (4):460–465

[81] Silverman EP, Garvan C, Shrivastav R, Sapienza CM. Combined modality treatment of adductor spasmodic dysphonia. J Voice. 2012; 26(1):77–86

[82] Sulica L, Louis ED. Clinical characteristics of essential voice tremor: a study of 34 cases. Laryngoscope. 2010; 120(3):516–528

[83] Filip P, Lungu OV, Manto MU, Bareš M. Linking essential tremor to the cerebellum: physiological evidence. Cerebellum. 2016; 15(6):774–780

[84] Sinclair CF, Gurey LE, Blitzer A. Neurological and neuromuscular diseases of the larynx. In: Fried MP, Tan M, eds. Clinical Laryngology. New York: Thieme Medical Publishers; 2015

[85] Darley FL, Aronson AE, Brown JR. Differential diagnostic patterns of dysarthria. J Speech Hear Res. 1969; 12(2):246–269

[86] Braak H, Del Tredici K. Invited Article: Nervous system pathology in sporadic Parkinson disease. Neurology. 2008; 70(20):1916–1925

[87] Del Tredici K, Braak H. Lewy pathology and neurodegeneration in premotor Parkinson's disease. Mov Disord. 2012; 27(5):597–607

[88] Sapir S. Multiple factors are involved in the dysarthria associated with Parkinson's disease: a review with implications for clinical practice and research. J Speech Lang Hear Res. 2014; 57(4):1330–1343

[89] Blumin JH, Pcolinsky DE, Atkins JP. Laryngeal findings in advanced Parkinson's disease. Ann Otol Rhinol Laryngol. 2004; 113(4):253–258

[90] Baker KK, Ramig LO, Luschei ES, Smith ME. Thyroarytenoid muscle activity associated with hypophonia in Parkinson disease and aging. Neurology. 1998; 51(6):1592–1598

[91] Zarzur AP, Duprat AC, Shinzato G, Eckley CA. Laryngeal electromyography in adults with Parkinson's disease and voice complaints. Laryngoscope. 2007; 117(5):831–834

[92] Belafsky PC, Postma GN. Vocal fold augmentation with calcium hydroxylapatite. Otolaryngol Head Neck Surg. 2004; 131(4):351–354

[93] Watts CR. A retrospective study of long-term treatment outcomes for reduced vocal intensity in hypokinetic dysarthria. BMC Ear Nose Throat Disord. 2016; 16:2

[94] Mahler LA, Ramig LO, Fox C. Evidence-based treatment of voice and speech disorders in Parkinson disease. Curr Opin Otolaryngol Head Neck Surg. 2015; 23(3):209–215

[95] Levitt JA. Case study: the effects of the "SPEAK OUT! ®" Voice Program for Parkinson's disease. Int J Appl Sci Technol. 2014; 4(2):20–28

[96] Ahmed J, Ghufoor K. Premalignant lesions of the larynx. In: Kirtane MV, de Souza CE, Bhattacharyya AK, Nerurkar NK, eds. Laryngology. New York: Thieme Medical Publishers; 2014

[97] Karatayli-Ozgursoy S, Pacheco-Lopez P, Hillel AT, Best SR, Bishop JA, Akst LM. Laryngeal dysplasia, demographics, and treatment: a single-institution, 20-year review. JAMA Otolaryngol Head Neck Surg. 2015; 141 (4):313–318

[98] Weller MD, Nankivell PC, McConkey C, Paleri V, Mehanna HM. The risk and interval to malignancy of patients with laryngeal dysplasia; a systematic review of case series and meta-analysis. Clin Otolaryngol. 2010; 35(5):364–372

[99] Isenberg JS, Crozier DL, Dailey SH. Institutional and comprehensive review of laryngeal leukoplakia. Ann Otol Rhinol Laryngol. 2008; 117(1):74–79

[100] Siegel RL, Miller KD, Jemal A. Cancer statistics, 2015. CA Cancer J Clin. 2015; 65(1):5–29

[101] English GM. Malignant Neoplasms of the Larynx. New York: Harper & Row; 1976

[102] O'Rourke A, Postma GN. Laryngopharyngeal reflux. In: Fried M, Tan M, eds. Clinical Laryngology. New York: Thieme Medical Publishers; 2015

[103] Baken RJ. The aged voice: a new hypothesis. J Voice. 2005; 19(3):317–325

[104] Roy N, Stemple J, Merrill RM, Thomas L. Epidemiology of voice disorders in the elderly: preliminary findings. Laryngoscope. 2007; 117(4):628–633

[105] Lagorio LA, Carnaby-Mann GD, Crary MA. Treatment of vocal fold bowing using neuromuscular electrical stimulation. Arch Otolaryngol Head Neck Surg. 2010; 136(4):398–403

[106] Ramig LO, Gray S, Baker K, et al. The aging voice: a review, treatment data and familial and genetic perspectives. Folia Phoniatr Logop. 2001; 53(5):252–265

[107] Sauder C, Roy N, Tanner K, Houtz DR, Smith ME. Vocal function exercises for presbylaryngis: a multidimensional assessment of treatment outcomes. Ann Otol Rhinol Laryngol. 2010; 119(7):460–467

[108] Ziegler A, Verdolini Abbott K, Johns M, Klein A, Hapner ER. Preliminary data on two voice therapy interventions in the treatment of presbyphonia. Laryngoscope. 2014; 124(8):1869–1876

[109] Benninger MS, Hanick AL, Nowacki AS. Augmentation autologous adipose injections in the larynx. Ann Otol Rhinol Laryngol. 2016; 125(1):25–30

[110] Davids T, Muller S, Wise JC, Johns MM, III, Klein A. Laryngeal papillomatosis associated dysplasia in the adult population: an update on prevalence and HPV subtyping. Ann Otol Rhinol Laryngol. 2014; 123(6):402–408

[111] Patel SA, Merati AL. Benign tumors of the larynx. In: Fried M, Tan M, eds. Clinical Laryngology. New York: Thieme Medical Publishers; 2015

[112] Shi ZP, Wang CH, Lee JC, Lin YS. Cidofovir injection for recurrent laryngeal papillomatosis. J Chin Med Assoc. 2008; 71(3):143–146

[113] Galván CA, Guarderas JC. Practical considerations for dysphonia caused by inhaled corticosteroids. Mayo Clin Proc. 2012; 87(9):901–904

[114] Abaza MM, Levy S, Hawkshaw MJ, Sataloff RT. Effects of medications on the voice. Otolaryngol Clin North Am. 2007; 40(5):1081–1090, viii

[115] Hartnick C, Setlur J. Pediatric laryngology. In: Fried M, Tan M, eds. Clinical Laryngology. New York: Thieme Medical Publishers; 2015

[116] Rousseau B, Hirano S, Chan RW, et al. Characterization of chronic vocal fold scarring in a rabbit model. J Voice. 2004; 18(1):116–124

[117] Carroll LM. Voice therapy. In: Fried M, Tan M, eds. Clinical Laryngology. New York: Thieme Medical Publishers; 2015

[118] Ford CN, Inagi K, Khidr A, Bless DM, Gilchrist KW. Sulcus vocalis: a rational analytical approach to diagnosis and management. Ann Otol Rhinol Laryngol. 1996; 105(3):189–200

[119] Giovanni A, Chanteret C, Lagier A. Sulcus vocalis: a review. Eur Arch Otorhinolaryngol. 2007; 264(4):337–344

[120] Vertigan AE, Theodoros DG, Gibson PG, Winkworth AL. The relationship between chronic cough and paradoxical vocal fold movement: a review of the literature. J Voice. 2006; 20(3):466–480

[121] Ludlow CL. Central nervous system control of the laryngeal muscles in humans. Respir Physiol Neurobiol. 2005; 147(2–3):205–222

[122] Sugumaran M, Altman KW. Cough and the unified airway. In: Fried M, Tan M, eds. Clinical Laryngology. New York: Thieme Medical Publishers; 2015

[123] Bellanti JA, Tutuncuoglu SO, Azem M, MacDowell-Carneiro AL, Wallerstedt DB. Persistent cough: differential diagnosis. Allergy Asthma Proc. 2000; 21 (5):307–308

[124] Hartley NA, Petty BE, Johnson B, Thibeault SL. Comparative analysis of clinical profile: chronic cough vs paradoxical vocal fold motion. Respir Med. 2015; 109(12):1516–1520

[125] Vertigan AE, Gibson PG. The role of speech pathology in the management of patients with chronic refractory cough. Lung. 2012; 190(1):35–40

Suggested Readings

[1] Baken RJ. The aged voice: a new hypothesis. J Voice. 2005; 19(3):317–325

[2] Blitzer A. Spasmodic dysphonia and botulinum toxin: experience from the largest treatment series. Eur J Neurol. 2010; 17 Suppl 1:28–30

[3] Branski RC, Verdolini K, Sandulache V, Rosen CA, Hebda PA. Vocal fold wound healing: a review for clinicians. J Voice. 2006; 20(3):432–442

[4] Cohen SM, Kim J, Roy N, Asche C, Courey M. Prevalence and causes of dysphonia in a large treatment-seeking population. Laryngoscope. 2012; 122 (2):343–348

[5] Dietrich M, Verdolini Abbott K, Gartner-Schmidt J, Rosen CA. The frequency of perceived stress, anxiety, and depression in patients with common pathologies affecting voice. J Voice. 2008; 22(4):472–488

[6] Gray SD, Hammond E, Hanson DF. Benign pathologic responses of the larynx. Ann Otol Rhinol Laryngol. 1995; 104(1):13–18

[7] Hillman RE, Holmberg EB, Perkell JS, Walsh M, Vaughan C. Objective assessment of vocal hyperfunction: an experimental framework and initial results. J Speech Hear Res. 1989; 32(2):373–392

[8] Roy N. Assessment and treatment of musculoskeletal tension in hyperfunctional voice disorders. Int J Speech-Language Pathol. 2008; 10(4):195–209

[9] Roy N. Differential diagnosis of muscle tension dysphonia and spasmodic dysphonia. Curr Opin Otolaryngol Head Neck Surg. 2010; 18(3):165–170

3 The Voice Diagnostic: Initial Considerations, Case History, and Perceptual Evaluation

Summary

This chapter reviews several key issues that must be considered by the voice clinician before initiating a voice diagnostic protocol. These issues include consideration of the organization and necessary content of the voice diagnostic protocol, a discussion of the meaning of "normal/typical" versus "abnormal/atypical" voice, and awareness of various forms of bias that must be minimized during the diagnostic process. Following discussion of these aforementioned considerations, this chapter focuses on a description of two of the necessary elements of the voice diagnostic: case history examination and perceptual evaluation of voice. Key elements of the case history examination will be described, and detailed information regarding the process of auditory-perceptual evaluation of the voice will be provided. Finally, methods of documenting patient self-perception regarding the possible debilitating effects of dysphonia will be detailed.

Keywords: voice evaluation, voice diagnostic, auditory-perceptual evaluation of voice, dysphonia, voice handicap

3.1 Learning Objectives

At the end of this chapter, readers will be able to
- Identify the necessary components and organization of the voice diagnostic protocol.
- Define the meaning of "normal/typical" versus "abnormal/atypical" voice.
- Identify and describe the key elements of the case history examination as conducted with potentially voice-disordered patients.
- Describe terminology and rating procedures associated with the auditory-perceptual evaluation of pitch, loudness, duration, and quality of voice.
- Describe the role of self-perception of voice handicap scales in the voice diagnostic.

3.2 Organization of the Clinical Voice Evaluation

In the following four chapters, we will describe the basic process for assessment and diagnosis of voice as carried out by the speech–language pathologist/voice therapist/vocologist. We refer to the assessment process as the *voice diagnostic protocol*, which comprises three primary areas: (1) preliminary information and case history, (2) perceptual analysis of voice, and (3) instrumental analysis of vocal function.[1] The processes and analyses described in this current chapter will focus on relatively low cost methods associated with the collection, analysis, and interpretation of preliminary information, case history, and auditory-perceptual analysis of voice. In clinical practice, these procedures will be augmented by acoustic methods used to obtain measurements related to characteristics such as the pitch, loudness, and quality of voice, aerodynamic methods such as the direct measurement of pressure

and flow, and laryngeal visualization via endoscopy. Acoustic, aerodynamic, and endoscopic methods are described in following chapters.

A complete voice diagnostic protocol will lead to accurate diagnosis and subsequent treatment planning when it is composed of multidimensional assessments. The clinician may question why we need multiple procedures such as acoustic analyses or laryngeal visualization if we have clearly perceived a characteristic such as breathiness in the voice during a perceptual assessment. Alternatively, if the physician or clinician has visualized the vocal folds, why do we need any other analyses? In answer to these questions, the clinician must understand that *structure* does not always dictate *function* or vice versa. It is very possible that a patient may have an essentially normal looking larynx and associated structures and yet have a very severe dysphonia (e.g., spasmodic dysphonia). In turn, it is also possible for a patient to have a significant structural or physiological change to the laryngeal structures and still have a relatively functional voice (e.g., patient who has a unilateral vocal fold paralysis in which the vocal fold is fixated at the midline of the glottis). In addition, it must always be remembered that *a vast number of different voice disorders can have very similar perceptual, acoustic, and aerodynamic characteristics*—perceptual and indirect acoustic/aerodynamic tasks alone would not be able to clearly define and describe the underlying condition responsible for the change in voice. Therefore, a complete profile of the voice is generated from a voice diagnostic protocol that incorporates at least four distinct areas, as illustrated in ▶ Fig. 3.1: (1) collection of preliminary and case history information; (2) perceptual analyses, including both the auditory-perceptual judgement of the clinician and the self-perception of the patient; (3) indirect measures of the acoustic and aerodynamic characteristics of voice; and (4) direct visualization of the larynx and phonatory structures. *Direct* evaluation indicates that the evaluation involves seeing the structure or actual activity (e.g., visualization of apparent vocal fold vibration during a laryngeal stroboscopic exam) or measurement of some characteristic of an activity in very close proximity to its source (e.g., measurement of airflow via a pneumotachograph). *Indirect* evaluation involves the analysis of some by-product of an activity (e.g., evaluation of the perceptual or acoustic characteristics of the voice signal produced by vocal fold vibration; estimation of airflow using a patient's vital capacity and maximum phonation time data).

3.3 Assessment versus Evaluation versus Diagnosis

An *assessment* may be described as a general process of gathering data to evaluate an examinee. The clinician will take the information from various sources including case history interview, test data, and measurement measures, and pull it all together into a cohesive whole. The *assessment* is a systematic method of obtaining information from tests and other sources,

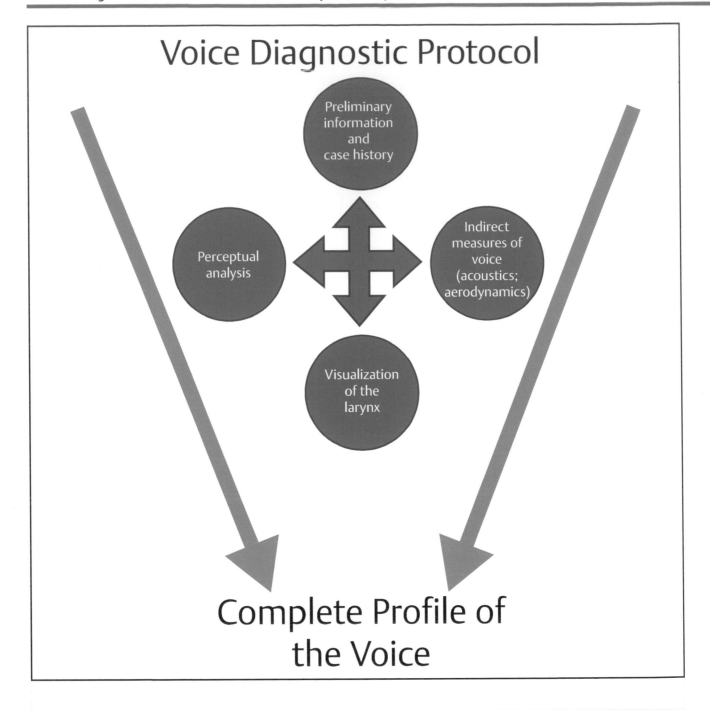

Fig. 3.1 Diagram of the interrelationship between case history, perceptual evaluation, indirect measures of voice, and laryngeal visualization used in the voice diagnostic protocol. The result of the protocol will be a complete and comprehensive profile of the patient's vocal function.

used to draw inferences about our patient.[2] In contrast, the various tests and procedures that are included in the assessment are our methods of *evaluation*, with our tests being evaluative procedures in which a sample of an examinee's behavior may be obtained, evaluated, measured, and scored using a standardized process.[2] Finally, once our assessment (composed of all of the evaluative procedures or tests) has been completed, we will finally make a statement or conclusion about the testing and other information gathering that was part of the overall assessment process—this is our *diagnosis.* Whether the assessment includes

tests that ask a specific question or obtain a focused measurable characteristic of the patient's voice, the diagnostic process involves gathering information and modifying the probability of a diagnosis in the light of that information.[3] "Diagnosis requires placing measurements and other observational data into context and perspective in order to decide whether a problem exists and to differentiate one problem from others which may have similar performance aspects."[4]

The term *diagnostic* has been specifically used to indicate that the outcome of this process will be based on a synthesis and application of information from diverse areas all dealing with aspects of voice function, such as anatomy and physiology, acoustics, perception, psychometrics, and knowledge of norms and testing techniques.[5] In particular, the final diagnosis should also be *differential* in nature. *Differential diagnosis* takes into account all significant variables contributing to the disorder and attempts to differentiate the presenting problem from related or dissimilar problems.[6] As such, the voice diagnostic protocol is the *modus operandi* by which information gathered from case history, perceptual, acoustic, aerodynamic, and endoscopic information is synthesized to produce a differential diagnosis.

3.3.1 Considerations Before Entering into the Voice Diagnostic

There are a number of basic but essential parameters that must be defined and understood by the voice clinician before entering into the diagnostic. First, what do we mean by "typical/normal" versus "disordered" voice? Fex states that "Normal voice quality is a conception based on subjective opinion, may vary with different cultures, and certainly is difficult to define; a vast number of people are supposed to have normal but nevertheless individually differentiated voice" (p. 155).[7] Defining "normal" or "typical" voice is difficult since there are a number of characteristics (age, sex, racial type, body size/type, etc.) that influence normal voice type and quality. Through our life experience, we are exposed to the vast range of normal/typical voices and, thereby, develop an internal gauge by which normal/typical is judged. With this in mind, we may state that *a voice is normal/typical if it does not deviate substantially from our internal gauge of parameters such as pitch, loudness, quality, and duration*.[1] This definition predicates that the clinician has a good understanding of normal/typical variations in voice associated with the effects of the aforementioned parameters of age, sex, racial type, etc.

Second, when a voice is perceived as deviating from normal/typical expectations, it may be characterized as being disordered or *dysphonic*. The term *dysphonia* literally means "abnormal/difficult/impaired voice." Of course, there is a wide variation in *types of dysphonia*; so, we must consider what the primary voice disorder types are by which we may categorize the dysphonic voice. In a previous chapter, we have discussed categories such as functional/behavioral versus organic. In addition, in the subsequent pages, specific categorical terminology will be provided by which commonly observed voice characteristics used to describe pitch, loudness, and voice quality are described.

Finally, identifying a dysphonia and categorizing it as a particular type is not enough—we must also describe the *severity* of the disorder/dysphonia. *Severity* is, perhaps, one of the most (if not most) important factors in determining why the patient has presented himself or herself before us and in determining if our treatment(s) have had any effect on the patient. When gauging the severity of the presenting voice disorder, we must recognize that the voice impairment is (1) multidimensional in nature (i.e., composed of numerous characteristics that may be weighted differently by different judges[8,9]) and (2) may impact the speaker's functional ability to communicate and obtain employment.[9] Several ways in which the severity of the presenting dysphonia can be communicated will be provided.

3.3.2 What Do We Do During a Voice Diagnostic?

As shown in ► Fig. 3.1, a number of different evaluation procedures are necessary to completely assess vocal function and arrive at a logical diagnostic decision. Based on time available to the clinician, insurance company regulations, and other factors, it may not be possible to complete all evaluation procedures in a single visit. In our experience, we have typically separated the diagnostic into two sets of procedures that combine to form the complete evaluation (► Table 3.1). These sets include (1) an initial exam which includes gathering preliminary information and conducting case history, perceptual evaluation of the voice, and laryngeal visualization and (2) a second examination in which behavioral voice evaluation and laryngeal function study are completed including acoustic and aerodynamic analyses (indirect measures of voice). In this second set of evaluation procedures, a series of trial diagnostic therapy tasks may also be conducted depending on the presenting case. The order of these two sets of evaluation procedures may be reversed depending on the order of referral (e.g., in some settings, the laryngeal visualization examination may occur after the voice evaluation and laryngeal function analysis). In this chapter, we will focus on gathering important preevaluation information, case history format and key components, and perceptual evaluation of the voice. Subsequent chapters will describe the evaluation procedures included in laryngeal visualization, acoustic, and aerodynamic analyses.

3.3.3 Preevaluation Information

Before meeting with their patient, the clinicians should attempt to gather pertinent background information that may be beneficial in determining the possible etiology and contributing factors to the patient's possible disorder, as well as review information on previous evaluation(s) and past or current treatment methods that the patient may have received. Immediate access to information about the prospective patient may be affected by the setting in which one works, with the range of initial information extending

Table 3.1 By necessity, the evaluation procedures incorporated into the voice diagnostic protocol are often administered over multiple sessions. The procedures in set I versus set II are those recommended by the authors, but may be varied at the choice of the voice clinician.

The voice diagnostic protocol	
Evaluation set I	Evaluation set II
Gather preliminary information chart review	Voice recordings and acoustic analyses for objective measures related to pitch, loudness, and quality
Case history interview	Aerodynamic measures that relate to respiratory phonatory capacity and control
Perceptual evaluation of voice (including auditory-perceptual evaluation and ratings of patient self-perception)	Trial diagnostic therapy tasks (if necessary)
Laryngeal visualization (stroboscopy)	

from simple referral slips with limited information about the patient's condition to extensive information obtained from medical charts and reports. A review of this preliminary information may inform initial suspicions regarding possible etiological factors, which often helps the clinician to develop a clinical hypothesis regarding a potential voice disorder (e.g., behavioral in nature due to vocal abuse/misuse vs. those associated with an underlying disease process). This hypothesis may be either accepted or rejected following the completion of a voice diagnostic profile. Complete consideration of possible etiological factors is essential, as attempting to treat a patient's current voice symptoms without a hypothesis of why the voice disorder developed may result in temporary voice change but will be ineffective in reducing the probability of disorder recurrence.

In certain cases, the clinician may already have access to chart history or to a completed case history form. Review of this information should be focused on evidence pertinent to the cause or maintenance of a voice or speech disorder. If the clinician cannot clearly answer why a question is being asked or why a piece of information is being included in a description of the patient's history, then the question or piece of information should not be included. The following are examples of information that are typically reviewed:

- Previous diagnoses including postnasal drainage, history of reflux, hypertension, and respiratory disorder.
- Any systemic disorder that may affect the respiratory and/or laryngeal mechanisms such as neurological disease and cancer of various forms should be noted.
- Significant injuries to the head, neck, chest regions, as well as any history of surgeries in these regions should also be identified.
- Surgical procedures that may have involved *intubation* (the passage of a tube through the nose or mouth into the trachea for maintenance of the airway during anesthesia).
- The presence of hearing deficits that may be related to vocal dysfunction.
- The chart history should also be reviewed for the previous physician's examination note, as well as the results of previous tests and procedures that involve the phonatory mechanism such as modified barium swallow and endoscopy.

It is essential that the clinician maintain an open mind regarding the possible etiological information gathered from the patient's chart history. While background information facilitates an initial hypotheses regarding the patient's condition and underlying deficits, the clinician must also be wary of bias toward a particular clinical hypothesis before the actual collection of patient *signs* (i.e., observed phenomenon by the clinician) and *symptoms* (i.e., patient descriptions that may not be verifiable) have taken place in the diagnostic session.[1] There are various forms of *bias* that may predispose the clinician to select a particular diagnosis regardless of the actual data observed. Croskerry described several forms of cognitive dispositions to respond (CDRs) that may lead to diagnostic error[10]:

- *Anchoring bias*—locking on to a diagnosis too early and failing to adjust to new information.
- *Availability bias*—thinking that a similar recent presentation is happening in the present situation.
- *Confirmation bias*—looking for evidence to support a preconceived opinion rather than looking for information to prove

oneself wrong. This often leads to *premature closure* in which the clinician has "jumped" to a conclusion regarding the patient's condition.
- *Diagnosis momentum*—accepting a previous diagnosis without sufficient skepticism.
- *Premature closure*—similar to "confirmation bias" but "jumping to a conclusion."

The clinician must balance the possibilities presented by background information with the realities of the actual diagnostic session. The background information should spur the clinician on to develop clinical hypotheses, carry out any necessary research regarding the patient's condition before evaluating the patient, and prepare any special tests that may need to be carried out (e.g., although we are focusing on voice evaluation, voice disorders may coexist with other communicative deficits that may also need to be evaluated).[1] However, the clinician must always be wary of clinical bias and be prepared for the possibility that the patient may have characteristics that are quite different than background information has led us to believe.

3.4 Key Content of the Case History

The diagnostic session typically starts with the gathering of background information and significant information regarding the patient's possible voice problem(s) in the case history interview. The following key areas should be explored with the patient[1]:

- The nature of the problem.
- Development of the problem.
- Variability versus consistency.
- Description of voice use.
- Effects of dysphonia on the patient.
- Health status and possible causes.

It is our view that, rather than carrying out a "form-filling" exercise, it is best to incorporate these issues into a conversation with the patient/caregiver. A brief conversation that covers most, if not all, of the subsequent areas of questioning not only gathers focused case information in an efficient manner (in our experience, generally within 5–10 minutes at most) but also allows for extended conversation in which the clinician has multiple opportunities to observe the pitch, loudness, quality, and durational characteristics of the patient's voice, as well as observe the patient themselves (e.g., signs of stress/anxiety, presence of tremors) in a typical conversational setting.

3.4.1 The Nature of the Problem

The starting point of the voice diagnostic interview is often described as an assessment of the *nature of the problem* (i.e., what is the problem and what are its characteristics). The patient's description of the characteristics of his or her voice problem(s) allows for a description of the disorder as the patient perceives it.[11] In describing the nature of the problem, the patient may describe the voice problem that will correspond closely to the perceptions of the clinician (e.g., "My voice has had a raspy sound to it for the last few weeks"; "My voice cuts out."). However, it is also common that the patient's description of the nature of the problem is at odds with previously gathered case history information and/or the perceptions of the clinician. These discrepancies may be due to factors such as (1) patients misunderstanding of their problems (i.e., reflecting a possible lack of awareness of their disorder), (2) an inability of the patient to deal realistically with their voice deficits, (3) intermittent voice problems with variable characteristics that may not be in evidence at the time of the interview, or (4) a voice problem that has changed considerably since first documented via previous evaluation.[1,11]

We suggest that the clinician start the diagnostic interview with a general open-ended question such as "*What can I do for you today?*" or "*Can you tell me why you are here today?*" Beginning the interview with this form of question provides the patient with the opportunity to describe the possible voice problem(s) in his or her own words, independent of any clinician bias that may be present. The patient quite often will relate important information that is not present in the patient chart history, and therefore, it is important that we allow the patient the opportunity and time to describe the problems they have been experiencing. In addition, since the use of an open-ended question requires the patient to provide a more extended response, the clinician is provided with the opportunity to observe some of the perceptual characteristics of the voice. Auditory-perceptual judgments regarding the patient's voice characteristics are often the first signs (i.e., observable and verifiable characteristics) collected by the clinician during the voice diagnostic. As the patient is speaking, the clinician is also provided with the opportunity to visualize features that may be accompanying the patient's speech/voice characteristics which can provide insight into possible underlying causes or contributory factors (e.g., excessive tension in the paralaryngeal region, limited oral movements, rigidity in the mandibular region, or tremors). In addition, attention to the patient's communication patterns can inform the development of hypotheses regarding personality traits and the relationship of those traits to the perceived voice characteristics and patient symptoms (e.g., introverted vs. extroverted personality).

While it is hoped that the patient will freely impart information regarding their voice problem(s), some patients will need to be cued toward revealing the nature of their deficits. As an example, the patent may respond to the clinician's introductory open-ended question of "Can you please tell me why you are here today?" with a very vague "I have been having trouble speaking lately." The clinician may then have to lead the patient with a question that cues certain necessary responses such as, "*Do you have trouble with the way your voice sounds, the ability to form sounds with your lips and tongue, or in finding the right words to say?*" Hopefully, this cued question will elicit a more focused response from the patient such as "The way my voice sounds," followed by a further clinician cue such as "*Can you describe for me how your voice sounds when you are having trouble speaking?,*" resulting in the patient stating, "It sounds hoarse." In this example, the clinician guided the patient to a more descriptive and informative response that verifies the probable presence of a voice disorder. If the patient is still unable to provide a reasonable description of the problems he or she has been experiencing, the clinician may also ask if the way the voice sounds today (i.e., during the interview) is the way the voice sounds when he or she is having the voice problems, or ask if the patient can demonstrate the disordered voice. The clinician should also be prepared to demonstrate various voice types themselves (e.g., breathiness and strain) as a means of eliciting the possible nature of the voice dysfunction from the patient.

In addition to the nature of the patient's specific voice problem, the clinician should be aware that other related symptoms may provide important insight into the eventual diagnosis. Several neurological and stress-related symptoms may be associated with voice problems as etiological factors or as contributing factors. Examples include the presence of possible dysphagia, nasal regurgitation of food and liquids, weakness (either bilateral or unilateral) in other parts of the body, neurologically related speech and language deficits, characteristics of increased musculoskeletal tension, increased fatigue, frequent heartburn, and dryness in the mouth and throat.[1]

3.4.2 Development of the Problem

After initial questioning about the nature of the voice problem, a logical transition is to investigate the development of the problem through questions such as "*How long have you had this problem?*" or "*When did you first notice your voice problem(s)?*" The onset of the disorder may be characterized as (1) long duration, gradual onset versus (2) sudden onset. Long duration, gradual onset disorders generally do not have a specific date or episode of onset that the patient can recall. Various types of voice disorders (organic and functional) may develop over weeks, months, or years, including those associated with conditions such as vocal abuse and progressive neurological diseases.[12] In certain cases, patients who have had a slow, gradual onset to their voice problem may show less concern about their voice and/or less overall effect on their daily life because they have learned to cope with and compensate for their deficits. **Because gradually developing dysphonias are often observed in patients with long duration, habituated vocal abuse, these patients may have a poorer overall prognosis for voice/behavior change.**[13]

In contrast to gradual onset disorders, those disorders with acute, sudden onset are often more disturbing to the patient, and often pose a severe disruption in both the ability to carry out daily activities and, possibly, overall health status.[13] With sudden onset dysphonias, the patient may be able to describe the date and details of onset with great detail. A variety of conditions with potential negative effects on voice may develop over a very short time (1–2 days or less), including

- Severe laryngitis.
- Neurological insult (e.g., cerebrovascular accident, closed head injury).
- Laryngeal trauma (external [e.g., blunt trauma to the neck region] or internal [e.g., sudden trauma to the vocal fold mucosa from a singular shouting/screaming episode]).
- Iatrogenic surgical injury (e.g., vocal fold paresis resulting from thyroid surgery. vocal fold ulceration resulting from intubation).

In addition, sudden voice change in the absence of signs or symptoms suggestive of organic pathological condition is often a key component in the diagnosis of psychogenic dysphonias (e.g., conversion reaction).[12]

3.4.3 Variability versus Consistency

Information regarding disordered voice characteristics that have been variable or have shown degrees of fluctuation over time versus those that have been relatively consistent may be an important factor in discerning voice disorder type. Disordered voices that periodically return to normal or near-normal characteristics **may be functional in nature** and may be due to underlying variations in vocal fold swelling and stiffness. In those conditions in which dysphonia fluctuates, it is important to question the patient regarding the conditions that are associated with either positive or negative voice change (environmental effects; effects of vocational, social, recreational situations; specific periods of the day associated with poor vs. improved voice).[1] In addition, factors such as personal habits (smoking, alcohol use), work conditions, or medical conditions may affect the variability of a voice disorder. Periods of emotional stress (personal, familial, work related) may also cause the voice to worsen. Highly variable voice characteristics have been associated with a variety of dysphonic conditions[1,5,12,13]:

- Hyperfunctional patients often report improved voice function earlier in the day, with increasing dysphonia with increased voice use.
- Voice quality that is worse in the morning versus later in the day may be a symptom of postnasal drip (PND) or laryngopharyngeal reflux (LPR). An accompanying symptom of PND and/or LPR is excessive throat clearing first thing in the morning.
- Functional voice disorders associated with psychosomatic conditions often report considerable variability in their vocal function.
- Dysphonias related to vocal fold swelling and stiffness will often be worse as the day progresses and improve with reduced voice use.

In contrast to those with variable voice characteristics, many disorders that have underlying neurological dysfunction or definitive changes in vocal fold structure (e.g., mass lesions) generally result in fairly consistent dysphonias that do not show considerable spontaneous improvement.[11] Of course, there will be exceptions to this view, such as with the case of myasthenia gravis (a deficit of neural transmission affecting the myoneural junction) which may be highly variable over time, with patients showing progressive weakness with muscle use, followed by periods of improvement after rest.

3.4.4 Description of Voice Use

Many voice disorders arise from the manner in which the patient uses the phonatory mechanism (i.e., functional dysphonias). Therefore, it is essential that a comprehensive description of how the patient uses his or her voice in various situations is obtained by the voice therapist. The identification of the patient's potential vocal abuse, misuse, and overuse in various vocational, social, and recreational settings is essential, with these various situations often the cause of many functional voice problems.[12,13] The clinician must determine the daily vocational and recreational vocal demands on the patient and determine whether the patient must use voice under adverse conditions. The development of voice disorders has been associated with several types of voice use and/or setting, including

- Work settings that require the patient to use his or her voice for their livelihood (i.e., professional voice users) may potentially lead to the development of voice disorders, particularly if these patients have not had any professional voice training.[12]
- Social settings such as gatherings at parties or in bars may present a vocally abusive environment (voice production in excessive background noise) with potential to elicit phonotrauma.
- Hyperfunctional phonation that is potentially damaging to the vocal fold mucosa may accompany strenuous exercise and sporting events for both spectator and participant.[12]
- Singing in various situations (choir, theater, recreational musician) presents a potentially phonotraumatic condition (e.g., high-intensity voice in the presence of high levels of background noise; possibly under adverse conditions such as singing in bars in a smoky atmosphere, poor monitors, etc.) for many vocalists, particularly if they have not had professional voice training.[1]

Because it is not always possible for the clinician to directly observe the patient in all the aforementioned situations, the patient may be encouraged to describe and possibly demonstrate the voice use in these various settings for the clinician.[13]

3.4.5 Effects of Dysphonia on the Patient

Regardless of the clinician-perceived severity of the patient's dysphonia, a voice disorder that the patient feels affects their vocation or draws negative reactions from others will be of more concern to the patient than a voice disorder that does not adversely affect daily life. We have seen patients with very mild dysphonias who have described potentially drastic effects on their daily lives (e.g., teachers, singers), as well as patients with perceptually severe dysphonias who have demonstrated very little concern (particularly once any potentially life-threatening disorder has been ruled out). Our observations are consistent with Colton and Casper who stated that, "*the severity of the (patient's) reaction is not always proportional to the severity of the voice problem*" (p. 190).[12] For those who do describe a debilitating effect on their daily lives, feelings of stress, anxiety, and development of possible negative psychological outlook may arise because of the dysphonia or from the reactions of others.[1,11] These negative psychological reactions can have their own exacerbating effect on any presenting voice disorder.

The perceived effect of a dysphonia on the patient also has implications for prognosis. In many cases, those who describe a particularly adverse effect on their lifestyles may be more motivated to participate in and follow through with treatment goals and recommendations. In contrast, those patients who demonstrate little concern or awareness of their particular voice disorder are often less motivated to follow through with treatment recommendations and may have a poorer prognosis for improvement. When asked about the effects of the dysphonia, some patients may be apprehensive about discussing what may be a potentially humiliating effect on their lifestyle. However, the clinician should ensure that expressions of denial regarding effects of the dysphonia are fully explored.[11,12]

3.4.6 Health Status and Possible Causes

Since voice characteristics reflect not only the emotional state and personality of the patient but also the overall physical status, the patient's current health history, as well as any particularly pertinent information from the preevaluation chart review, should be assessed to determine any possible relationship to the presenting voice disorder.[12] A brief review of current health history should be a part of the case history interview, as complete details of the patient's health history may either be absent from the patient's chart details or may have changed since their most recent examination. The voice clinician is particularly interested in health history in the following areas[1]:

- Current health status (including recent illness, injuries, and surgical or other medical procedures).
- Injuries or trauma to the upper chest, head, and/or neck region.
- Neurological problems.
- Respiratory deficits.
- Allergy-related problems.
- History of frequent upper respiratory tract infections.
- Surgeries involving the head, neck, or upper chest region, as well as any procedures in which the patient may have been intubated.
- Smoking, alcohol use, illicit drug use.
- Ingestion of caffeinated beverages (coffee, tea, soft drinks).
- Use of prescription and over-the-counter medications (e.g., antihistamines, decongestants, diuretics).
- Endocrine imbalances.
- Previous occurrences of voice dysfunction or "loss" of the voice.
- Hydration status—degree of internal hydration may affect the viscosity of mucus secretions and aids in lubrication of the vocal fold cover.[14] A well-lubricated cover protects the vocal fold during the vibratory cycle and aids in heat dissipation. Ingestion of six 8-ounce glasses of water or fruit juice per day is generally recommended.
- Psychological issues with a particular focus on sources of stress and anxiety.

In this stage of our discussion with the patient, we should also ask (if it has not already been stated) what the patient believes may have been the possible cause(s) of the voice problem(s). A comparison of possible causes described by referral sources (e.g., physician, previous speech–language pathologist) versus those possible causes described by the patient may reflect on the knowledge and insight the patient has regarding his or her voice problem. Differing views on the possible cause of a voice disorder between the patient, referral sources, and family members may reflect (1) an inability to adequately understand what may have been previously explained to the patient, (2) the patient's inability to recognize possible underlying causes of the voice problem, or (3) an inability to accept and cope with the problem.[1] Differences between the patient's perceptions of what has caused the voice problem versus opinions offered by referral sources may have to be addressed if the patient is to gain awareness and recognition of the underlying cause(s) of their dysphonia and develop a positive prognosis for improvement in voice therapy.[11]

3.4.7 Auditory-Perceptual Evaluation of Voice

As we are leading the patient through our case history examination and documenting the aforementioned key areas of questioning, it is essential that we are also listening to and documenting the perceptual characteristics of the patient's voice. The term *perceptual evaluation* is recommended by the Voice Committee of the International Association of Logopedics and Phoniatrics (IALP) and entails a comparison between the characteristics of the voice of the speaker and those that are considered as normal or typical for the listener.[15] Since we are focused on the audible characteristics of the voice, many expand this term to *auditory-perceptual evaluation*. Clinicians and researchers believe that this form of perceptual evaluation is an essential component of voice assessment, diagnosis, and treatment for the following reasons[16]:

1. Perceptual evaluation methods are available to all clinicians and may provide a global measure of vocal performance.
2. The perceived characteristics of the voice are quite often the reason that a patient has presented themselves or has been referred for the voice diagnostic in the first place.
3. The perceived characteristics of the voice present a primary gauge by which therapy recommendations will be made and success in therapy will be evaluated.
4. Measures and observations obtained via acoustic, aerodynamic, and laryngeal visualization will be related and often interpreted in light of the perceptual characteristics of the voice.

Previously, we had stated that a voice is normal/typical if it does not deviate substantially from our internal gauge of parameters such as pitch, loudness, quality, and duration.[1] If the voice that we are listening to deviates from this definition, it is abnormal/atypical. In the next section, we will describe some of the methods by which various voice types and their severity are documented and describe in more detail commonly observed typical and atypical auditory-perceptual voice characteristics.

Methods for Rating the Type and Severity Voice Disruption

Because disordered voice is multidimensional (i.e., composed of numerous characteristics including pitch, loudness, duration, and quality), it is necessary to communicate what category or type of voice disruptions we are observing, as well as the severity of the observed disruption. Of these two components (category/type of vocal disruption vs. severity of vocal disruption), accurate descriptions of severity can be the most difficult for many clinicians. When we judge the severity of a disorder, we are recognizing that the condition may exist along a continuum. This continuum extends in growing proportions from an absence or minor amount of the observed deviant voice characteristic to an extreme amount. The lower end of this continuum should be acknowledged as being a "minimal" level, because even normal voice signals are not necessarily perfect. On the other end of the continuum, an extreme level of voice deviation has a significant effect on patient and listener alike and often prevents phonatory function.

When documenting and communicating the perceptual characteristics of the voice, the clinician should select a method of describing and rating voice characteristics that is complex enough to portray the multidimensional nature of voice quality deviation and yet be understandable enough that (1) clinicians may easily learn and use the system with limited training and (2) results may be communicated easily among colleagues and other professionals. **Because the perceptual characteristics of the voice may differ depending on the context in which the voice sample is elicited, it is recommended that the clinician describe voice characteristics in both sustained vowel** (e.g., repetitions of the vowel /a/) **and standardized speech and/or reading contexts** (e. g., portions of "The Rainbow Passage"; counting). These contexts will augment the perceptual descriptions of voice obtained during the case history conversation. Here are three commonly used methods for documenting the perceptual evaluation of the voice:

Categorical Ratings

In this method, voice samples are assigned to discrete categories such as mild, moderate, severe. The following severity terminology attempts to incorporate a number of the possible diverse effects of dysphonia[1]:

Mild

While the listener experienced in the perceptual characteristics of the disordered voice would consider the voice abnormal/atypical, the lay listener may consider the voice to be only unusual in nature. The voice characteristic is not distracting, and the ability to effectively communicate is not affected. The dysphonia has a minimal effect on phonation.

Moderate

Dysphonia is more prominent, and both trained and untrained listeners would consider the voice abnormal. There may be intermittent periods in which the voice characteristic is highly distracting. The ability to effectively communicate is noticeably affected under certain conditions (e.g., noisy environments). The dysphonia may occasionally cause substantial disruption to phonation (i.e., phonation ceases or becomes highly effortful).

Severe

Both trained and untrained listeners would consider the voice extremely abnormal. The voice characteristic is highly distracting. The ability to effectively communicate is consistently affected. The dysphonia may cause phonation to be mainly absent (i.e., aphonic) or extremely effortful.

Using these categories of severity, the clinician may state (e.g., in the impressions section of their diagnostic report) whether the voice is typical or dysphonic, if dysphonic, the severity of the dysphonia and the type of dysphonia present. As examples, a report may state that, "*The patient presents with dysphonia characterized by mild breathiness*" or, alternatively, "*The patient presents with moderate strain*," where the presence of dysphonia is assumed.

Equal-Appearing Interval Scales

The severity of a perceived voice characteristic is assigned a number (the range of numbers varies), with the higher numbers representing increased severity and perceived deviation

Table 3.2 Description of the parameters of the GRBASI scale

Parameter	Description
G	*Grade*: a summary rating of the severity of dysphonia as a whole (i.e., an overall impression of the voice)
R	*Roughness*: coarse, gravelly, low-pitched noise. Related to irregularity of vocal fold vibration
B	*Breathiness*: airy, whispery voice due to audible detection of airflow through the glottis. Related to hypoadduction of the vocal folds
A	*Asthenia*: weak voice
S	*Strain*: impression of effortful, hyperfunctional voice. Related to excessive muscular effort and glottal/supraglottal constriction
I	*Instability*: fluctuation/variation vocal characteristics such as pitch, loudness, and quality

Notes: Each parameter is rated on a 0 to 3 scale where 0 is normal, 1 is a slight degree, 2 is a medium degree, and 3 is a high degree.

from the normal/typical voice. The assumption of these scales is that they are linear with each interval representing an equal increment in the characteristic being measured or described (e.g., the difference/distance between an adjoining set of values [e.g., 0–1] is the same as any other adjoining set of values [e.g., 1–2]). A commonly used example of this type of equal-appearing interval (EAI) scale is the GRBAS scale (**Table 3.2**). The GRBAS scale was developed by the Japanese Society of Logopedics and Phoniatrics, which gives scores of 0, 1, 2, or 3 for the grade of hoarseness (roughness, breathiness, asthenia, and strain), where 0 is normal, 1 is a slight degree, 2 is a medium degree, and 3 is a high degree.[17] This scale has also been extended to the GRBASI (or GIRBAS) by adding a rating for instability to reflect fluctuation of voice quality over time.[18]

Visual Analog Scales

Instead of scaling the voice by use of specified incremental levels of voice disruption (as in EAI scales), visual analog scales (VASs) provide the judge with an undifferentiated line on which a mark is placed to indicate the level of voice severity or deviation. Generally, only the extremes of the line are labeled (e.g., minimal vs. extreme). The use of this type of scaling procedure may be helpful in reducing bias in the rating process.

An application of the VAS method is found in the *Consensus Auditory-Perceptual Evaluation of Voice* (CAPE-V) scale. The CAPE-V was developed to help standardize clinical auditory-perceptual assessment of voice and to describe the severity of perceptual attributes in a manner that would facilitate communication among clinicians.[19] The CAPE-V elicits sustained vowels as well as connected speech productions in both sentence reading and spontaneous speech. This tool provides specific sentence contexts developed to assess different elements of vocal quality:

- Sentence 1 ("**The blue spot is on the key again**") may be used to examine the coarticulatory influence of vowels /a/, /i/, and /u/ on voice quality.
- Sentence 2 ("**How hard did he hit him**?") assesses soft glottal attacks and voiceless to voiced transitions.

Consensus Auditory-Perceptual Evaluation of Voice (CAPE-V)

Vocal Tasks

- **Sustained vowels**
  - /a/
  - /i/
- **Six sentences**
  - The blue spot is on the key again.
  - How Hard did he hit him?
  - We were away a year ago.
  - We eat eggs every Easter.
  - My mama makes lemon muffins.
  - Peter will keep at the peak.
- **Spontaneous speech**

Perceptual Domains - 100mm scale

- **Overall severity**
- **Roughness**
- **Breathiness**
- **Strain**
- **Pitch**
- **Loudness**

Fig. 3.2 Structure of the CAPE-V perceptual assessment. The examiner listens to elicited sustained vowels, six sentences (read or repeated by the patient), and conversational speech before rating six perceptual domains on a 100-mm visual analog scale. Additional comments on voicing behaviors (e.g., diplophonia, glottal fry, and falsetto) may be added to the assessment. A CAPE-V form can be downloaded from http://www.asha.org/Form/CAPE-V/, and may also be obtained from Kempster et al.[19]

- Sentence 3 ("**We were away a year ago**") is an all voiced sentence that allows for the observation of the ability to maintain voicing in a variable context, as well as for the observation of possible voice stoppages/spasms.
- Sentence 4 ("**We eat eggs every Easter**") includes vowel-initiated words that may elicit hard glottal attacks.
- Sentence 5 ("**My mama makes lemon jam**") includes numerous nasal consonants important in certain types of voice therapy (e.g., resonant voice therapy), as well as may be used to assess the presence of hyponasal resonance imbalance.
- Sentence 6 ("**Peter will keep at the peak**") provides a useful context for assessing pressure consonant production and possible hypernasal resonance imbalance or nasal air emission. Voice characteristics are also assessed in conversational speech.

The CAPE-V involves rating overall severity of dysphonia, roughness, breathiness, strain, pitch, and loudness using 100 mm VAS. While the CAPE-V incorporates a VAS, it is actually a hybrid scale since it also includes indicators for mildly deviant (MI), moderately deviant (MO), and severely deviant (SE) ratings. The clinician is asked to observe and describe possible task-dependent differences in vocal performance between the three CAPE-V contexts (sustained vowels, elicited sentences, and conversational speech). A summary of the key content of the CAPE-V is provided in ▸ Fig. 3.2, and the form may be downloaded from http://www.asha.org/Form/CAPE-V/.

3.4.8 Commonly Used Terminology to Describe Voice Characteristics

The human voice (and for that matter, any sound) can be described in terms of four perceptual characteristics: *pitch, loudness, duration, and quality*. These same terms are the key perceptual characteristics of the voice that may become disrupted or which will deviate from our normal/typical expectations when a patient has a disordered voice.

Pitch

Most people can identify a "high" note versus a "low" note when listening to a musical or singing passage, and this "high" or "low" distinction is based on the perception of the *pitch* of the voice or instrument that he or she is listening to.[1] **Pitch** is the auditory perception of the fundamental rate of vibration of some sound-producing source. Because the pitch of the voice is a direct result of changes in factors such as (1) elasticity, (2) mass, and (3) the length of the vocal folds, the voice clinician may be able to develop hypotheses regarding the underlying structural condition of the vocal folds from the perception of the patient's vocal pitch and his or her knowledge of normal/typical pitch levels. **The typical sound wave measurement that corresponds to pitch is the measurement of *frequency*.** In contrast to pitch, frequency is the objective measurement of the fundamental rate of vibration (i.e., a measurement of the number of cycles of vibration per second). The assessment of pitch and frequency is an essential aspect of the voice evaluation.

Perceptual analysis of pitch generally focuses on descriptions of (1) habitual pitch level, (2) pitch variability and stability, and (3) total pitch range. The following terminologies have been used to describe these various aspects of vocal pitch:

Habitual Pitch

The *habitual pitch* has been defined as the pitch that the patient uses most often in everyday speech[11] and is the pitch level around which normal pitch inflections/variations occur.[20] Boone and McFarlane[13] state that the habitual pitch corresponds to the *modal pitch level* (i.e., the most frequently used pitch), whereas Case[20] indicates that habitual pitch is synonymous with the *average pitch level*.

Colton and Casper indicate that the assessment of the habitual pitch level should focus on whether the pitch level is appropriate for the patient's age and gender.[12] The determination of "normal" habitual pitch level is clearly related to knowledge of several key patient characteristics (age and gender, body size/type, and race) other than the characteristics of the voice itself.[6] When gauging the normality of pitch, it appears that we make a mental/internal comparison between the perceived pitch level and our expectations (gained through experience) for the person's/speaker's age, gender, etc. When the speaker's pitch level does not fall within our expected range, an abnormal pitch level is perceived. In addition, listener's confusion as to age and gender may also occur.

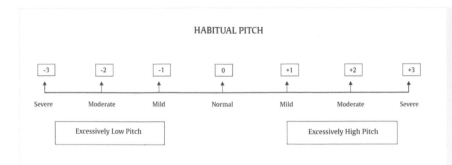

Various rating scales are available for rating habitual pitch level. As an example, Awan described a seven-point equal-interval scale with the central point of the scale rated as "0" (i.e., no substantial difference from normal expectations), with ratings of high pitch (positive numbers) and low pitch (negative numbers) rated on either side of normal (▸ Fig. 3.3).[1] Definitions for mild, moderate, and severe are those presented previously in this chapter.

Alternatively, habitual pitch level may be rated using the pitch scale of the CAPE-V form, with the nature of the abnormality (e.g., abnormally high vs. low) described by the clinician and the severity of the disruption identified on a 100-mm VAS with normal pitch level rated toward the extreme left end of the scale and increasing levels of pitch disruption rates toward the right end of the scale.[19]

Pitch Variability and Stability

In addition to the habitual pitch level, the voice clinician should make determinations of the patient's capability to vary/change pitch levels during speech, as well as the patient's ability to control the vocal pitch. Normal continuous speech production may incorporate a relatively wide range of pitch variation (a range of approximately 4–10 musical notes/semitones).[21] These pitch variations make up the normal intonation patterns of speech. Intonation patterns include pitch variations that are used linguistically to vary the meaning of utterances.[12]

Increases in pitch level may be used to indicate a particularly informative linguistic unit within the utterance or an interrogative/questioning statement; decreases in pitch often accompany unstressed syllable production and the end of declarative statements. The use of pitch variability/intonation patterns allows for more interesting and expressive communication. Continuous speech production that lacks pitch variability (referred to as *monopitch*—a "single" pitch level) may be perceived as dull and uninteresting. If pitch variability (either too little or too much) draws attention to itself, it may be abnormal.[5] In addition, there is evidence that reduced pitch variability and intonation patterns may decrease the intelligibility of the utterance, because the rise and fall of the normal pitch contour direct the attention of the listener to the content words of an utterance.[22]

An important aspect of pitch variability that must be attended to by the voice clinician is the presence of pitch instability or the lack of control of vocal pitch. This type of pitch instability is relatively easily perceived by the clinician (macroscopic) and should not be confused with the relatively microscopic cycle-to-cycle pitch instabilities measured in *jitter* (see section "Vocal Quality in

Normal versus Disordered Individuals" and Chapter 4 of this book). Pitch instability may be perceived as a "shakiness" in the voice or observed as unexpected pitch changes/variations during conditions in which we would expect pitch to remain relatively stable. Three commonly observed forms of pitch instability in which it is most common to observe a rapid pitch change/break upward. This may occur if the speaker is using an inappropriately low pitch during speech, if a patient attempts to sustain a high-pitch modal register phonation that rapidly shifts into falsetto, or may occur during sudden hard onset loud voice productions (e.g., an abrupt shout).[5] **Diplophonia** is a condition in which the listener may perceive the simultaneous production of two pitches in the voice signal. Diplophonia is attributed to the differential vibration of two different sound sources with different mass/length/tension characteristics.[11] Monsen observed that the diplophonic voice was characterized by alternating pitch periods rather than simultaneous production of different pitches and attributed diplophonia to irregularities in glottal vibration pattern in which alternating glottal periods were slightly different in period or shape.[23] Although diplophonia is being discussed as a pitch deviation, it should be noted that this characteristic often gives the impression of roughness in the voice. **Vocal tremor** is a form of pitch variability defined as a rhythmic variation in pitch (and often loudness) during conditions in which steadiness of pitch would be expected. This characteristic is most evident during the production of sustained vowels.

Awan described a seven-point equal-interval scale with the central point of the scale rated as "0" (i.e., no substantial difference from normal expectations), with ratings of increased pitch variability (positive numbers) and reduced pitch variability (negative numbers) rated on either side of normal (▸ Fig. 3.4).[1] Definitions for mild, moderate, and severe are those presented previously in this chapter. The clinician should note the type of sample that the description of pitch variability pertains to. It is recommended that ratings of pitch variability as used during intonation be obtained from continuous speech samples. In contrast, the ability to maintain a steady pitch production is best observed during a sustained vowel sample.

The pitch scale found in the CAPE-V form could also be used to indicate the severity of pitch variability dysfunction, and could be labeled as "low/reduced pitch variability" or "high/excessive pitch variability." A section labeled "Additional features" provides a space in which the clinician may specifically describe examples of atypical pitch variability such as tremor, pitch instability, and diplophonia.

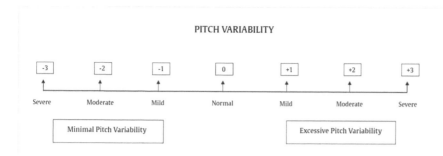

Fig. 3.4 Example scale for the auditory-perceptual rating of pitch variability.

Total Pitch Range

Another important aspect of pitch determination is the assessment of the total pitch range of the patient (a.k.a., vocal range, total phonational range). This entails an assessment of the range between the lowest pitch in modal register to the highest pitch in falsetto. Total pitch range has been said to provide an important index of laryngeal health and is often one of the first parameters of vocal capability adversely affected in voice disorders.[20]

3.4.9 Vocal Pitch in Normal versus Disordered Patients

As we have previously stated, the speaking pitch of the voice primarily depends on the age, gender, and body stature of the patient (e.g., skeletal size). The normal vocal pitch should be an appropriate match for the presenting speaker and should not present any age or gender confusion for the listener. In normal voice speakers, there is generally a great deal of similarity in male and female voices from birth until the onset of puberty. The pitch of the voice in both sexes gradually lowers from infancy to the point of onset of puberty.[24]

Definitive pitch distinctions between the sexes begin during puberty and continues throughout adolescence. As males and females progress through puberty (often from ages 8 to 13 years, marked by the onset of secondary sex characteristics[25]), both genders will exhibit a lowering of the pitch of the voice, although the lowering is generally not as drastic in the female as the male.[26] In females, the vocal pitch lowers in the vicinity of one octave from birth to adulthood versus approximately two octaves in males. This lowering may be attributed to changes in vocal fold length, with the length of the male vocal fold increasing approximately 4 to 8 mm from puberty to adulthood, and the female vocal fold increasing approximately 1 to 3.5 mm.[27] Complete mutation of voice takes place within approximately 3 to 6 months, during which time the neck lengthens and the larynx descends and grows in size. In many cases, the adult habitual pitch level has been achieved by the age of 14 to 15 years; however, slight "deepening " of the voice may accompany other growth changes within the vocal tract that affect vocal tract resonances rather than the vibratory frequency of the vocal folds.

As normal speakers enter into *senescence* (i.e., the process of aging, often marked by a gradual deterioration of bodily functions), age-related changes in the speech mechanism may include increased stiffness of respiratory and laryngeal structures, muscle and nervous system degeneration, reduced speed of neural transmission, and reduction in vocal tract mucous production.[28] As the female approaches and then goes through menopause, it has been observed that the pitch of the voice may lower.[29,30] This lowering has been associated with factors such as hormonal changes and edema.[31,32]

In contrast to the female, the male vocal pitch and F_0 appear to remain relatively stable throughout adulthood. However, there have been studies that indicate that some men may experience a rise in the pitch of the voice during senescence.[32,33,34] It has been hypothesized that pitch and frequency elevation in the elderly male voice may be due to changes in vocal fold tissue mass and/or an imbalance between cricothyroid and thyroarytenoid muscle forces.[34] It should be noted that the magnitude of any possible effect of aging on vocal pitch level may vary tremendously from person to person[35] and appears to be more strongly related to physiological age (e.g., overall physical condition) rather than chronological age.[36]

The ability to produce steady, controlled pitch levels or to purposefully vary pitch for intonation or singing purposes also varies across the age span. Poor control of vocal pitch in the infant voice has been said to reflect a low level of neuromuscular coordination and limited ability to control the tension of the vocal folds.[12] Pitch instability has been mentioned as one of the main characteristics of the adolescent voice, with this observation particularly true for the male adolescent voice. Pitch instability during adolescence has been attributed to differential development between gradual nervous system control and relatively rapid peripheral speech mechanism growth.[37] Pitch instability has also been reported as a possible characteristic of the senescent voice. It has been speculated that as we age, decrements in motor/sensory control of the speech mechanism may occur which may result in a "shaky" or even tremulous voice.[28,38,39]

The pitch range (both in continuous speech and in total phonational range) has also been reported to vary considerably with age. Although the physiological range of the voice (i.e., the range encompassing all possible vocal pitches and including vegetative and emotional voice use as in crying, screaming, etc.) may be relatively stable across the life span, the actual useable or musical range of the voice appears to be restricted somewhat during childhood.[27] As males and females move through puberty and into adulthood, the range of useable vocal pitches will extend to approximately two to three octaves, with pitch range again becoming somewhat restricted in the senescent voice.

In the disordered voice, changes in the effective mass, length, and stiffness/tension characteristics of the vocal folds may very well result in changes in the perceived pitch of the voice. As an example, we may expect that a disorder that involves an additive lesion to the vocal fold(s) would increase the effective mass of the fold(s) and, therefore, result in a decreased vocal pitch level. However, we must remember that there is a complex interaction between the effective mass, length, and stiffness/tension characteristics we have mentioned. In this example of a vocal fold lesion, there may also be an increase in stiffness of the vocal fold tissue. Now the actual effect of the additive lesion on vocal pitch becomes questionable, and the pitch level of the patient may be relatively unaffected or even increase. The point being made is that the interaction of the physical determinants of vocal frequency is a complex one, and the possibility of highly variable effects on vocal pitch should be kept in mind as we look at some of the possible effects of various disordered states.

Mass Lesions and Distributed Tissue Change

Lesions (e.g., nodules, polyps, tumors) or added mass (e.g., edema) that develop on or within the vocal fold tissue may have several variable effects on the pitch of the voice. A lowering of the habitual pitch may occur secondary to vocal fold trauma and/or irritation due to increased mass of the vocal folds (e.g., as in cases of edema and mass lesion development).[13,40,41] In contrast, habitual pitch may be increased because of increased stiffness of the fold(s) and compensatory increased laryngeal tension, or be unaffected by the presence of laryngeal tissue changes.[1,42] The presence of mass lesion(s) may also result in increased pitch variability (e.g., diplophonia, pitch breaks) because of altered vibratory characteristics.[5] In addition, monopitch and decreased total pitch range may be observed because of restricted range of lengthening/tensing motion within the vocal folds.[13]

Smoking is one of the most common forms of vocal abuse and is associated with the development of additive mass conditions such as chronic edema, precancerous conditions such as leukoplakia, and laryngeal carcinomas. Substantial lowering of habitual pitch is a frequent effect of Reinke's edema, a condition in which fluid is retained within the spaces between the mucosal cover and the various layers of the lamina propria, resulting in a distension of the mucosal layer, a thickening of the vocal folds and the connective tissue, and an overall increase in vocal fold mass. In addition, increased pitch variability during sustained voicing and a reduction in total pitch range have also been observed.[43,44]

Neurological Disturbance

Damage to the neuromotor system because of disease or trauma may result in dysarthrias. Dysarthric effects on the pitch characteristics of the voice have been described by a number of sources.[5,12,13,40,45,46] A lowering of the habitual pitch may be observed in hypotonic states (e.g., flaccidity) versus a possible raising of vocal pitch level in hypertonic states (e.g., spasticity). In addition, pitch range and variability may also be affected in dysarthria, with monopitch and restricted pitch range reported in ataxia and Parkinson's disease,[45,47,48] superior laryngeal nerve disruption,[27] and vocal fold paralysis.[13] In contrast, excessive pitch variability has been reported in conditions in which hypertonicity, lack of coordination of muscular activity, or in which sudden, uncontrolled muscular contractions may occur (e.g., spasticity, ataxia, and hyperkinetic states). Rhythmic variations in pitch (particularly noticeable during a sustained vowel production) are characteristic of vocal tremor associated with motor disruptions such as ataxia and spasmodic dysphonia (often acknowledged as a type of focal dystonia and hyperkinetic state).

Muscle Tension Dysphonias/Hyperfunctional Voice

Increased muscle tension within the intrinsic or extrinsic vocal musculature may result in changes in vocal pitch level. Increased laryngeal muscle tension may be of functional or organic origin (e.g., due to underlying organic neurological disturbance such as spasticity). In functional cases, the increased tension may occur because of factors such as emotional stress (e.g., someone trying to speak when they are about to cry will characteristically experience tension in the laryngeal region and increased pitch level), habitual use of an inappropriate pitch level, muscular compensation during periods of vocal fatigue, or retained compensatory activity after some previous organic disturbance (e.g., laryngitis). Although increased pitch is most commonly associated with excessive tension, decreased pitch may also be observed in this condition, possibly due to increased tension being localized to the thyroarytenoid/vocalis muscle(s), resulting in shorter, more massive folds, and/or (2) compression of the vocal folds due to anterior-posterior squeezing of the larynx.[49]

Puberphonia/Mutational Falsetto

As males move from childhood to adulthood via puberty, a substantial lowering of the pitch of the voice is generally observed. In some cases, disturbed mutation may occur in which the male individual retains a childlike, higher pitched voice after puberty, resulting in a voice versus age mismatch and pitch abnormality. Luchsinger and Arnold classified disturbed mutation in boys into three clinical forms: (1) delayed mutation, (2) prolonged mutation, and (3) incomplete mutation. In all three forms, the voice is characterized by high pitch, chronic hoarseness, and pitch breaks.[50] The continued use of the high pitch level of childhood is called *mutational falsetto* or *puberphonia*.[12] Cases of puberphonia are often confirmed by the presence of normally developing secondary sex characteristics, an otherwise normal speech/vocal mechanism, and the demonstrated capability to produce the expected lower pitch level.[25] Although puberphonia/mutational falsetto is most commonly reported for male patients, the condition may also affect females. However, the pitch abnormality in females may be less noticeable compared with the male condition, because the female voice does not undergo as drastic a shift in pitch level as the male voice.

Psychological Disorders

Emotional expressiveness (i.e., *affect*) is certainly communicated via the pitch of the voice. Severe reduction in emotional expressiveness (i.e., *flat affect*) has been noted in psychological states such as schizophrenia and severe clinical depression, resulting in substantially reduced pitch variability and monotone/monopitch voice.[40,51]

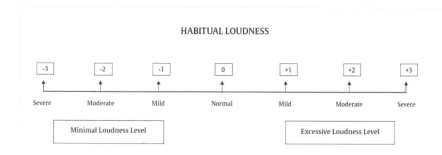

Fig. 3.5 Example scale for the auditory-perceptual rating of habitual loudness.

Deafness/Hearing Impairment

The hearing mechanism plays an important role in acquiring volitional control over various parameters of phonation, including the control of the pitch characteristics of the voice. Monsen reported that the type of intonation contour used by the hearing-impaired individuals appeared to be a key characteristic in differentiating hearing impaired from normal individuals and in differentiating better from poorer deaf speakers, with some hearing-impaired individuals observed to produce flat intonation patterns and others producing highly variable intonation during speech.[23] Monsen indicated that the deviant intonation patterns observed may be due to poor control over respiratory supply and vocal fold tension.

3.4.10 Loudness

A sound wave is typically produced due to disturbances in the air that are received and interpreted by the hearing mechanism. **Loudness** is the perceptual attribute that corresponds to the magnitude of these pressure disturbances, and most of us are able to easily distinguish between varying degrees of quieter and louder sounds.[42] As with the perceptual characteristic of pitch, the perception and categorization of differences in vocal loudness may help us develop hypotheses about the underlying phonatory mechanism, as loudness relates not only to the degree of respiratory force but also to the amplitude of vocal fold vibration.[52] In addition, vocal loudness is affected by (1) glottal resistance to the expiratory airstream and (2) the rate of airflow change at the moment of vocal fold closure.[12] Therefore, the evaluation of vocal loudness is essential because it provides us with information about the coordination between phonatory and respiratory mechanisms.[1] The perceptual assessment of loudness generally focuses on the same three parameters that were used in pitch evaluation: (1) habitual loudness, (2) loudness variability, and (3) loudness range.

Habitual Loudness

Habitual loudness is analogous to the most commonly used loudness or average loudness level. No single loudness level would be considered normal. Instead, the habitual loudness level should be appropriate for the speaking situation. Prater and Swift indicated that the habitual loudness level should be loud enough to be heard over background noise but not be so loud that it brings discomfort or distraction to the listener.[11] Abnormal habitual loudness level is found in speakers who use vocal loudness/intensity levels conspicuously higher or lower than typical for a particular speaking situation.[6]

Because the appropriate level of vocal loudness differs depending on the situation and environment in which voice is to be used, it has been suggested that the clinician should evaluate the habitual vocal loudness under various conditions such as in background noise or at different proximities (e.g., from a conversational distance [1–3 ft] vs. 10–15 ft away).[11] Once a judgment is made regarding the patient's habitual loudness level, the result may be reported using a seven-point EAI scale as described by Awan (▶ Fig. 3.5).[1]

In the scale represented in ▶ Fig. 3.5, the central point is zero (i.e., no substantial difference from normal expectations), with ratings of excessively loud voice (positive numbers) and ratings of excessively low vocal loudness (negative numbers) rated on either side of the normal expectation point. Definitions for mild, moderate, and severe are the same as those previously presented. Alternatively, habitual loudness may be rated using the loudness scale of the CAPE-V form, with the nature of the abnormality (e.g., abnormally high vs. low) described by the clinician and the severity of the disruption identified on a 100-mm VAS as previously described for habitual pitch.

Loudness Variability

Normal stress/syllabic patterns require the use of loudness variability. A stressed word or syllable is generally produced with an increase in perceived loudness. Loudness variations are an important aspect of *prosody*, the physical attributes of speech that are used to alter or accentuate the linguistic nature of an utterance. When a patient speaks with little or no fluctuation in loudness, the result may be a "boring, colorless voice."[11] This type of voice has been referred to as *monotone*[11] or as displaying *monoloudness*[12] and may reflect the personality characteristics of the speaker or some underlying disruption with the control of vocal loudness.

In addition to loudness variations as applied to suprasegmentals, *loudness instability* is also an aspect of variability that must be attended to by the clinician. Abrupt changes in loudness may be observed during *phonation breaks*, which are periods in which the vocal folds cease to vibrate during situations of intended voicing. In *vocal tremor*, rhythmic variations in loudness (as well as pitch) are observed, particularly during the production of sustained vowels. In addition, vocal loudness should be controlled throughout an utterance and not decrease noticeably at the end of a sentence.

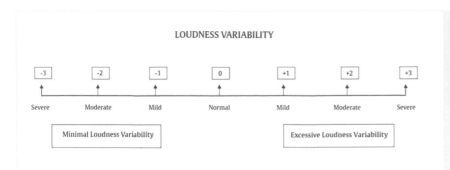

Fig. 3.6 Example scale for the auditory-perceptual rating of loudness variability.

Loudness variability may be rated on a seven-point equal-interval scale as described by Awan, in which the central point of the scale is rated as "0" (i.e., no substantial difference from normal expectations), and ratings of increased loudness variability are given positive ratings and reduced loudness variability negative ratings (▶ Fig. 3.6).[1] Definitions for mild, moderate, and severe are those presented previously in this chapter. The clinician should note the type of sample that the description of loudness variability pertains to, with ratings of loudness variability as used during prosodic patterns obtained from continuous speech samples versus the ability to maintain a steady loudness level observed during a sustained vowel sample.

The severity of the observed loudness variability dysfunction may also be communicated using the loudness scale found in the CAPE-V form, and could be labeled as "low/reduced loudness variability" or "high/excessive loudness variability."

Loudness Range

The *loudness range* (a.k.a, *dynamic range*), from minimal to maximal levels, is also an important aspect of loudness evaluation.[5] The assessment of loudness range is believed to be an essential aspect of vocal evaluation because voice production at different loudness levels assesses the function and interaction of all components (respiratory, laryngeal, and supralaryngeal/articulatory) of the speech mechanism. It is generally considered that vocal dysfunction will reduce the available loudness/intensity range.[52] Andrews stated that observations of voice characteristics such as the presence of voice/phonation breaks and quality changes at different levels should be noted during the evaluation of loudness range.[3]

3.4.11 Vocal Loudness in Normal versus Disordered Individuals

As with vocal pitch, characteristics such as age, gender, and body stature may have a substantial effect on the loudness of the voice. Normal vocal loudness is particularly related to respiratory driving forces and should be adequate enough that the voice may be heard over background noise and provide the capability to vary loudness for various situations (e.g., quiet, confidential voice to loud singing or shouting).[1]

Habitual loudness and the capability to vary vocal loudness are expected to change throughout the lifespan. Because of their smaller respiratory capacities, it may be expected that the vocal loudness level of the childhood voice would be somewhat lower than that observed in adulthood and/or that children may have

to expend more respiratory effort to achieve the same loudness level as adults.[53] During adolescence, dynamic range expands due to increases in physical stature and increased respiratory capacity.[54] A review of research studies dealing with the effects of advanced age on loudness of the voice is somewhat ambiguous. While some reports have indicated that overall vocal loudness level and total dynamic range may be restricted in elderly persons,[55,56] others have concluded that laryngeal senescence in healthy persons may not be significant enough to affect phonatory parameters such as vocal loudness level.[53]

When considering the disordered voice, it is clear that a variety of voice disorders that affect respiratory and/or laryngeal valving capability may adversely affect vocal loudness and/or dynamic range.

Mass Lesions and Distributed Tissue Change

Several authors have stated that reduced speaking loudness and reduced dynamic range may accompany mass lesions of the vocal folds and associated laryngeal inefficiency.[11,13,40] Although the patient may be observed to have decreased vocal loudness, the clinician should consider that many mass lesions (e.g., vocal nodules and polyps) are a consequence of vocal abuse in which excessive loudness/excessive effort was the habitual speaking style of the patient before the disorder developed.[5] While some patients with mass lesions will present with reduce loudness voices, others may only be able to initiate and maintain phonation while using louder rather than softer voices, and thus a louder voice that often fatigues as the day progresses may be observed.[17,40] In addition to changes in speaking loudness levels, uncontrolled loudness variability (e.g., loudness level "trailing off" at the end of a sentence), limited loudness variation (*monoloudness*), and variable loudness due to phonation breaks may also be observed.[5,27]

Neurological Disorders

Various neurologically based disorders may affect the ability to generate adequate respiratory force and/or build up subglottal pressure by means of laryngeal valving. The result may be disruptions in the ability to control habitual loudness levels and dynamic range. Several authors have stated that speaking loudness levels may be reduced in neurological disorders such as Parkinsonism and bulbar palsy (flaccidity).[11,26,27,45] The decreased vocal loudness observed in Parkinsonism has been attributed to bowing of the vocal folds or other forms of glottal incompetence in combination with reduced expiratory volumes for speech secondary to limited thoracic excursion and difficulty coordinating respiratory and laryngeal systems.[57] In contrast, certain neurological conditions (e.g., spasticity, dystonias, multiple sclerosis) may result in inappropriately loud "booming" voices due to respiratory and/or vocal hyperfunction.[5,11,45]

An inability to vary loudness during typical prosodic patterns may also be observed in a variety of neurological conditions. Reduced loudness variability is often referred to as *monoloudness* and was identified by Darley et al as one of the primary deviant speech dimensions in spastic, ataxic, and both hypokinetic and hyperkinetic dysarthrias.[45] In contrast, excessive variations in loudness level may be observed in certain hyperkinetic states (e.g., choreas, dystonias, and vocal tremor).[40,45]

Muscle Tension Dysphonias/Hyperfunctional Voice

The presence of excessive tension in the vocal musculature and/or excessive use of the voice may have variable effects on vocal loudness. As previously stated, many hyperfunctional voices initially present with excessive loudness levels during speech, followed by periods of reduced vocal loudness as a result of vocal fatigue. In addition, dynamic range may be reduced in cases of excessive tension and elevated larynx.[40]

Psychologically Based Voice Disorders

Vocal loudness may be reduced in patients with psychological disorders and personality disturbances such as inferiority complex and withdrawal.[11,13,26] In addition, monoloudness may be observed in cases of depression.[5,11,26,40]

Hearing Impairment/Deafness

Several authors have indicated that acquired hearing impairment may result in changes in habitual loudness levels,[11,26,40] with the observed vocal loudness level related to the type and severity of hearing loss experienced by the patient.[41] In sensorineural losses, both air and bone conductions are detrimentally affected, with some patients tending toward an abnormally loud voice as compensation. In contrast, a conductive loss may result in a reduced loudness, abnormally soft voice, since the patient may "hear" their own voice quite well (because of adequate bone conduction) and therefore believes that they are producing an acceptable vocal loudness when the voice is actually too quiet for the speaking situation.

3.4.12 Duration

The **duration** of a sound deals with the perception of how long in time the sound is sustained. Most of us would easily be able to distinguish between a "short" tone and a "long" tone. During voice production, whether during continuous speech or sustained vowel production (e.g., in singing), normal phonatory function may be sustained briefly (e.g., only during the brief central vowel production in single word production of "coat") or for long duration (e.g., in longer **phrases** or singing **passages**). These capabilities reflect the precisely coordinated function of the respiratory and phonatory mechanisms. In particular, to extend the duration of phonatory activity during speech production or singing, the speaker must be able to generate an increase

in inspiratory air (slight to substantial depending on the intended duration of production); control the outgoing (expiratory) airstream using *checking action* (activity in which inspiratory muscle forces are used to counteract or "check" passive expiratory forces[58]); and adduct and approximate the vocal folds at the midline of the glottis in coordination with the outgoing airstream to generate the subglottal pressure required to put the vocal folds into vibration. However, if the ability to generate and control the outgoing airstream is disrupted, the following noticeable effects on voice and speech production may be observed:

- An inability to put the vocal folds into vibration, resulting in aphonia or intermittently aphonic productions.
- An inability to maintain appropriate duration of respiratory/phonatory function, resulting in inappropriate phrase length and inappropriate breath groups. The patient needs to breathe (inspire) more frequently, resulting in fewer words or syllables per breath groups (inappropriately short utterances) and/or inappropriate breath groups (i.e., pauses for inspiration occur at illogical places in the utterance).
- Effortful speech and vocal strain as a result of excessive muscular force to compensate for poor respiratory/phonatory control and function. In the absence of adequate respiratory support, the patient attempts to build subglottal pressure and sustain voicing by increased musculoskeletal tension and hyperfunctional voice. For those who continue speaking on a limited expiratory supply, speaking on residual air often leaves the listener with the impression of a strained voice quality.
- Eventual fatigue.

Beyond observing our patient in conversational speech, it has been suggested that one way in which the clinician can focus on the patient's ability to control and coordinate expiratory and phonatory function is by having the patient read as much of a standard passage as possible on one breath at a typical reading rate governed by a metronome beat (**normal adult speaking rate is approximately 150–200 words per minute or approximately 3–5 syllables per second**).[46] The number of words and the length of time (in seconds) that the patient is able to read on the single breath should be recorded.[11] In addition to number of words and sample time, Prater and Swift also stated that (1) the respiratory pattern and (2) the degree of phonatory control (hypofunctional, hyperfunctional, etc.) should be noted during the task. *Respiratory pattern* refers to one of three commonly observed forms of breathing patterns observed during speech/voice production:

Thoracic Breathing

This type of breathing pattern is characterized by expansion of the midthoracic region (chest expansion). This is a commonly used breathing pattern that should be adequate to support most speaking situations.

Diaphragmatic-Abdominal Breathing

Diaphragmatic-abdominal breathing is a mechanically efficient form of breathing that allows for the greatest exchange of air during the respiratory cycle.[11] In this breathing pattern, thoracic enlargement is achieved by expansion of the lower thoracic and abdominal cavities during inspiration with relatively little noticeable upper chest movement.[59] The breathing pattern is particularly useful for those who make heavy demands on the respiratory system for singing, acting, etc., and may also be used as a voice treatment exercise used to encourage efficiency of vocal function.

Clavicular Breathing

In otherwise healthy individuals, this type of breathing pattern should be avoided as it results in a weak, shallow inspiration and, therefore, poor respiratory support for speech and voice. This type of breathing pattern mainly uses the secondary/accessory muscles of respiration (upper thoracic and neck muscles such as the scalenes and the sternocleidomastoid) to elevate the shoulders and upper chest during inspiration.[13] In addition, because many of these muscles course in the vicinity of the larynx, overuse of these muscles may effect an increase in laryngeal tension and may be a component of hyperfunctional voice use.[5,11]

As stated, observations of durational control during speech/voicing may be obtained from conversational speech, as well as from a standard reading. In particular, the clinician should rate utterance length. The durational characteristics of the utterance may be communicated on a seven-point scale as suggested by Awan.[1] Note that in this particular scale (▶ Fig. 3.7), the central point of the scale is zero (i.e., no substantial difference from normal expectations), with positive numbered ratings used for the observation of utterance duration beyond the point of expected respiratory replenishment, and negative numbered ratings used for the observation of inappropriately short breath groups. Definitions for mild, moderate, and severe are the same as previously presented. In addition to noting the length of utterance in relation to expected point of inspiration, the clinician should also note perceptions of tension/effort (often observed on the positive side of the scale) and signs of laryngeal hypofunction (often observed on the negative side of the scale [e.g., breathy voice]). *Inhalatory stridor* (excessive noise during inspiration)[11] is a particularly important observation, because it is associated with narrowing/stenosis of the airway.[12] While the CAPE-V does not include a specific rating scale for the durational aspects of voice, there are two blank scales provided that could be utilized for this rating.

3.4.13 Control of Voicing Duration in Normal versus Disordered Individuals

Typical speakers are able to produce multiple words easily on one breath without evident strain or effort (e.g., the sentence "The rainbow is a division of white light into many beautiful colors" is commonly produced on a single breath and is composed of 20 syllables/12 words). However, patients who present with disruptions of respiratory capacity or control maybe observed to have inappropriately short breath or may have to strain to complete an utterance without replenishing the air supply. The following are examples of potential patient groups who may have difficulty controlling the duration of voicing during speech production:

Patients with Reduced Respiratory Capacities

The following patient groups may have reduced respiratory capacities that influence their ability to sustain speech/voice production[1,46]: (1) patients with pulmonary diseases such as severe asthma, emphysema, and tuberculosis that increase airway resistance; (2) patients with diseases such as asbestosis, pneumonia, and lung cancer that reduce the elasticity and compliance of the lungs and chest wall; (3) patients who may be using inefficient breathing patterns (shallow breathing or clavicular breathing); (4) patients with neuromuscular disorders may also present with reduced respiratory capacity (e.g., shallow inhalations, poor respiratory postures, uncoordinated inspiratory-expiratory patterns, and rigidity of the respiratory musculature may also result in reduced capacity in all major groups of dysarthria).

Mass Lesions and Distributed Tissue Change

Control of airflow from the lungs occurs primarily at the glottis via vocal fold contact during voicing. Hypoadduction of the folds (i.e., reduced vocal fold contact during voicing) is associated with breathy voice quality, rapid expenditure of air, short breath groups, and decreased duration of sustained vowel productions.[11,27] Many pathological conditions involving mass lesion development result in ineffective vocal fold closure during voicing, subsequent air escape (i.e., increased mean airflow rate) and possible difficulty in controlling the duration of voicing.

Neurological Disorders

Those neurological disorders resulting in hypoadduction and hypofunctional voice (e.g., cases of vocal fold paralysis) and/or insufficient respiratory function and/or incoordination of inspiratory/expiratory function may be expected to have short breath groups and decreased duration of sustained vowel productions. It is also possible that patients who show incoordination of inspiratory/expiratory function may also prolong speech and voice for too long without replenishing the air supply, resulting in strained and effortful voice production.

Fig. 3.7 Example scale for the auditory-perceptual rating of control of voicing duration.

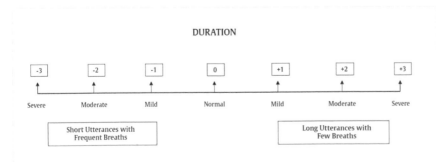

3.4.14 Quality

Characterization of voice *quality* is one of the key facets of perceptual assessment of the voice and an integral aspect of any voice evaluation. The term *quality* may be defined simply as a distinguishing characteristic. When used to describe the human voice, we can think of *quality* as referring to the characteristic of a voice that distinguishes it from other voices of similar pitch, loudness, and duration. In musical terms, quality is somewhat analogous to *timbre*. Voice quality is one of the means by which we are able to distinguish between people of similar age and gender, even though they may be speaking with similar pitch and loudness. Quality is also one of the key parameters we will use to perceptually discriminate the normal from the disordered voice. We will see that, acoustically, vocal quality disruptions have been associated with disturbance or *perturbation* to the highly periodic vibration of the vocal folds during voiced contexts such as sustained vowel productions. In addition, vocal quality disruptions have also been associated with changes to the spectral characteristics of the acoustic voice waveform.

While a wide variety of terms have been used in the voice literature to describe dysphonic voice qualities (e.g., *creaky, tense, unstable, lax, guttural, husky*), several terms have been consistently used to describe the voice qualities often observed in disordered voice.

Breathiness

The *breathy* voice is commonly perceived as a *whispery* or *airy* voice. Although we will discuss breathiness as a common attribute of disordered voices, a slight amount of breathy voice may be observed in the normal female voice and may be a social marker of female gender emulated by others.[60,61] In addition, softer, gentle voices are often produced with a breathy component and may be perceived as having a pleasant quality. Physiologically, the term *breathiness* is associated with *hypoadduction* of the vocal folds (i.e., lack of vocal fold adduction or closure) and refers to the audible detection of airflow through the glottis during phonation (i.e., the escaping airflow is often combined with vocal fold vibration). At its extreme, the breathy voice becomes similar to a whisper in which the vocal folds cease to vibrate and only the aperiodic/noise of turbulent, escaping air remains. In these instances, the attempted voice production is referred to as *aphonia*.

Roughness

Unlike the breathy voice, the *rough* voice is typically perceived as unpleasant, and has been described in terms such as *coarse, gravelly,* and *low-pitched noise*. Rough voices are also associated with *diplophonia* in which two different pitches are produced simultaneously. Physiologically, the rough voice is often associated with irregularity of vocal fold vibration, and this irregular vibration tends to result in low-frequency noise components[8,62,63] and alternating glottal periods that are slightly different in period or shape.[23]

Hoarseness

A number of authors have concluded that hoarseness is probably the most common term used by laypersons and professionals alike to describe disordered voice.[1,13] However, to be specific, the term *hoarseness* is used to describe a voice that has both breathy and rough qualities simultaneously. Therefore, hoarseness originates from a combination of irregularity of vocal fold vibration and turbulent airflow through the glottis.[1,64] This voice quality may arise, for example, in a patient with a unilateral vocal fold lesion that results in irregular vibration (*roughness*) and also prevents the vocal folds from effectively adducting (*breathiness*). In some cases, one of the combined characteristics will predominate, resulting in *breathy hoarseness or rough hoarseness*. In addition, the hoarse voice may also be characterized as *dry* versus *wet*, in which *wet hoarseness* is related to the presence of secretions at the vocal fold level.[1,13]

Harshness

The harsh voice is also commonly perceived as an unpleasant voice and associated with terms such as *strident* and *rasping*.[62,65,66] In terms of underlying physiology, the harsh voice is often associated with *hyperadduction* (i.e., excessive vocal fold adduction or closure) of the vocal folds and/or supraglottal vocal tract. Acoustically, harsh voices tend to have high-frequency noise.

Strain

The strained voice is one which is associated with the impression of vocal effort and a hyperfunctional state of phonation.[8,17] Strained voices are also often observed to be higher pitched. Vocal effort and strain may be observed in both hypoadductive and hyperadductive states if the speaker uses increased muscular force and tension in the attempt to produce phonation, and is often associated with voice produced with excessive supraglottal constriction.

Instability

This term refers to fluctuation in voice quality over time.[8,16] Rather than a consistent disruption, the vocal quality disruption in the unstable voice is *intermittent* (e.g., intermittent breathiness or roughness) and may occur only during certain forms of voice use (e.g., louder voice production). Andrews also uses the term instability in describing tremor, which occurs intermittently on vowels and during sentences versus constant occurrences of the deviation.[40]

The quality of the voice may be rated on a seven-point interval scale as described by Awan (► Fig. 3.8). Commonly observed voice quality disruptions of breathiness, hoarseness, and roughness may be identified at the top of the scale, and the severity terminologies (mild, moderate, and severe) are similar to that previously provided in this chapter.

Alternatively, the severity of commonly observed dysphonic quality types may be communicated using the scales for roughness, breathiness, and strain found in the CAPE-V form. A section labeled "Additional features" provides a space in which the clinician may specifically describe examples of vocal quality disruption such as asthenia (weak voice), wet/gurgly voice, and diplophonia (often associated with the perception of roughness).

3.4.15 Vocal Quality in Normal versus Disordered Individuals

As with previous vocal parameters such as pitch and loudness, the quality of the normal voice lies on a continuum that may

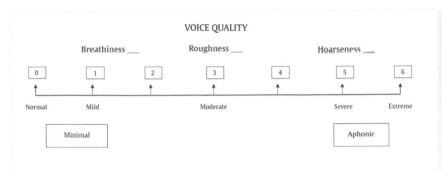

Fig. 3.8 Example scale for the auditory-perceptual rating of vocal quality.

range from excellent (i.e., one that appears to have professional training and good vocal tract excitement) to one that is adequate with no apparent pathology.[63] Though we generally expect that normal/typical voices do not have any distracting levels of characteristics such as breathiness, hoarseness, roughness, or strain, possible subtle differences in the anatomy and/or physiology of the sexes or functional changes in the larynx and general sensorimotor deficits with increased age may produce variations in voice quality even in otherwise vocally healthy individuals. For example, there has been some indication that perceived voice quality may be affected by the sex of the individual. Extremely low-pitch voice in some males may occasionally be perceived as rough,[67,68] while perceived breathiness in the female voice may be an important gender marker.[60,61] In addition, the senescent voice may be perceived as hoarse, breathy, "tense," or "crackly."[32,39,69] As with the previous discussion of possible changes in pitch with senescence, voice quality deviation is not a necessary characteristic feature of aging, and heterogeneity of the aging process as it affects voice function is to be expected.

Of course, voice quality deviations are often a key characteristic of dysphonia. The following are examples of potential patient groups that have been observed to frequently present with various types of voice quality disturbances:

Mass Lesions and Distributed Tissue Change

Changes in the characteristics of the vocal fold tissues (e.g., by means of a pathological lesion or from edema) may have substantial effects on phonation: (1) the lesion may cause irregular vocal fold vibration (particularly if the lesion or tissue change is unilateral or asymmetric) associated with perceived roughness and/or (2) the presence of lesion or tissue change may affect the ability to adequately approximate the vocal folds during phonation, resulting in excessive airflow and perceived breathiness. If both rough and breathy characteristics are produced simultaneously, the result will be a hoarse voice quality. Therefore, a wide variety of different forms of mass lesion and/or tissue change may be associated with breathiness, roughness, or hoarseness including irregularities of the vocal fold margins, mass lesions (e.g., nodules, polyps), and vocal fold edema.

When the presence of mass lesions or tissue change results in glottal incompetence, it may be expected that the degree of perceived breathiness will be related to the degree of incomplete vocal fold closure. However, the degree of breathiness may also be influenced by the loudness of voice production (increased breathiness with decreased loudness of phonation) or by laryngeal conditions that may result in increased turbulence in transglottal airflow.[40,52,70]

Neurological Disorders

Various dysarthric states have been described as being characterized by accompanying vocal quality disturbances, including upper motor neuron disorders such as spasticity (strained-strangled harshness); hypokinetic states such as Parkinsonism (rigidity in the laryngeal musculature may result in strained or harsh voice quality; vocal fold bowing may result in breathiness); hyperkinetic states such as chorea (uncontrolled contractions may result in harsh/strained-strangled quality, although sudden changes between harshness and breathiness/aphonia are also possible; severe tremors in focal dystonias such as spasmodic dysphonia may result in voice arrest); ataxia (harshness, hoarseness, and tremor have been described); and lower motor neuron disruptions resulting in flaccidity (breathiness, roughness, and hoarseness have all been described).[12,45,46]

Muscle Tension Dysphonias/Hyperfunctional Voice

In cases in which the patient uses excessive effort and muscular tension during voice production, hyperadduction of the vocal folds may result. The perceived voice quality in these cases is often strain or harshness. As with breathiness, the strained or harsh voice may be observed in a variety of voice disordered patients, including those with personality attributes and conflicts; pharyngeal and/or glottal constriction secondary to vocal abuse/misuse; neurological disorders such as spasticity and focal dystonia/spasmodic dysphonia; and those with poor respiratory support for voice production.[11,40,52,62] Hyperfunction and laryngeal rigidity may be combined with conditions such as vocal fatigue and *myasthenia larynges* (functional vocal fold bowing) to result in variable voice quality deviations (breathiness, roughness, and hoarseness).

Hearing Impairment/Deafness

The presence of moderate-to-severe hearing loss during the developmental acquisition of speech and voice may affect the ability to control normal vocal quality. Breathiness, diplophonia and roughness, and effortful "tense," "strained," or "metallic" voice have been noted as possible vocal quality disruptions in a number of hearing-impaired patients.[23,71]

3.4.16 Limitations of Perceptual Evaluation of Voice

Though the importance and necessity of perceptual description of the voice cannot be overstated, the clinician should be aware of a number of factors that are involved with the perceptual assessment of the voice that may make the process prone to validity and reliability issues[1,16]:

1. Perceptual assessment of the voice appears to be affected by problems of scale validity and reliability.
2. Perceptual assessment does not necessarily provide an awareness of the physiological details that result in the acoustic product.
3. Perceptual quality may be difficult to characterize and communicate via quantified results and, therefore, may not be as credible as numerical test procedures. In this regard, results of perceptual assessment may not be sufficient for medicolegal purposes.

3.5 Self-perception of Voice Handicap

While it is essential that we describe the auditory-perceptual characteristics of the patient's voice, it is also important that we also gauge the patent's perception of how the possible vocal dysfunction may be affecting their daily lives. The manner and degree in which a voice disorder affects the patient may provide an indication of (1) the patient's self-awareness of the presence of disorder, (2) the possible level of stress and anxiety on the patient, and (3) the potential degree of patient motivation toward following through on treatment recommendations.

Measures of phonatory function such as listener ratings of dysphonia severity, acoustic, and aerodynamic measures are considered *impairment*-level measures.[72] In contrast, *disability* refers to the impact on performance due to the impairment, and *handicap* is the impact of the impairment or disability on social, environmental, or economic functioning. As an example, if a schoolteacher with unilateral vocal fold paralysis cannot speak loudly enough to be heard in the classroom, the teacher could be considered to have a form of disability. If the same teacher is forced to leave the teaching profession because of an inability to project the voice, the occupational, economic, and social effects are regarded as handicaps. Clearly, documenting these forms of disability and handicap can be useful in understanding the full extent of how vocal dysfunction affects the patient.

The increased diagnostic emphasis on better understanding and assessing the impact of a voice disorder on an individual's quality of life has led to the development of a number of patient-based instruments. including the **Voice Handicap Index**[73] (VHI), **Voice-Related Quality of Life**[74] (V-RQOL), the **Voice Activity and Participation Profile**,[75] and the **Voice Symptom Scale**.[76] Branski et al provided a complete review of these instruments and their development.[77] Of these instruments, the VHI is one of the most studied and popular (▶ Fig. 3.9).[73] The VHI is a psychometrically validated tool developed for the measurement of the psychosocial handicapping effects of voice disorders. According to the test authors, the VHI can be used to assess the patient's judgment about the relative impact of their voice disorder on daily activities and

also be used as a component of measuring the functional outcomes of behavioral, medical, and/or surgical treatments of voice disorders. The VHI is a questionnaire designed to subjectively measure the patient's degree of voice handicap. This instrument asks respondents to rate the degree to which their quality of life is affected by their voice disorder by selecting a number on a severity scale graded from 0 to 4 (never to always) for each item on the questionnaire. The VHI contains 30 total items including 10 items in each of three domains: emotional, physical, and functional handicap. Possible scores range from 0 to 120, with a score of 120 being the most severely handicapped.

A number of studies have reported on VHI cutoff scores that may be used to categorize patients with and without substantial degrees of voice handicap:

- Behrman et al[78]: These authors obtained VHI data based from 100 normal adults (50 females and 50 males) and reported a mean VHI score of 9.3 (SD = 11.2, range: 0–19). The 95% confidence interval was 2.2, which indicated that 95% of the sample would have a mean between 7.1 and 11.5. These authors suggested that the upper limit of 11.5 may be used as a VHI cutoff score.
- Niebudek-Bogusz et al[79]: These authors reported on VHI scores in 165 voice disordered patients (147 females and 18 males) and 65 individuals with normal voice (54 females and 11 males). A VHI cutoff score of 12 (98% sensitivity and 95% specificity) was observed to effectively categorize normal versus disordered cases.
- Moradi et al[80]: VHI scores in 80 patients with dysphonia (40 males and 40 females) and 80 individuals without voice disorders (40 males and 40 females) were examined. A VHI score of 14.5 was reported to identify existence versus nonexistence of voice disorders (92% sensitivity and 95% specificity).

The VHI and other self-report symptom questionnaires have been useful in clinical situations to monitor progression of disorders and changes resulting from interventions.[81] Several research studies have noted a decline on the VHI scores following treatment, suggesting that intervention improves how patients view their quality and functioning of life.[59,82,83]

3.5.1 The Role of Quality of Life/Handicap Scales versus Auditory-Perceptual Evaluation of Voice

Self-perception scales like the *VHI* help assess quality of life and the impact of the impairment or disability on social, environmental, or economic functioning. In contrast, auditory-perceptual evaluation of voice is an impairment-level measure that assesses the specific impact of a disease/disorder on bodily function. The practitioner should be aware that, in clinical practice, it is not uncommon for two patients with similar levels of impairment to perceive different levels of handicap or vice versa. As an example, the degree of handicap experienced by someone with a breathy voice secondary to vocal nodules who uses their voice as the primary tool of trade (e.g., teacher, actor, clergy, broadcaster, politician, salesperson) likely differs substantially from a nonprofessional voice user even though these two individuals may share similar levels of impairment (as determined by auditory-perceptual ratings of voice type

Name_____ Date_____

Voice Handicap Index (VHI)
(Jacobson, Johnson, Grywalski, *et al.*)

Instructions: These are statements that many people have used to describe their voices and the effects of their voices on their lives. Check the response that indicates how frequently you have the same experience.

	Never	Almost Never	Sometimes	Almost Always	Always
F1. My voice makes it difficult for people to hear me.					
P2. I run out of air when I talk					
F3. People have difficulty understanding me in a noisy room					
P4. The sound of my voice varies throughout the day.					
F5. My family has difficulty hearing me when I call them throughout the house.					
F6. I use the phone less often than I would like.					
E7. I'm tense when talking with others because of my voice.					
F8. I tend to avoid groups of people because of my voice.					
E9. People seem irritated with my voice.					
P10. People ask, "What's wrong with your voice?"					
F11. I speak with friends, neighbors, or relatives less often because of my voice.					
F12. People ask me to repeat myself when speaking face-toface.					
P13. My voice sounds creaky and dry.					

Fig. 3.9 Example of the Voice Handicap Index (VHI) rating scale. Scoring rubric is (Never = 0; Almost Never = 1; Sometimes = 2; Almost Always = 3; Always = 4). Question prefixes stand for domains of functional (F), physical (P), and emotional (E).

	Never	Almost Never	Sometimes	Almost Always	Always
P 14. I feel as though I have to strain to produce voice					
E15. I find other people don't understand my voice problem.					
F16. My voice difficulties restrict my personal and social life.					
P17. The clarity of my voice is unpredictable.					
P18. I try to change my voice to sound different.					
F19. I feel left out of conversations because of my voice.					
P20. I use a great deal of effort to speak.					
P21. My voice is worse in the evening.					
F22. My voice problem causes me to lose income.					
E23. My voice problem upsets me.					
E24. I am less out-going because of my voice problem.					
E25. My voice makes me feel handicapped.					
P26. My voice "gives out" on me in the middle of speaking.					
E27. I feel annoyed when people ask me to repeat.					
E28. I feel embarrassed when people ask me to repeat.					
E29. My voice makes me feel incompetent.					
E30. I'm ashamed of my voice problem.					

****

P_____F_____E_____   Total_____

(Never = 0 points; Almost Never = 1 point; Sometimes = 2 points; Almost Always = 3 points; Always = 4 points)

Fig. 3.9 (Continued)

and severity). This is because impairment-level measures such as auditory-perceptual ratings of voice do not consider the context of the person who suffers with the voice disorder, and relatively small changes (either negative or positive) in voice can have significant effects on quality of life depending on personal factors (and vice versa). Therefore, it should not be surprising that decontextualized, impairment-level descriptions and measures of voice may not necessarily correlate well with quality-of-life measures like the VHI. Instead, impairment-level measures (such as auditory-perceptual ratings of voice, as well as instrumental evaluation methods to be discussed in subsequent chapters) and quality-of-life measure such as the VHI should be seen as providing relatively unique, meaningful, and complementary information that helps form the voice diagnostic protocol and result in a complete profile of this patient's vocal function.[72]

3.6 Conclusion

This chapter has summarized the basic process for behavioral and qualitative assessment of voice, an essential part of a comprehensive voice diagnostic protocol. The behavioral and qualitative assessment included (1) information from previous healthcare assessments, (2) client history information, (3) auditory-perceptual assessments of vocal function, and (4) self-assessments of vocal handicap. We have provided the reader with clinical expectations for these behavioral and qualitative assessments in healthy and impaired populations.

A complete voice diagnostic protocol includes additional steps that utilize instrumentation to perform quantitative assessments of vocal function. The next chapter will review the rationale and procedures for conducting the acoustic assessment of voice. Key concepts associated with acoustic instrumentation, recording procedures, and analysis of evidence-based acoustic measures correlating with perceptions of dysphonia will be discussed. In particular, we will describe the relationship between acoustic measurements and underlying physiology in normal and impaired populations specific to domains of frequency, intensity, and voice quality.

Clinical Case Study: Vocal Nodules

Mrs. Granger is a 31-year-old woman who has experienced dysphonia for 8 months. Her current symptoms began to form gradually after spending the summer as a vocal coach at a singing camp. The camp required heavy vocal demands on a daily basis including singing and loud speaking. Over the past 2 weeks of the camp, she noticed a sudden onset of a change in her voice (it started one morning and then got worse over the next 2 weeks), which she characterized as a lower speaking pitch, a loss of her upper frequency range when singing, and vocal fatigue when speaking or singing for an extended amount of time. The problem has affected her job as a high school voice (singing) teacher, which requires her to work with individuals and small groups throughout the day. She reports that her voice quality is beginning to further deteriorate when speaking and singing, and that she is no longer able to hold notes in the upper part of her register.

She was evaluated by an otolaryngologist 3 weeks ago who diagnosed her with vocal nodules.

Mrs. Granger has a college degree in voice and she continued professional voice lessons after college for 3 years. Prior to the onset of the current problem, she participated in an amateur band on weekends performing contemporary music (pop, soft rock). Due to her problems, she has stopped performing. She has no history of voice problems prior to the current issues, is a nonsmoker, and drinks at least five glasses of water per day and two cups of green tea during the day, but no other caffeinated beverages. She is not currently taking any medications and has no priory history of surgeries.

Part 1
1. For purposes of differential diagnoses, what other questions would be informative to ask this patient?
2. Based on the patient's age, gender, and vocal use history, what clinical hypotheses would you develop with regard to the potential diagnosis (e.g., functional, organic, or neurological—and why)?
3. If the information above was obtained from the history portion of the voice evaluation, describe the subsequent process of voice evaluation—what will you be doing and why?

Part 2
Laryngeal videostroboscopy revealed a large unilateral polyp at the mid-membranous (anterior 1/3 to posterior 2/3 juncture) portion of the true vocal fold, with a contralateral reactive lesion. The polyp is broad based with prominent blood vessels surrounding it. The contralateral lesion appears edematous and translucent.

Study the following webpage:
http://www.voicemedicine.com/polyp.htm
1. Describe a theory which explains why polyps form.
2. What does it mean that a polyp is a "benign" laryngeal lesion?
3. Does the patient's description of the onset of her voice problem fit with the description of time-course for onset of polyps described on voicemedicine.com?
4. What is the recommended initial form of treatment for this lesion, and why?

Part 3
Read the following article:
   Nunes RB, Behlau M, Nunes MB, Paulino JG. Clinical diagnosis and histological analysis of vocal nodules and polyps. Braz J Otorhinolaryngol 2013;79(4):434–434.[84]
1. What is one explanation for why nodules are formed instead of polyps?
2. How does this explanation inform our understanding of why polyps might be more resistant to voice therapy than nodules?
3. Once you have confirmed the diagnosis, how might you present (explain) the treatment options to the patient based on the information you have learned from this case study?

Review the following case studies:
   http://voicedoctor.net/media/overdoer/central/polyps

3.7 Review Questions

1. Which of the following voice evaluation procedures is a *direct* form of evaluation?
   a) Voice Handicap Index.
   b) CAPE-V ratings of roughness, breathiness, and strain.
   c) Case history examination.
   d) Laryngeal stroboscopic examination.
   e) None of the above.

2. A voice is normal/typical if it does not deviate substantially from our internal gauge of parameters such as
   _____.
   a) Loudness.
   b) Quality.
   c) Pitch.
   d) Articulation.
   e) a, b, and c.

3. The voice clinician decides to go ahead with a treatment plan for vocal nodules even though, following further voice evaluation, the patient has no signs or symptoms obtained via case history and perceptual evaluation consistent with the diagnosis. This may be an example of _____.
   a) Diagnosis momentum.
   b) Anchoring bias.
   c) Confirmation bias.
   d) Premature closure.
   e) Availability bias.

4. Which of the following is associated with poor voice quality and excessive throat clearing first thing in the morning?
   a) Postnasal drip.
   b) Laryngopharyngeal reflux.
   c) Hyperfunctional voice use.
   d) Psychosomatic conditions.
   e) a and b.

5. Why is auditory-perceptual evaluation of voice a necessary and valuable component of the voice diagnostic?
   a) Perceptual evaluation methods are available to all clinicians.
   b) The perceived characteristics of the voice are often the reason that a patient has presented themselves or has been referred for in the first place.
   c) The perceived characteristics of the voice present a gauge by which the success of therapy will be evaluated.
   d) Perceptual evaluation provides a direct method of laryngeal evaluation.
   e) a, b, and c.

6. The term used to describe the pitch level around which normal pitch inflections/variations occur and is used most often in everyday speech is _____.
   a) Habitual pitch.
   b) Monopitch.
   c) Intonation.
   d) Tremor.
   e) All of the above.

7. The perceptual attribute that corresponds to the magnitude of sound pressure disturbances is
   _____.
   a) Quality.
   b) Pitch.
   c) Loudness.

d) Duration.
   e) All of the above.

8. A respiratory pattern that results in a weak, shallow inspiration and mainly uses the secondary/accessory muscles of respiration is _____.
   a) Thoracic breathing.
   b) Clavicular breathing.
   c) Diaphragmatic-abdominal breathing.
   d) Inhalatory stridor.
   e) a or b.

9. A disordered voice quality that is often described as "gravelly" and is associated with irregularity of vocal fold vibration is _____.
   a) Strain.
   b) Breathiness.
   c) Monopitch.
   d) Roughness.
   e) None of the above.

10. Which of the following evaluation procedures is not an *impairment-level* measure?
   a) Auditory-perceptual evaluation of voice.
   b) Acoustic analysis methods.
   c) The Voice Handicap Index.
   d) Aerodynamic measurement.
   e) Laryngeal stroboscopy.

3.8 Answers and Explanations

1. Correct: Laryngeal stroboscopic examination (**d**).
   (**d**) Of the possible answers, only laryngeal stroboscopy provides a direct (i.e., at the source) visualization and explicit information about laryngeal structures and vibratory characteristics. However, it should be remembered that a complete profile of the patient's voice requires not only a visualization and description of laryngeal structures but also an evaluation and description of the output and by-products of laryngeal-phonatory function such as the auditory-perceptual description of the voice signal, the objective acoustic measurement of the voice signal, and the interpretation of information provided via case history examination. (**a, b, c**) The VHI, CAPE-V ratings, and case history examination information are based on the by-products of laryngeal phonatory function (e.g., the perception of breathiness or strain, the patient's self-perception of the emotional effects of their possible voice disorder, the patient's description of the variability vs. consistency of their voice problem). While in many cases these indirect forms of evaluation will be related to a particular structural or functional deficit, a complete profile of the voice is incomplete without direct laryngeal evaluation (e.g., the perception of breathiness tells us that air is escaping between the vocal folds during phonation—the perception does not tell us why it is escaping).

2. Correct: a, b, and c (**e**).
   (**e**) Any sound (including that produced during phonation) can be characterized perceptually in terms of pitch, loudness, quality, and duration. As we have experienced voices from numerous people, we have developed an internal gauge as to what is typical or expected for these parameters for different ages, sexes, races, etc. If a perceived voice matches our expectations for these parameters, we will deem it "normal"

or "typical." (**d**) "Articulation" is a term used to describe (primarily) supraglottal (i.e., above the glottis) activity of structures such as the tongue, lips, and mandible that transforms airflows and pressures into recognizable vowels, stop-plosives, fricatives, etc. Supraglottal articulation is somewhat independent of laryngeal phonatory function (e.g., whispered, aphonic speech can still be articulated to produce a completely intelligible message). Therefore, "articulation" is not a consideration when judging the normality of voice production.

3. Correct: diagnosis momentum (**a**).

(**a**) Diagnosis momentum occurs when the clinician accepts a previous diagnosis without sufficient skepticism. We must always be aware of accepting information regarding explanations based solely on authority, and it may occur that a clinician accepts a previous diagnosis because "Dr. %$#& said so." However, we must remember that (1) previous diagnoses can be fallible, (2) the patient's presenting condition may have changed from a previous examination, and (c) blindly accepting a previous diagnosis negates the potential value of the detailed information we are attempting to gather via our own diagnostic protocol. Therefore, while we should certainly take information from previous examinations as part of our initial diagnostic considerations, we must be open to the possibility that a change in diagnosis may be recommended based on the information that we will gather. (**b, c, d, e**) Besides diagnosis momentum, other forms of clinical bias must be avoided so that the clinician does not "jump to conclusions" regarding the patient's diagnosis. The final diagnosis for the presenting voice problem must follow a synthesis of information gathered from case history, perceptual, acoustic, aerodynamic, and endoscopic information.

4. Correct: a and b (**e**).

(**e**) Postnasal drainage and/or laryngopharyngeal reflux are both conditions that may result in overnight laryngeal irritation. As the patient is in a supine position during sleeping, mucus from the nasal cavities may drain downward and pool in the laryngopharyngeal region. Alternatively, for some patients the supine position is one in which acid reflux is able to move upward toward the laryngopharyngeal region and may also result in laryngeal irritation. In both cases, the patient may describe poor voice quality and excessive throat clearing first thing in the morning. (**c**) Hyperfunctional voice use often results in some combination of phonotrauma and fatigue as the day progresses. Patients will often describe that voice quality worsens as the day progresses and improved voice follows extended voice rest. (**d**) Voice disorders that have a psychogenic/psychosomatic cause are variable in their occurrence and may be associated with particular periods of stress or conflict.

5. Correct: a, b, and c (**e**).

(**e**) Auditory-perceptual evaluation has been, and will continue to be, a standard tool for the voice diagnostic. Regardless of whether they have access to instrumental forms of voice analysis (e.g., stroboscopy; acoustic analysis equipment), all speech pathologists and vocologists are able to use a combination of their auditory perception and their knowledge of what certain auditory characteristics reveal about voice

function to describe the patients voice. In addition, though they may not have extensive knowledge regarding the auditory-perceptual characteristics of voice, lay patients are often presenting themselves for the diagnostic based on their or someone else's perception of their voice. Finally, when a patient is treated for a voice disorder, the success of any medical, surgical, or behavioral voice treatment is often gauged by the degree of positive change in the auditory-perceptual characteristics of the patient's voice. (**a, b, c, d**) Auditory-perceptual evaluation of voice is based on our interpretation of the perceived acoustic signal produced by the patient's speech/voice mechanism and is therefore an indirect form of voice evaluation. Though auditory perceptions along with knowledge of underlying vocal anatomy and physiology often result in quite accurate hypotheses regarding potential vocal pathology, they are not a form of direct evaluation in which the larynx is visualized.

6. Correct: Habitual pitch (**a**).

(**a**) Habitual pitch (a.k.a., modal pitch level; average pitch level) is the pitch used most commonly by the patient in day-to-day voice use. (**b**) Monopitch refers to continuous speech production that lacks pitch variability. (**c**) Intonation refers to pitch variations that are used linguistically to vary the meaning of utterances. (**d**) Tremor refers to rhythmic variation in pitch and/or loudness. While some tremors can be purposeful (e.g., vibrato as observed in some singing voices), vocal tremor is also associated with motor disruptions such as ataxia and spasmodic dysphonia.

7. Correct: Loudness (**c**).

(**c**) A sound wave is typically produced due to disturbances in the air that are received and interpreted by the hearing mechanism. If the magnitude or amplitude of these disturbances is relatively small, we will interpret this as a quiet sound versus those with large amplitude/magnitude disturbances which will be perceived as louder sounds. Therefore, the interpretation of sound pressure magnitude is *loudness*. (**a**) *Quality* refers to the characteristic of a sound that distinguishes it from other sounds of similar pitch, loudness, and duration, and is associated with the spectral characteristics of the acoustic voice waveform. (**b**) *Pitch* is the auditory perception of the fundamental rate of vibration of some sound-producing source. (**d**) The *duration* of a sound deals with the perception of how long in time the sound continues or is produced.

8. Correct: Clavicular breathing (**b**).

(**b**) Clavicular breathing mainly uses the upper thoracic and neck muscles such as the scalenes and the sternocleidomastoid to elevate the shoulders and upper chest during inspiration and, therefore, results in a weak, shallow inspiration and poor respiratory support for speech and voice. (**a**) Thoracic breathing is a commonly used breathing pattern characterized by expansion of the midthoracic region (chest expansion). (**c**) Diaphragmatic-abdominal breathing uses expansion of the lower thoracic and abdominal cavities during inspiration to achieve thoracic enlargement and is felt to be a highly efficient pattern of respiration. (**d**) Inhalatory stridor is an audible noise perceived during inhalations, typically caused by narrowing/stenosis or possible partial blockage of the glottis.

9. Correct: Roughness (**d**).

(**d**) Roughness is typically perceived as an unpleasant voice, and has been described in terms such as *coarse*, *gravelly*, and *low-pitched noise*. Physiologically, the rough voice is often associated with irregularity of vocal fold vibration, low-frequency spectral noise, and alternating glottal periods that are differ in period or shape. (**a**) Strain is associated with the impression of vocal effort, higher pitched voice, and a hyper-functional state of phonation. (**b**) Breathiness is commonly perceived as a whispery or airy voice, is associated with hypoadduction of the vocal folds, and refers to the audible detection of airflow through the glottis during phonation. (**c**) Monopitch refers to continuous speech production that lacks pitch variability.

10. Correct: The Voice Handicap Index (**c**).

(**c**) The Voice Handicap Index is a quality-of-life measure developed for the measurement of the psychosocial handicapping effects of voice disorders. (**a, b, d**) Auditory-perceptual ratings of voice, acoustic analyses, aerodynamic analyses, and laryngeal stroboscopy are all examples of impairment-level measures that assess the specific impact of a disease/disorder on bodily function. Impairment-level measures are not necessarily strongly correlated with measures of quality of life.

References

[1] Awan S. The Voice Diagnostic Protocol: A Practical Guide to the Diagnosis of Voice Disorders. Austin, TX: Pro-Ed Inc.; 2001

[2] American Educational Research Association. American Psychological Association, & National Council on Measurement in Education & Joint Committee on Standards for Educational and Psychological Testing. Standards for Educational and Psychological Testing. Washington, DC: American Educational Research Association; 2014

[3] Willis BH. Spectrum bias–why clinicians need to be cautious when applying diagnostic test studies. Fam Pract. 2008; 25(5):390–396

[4] Peterson H, Marquardt T. Appraisal and Diagnosis of Speech Language Disorders. New Jersey: Prentice Hall Inc.; 1990

[5] Haynes W, Pindzola R, Emerick L. Diagnosis and Evaluation in Speech Pathology. New Jersey: Simon and Schuster Co.; 1992

[6] Weinberg B. Diagnosis of phonatory based voice disorders. In: Meitus I, Weinberg B, eds. Diagnosis in Speech Language Pathology. Baltimore, MD: University Park Press; 1983:151–182

[7] Fex S. Perceptual evaluation. J Voice. 1992; 6(2):155–158

[8] de Krom G. Consistency and reliability of voice quality ratings for different types of speech fragments. J Speech Hear Res. 1994; 37(5):985–1000

[9] Higgins MB, Chait DH, Schulte L. Phonatory air flow characteristics of adductor spasmodic dysphonia and muscle tension dysphonia. J Speech Lang Hear Res. 1999; 42(1):101–111

[10] Croskerry P. The importance of cognitive errors in diagnosis and strategies to minimize them. Acad Med. 2003; 78(8):775–780

[11] Prater R, Swift R. Manual of Voice Therapy. Boston, MA: Little, Brown and Company; 1984

[12] Colton R, Casper J. Understanding Voice Problems: A Physiological Perspective for Diagnosis and Treatment. Baltimore, MD: Williams and Wilkins; 1996

[13] Boone D, McFarlane S. The Voice and Voice Therapy. 4th ed. New Jersey: Prentice Hall Inc.; 1988

[14] Stemple J. Voice Therapy: Clinical Studies. St. Louis, MO: Mosby Year Book, Inc.; 1993

[15] Bless D, Baken R. Assessment of voice (special article). Journal of Voice. 1992; 6:95–97

[16] Orlikoff R, Dejonckere PH, Dembowski J, et al. The perceived role of voice perception in clinical practice. Phonoscope. 1999; 2:89–104

[17] Hirano M. Psycho-acoustic evaluation of voice: GRBAS scale for evaluating the hoarse voice. In: Clinical Examination of Voice. Wien: Springer-Verlag; 1981

[18] Dejonckere PH, Remacle M, Fresnel-Elbaz E, Woisard V, Crevier-Buchman L, Millet B. Differentiated perceptual evaluation of pathological voice quality:

[19] Kempster GB, Gerratt BR, Verdolini Abbott K, Barkmeier-Kraemer J, Hillman RE. Consensus auditory-perceptual evaluation of voice: development of a standardized clinical protocol. Am J Speech Lang Pathol. 2009; 18(2):124–132

[20] Case J. Clinical Management of Voice Disorders. Texas: Pro-Ed Inc.; 1996

[21] Awan SN. Superimposition of speaking voice characteristics and phonetograms in untrained and trained vocal groups. J Voice. 1993; 7(1):30–37

[22] Laures JS, Weismer G. The effects of a flattened fundamental frequency on intelligibility at the sentence level. J Speech Lang Hear Res. 1999; 42(5):1148–1156

[23] Monsen RB. Acoustic qualities of phonation in young hearing-impaired children. J Speech Hear Res. 1979; 22(2):270–288

[24] Kent RD. Anatomical and neuromuscular maturation of the speech mechanism: evidence from acoustic studies. J Speech Hear Res. 1976; 19(3):421–447

[25] Pedersen MF, M, ø, ller S, Krabbe S, Bennett P. Fundamental voice frequency measured by electroglottography during continuous speech. A new exact secondary sex characteristic in boys in puberty. Int J Pediatr Otorhinolaryngol. 1986; 11(1):21–27

[26] Murry T. Phonation: assessment. In: Lass N, McReynolds L, Northern J, Yoder D, eds. Speech Language, and Hearing. Vol II. Philadelphia, PA: W. B. Saunders Company; 1982:477–488

[27] Aronson AE. Clinical Voice Disorders: An Interdisciplinary Approach. 3rd ed. New York: Thieme Medical Publishers, Inc.; 1990

[28] Kahane JC. Age-related changes in the peripheral speech mechanism: structural and physiological changes. Proceedings of the Research Symposium on Communication Sciences and Disorders and Aging, No. 19, 75–87; 1990

[29] Awan SN, Mueller PB. Speaking fundamental frequency characteristics of centenarian females. Clin Linguist Phon. 1992; 6(3):249–254

[30] Perkins W. Assessment and treatment of voice disorders: state of the art. In: Costello J, ed. Speech Disorders in Adults. San Diego, CA: College Hill Press; 1985

[31] Gilbert HR, Weismer GG. The effects of smoking on the fundamental frequency of women. Journal of Linguistic Research. 1974; 3(3):225–231

[32] Honjo I, Isshiki N. Laryngoscopic and voice characteristics of aged persons. Arch Otolaryngol. 1980; 106(3):149–150

[33] Hollien H, Shipp T. Speaking fundamental frequency and chronologic age in males. J Speech Hear Res. 1972; 15(1):155–159

[34] Shipp T, Qi Y, Huntley R, Hollien H. Acoustic and temporal correlates of perceived age. J Voice. 1992; 6(3):211–216

[35] Morris RJ, Brown WS, Jr. Age-related differences in speech intensity among adult females. Folia Phoniatr Logop. 1994; 46(2):64–69

[36] Ramig LA, Ringel RL. Effects of physiological aging on selected acoustic characteristics of voice. J Speech Hear Res. 1983; 26(1):22–30

[37] Boltezar IH, Burger ZR, Zargi M. Instability of voice in adolescence: pathologic condition or normal developmental variation? J Pediatr. 1997; 130 (2):185–190

[38] Caruso AJ, Mueller PB, Xue A. Relative contributions of voice and articulation to listener judgements of age and gender: preliminary data and implications. Voice. 1994; 3:1–9

[39] Mueller PB. Voice ageism. Contemp Issues Commun Sci Disord. 1998; 25:62–64

[40] Andrews M. Manual of Voice Treatment: Pediatrics through Geriatrics. San Diego, CA: Singular Publishing Group, Inc.; 1995

[41] Dworkin J, Meleca R. Vocal Pathologies: Diagnosis, Treatment, and Case Studies. San Diego: Singular Publishing Group, Inc.; 1997

[42] Baken RJ. Clinical Measurement of Speech and Voice. Boston: Little Brown and Company; 1987

[43] Awan S, Knych C. Acoustic characteristics of the voice in young adult smokers. In: Windsor F, Kelley L, Hewlett N, eds. Themes in Clinical Phonetics and Linguistics. Mahwah, NJ: Lawrence Erlbaum & Associates; 2002:449–458

[44] Hewlett N, Topham N, McMullen C. The effects of smoking on the female voice. In: Ball MJ, Duckworth M, eds. Advances in Clinical Phonetics. Philadelphia, PA: John Benjamins Publishing Company; 1996:227–235

[45] Darley FL, Aronson AE, Brown JR. Motor Speech Disorders. Philadelphia, PA: W. B. Saunders Company; 1975

[46] Dworkin JP. Motor Speech Disorders: A Treatment Guide. St. Louis, MO: Mosby Year Book; 1991

[47] Dromey C, Ramig LO, Johnson AB. Phonatory and articulatory changes associated with increased vocal intensity in Parkinson disease: a case study. J Speech Hear Res. 1995; 38(4):751–764

[48] Kent RD, Rosenbek JC. Prosodic disturbance and neurologic lesion. Brain Lang. 1982; 15(2):259–291

[49] Morrison MD, Rammage LA. Muscle misuse voice disorders: description and classification. Acta Otolaryngol. 1993; 113(3):428–434

[50] Luchsinger R, Arnold G. Physiology and pathology of respiration and phonation. In: Luchsinger R, Arnold G, eds. Voice-Speech-Language. Clinical Communicology: Its Physiology and Pathology. Belmont: Wadsworth Publishing Co.; 1965

[51] Leff J, Abberton E. Voice pitch measurements in schizophrenia and depression. Psychol Med. 1981; 11(4):849–852

[52] Bless D, Hicks D. Diagnosis and measurement: assessing the "whs" of voice function. In: Brown W, Vinson B, Crary M, eds. Organic Voice Disorders Assessment and Treatment. San Diego, CA: Singular Publishing Group; 1996:119–170

[53] Sapienza CM, Stathopoulos ET. Respiratory and laryngeal measures of children and women with bilateral vocal fold nodules. J Speech Hear Res. 1994; 37(6):1229–1243

[54] Komiyama S, Watanabe H, Ryu S. Phonographic relationship between pitch and intensity of the human voice. Folia Phoniatr (Basel). 1984; 36(1):1–7

[55] Morris RJ, Brown WS, Jr. Age-related differences in speech variability among women. J Commun Disord. 1994; 27(1):49–64

[56] Mueller PB. The aging voice. Semin Speech Lang. 1997; 18(2):159–168, quiz 168–169

[57] Countryman S, Hicks J, Ramig LO, Smith ME. Supraglottal hyperadduction in an individual with Parkinson disease: a clinical treatment note. Am J Speech Lang Pathol. 1997; 6(4):74–84

[58] Zemlin W. Speech and Hearing Science: Anatomy and Physiology. Englewood Cliffs, NJ: Prentice-Hall Inc.; 1988

[59] Bouwers F, Dikkers FG. A retrospective study concerning the psychosocial impact of voice disorders: Voice Handicap Index change in patients with benign voice disorders after treatment (measured with the Dutch version of the VHI). J Voice. 2009; 23(2):218–224

[60] Andrews ML, Schmidt CP. Gender presentation: perceptual and acoustical analyses of voice. J Voice. 1997; 11(3):307–313

[61] Klatt DH, Klatt LC. Analysis, synthesis, and perception of voice quality variations among female and male talkers. J Acoust Soc Am. 1990; 87(2):820–857

[62] Askenfelt AG, Hammarberg B. Speech waveform perturbation analysis: a perceptual-acoustical comparison of seven measures. J Speech Hear Res. 1986; 29(1):50–64

[63] Eskenazi L, Childers DG, Hicks DM. Acoustic correlates of vocal quality. J Speech Hear Res. 1990; 33(2):298–306

[64] Omori K, Kojima H, Kakani R, Slavit DH, Blaugrund SM. Acoustic characteristics of rough voice: subharmonics. J Voice. 1997; 11(1):40–47

[65] Gelfer MP. A multidimensional scaling study of voice quality in females. Phonetica. 1993; 50(1):15–27

[66] Fairbanks G. Voice and Articulation Drillbook. 2nd ed. New York: Harper & Row; 1960

[67] Coleman RF. Effect of median frequency levels upon the roughness of jittered stimuli. J Speech Hear Res. 1969; 12(2):330–336

[68] Davis SB. Acoustic characteristics of normal and pathological voices. ASHA Reports; 1981:11:97–115

[69] Ryan WJ, Burk KW. Perceptual and acoustic correlates of aging in the speech of males. J Commun Disord. 1974; 7(2):181–192

[70] S, ö, dersten M, Lindestad PA. Glottal closure and perceived breathiness during phonation in normally speaking subjects. J Speech Hear Res. 1990; 33(3):601–611

[71] Thomas-Kersting C, Casteel RL. Harsh voice: vocal effort perceptual ratings and spectral noise levels of hearing-impaired children. J Commun Disord. 1989; 22(2):125–135

[72] Awan SN, Roy N, Cohen SM. Exploring the relationship between spectral and cepstral measures of voice and the Voice Handicap Index (VHI). J Voice. 2014; 28(4):430–439

[73] Jacobson B, Johnson A, Grywalski C, et al. The voice handicap index (VHI): development and validation. Am J Speech Lang Pathol. 1997; 6(3):66–70

[74] Hogikyan ND, Sethuraman G. Validation of an instrument to measure voice-related quality of life (V-RQOL). J Voice. 1999; 13(4):557–569

[75] Ma EP, Yiu EM. Voice activity and participation profile: assessing the impact of voice disorders on daily activities. J Speech Lang Hear Res. 2001; 44(3):511–524

[76] Portone CR, Hapner ER, McGregor L, Otto K, Johns MM, III. Correlation of the Voice Handicap Index (VHI) and the Voice-Related Quality of Life Measure (V-RQOL). J Voice. 2007; 21(6):723–727

[77] Branski RC, Cukier-Blaj S, Pusic A, et al. Measuring quality of life in dysphonic patients: a systematic review of content development in patient-reported outcomes measures. J Voice. 2010; 24(2):193–198

[78] Behrman A, Rutledge J, Hembree A, Sheridan S. Vocal hygiene education, voice production therapy, and the role of patient adherence: a treatment effectiveness study in women with phonotrauma. J Speech Lang Hear Res. 2008; 51(2):350–366

[79] Niebudek-Bogusz E, Kuza, ń, ska A, Woznicka E, Sliwinska-Kowalska M. Assessment of the voice handicap index as a screening tool in dysphonic patients. Folia Phoniatr Logop. 2011; 63(5):269–272

[80] Moradi N, Pourshahbaz A, Soltani M, Javadipour S. Cutoff point at voice handicap index used to screen voice disorders among Persian speakers. J Voice. 2013; 27(1):130.e1–130.e5

[81] Deary IJ, Webb A, Mackenzie K, Wilson JA, Carding PN. Short, self-report voice symptom scales: psychometric characteristics of the voice handicap index-10 and the vocal performance questionnaire. Otolaryngol Head Neck Surg. 2004; 131(3):232–235

[82] Rosen CA, Murry T, Zinn A, Zullo T, Sonbolian M. Voice handicap index change following treatment of voice disorders. J Voice. 2000; 14(4):619–623

[83] Roy N, Gray SD, Simon M, Dove H, Corbin-Lewis K, Stemple JC. An evaluation of the effects of two treatment approaches for teachers with voice disorders: a prospective randomized clinical trial. J Speech Lang Hear Res. 2001; 44(2):286–296

[84] Behlau M, Madazio G, Feijó D, Pontes P. Avaliação de voz. In Voz: O Livro do Especialista. Vol. 1 Rio de Janeiro: Revinter; 2001:85–245

Suggested Reading

[1] Awan S. The Voice Diagnostic Protocol: A Practical Guide to the Diagnosis of Voice Disorders. Austin, TX: Pro-Ed Inc.; 2001

[2] Bless D, Hicks D. Diagnosis and measurement: assessing the "whs" of voice function. In: Brown W, Vinson B, Crary M, eds. Organic voice disorders assessment and treatment. San Diego, CA: Singular Publishing Group; 1996:119–170

[3] Kempster GB, Gerratt BR, Verdolini Abbott K, Barkmeier-Kraemer J, Hillman RE. Consensus auditory-perceptual evaluation of voice: development of a standardized clinical protocol. Am J Speech Lang Pathol. 2009; 18(2):124–132

[4] Ma EP, Yiu EM. Voice activity and participation profile: assessing the impact of voice disorders on daily activities. J Speech Lang Hear Res. 2001; 44 (3):511–524

4 Acoustic Analysis of Voice

Summary

This chapter reviews acoustic analysis methods that have been used to provide objective correlates of vocal pitch, loudness, and quality. Information regarding required equipment (e.g., microphone, amplifier, and software information) and a review of the basics of digital sound recording necessary for high-quality voice recordings are provided. Once elicited voice recordings are obtained, commonly used measures of vocal *frequency* correlate with the perception of vocal pitch, and include *mean speaking fundamental frequency* (mean F_0), the *average variability of the vocal F_0* (F_0 standard deviation and F_0 coefficient of variation), and the *total phonational range* (often reported in semitones). Commonly used measures of vocal sound level (a.k.a. vocal intensity) correlate with the perception of vocal loudness, and include the *mean or modal sound level/intensity* and the *dynamic range* (i.e., the range from the lowest sound level/intensity to the greatest sound level/intensity). Correlates of atypical forms of vocal quality (such as breathiness or roughness) include measures of *perturbation* (including jitter, shimmer, and harmonics-to-noise ratio) and measures obtained from the *cepstrum* such as the *cepstral peak prominence*. Finally, a number of *multivariate forms of voice analysis* that combine multiple acoustic measures of voice are also discussed.

Keywords: vocal frequency, fundamental frequency (F_0), speaking fundamental frequency, F_0 standard deviation, F_0 coefficient of variation, vocal sound level, vocal intensity, voice quality, perturbation measures, cepstrum

4.1 Learning Objectives

At the end of this chapter, readers will be able to
- Understand the rationale, benefits, and limitations of measures of voice obtained using acoustic analysis.
- Identify the necessary equipment and recording procedures necessary for high-quality audio recordings of the voice.
- Describe how the commonly used measures of vocal frequency are obtained and how they relate to the perceived pitch of the voice in typical and dysphonic individuals.
- Describe how the commonly used measures of vocal sound level/intensity are obtained and how they relate to the perceived loudness of the voice in typical and dysphonic individuals.
- Describe how the traditionally used perturbation measures relate to atypical/dysphonic vocal qualities and understand key limitations with these measures.
- Describe the observed benefits of measures obtained via cepstral analyses with dysphonic voices in both sustained vowel and continuous speech contexts.
- Describe several multivariate methods of voice analysis (including the *Cepstral Spectral Index of Dysphonia [CSID]* and the *Dysphonia Severity Index*) and the potential benefits of these measures versus univariate (i.e., single variable) measures.

4.2 Introduction to Acoustic Analyses of Voice

In the previous chapter, we have described the initial stages of the voice evaluation process in which the perceptual description of the patient's voice holds a necessary and essential place as a voice evaluation measure for both the clinician and the patient. However, we have also stated key limitations with auditory-perceptual evaluation of voice including inter-clinician differences and biases that may result in problems of scale validity and reliability. Auditory-perceptions may also be difficult to characterize and may not be as credible as numerical test procedures. In addition, since **one of the fundamental decisions made in any diagnostic is one of "normal/typical" versus "abnormal/atypical,"** we must recognize that perceptual judgments alone do not allow for objective comparison with normative groups.[1] In making these diagnostic comparisons, it is common to compare our current patient to the average performance and average deviation of a target sample. Unfortunately, perceptions cannot be compared with measurable norms in any valid manner.

These aforementioned issues may be addressed by incorporating *instrumental measures* into our assessment procedures. Instrumental measures are typically obtained using electronic or computer-based equipment.[2] Because the environment in which speech–language pathologists practice continually and rapidly evolves, ever greater sophistication from the clinician is demanded in terms of our evaluation methods and procedures, and this includes the expanding use of instrumental procedures. In addition, the demands of effective health care delivery and reimbursement issues have required the voice clinician to quantify patient characteristics both in diagnosis and through the course of therapy via instrumental measures. Instrumental measures can also help guide and support overall clinical judgments and allow for the comparison of vocal performance to appropriate normative data. If clinical experience, expertise, and perceptual judgments form the foundation of diagnostic hypotheses, then instrumental measures are a key factor in the acceptance or rejection of these hypotheses.[1]

4.2.1 Rationale for Acoustic Methods

There are many forms of instrumental measures that may be used to describe the voice signal and underlying vocal function. However, it is our view that the choice of acoustic analysis methods presents several **distinct advantages** for the voice clinician[1]:

1. **Clinician experience and familiarity**: Since all certified speech–language pathologists must have acquired knowledge and skills in basic speech science and acoustic methods as part of their academic training, key acoustic analysis concepts and measures (e.g., period, frequency) will be relatively familiar to the clinicians using them.
2. **Noninvasive**: Because acoustic methods are noninvasive, they may be used with ease, comfort, and familiarity with all patients by any clinician.

3. **Readily available and relatively low cost**: Key components necessary for high-quality computerized acoustic analysis are readily available to most clinicians in their own desktop or laptop computers. In addition, high-quality acoustic analysis software (both freely available and commercial) is widely available. The addition of a good-quality microphone and possible preamplifier make a high-quality acoustic analysis setup available for a fraction of the cost of other instrumental voice analysis methods.

4. **Correspondence with the underlying physiology of voice disorders**: Because the acoustic signal is determined, in part, by movements of the vocal folds, "there is a great deal of correspondence between the physiology and acoustics, and much can be inferred about the physiology based on acoustic analysis."[3] It must be noted that the relationships between phonatory physiology and acoustics are certainly not perfect. The voice signal "is a complex product of the nonlinear interaction between aerodynamic and biomechanical properties of the voice production system."[4] Because this interaction is nonlinear, accurate predictions regarding underlying phonatory physiology cannot always be made on the basis of the acoustic signal alone. However, when acoustic analysis results are placed within the context of a complete *voice diagnostic protocol*, very powerful inferences may be made.

5. **Good applicability to future therapy**: Acoustic methods lend themselves well to both diagnostic procedures and treatment methods. It has been our experience that most patients, even relatively young children, are able to easily understand (in a simple, but effective manner) many of the measures displayed in voice analysis programs (e.g., jitter values "should go down"; F_0 values "should go up"; displayed F_0 contours should flatten or become more variable, depending on the context). In this way, acoustic methods provide a valuable link between the voice diagnostic and voice therapy.

6. **Wide body of literature**: Acoustic analysis methods have an extensive history of use with a wide range of voice-disordered populations. This provides the clinician with a vast body of literature that may be accessed to aid in the interpretation of diagnostic findings.

It is important to recognize that, while acoustic measures have been used as effective indices of dysphonia severity and even voice quality type (i.e., breathy, hoarse, rough voices), acoustic methods have been largely ineffective in specifying *disorder type* (e.g., paralysis vs. mass lesion vs. functional disorder). *Since the perceptual and acoustic characteristics of functional versus organic voice disorders are often quite similar in nature, it is additional key evaluation components (e.g., case history; laryngeal visualization) of the voice diagnostic that often provide important information by which differential diagnosis may be achieved.*

4.3 Necessary Requirements for High-Quality Audio Recordings of the Voice

In this section, we will describe valuable acoustic measures that will be used to supplement our auditory-perceptual impressions of the voice and to provide key objective measures that we may use to both validate and guide our diagnostic impressions. We will see that for each of the previously described perceptual impressions of the voice signal such as pitch, loudness, and quality, there are corresponding objective acoustic correlates that may be readily measured from the recorded voice sound wave. However, prior to exploring some of these acoustic voice analysis methods, we will review some of the necessary requirements for high-quality audio recordings of the voice, including

- Choice of software.
- Good-quality microphone.
- Analog-to-digital (A-to-D) recording interface.
- Speakers or headphones for signal playback.

4.3.1 Voice Analysis Software

There are several very good programs available for voice analysis (both free and commercial). Examples of free recording and analysis programs include **Praat**[5] and **SpeechTool**.[6] Examples of commercial programs designed for voice analysis include programs such as **Computerized Speech Lab** and **Multi-Speech**[7] and **lingWaves**[8] (see ▶ Fig. 4.1 for representative screenshots from these aforementioned programs).

The potential users of these programs should be aware that there are pros and cons to the use of free versus commercial

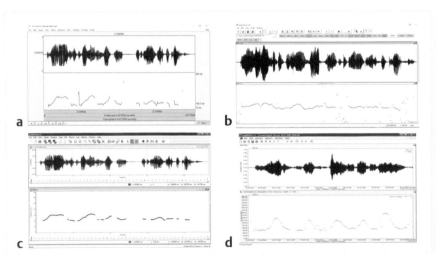

Fig. 4.1 Example screenshots of sound wave display and associated fundamental frequency contour in **(a)** Praat, **(b)** SpeechTool, **(c)** Multi-Speech, and **(d)** lingWaves.

software. In the case of free software, *the pro* is obvious—**the costs** involved to put together a high-quality voice recording and analysis system using free software (e.g., Praat) can be relatively low (certainly < $500). However, *the primary con is that support for installation, maintenance, and use of the software and associated hardware is minimal* and will primarily depend on the troubleshooting skills of the user. In contrast, *commercial systems* are often *fully customer-supported* via live service and/or phone and internet support. In addition, it is generally to the interest of commercial entities to offer *consistent upgrades to software*, to provide *highly compatible software and hardware packages, and to organize and support presentations and workshops that demonstrate effective product use*. Of course, the costs for a commercial hardware/software system can be *relatively costly* (though still considerably less than the costs of aerodynamic or laryngeal imaging systems also used in voice evaluation). The clinicians will have to decide which option is best for them based on their experience, daily needs, and time available for the necessary "learning curve" required to use whatever software/hardware system they choose or are provided for acoustic analysis of voice.

4.3.2 Microphone and Preamplifier

A microphone transduces the analog (i.e., the continuously variable signal as it occurs in the natural world) acoustic sound wave into an electrical audio waveform. This waveform will then be captured for analysis and playback. Microphones may be handheld (▶ Fig. 4.2) or head-mounted (▶ Fig. 4.3), with the *head-mounted microphone preferable* since a consistent mouth-to-microphone distance and positioning may be easily maintained.

While mouth-to-microphone distance is not essential for consistent measures of vocal frequency, *a consistent distance is essential when attempting to make measures that correlate with vocal loudness*. For a headset microphone, a position of approximately *4 to 10 cm from the lips at a 45-degree angle*[9] is

suggested to obtain a high-quality voice signal with limited background noise and with avoidance of excessive noise from production of plosive sounds.[10] Microphones may be *omnidirectional* (receives signals from all directions with similar sensitivity) or *unidirectional* (highly sensitive from a single direction). The microphone should also have a relatively *flat frequency response* (i.e., variation of < 2 dB) across the spectral frequency range of the voice, with particular focus on flat response between approximately 50 to 8,000 Hz, and should have a *dynamic range* wide enough to capture both quietest and loudest voice productions.

The electrical signals produced by microphones are extremely small amplitude signals and generally should be preamplified. A *preamplifier* (▶ Fig. 4.2) is an electronic device that amplifies a weak signal. With lower cost microphones that will plug directly into the computer (via USB or 1/8th inch phono jack), the preamplifier is built into the computer audio interface. With higher quality microphones, an external preamplifier will be necessary to accept the microphone **XLR plug** (often a circular connector with three pins; ▶ Fig. 4.2). In addition, the preamplifier may also provide power (referred to as **phantom power**) necessary for certain high sensitivity microphones called *condenser* microphones. The preamplifier will generally have a gain control that may be adjusted so that the levels of the loudest phonations are not distorted and clipped and quiet phonations are raised above any background noise. Many current computer audio interface preamplifiers will provide an output that will connect to either the audio input of your computer interface (typically receives a 1/8th inch phono jack) or to the USB port of your computer via a USB cable. For a summary of microphone and preamplifier characteristics, see the studies by Svec and Granqvist and Patel et al.[9,11]

4.3.3 Digital Recording Basics

Once we have acquired our microphone and (if necessary) external preamplification hardware, we are almost ready to record

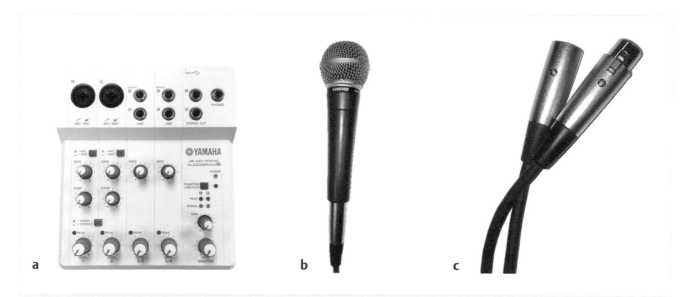

Fig. 4.2 Examples of a **(a)** microphone preamplifier (Yamaha AUDIOGRAM3 Computer Recording interface), **(b)** a handheld dynamic microphone (Shure SM58), and **(c)** an XLR microphone cable.

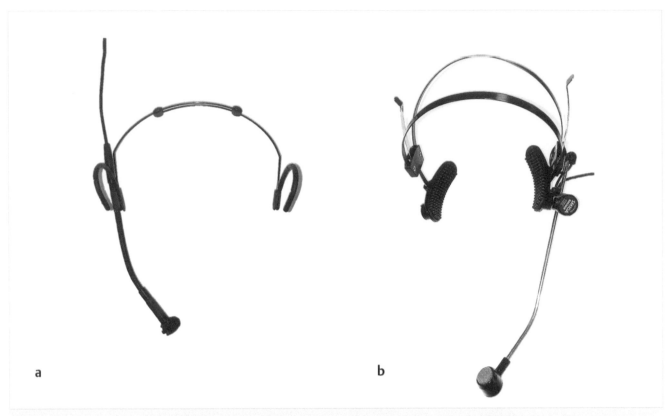

Fig. 4.3 Examples of **(a)** a condenser headset microphone (AKG C-520) and **(b)** a dynamic headset microphone (Shure SM10A).

our patient's voice signal into the computer. When a voice/speech signal is recorded for computer analysis, it must be converted into a data format that the computer can manipulate. This procedure is known as ***analog-to-digital (A-to-D) conversion***. In this process, the sound wave is transformed into a series of numbers (i.e., *digits*) which represent the fluctuating amplitude of the signal over time. The number of times the amplitude of the sound wave is captured per second is referred to as the *sampling rate*.

Sampling Rate

When a sound is "sampled," we have a process analogous to taking a series of snapshots of some variable activity (e.g., someone running from one point to another); the more snapshots or samples we have over time, the more accurate the reproduction of the variable activity being observed. *Sampling rate refers to the number of samples (i.e., pieces of data) that will be captured per second* (in the case of sound waves, we will capture multiple measures of the changing amplitude of the sound wave per second). For sound recordings and reproduction, many thousands of samples are required per second if we are to obtain an accurate reproduction of the human voice sound wave. Therefore, prior to recording, the user should check the options or preferences of their recording software to select the sampling rate and the appropriate *channel* for recording (a single-mono channel is generally all that is required for voice recordings) (▶ Fig. 4.4).

The appropriate sampling rate for a particular signal is determined by the ***Nyquist Theorem***, which states that *the sampling rate should be at least two times the highest frequency of interest.*

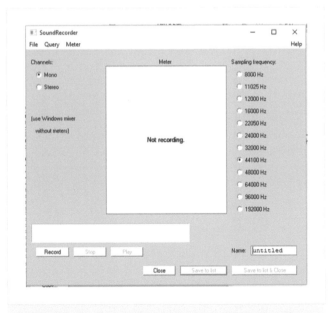

Fig. 4.4 Example of the sound recording application in *Praat*. The required number of channels (e.g., single-mono vs. dual-stereo) and the sampling rate/frequency should be selected prior to recording.

Since the normal hearing mechanism is expected to be sensitive to frequencies as high as approximately 20,000 Hz (i.e., 20 kHz), a sampling rate of approximately 2 × 20 kHz (40 kHz) or higher should capture the key acoustic characteristics (e.g., fundamental frequency (F_0), harmonics of the F_0, vocal tract resonances

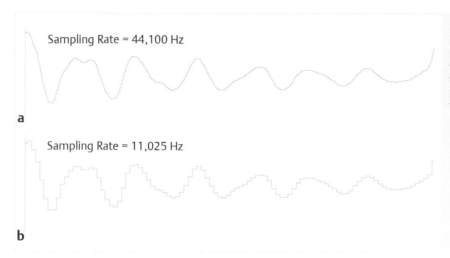

Fig. 4.5 Portion of a voice sound wave sampled at **(a)** 44,100 Hz (44.1 kHz) vs. **(b)** 11,025 Hz (≈11 kHz). While the general profile of the waveforms is similar, the digital representation of the sound wave is much more accurate when recorded at the higher sampling rate in **(a)** versus the lower sampling rate in **(b)**.

(formants), speech noise as observed in consonant productions, and noise as produced in disordered voice such as breathiness).[12] Sampling rates should be selected based on an understanding of the range of frequencies of interest in the signal being analyzed. While analysis of certain speech characteristics (e.g., vocal tract resonances/formants, analyses that focus on the vocal F_0 and lower harmonics) may be effectively analyzed using lower sampling rates such as 11 to 22 kHz, valid analysis of higher frequency spectral energy and/or rapid changes and perturbations in the voice signal will require higher sampling rates. Most computer external recording interfaces and internal sound cards are capable of recording the speech/voice wave at approximately 44 thousand samples per second (44.1 kHz/ 44,100 Hz) or higher. The 44.1 kHz sampling rate provides very accurate reproduction of the fluctuations of the sound waveform in time (▶ Fig. 4.5) and also provides a high-quality recording of similar quality to the sound reproduced on most music compact discs.

Quantization

While sampling rate is used to control time resolution, amplitude resolution is controlled via *quantization*. When an analog signal is quantized, the continuous amplitude variations are converted to discrete values or increments. The number of possible amplitude variations that can be measured are related to the number of *bits of resolution*. Bits of resolution are calculated using a base number of 2. As an example, 2^8 would give 256 levels of possible amplitude. Current A-to-D conversion methods generally use at least 16 bits of resolution (2^{16}), providing 65,536 possible amplitude levels (+32,768 to –32,768 amplitude increments).

Audio Format

There are many different methods or formats in which to save your recording. We want to make sure that we select an audio file format that has *no compression (e.g., do not use .mp3)*. Though convenient for simply listening to a recorded sound wave, *avoid saving your recordings in .mp3 or similar format*, since these formats often reduce the size of the saved data file by removing certain frequencies within the sound wave that may be of interest during acoustic analysis of the voice. The most common noncompressed format that will allow you to

analyze and play back your recording using a wide variety of voice analysis programs is the **.wav** format.

Appropriate Recording Quality and Signal Amplitude

In any type of speech/voice analysis, high-quality recordings are *essential*. Many of the acoustic analysis methods that are used to describe normal versus disordered voice production are essentially methods that quantify the degree of disturbance or perturbation in the voice signal. *Poorly recorded signals which contain significant background noise or are distorted by poor recording levels can result in invalid measurements.* During recording, some programs such as *Praat* will provide a colored volume unit (VU) meter to indicate the signal amplitude of the recording. With many colored VU meters, recorded signals should *peak in the high green/low yellow region and not be in the red region or have too weak/low recording level* (barely any movement of the VU meter). When signals exceed the available amplitude range and go "into the red," the recorded signal becomes "**clipped**" (i.e., the tops and/or bottoms of the waveform are clipped off)—in digital recording, this tends to result in an obvious harsh distortion to the signal on playback. Unfortunately, in avoidance of clipping, many will record signals using minimal recording levels which use only a small fraction of the available amplitude range—this results in signals that have a very *poor signal-to-noise ratio* (SNR; i.e., the noise inherent in any recording begins to compete with the actual signal). This is also a type of signal distortion that may result in invalid acoustic analysis results. As shown in ▶ Fig. 4.6, the recorded signal should fill the middle one-third to half of the available amplitude scale, resulting in a strong SNR and good representation of the amplitude variations of the signal while still leaving available dynamic range (i.e., "headroom") to capture occasional peaks in the recorded signal without clipping.

4.4 Key Acoustic Measurements Used in the Analysis of Voice

Now that we have reviewed some of terminology and processes involved in capturing a high-quality recording of our patient's voice, we will discuss several key acoustic measurements that

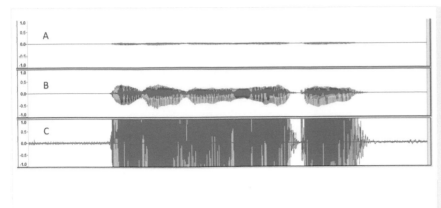

Fig. 4.6 Recordings of the sentence "We were away a year ago" at three different recording levels. In sound wave A, the recording level was too low, resulting in a signal that has a weak signal-to-noise ratio and poor representation of the waveform in the amplitude domain. In sound wave C, the recording level was too high, resulting in distortion of the sound wave by "clipping" (the tops and bottoms of the sound wave have been cut off since the recording amplitude has exceeded the range of the allowable amplitude resolution). In sound wave B, the recording level is just right—the recorded sound wave fills the approximate middle one third to half (≈ 33–50%) of the allowable amplitude range resulting in an excellent representation of the sound wave without clipping.

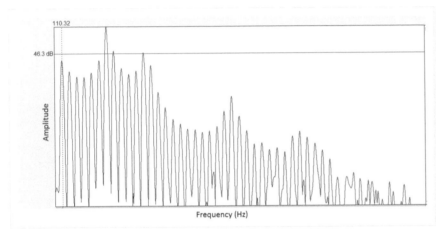

Fig. 4.7 Spectrum of a portion of a highly periodic voice waveform. The first significant peak in the spectrum is often the fundamental frequency (F0—a.k.a. the first harmonic). In this example, the $F_0 \approx 110$ Hz and higher frequency harmonics that occur at integer multiples (i.e., whole number multiples) of the F_0 are also observed. Therefore, the frequency spacing between the harmonics is also equal to the F_0.

provide objective correlates to the perceptual attributes of vocal pitch, loudness, and quality. Many of these measures have been recently identified and described as essential in forming a minimal set of acoustic measures used in the instrumental assessment of voice.[11]

4.4.1 Measures of Vocal Frequency

The categorization of typical or disordered voice in terms of *pitch* (a psychoacoustic scale that allows for the ordering of sounds from "low" to "high") is an essential part of the conventional voice diagnostic.[13] An objective and measurable correlate of pitch is *frequency* (Hz), with the *fundamental frequency* (F_0) generally appearing as the lowest harmonic frequency in the voice signal and may be observed in the spectrum of the voice signal as the frequency spacing between the harmonics (▶ Fig. 4.7).

How do we measure the F_0 of the voice signal? We know that, during the vibratory cycle, the adducted vocal folds are put into oscillation/vibration by the expiratory airstream, and the pitch of the sound produced is related to the number of vocal fold oscillations/cycles of vibration per unit time. The term *frequency* (typically measured in Hertz [Hz]) refers specifically to the measurement of the number of cycles of vibration per second. While the **fundamental frequency** (F_0) of the voice may be identified from the frequency location of the lowest harmonic peak in the spectrum, as well as via the frequency spacing between the spectral harmonics, the identification of vocal F_0 is calculated from

the sound wave by estimating the *period* (i.e., the time it takes to complete a cycle of vibration) of the cycles of vibration being analyzed (▶ Fig. 4.8).

While it is possible to measure the period (and convert to frequency) for each visible cycle of vibration in a sound wave, we typically use computer programs to do these calculations in a much more efficient manner. Estimations of the vocal period may be computed from the digitized voice signal using various methods such as *peak picking* (measurement of the period of the cycle as the time interval between two consecutive peak amplitudes), *zero-crossings* (measurement of the period of the cycle as the difference between two consecutive zero-crossing points, often defined as the amplitude closest to zero immediately preceding the peak amplitude of the cycle), *waveform matching* (determine the period by computation of the point at which the mean squared error between the two adjacent cycles is minimized), and *autocorrelation* (determines the period by identifying the repeating pattern of vibration via correlation). Once the period of a cycle (or average period within a specified duration of the sound wave) is identified, the frequency may be easily computed from reciprocal of period (in seconds)

$$(i.e., Frequency\ (Hz) = \frac{1}{Period\ (s)}).$$

As you will see, changes and/or differences in vocal pitch and frequency are associated with factors such as typical aging, sex, and body type. In addition, changes in pitch and frequency are also frequently reported as characteristics of disordered voice.

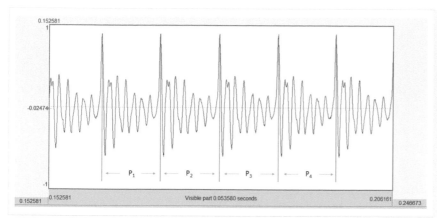

Fig. 4.8 A portion of a highly periodic voice waveform. Four cycles of vibration are shown. The time it takes to complete a cycle of vibrating is referred to as the period (P). The inverse of the period (in seconds) is the frequency (i.e., frequency [Hz] = 1/(Period (s))). Successive estimates of the period and frequency can be averaged to estimate the mean fundamental frequency (F_0). In this example, the mean period is 0.00907 and the mean F_0 is 110.25 Hz.

Measures of vocal frequency are particularly important to obtain because the complexity of the disordered voice signal may lead to inaccurate judgments of pitch. Because the fundamental frequency of the voice is a direct result of changes in factors such as (**1**) elasticity or tissue stress, (**2**) effective length, and (**3**) (to a degree) the effective vibratory mass of the vocal folds, the speech-language pathologists may discern key insights in reference to the function of the phonatory mechanism from their evaluation.[14] As a result, fundamental frequency measures, and in particular measures of the *mean fundamental frequency*, are the most frequently reported measures obtained in voice evaluation protocols. The following minimal set of vocal frequency measures have been demonstrated to be effective in the description of both typical and atypical/disordered voice production.[11]

Mean Speaking Fundamental Frequency (Mean F_0)

The measurement of mean fundamental frequency (*mean F_0*) during speech production (often referred to as the *mean speaking F_0* or *speaking fundamental frequency [SFF]*) is the average of the fundamental frequency estimates across the entire acoustic signal or portion of signal being analyzed and is generally reported in **Hertz** (**Hz**). This measurement approximates the perception of habitual pitch.[15] Because mean F_0/SFF is a useful correlate of vocal pitch, this measurement is useful in objectively documenting the appropriateness of pitch level for a patient's age, sex, race, etc.

It is best to make the measurement of mean F_0/SFF from a sample of reading or spontaneous speech (i.e., a continuous speech sample), with commonly used samples including portions of "the Rainbow Passage"[16] or CAPE-V sentences.[17] Zraick et al have indicated that it is best to make this measurement from a continuous speech sample of at least 5 seconds in duration (e.g., second and third sentences of the Rainbow Passage; combined CAPE-V sentence productions).[18] As always, procedures should be standardized so that the same procedures/instructions are provided both inter-subject and intra-subject (e.g., if used for tracking progress).

It has been recommended that, when using a reading sample, we ask our patient to read an entire passage (e.g., the entire first paragraph of "the Rainbow Passage"), but we will record and analyze an embedded or central portion of the passage (e.g., second or second and third sentences of the passage). Use of an embedded portion of a larger passage helps retain the naturalness of the patient's speaking style while avoiding possible initial or final sentence effects, and also provides a sample of speech production that tends to correlate well with longer productions while keeping storage requirements for digitized speech samples at a manageable level.[19] The reading of a standard passage is generally useable for most patients. However, when working with patients who may not be able to read effectively (e.g., very young children, those with linguistic deficits, or patients with visual deficits), a sample may be elicited by means of sentence repetition, counting, or picture description tasks.

Based on a review of literature and the clinical experience of these authors, the following general expectations for mean F_0/SFF in nondysphonic individuals are suggested:

- **Infants**: 400 to 600 Hz (both males and females).
- **Children**: 250 to 300 Hz (both males and females).
- **Adults**: Males, 100 to 150 Hz; females, 180 to 230 Hz.
- **Senescent adults**: Possible increases in the mean F_0 of the male voice; possible decreases in the mean F_0 of the postmenopausal female voice.

▸ Table 4.1 provides representative examples of mean F_0/SFF obtained from various literature sources.

Fundamental Frequency Standard Deviation, Pitch Sigma, and F_0 Coefficient of Variation (F_0 CV/vF_0)

The F_0 standard deviation (F_0 SD, reported in Hz) is a measure of average F_0 variability and is a useful correlate of expected variations in pitch level during speech production, as well as the ability to produce a steady pitch sustained vowel production. When measured from a *continuous speech samples*, the F_0 SD is a useful measure in documenting the **intonation capability** (i.e., purposeful variations in pitch used to express linguistic intent). When measured in a *steady pitch sustained vowel* context, the F_0 SD is a valuable measure of **pitch stability or instability**. When measured in the context of sustained vowel production, the F_0 SD has been referred to as a measure of *long-term instability*, in which variations in frequency occur more slowly than the glottal vibration itself.[46]

Although F_0 SD may be reported in Hz, it is necessary to normalize the average variation for different mean F_0s (e.g., adult males vs. females). One such method is to convert the F_0 SD into

Table 4.1 Examples of mean F_0/SFF from various literature sources

Author	Gender	No. of subjects	Age	Mean and SD	Range
Fitch[20]	M	100	M = 19:6	116.65 (1.05 T)	85.0–155.0
	F	100	M = 19:5	217.00 (0.85 T)	165.0–255.0
Hollien and Jackson[21, a]	M	157	17:9–25:8 (M = 20:3)	123.3 Hz	90.5–165.2
Hollien and Shipp[22]	M	25	20–29	119.5	N/A
	M	25	30–39	112.2	N/A
	M	25	40–49	107.1	N/A
	M	25	50–59	118.4	N/A
	M	25	60–69	112.2	N/A
	M	25	70–79	132.1	N/A
	M	25	80–89	146.3	N/A
McGlone and McGlone[23]	F	10	7:6–8:6	275.8 (0.6 T)	N/A
Horii[24]	M	65	26–79 (M = 54.1 y)	112.5 (17.3)	84–151
Honjo and Isshiki[25]	M	20	69–85	162.0 (30.7)	N/A
	F	20	69–85	165.0 (32.5)	N/A
Hudson and Holbrook[26, b]	M_B	100	18–29	110.15 (16.21)	81.95–158.50
	F_B	100	18–29	193.10 (18.58)	139.05–266.10
Murry and Doherty[27]	M	5	55–71 (M = 63.8)	122.9	104.0–137.7
Stoicheff[28]	F	21	20–29 (M = 24.6)	224.3	192.2–275.4
	F	18	30–39 (M = 35.4)	213.3	181.0–240.6
	F	21	40–49 (M = 46.4)	220.8	189.8–272.9
	F	17	50–59 (M = 54.4)	199.3	176.4–241.2
	F	15	60–69 (M = 65.8)	199.7	142.8–234.9
	F	19	70 + (M = 75.4)	202.2	170.0–248.6
Bennett[29, c]	M	15	M = 8:2	234.0 (19.76)	204.0–270.0
	F	10	M = 8:2	235.0 (12.31)	221.0–258.0
	M	15	M = 9:2	226.0 (16.42)	198.0–263.0
	F	10	M = 9:2	222.0 (8.25)	209.0–236.0
	M	15	M = 10:2	224.0 (14.68)	208.0–259.0
	F	10	M = 10:2	228.0 (9.37)	215.0–239.0
	M	15	M = 11:2	216.0 (15.04)	195.0–259.0
	F	10	M = 11:2	221.0 (13.43)	200.0–244.0
Ramig and Ringel[30, d]	$M_{Y,G}$	8	26–35 (M = 29.5)	121.93 (1.91 ST)	N/A
	$M_{Y,P}$	8	25–38 (M = 32.3)	127.30 (2.61 ST)	N/A
	$M_{M,G}$	8	46–56 (M = 53.0)	118.36 (3.02 ST)	N/A
	$M_{M,P}$	8	42–59 (M = 52.6)	122.85 (2.17 ST)	N/A
	$M_{O,G}$	8	62–75 (M = 67.5)	125.98 (2.96 ST)	N/A
	$M_{O,P}$	8	64–74 (M = 69.1)	132.89 (2.43 ST)	N/A
Horii[19]	M	18	10–12	226.5 (20.5)	192.1–268.5
	F	18	10–12	237.5 (15.9)	198.1–271.1

Table 4.1 continued

Author	Gender	No. of subjects	Age	Mean and SD	Range
Moran and Gilbert[31]	M	2	24–29	152.0	137.0–167.0
	F	3	24–29	244.0	220.0–278.0
Pedersen et al[32]	M	19	8.7–12.9	273.0	N/A
	M	15	13.0–15.9	184.0	N/A
	M	14	16.0–19.5	125.0	N/A
Kent et al[33]	F	19	65–80 (M =71.8)	194.0 (6.0)	N/A
Shipp et al[34, e]	M_Y	10	21–35 (M=25.3)	120.67 (10.87)	103.54–139.08
	M_M	10	46–71 (M=57.7)	106.22 (2.27)	91.0–131.24
	M_O	10	77–90 (M=83.7)	149.23 (19.97)	116.39–187.57
Awan and Mueller[35]	F_Y	9	M = 21.18 (1.06)	207.67 (16.38)	186.0–230.0
	F_E	9	M = 101.7 (2.40)	176.92 (22.61)	135.35–210.33
Awan[36, f]	M	10	18–30 y	123.00 (12.54)	102.0–137.0
	F	10	18–30 y	206.60 (14.99)	186.0–230.0
Morris et al[37, g]	M	18	20–35	125.8 (11.1)	N/A
	M	14	40–55	117.2 (9.4)	N/A
	M	18	>65	130.1 (16.7)	N/A
Murry et al[38, h]	M_Y	9	20–35	137.0 (0.9 ST)	N/A
	M_O	6	59–73	139.0 (6.9 ST)	N/A
	F_Y	10	20–35	195.0 (1.2 ST)	N/A
	F_O	7	59–73	170.0 (2.3 ST)	N/A
Awan and Mueller[39, i]	M_W	15	5:1–6:3	240.07 (15.89)	211.89–263.06
	F_W	20	5:1–6:1	243.35 (22.17)	195.20–291.10
	M_B	18	5:0–6:0	241.31 (18.05)	204.94–274.35
	F_B	17	5:1–6:0	231.48 (14.99)	208.08–261.73
	M_H	16	5:1–6:0	248.99 (20.18)	219.16–287.51
	F_H	19	5:1–5:11	248.04 (14.45)	217.56–274.03
Morris[40, j]	M_W	15	M = 8.4 y (0.4)	213.0 (15.0)	N/A
		15	M = 9.4 y (0.3)	219.0 (18.0)	N/A
		15	M = 10.5 y (0.2)	220.0 (21.0)	N/A
	M_B	15	M = 8.3 y (0.4)	230.0 (22.0)	N/A
		15	M = 9.5 y (0.2)	217.0 (39.0)	N/A
		15	M = 10.6 y (0.2)	204.0 (37.0)	N/A
Awan[41]	F	10	18–30 (mean = 23.80 y)	200.85 (15.70)	N/A
	F	10	40–49 (mean = 43.40 y)	175.37 (11.18)	N/A
	F	10	50–59 (mean = 54.80 y)	167.66 (22.23)	N/A
	F	10	60–69 (mean = 65.20 y)	151.16 (18.30)	N/A
	F	10	70–79 (mean = 72.30 y)	156.08 (20.19)	N/A
Izadi et al[42]	M	100	18–45 (mean = 29.2 y)	122.48 (13.18)	N/A
	F	100	18–45 (mean = 31.6 y)	183.12 (26.5)	N/A

Table 4.1 continued

Author	Gender	No. of subjects	Age	Mean and SD	Range
Goy et al[43]	M	55	18–28 (mean =19.4)	128 (21)	N/A
	M	51	65–86 (mean =73.3)	127 (27)	N/A
	F	104	18–27 (mean =18.9)	251 (28)	N/A
	F	82	63–82 (mean =71.1)	211 (42)	N/A
Gelfer and Denor[44]	M & F	18	6 (mean = 6.33 y)	240.5 (34.0)	N/A
		22	7 (mean = 7.27 y)	252.9 (26.6)	N/A
		23	8 (mean = 8.29 y)	239.7 (29.5	N/A
		63	6–8	244.8 (30.0)	N/A
Cox and Selent[45]	M	10	20–29 (mean = 22.7 y)	121.48 (14.87)	N/A
	M	5	30–39 (mean = 34.6 y)	128.38 (12.07)	N/A
	M	6	40–49 (mean = 42.5 y)	117.16 (6.03)	N/A
	M	9	50–59 (mean = 55.11 y)	114.25 (14.63)	N/A
	M	5	60–69 (mean = 62.6 y)	112.95 (6.28)	N/A

Abbreviations: M, mean; N/A, not available; SFF, speaking fundamental frequency; T, tones; ST, semitones; y, years.
Notes:
a. Data from extemporaneous speech only.
b. Data from Black (B) subjects.
c. Longitudinal study - same male and female subjects studied over a 3 year period.
d. Young (Y), Middle age (M), and Old age (O) subjects in good (G) and poor (P) condition. Data from reading of a standard passage.
e. Young (Y), Middle-aged (M), and Old (O) subjects.
f. Data from nonsingers only.
g. Data from nonsingers only.
h. Young (Y) and older (O) subjects. Data from a standard reading passage averaged over three times daily on three different days.
i. Data from White (W), Black (B), and Hispanic (H) children.
j. Data from White (M_W) and Black (M_B) subjects (spontaneous speech data only).

pitch sigma, in which the average variation in Hz is converted to semitones. The conversion is accomplished using the following formula:

$$n = \frac{12\log_{10}(f_2/f_1)}{\log_{10}2} \text{ or } n = 39.86 \times \log_{10}(f_2/f_1)$$

where n is the number of semitones between the two frequency values, and f_2 is a higher frequency value and f_1 is a lower frequency value.

While pitch sigma may be useful for describing the perceived pitch variations purposefully used in speech production or singing, it is our view that the use of a perceptual semitone scale to represent the stability of pitch/F_0 production in sustained vowel contexts is less useful. In addition, the computation of semitones is relatively cumbersome. Instead, we prefer the use of an F_0 coefficient of variation (CV), in which the term *coefficient of variation* refers to the reporting of the average variation as a percentage of the mean value. By converting to a percentage of the mean (i.e. $\frac{F_0 \text{ standard deviation}}{\text{mean}F_0} \times 100$) we "normalize" F_0 variability for the comparison of different voice types. As an example, it is often observed that, *during continuous speech*, the F_0 SD is **minimally ≈ 10% of the mean speaking F_0.**[180] Therefore, for a male speaking with an F_0 of 120 Hz, we would expect an F_0 SD of approximately 12 Hz; for a child with an F_0 of 250 Hz, F_0 SD would be approximately 25 Hz. In this example, it appears clear that the child has substantially greater absolute F_0 variability (in Hz)

than the adult male (25 vs. 12 Hz). However, when converted to a CV, we would see that both subjects produce the same variability (10% of the mean). *An F_0 CV (a.k.a. vF_0) markedly less than 10% during speech production may be consistent with the perception of* **monopitch**.

In contrast to expectations in speech production, **if the patient is able to produce and control a stable, steady pitch during sustained vowel production, we will expect that the F_0 SD will be quite small in relation to the mean F_0, and the F_0 CV will tend to be less than 1% of the mean F_0.** Increased F_0 CV/ vF_0 in sustained vowels may reflect pitch instability, but also may reflect increased levels of noise and the tendency toward aperiodic voice production. This is because the F_0 estimates used in the computation of F_0 SD and F_0 CV are derived from estimates of cycle periods (remember, $\frac{1}{\text{Period (s)}} = Frequency\ [Hz]$. and if the ability to identify highly repetitive, cyclic patterns in the voice signal is disturbed, the F_0 computations will also be disturbed and increased variation in estimates of F_0 will occur. Therefore, an increased F_0 SD and F_0 CV in sustained vowel production may also be used as a correlate of quality disturbance (e.g., breathiness; roughness) as well as a correlate of pitch stability/instability.

The sustained vowel sample(s) we elicit for the measurement of F_0 SD and F_0 CV will also be used for several other acoustic measures specifically related to vocal quality. However, if we simply ask the subject or patient to hold out a vowel (say "ahhhh"), in the majority of cases, the patient will produce the

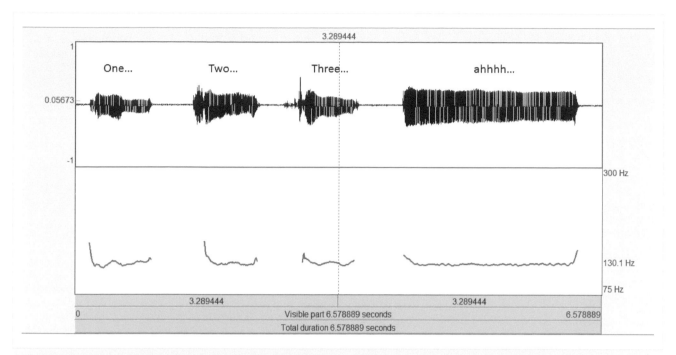

Fig. 4.9 Recorded sample of the sustained vowel /a/ elicited using the "1, 2, 3" method (upper window) and associated F_0 contour (lower window). Note that the F_0 level during the sustained vowel production is very similar to the F_0 produced during the chanted "1, 2, 3." Elicitation of a sustained vowel with this method tends to prevent atypically high F_0 productions.

vowel production at a substantially higher pitch level than their habitual speaking pitch. Instead, we would like this sustained vowel to have some reasonable similarity to the patient's habitual voice characteristics during their typical speech. The method that this book proposes is the "1, 2, 3" method of sustained vowel elicitation similar to that of Murry.[47] In this method, we ask our patient to "chant" the numbers "1, 2, 3," followed by a sustained vowel /a/ demonstration by the clinician is useful). Instructions may be as follows:

"I want you to chant the numbers 'one, two, three' followed by the vowel /a/ at a comfortable pitch and loudness, something like this":

→→→

"One, two, three, ahhhhhhhhhhhhhhhhh" (These words have a horizontal arrow over them to imply a flat intonation pattern; the vowel /a/ should be *sustained for 3 to 5 seconds*).

Sample 4.1 provides an audio example of a sustained vowel elicited using the "1, 2, 3" method and ▶ Fig. 4.9 shows the sound wave of the recorded sample and the associated F_0 contour. Note that the level of the F_0 contour for the sustained vowel is very similar to F_0 produced during the chanted "1, 2, 3."

Demonstrate the method and have your patient repeat it once without recording to make sure that they understand what he or she is to do. If you are satisfied that the patient understands the procedure, start your recording and have the patient repeat the sample three times. These three trials can all be captured in the same recording and saved for later analysis. Once your sample has been acquired, you will measure F_0 SD (as well as subsequent measures of jitter, shimmer, and HNR) on a central portion of the vowel (at least the central 1 second). If all three trials are similar in perceptual characteristics,

measures from the second trial will suffice for clinical purposes. If the voice quality deviation is intermittent and, perhaps, only affects one of the vowel samples, it is suggested that you compute your measurements on both a disrupted and nondisrupted sample to reflect the intermittent disturbance in your data.

The following are suggested general expectations for F_0 SD/F_0 CV in nondysphonic individuals:

- **Infants:** Increased F_0 SD and F_0 CV in sustained vowel production for infants and during puberty.
- **Adults:** F_0 CV is minimally ≈ 10% of the mean F_0 or higher in continuous speech, and pitch sigma is generally observed to be ≈ 2 to 4 STs. In sustained vowel production, we often observe F_0 CV to be ≈ 1% of the mean F_0 or less, and substantially less than 1 ST for pitch sigma.
- **Senescent adults:** Possible increases in F_0 SD, F_0 CV, and pitch sigma during both sustained vowel and continuous speech productions.

▶ Table 4.2 provides representative examples of F_0 SD obtained from various literature sources.

4.4.2 Examples of Mean F_0, F_0 Standard Deviation, and F_0 Coefficient of Variation Measurements Using Praat

The following examples were analyzed using *Praat*. The clinician may have recorded a new voice signal (in Praat, select **New | Record Mono Sound**) or may be analyzing a previously recorded voice sample (in Praat select **Open | Read from File**). The recorded or opened sound wave will be placed in the "Objects"

Table 4.2 Examples of F_0 standard deviation (SD) from various literature sources as reported in terms of F_0 coefficient of variation (vF_0; F_0, CV) and pitch sigma (F_0 SD reported in semitones—ST).

Author	Gender	No. of subjects	Age	Mean and SD	Range
Hollien and Jackson[21, a]	M	157	17:9–25:8 (M = 20:3)	1.6 T	0.5–2.5
Horii[24]	M	65	26–79 (M = 54.1)	2.41 ST (0.48)	1.46–3.54
Murry and Doherty[27, b]	M	5	55–71 (M = 63.8)	1.88 ST	1.0–3.2
Stoicheff[28]	F	21	20–29 (M = 24.6)	3.78 ST	N/A
	F	18	30–39 (M = 35.4)	3.92 ST	N/A
	F	21	40–49 (M = 46.4)	4.00 ST	N/A
	F	17	50–59 (M = 54.4)	4.33 ST	N/A
	F	15	60–69 (M = 65.8)	4.25 ST	N/A
	F	19	70 + (M = 75.4)	4.70 ST	N/A
Horii[48, c]	M	12	24–40	0.27 ST (0.09)	0.14–0.47
Linville and Fisher[49, V]	F	25	25–35	1.47 Hz (0.39)	0.84–2.39
		25	45–55	1.68 Hz (0.43)	1.08–2.69
		25	70–80	2.52 Hz (1.49)	1.06–8.05
Linville[50, d, V]	F	22	18–22 (M = 20.32; S.D. = 0.95)	0.11 ST (0.04)	0.05–0.33
Linville et al[51, V]	F	20	67–86 (M = 76.0; S.D. = 6.09)	0.34 ST (0.19)	0.10–0.74
Orlikoff[52, e]	M_Y	6	26–33 (M = 30.0)	0.96%	
	M_E	6	68–80 (M = 73.3)	2.19%	
Shipp et al[34, f]	M_Y	10	21–35 (M = 25.3)	1.76 ST (0.26)	1.34–2.30
	M_M	10	46–71 (M = 57.7)	2.25 ST (0.45)	1.61–3.08
	M_O	10	77–90 (M = 83.7)	2.60 ST (0.60)	2.08–3.85
Wolfe et al[53]	M & F	20	18–30	1.86 (1.89)	0.33–7.52
Awan and Mueller[39, g]	M_W	15	5:1–6:3	4.38 ST (1.78)	2.18–9.36
	F_W	20	5:1–6:1	5.59 ST (1.81)	2.92–8.98
	M_B	18	5:0–6:0	5.26 ST (1.44)	2.85–8.28
	F_B	17	5:1–6:0	5.03 ST (2.04)	2.64–10.71
	M_H	16	5:1–6:0	5.39 ST (2.59)	2.75–11.08
	F_H	19	5:1–5:11	4.64 ST (1.67)	2.53–9.64
Morris[40, h]	M_W	15	M = 8.4 y (0.4)	2.5 ST (0.9)	N/A
		15	M = 9.4 y (0.3)	1.9 ST (0.7)	N/A
		15	M = 10.5 y (0.2)	2.3 ST (0.8)	N/A
	M_B	15	M = 8.3 y (0.4)	2.1 ST (0.7)	N/A
		15	M = 9.5 y (0.2)	2.5 ST (0.9)	N/A
		15	M = 10.6 y (0.2)	3.2 ST (0.7)	N/A
Awan[1, i]	M	20	18–30	0.29 ST (0.09)	0.17–0.54
	F	20	18–30	0.22 ST (0.07)	0.13–0.45
Awan and Scarpino[54, R]	M	10	18–30	16.65%	N/A
	W	10	18–30	15.60%	N/A

Table 4.2 continued

Author	Gender	No. of subjects	Age	Mean and SD	Range
	C	10	5–9	13.01%	N/A
Awan[41, j]	F	10	18–30 (Mean = 23.80 y)	2.79 ST (1.07)	N/A
	F	10	40–49 (Mean = 43.40 y)	3.00 ST (1.19)	N/A
	F	10	50–59 (Mean = 54.80 y)	3.65 ST (1.13)	N/A
	F	10	60–69 (Mean = 65.20 y)	4.77 ST (1.21)	N/A
	F	10	70–79 (Mean = 72.30 y)	4.90 ST (0.72)	N/A
	M & F	10	5–6	0.29 ST (0.06)	0.20–0.37
Hema et al[55, V]	M	30	18–25	0.98%	
	F	30	18–25	0.97%	N/A
Petrović-Lazić et al[56]	F	21	21–61 (Mean = 47.57)	1.12% (0.44)	N/A
Aithal et al[57]	M	24	20–30	1.04% (0.50)	0.53–2.45
	F	24	20–30	0.84% (0.31)	0.40–1.64
Gelfer and Denor[44]	M & F	18	6 (Mean = 6.33 y)	1.96 ST (0.77)	N/A
		22	7 (Mean = 7.27 y)	2.24 ST (1.03)	N/A
		23	8 (Mean = 8.29 y)	1.96 ST (0.59)	N/A
		63	6–8	2.06 ST (0.82)	N/A

Notes: M, mean; R, rainbow; V, vowel.
a. Data from extemporaneous speech only.
b. Speech - Converted from tones.
c. Vowel - Data reported from modal register phonations and reported in semitones.
d. Data from the vowel /a/ only.
e. Vowel - Data from healthy young men (M_Y) and healthy elderly men (M_E).
f. Speech - Young (Y), Middle-aged (M), and Old (O) subjects.
g. Data from White (W), Black (B), and Hispanic (H) children.
h. Speech - Data from White (M_W) and Black (M_B) subjects (spontaneous speech data only).
i. Data for the vowel /a/ only.
j. Speech.

list—selection of the "*View& Edit*" button will provide a view of the sound wave and the ability to playback the recorded sound. Selection of *View | Show Analyses* will provide checkboxes—for these examples, select "*Show Pitch*" and "*Show Pulses.*"

The F_0 contour is computed automatically using the default settings in Praat once *View | Edit* is selected. However, selecting the *Pitch | Pitch Settings* will allow the user to select the analysis method (the autocorrelation method is recommended for F_0 analysis) and pitch range (please note that the use of the term "pitch" as per *Praat* is inaccurate and should be "frequency"). It is recommended that the pitch analysis range be set so that the low and high limits of the analysis will be approximately 100 to 150 Hz above the expected mean F_0 for the speaker. As an example, a pitch range of 100 to 300 Hz for typical young adult female speakers will tend to place the F_0 contour within the middle of the lower analysis window with variations within the F_0 contour nicely detailed. If the user selects a pitch range that is too large (e.g., 75–1,000 Hz), the F_0 contour will appear highly compressed with very little detail regarding fluctuations in the contour provided and the estimates of F_0 will be prone to error.

If the user selects a pitch range that is too narrow (e.g., 175–225 Hz for a typical adult female), errors in F_0 estimation will occur in which F_0s above or below the selected range may not be captured and F_0s above the higher limit may be measured at half of the actual F_0 or may result in estimation errors. It is important that the user of voice analysis software becomes familiar with key analysis parameters and always compares what they are seeing in the F_0 contour and measuring with their perception of the recorded voice sample and their knowledge regarding expectations for measured vocal parameters such as mean F_0.

To obtain various measurements of F_0 (e.g., mean, SD), the user will select *Pulses | Show Pulses*, use the mouse pointer to select the portion of the sound wave they want to analyze, and then select *Pulses | Voice Report* to view analysis statistics. The "pulses" are markers that identify the boundaries of each detected cycle of vibration (i.e., where a repetitive pattern starts and ends/repeats). ▶ Fig. 4.10 shows a magnified view of the syllable "rain" in the word "rainbow." The pulses can be observed marking each cycle of vibration in the sound

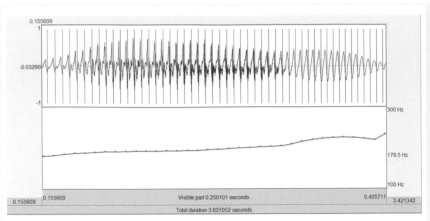

Fig. 4.10 Magnified view of the syllable "rain" in the word "rainbow." Each cycle of vibration in the sound wave (upper window) is marked with a blue line ("pulse") indicating the boundaries of each cycle. The time between pluses is the period, and the estimates of period are converted to estimates of frequency (lower window). When using Praat, pulses must be turned on to compute many statistical measures of the sound wave such as the mean F_0.

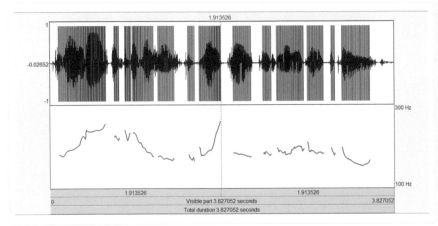

Fig. 4.11 Typical young adult female speaking the second sentence of the Rainbow Passage. The mean $F_0 = 193.11$ Hz and the F_0 standard deviation = 24.11 Hz (F_0 coefficient of variation = 12.45%). Praat analysis parameters: pitch range = 100 to 300 Hz; autocorrelation; voicing threshold = 0.60.

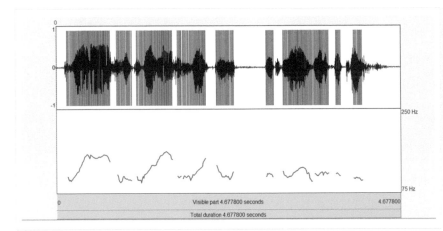

Fig. 4.12 Typical adult male speaking the second sentence of the Rainbow Passage. The mean $F_0 = 122.54$ Hz and the F_0 standard deviation = 17.98 Hz (F_0 coefficient of variation = 14.67%). Praat analysis parameters: pitch range = 75 to 250 Hz; autocorrelation; voicing threshold = 0.60.

wave. Estimates of *period* are computed from these pulses and then converted to estimates of *frequency*.

▶ Fig. 4.11 shows the sound wave and F_0 contour for a typical young adult female (age 22 years) speaking the second sentence of the Rainbow Passage (play **Sample 4.2** to hear the voice sample). The voice sample should be perceived as appropriate in pitch for a typical young adult female with expected intonation (i.e., pitch variations are not excessive and are not highly limited as in flattened intonation and monopitch). The intonation is viewed as fluctuations in the F_0 contour, with stressed syllables observed to have marked increases in F_0 (e.g., the syllable "rain"; the word "white")

and typical falling pitch and F_0 at the end of a noninterrogative sentence. In this example, the mean $F_0 = 193.11$ Hz, well within the expected range of 180 to 230 Hz for a young adult female. In addition, her F_0 SD = 24.11 Hz, resulting in a F_0 CV = 12.45%, reflecting typical F_0 variation in speech that is often observed to be greater than 10% of the mean F_0.

Sample 4.3 and ▶ Fig. 4.12 present the sound wave and F_0 contour for the second sentence of the Rainbow Passage produced by a typical adult male (25 years). The mean F_0 of 122.54 is very close to the midpoint of the typical expected range of 100 to 150 Hz. Again, intonation patterns are typical

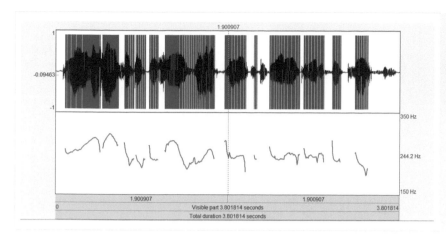

Fig. 4.13 Typical 5-year-old female speaking the second sentence of the Rainbow Passage. The mean $F_0 = 249.17$ Hz and the F_0 standard deviation = 20.11 Hz (F_0 coefficient of variation = 8.10%). Praat analysis parameters: pitch range = 150 to 350 Hz; autocorrelation; voicing threshold = 0.60.

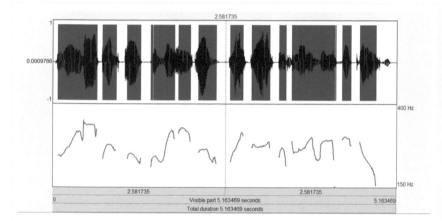

Fig. 4.14 Typical 5-year-old male speaking the second sentence of the Rainbow Passage. The mean $F_0 = 271.55$ Hz and the F_0 standard deviation = 34.36 Hz (F_0 coefficient of variation = 12.65%). Praat analysis parameters: pitch range = 150 to 400 Hz; autocorrelation; voicing threshold = 0.60.

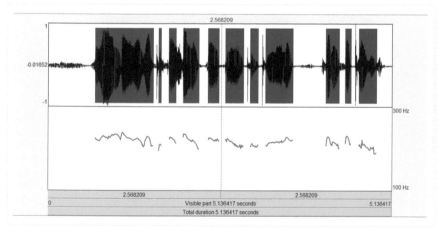

Fig. 4.15 Adult female (45 years old) with unilateral vocal fold paresis producing the second sentence of the Rainbow Passage. The mean $F_0 = 218.05$ Hz and the F_0 standard deviation = 9.69 Hz (F_0 coefficient of variation (CV) = 4.44%). The F_0 contour is relatively flat consistent with the perception of monopitch and the measurement of a substantially reduced F_0 CV (substantially < 10% minimum expected variation). Praat analysis parameters: pitch range = 100 to 300 Hz; autocorrelation; voicing threshold = 0.60.

with appropriate F_0 variation confirmed by the measured F_0 CV = 14.67%.

▶ Fig. 4.13 and **Sample 4.4** as well as ▶ Fig. 4.14 and **Sample 4.5** show the speech samples of a typical 5-year-old female and male, respectively. As expected, both child speakers have substantially higher mean F_0s than either of the previous adult speakers (mean $F_0 = 249.17$ Hz and 271.55 Hz). Note that, at this age, males and females often have very similar mean F_0s, and a male may very well have a higher mean F_0 than a female of the same age (as in this case). Though the female speaker has a somewhat smaller F_0 CV than our general expectation (8.10%),

her intonation is perceived as typical and not flattened, and may reflect a slightly limited range of F_0 variation or may simply reflect her reading style. The F_0 CV for the 5-year-old male speaker is at an expected level (12.65%).

Let us now look and listen to some dysphonic speech samples and examine some possible effects on mean F_0, F_0 SD, and F_0 CV. ▶ Fig. 4.15 and **Sample 4.6** represent a speech sample from a 45-year-old female who was diagnosed with unilateral vocal fold paresis post-thyroidectomy. Her voice was perceived as being initiated with audible breathing (inhalatory stridor) and having a weak, breathy quality and monopitch. The flattened F_0

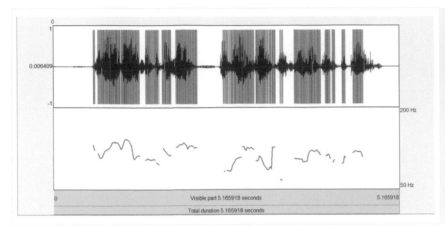

Fig. 4.16 Adult female (59 years old) chronic smoker with Reinke's edema producing the second sentence of the Rainbow Passage. The mean $F_0 = 114.55$ Hz and the F_0 standard deviation = 14.99 Hz (F_0 coefficient of variation = 13.08%). Praat analysis parameters: pitch range = 50 to 200 Hz; autocorrelation; voicing threshold = 0.60.

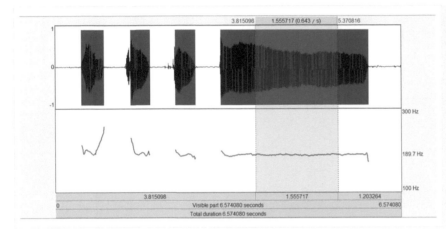

Fig. 4.17 Typical voice young adult female (24 years old) producing the sustained vowel /a/ ("ahhh"). Measures from a central portion of the vowel production showed a mean $F_0 = 189.68$ Hz and the F_0 standard deviation = 1.12 Hz (F_0 coefficient of variation = 0.59%). Praat analysis parameters: pitch range = 100 to 300 Hz; autocorrelation; voicing threshold = 0.60.

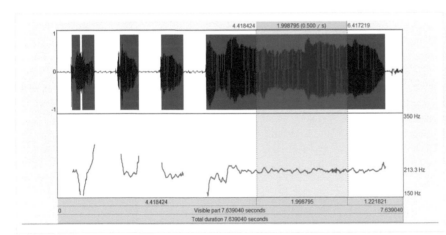

Fig. 4.18 Adult female (32 years old) with hyperfunctional, strained voice producing the sustained vowel /a/ ("ahhh"). Measures from a central portion of the vowel production showed a mean $F_0 = 213.28$ Hz and the F_0 standard deviation = 2.98 Hz (F_0 coefficient of variation = 1.40%). Praat analysis parameters: pitch range = 150 to 350 Hz; autocorrelation; voicing threshold = 0.60.

contour is evident, and the F_0 CV = 4.44% (mean $F_0 = 218.05$ Hz; F_0 SD = 9.69 Hz) provides a measured correlate of the perception of monopitch.

In ► Fig. 4.16 and **Sample 4.7**, the voice of a 59-year-old female chronic smoker with Reinke's edema is analyzed and heard. Her voice was perceived as mildly diplophonic with audible breathing, and particularly low in pitch. Her mean F_0 was measured at 114.55 Hz (F_0 SD = 14.99 Hz; F_0 CV = 13.08%). While mean F_0 may lower in some postmenopausal females, this F_0 is substantially reduced secondary to increased vocal fold mass and is lower than the mean F_0 of many adult male speakers.

Measures of F_0 SD and F_0 CV obtained from sustained vowel samples are useful measures of vocal stability. As observed in ► Fig. 4.17 and **Sample 4.8**, a steady pitch and loudness sustained vowel produced by a nondysphonic speaker should be produced with very little average variability and a CV that is typically less than 1% of the mean F_0 (mean $F_0 = 189.68$ Hz; F_0 SD = 1.12 Hz), F_0 CV = 0.59%). In contrast, ► Fig. 4.18 and **Sample 4.9** show the sustained vowel sample of an adult female with a strained, effortful voice quality. The F_0 instability observed in the F_0 contour is reflected in an increased F_0 SD and F_0 CV above our expected less than 1% threshold (1.40%). The patient produces a considerable

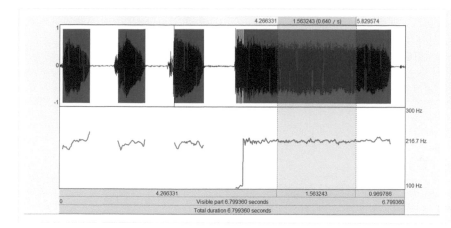

Fig. 4.19 Adult female (29 years) with breathy voice secondary to vocal nodules producing the sustained vowel /a/ ("ahhh"). Measures from a central portion of the vowel production showed a mean F_0 = 216.67 Hz and the F_0 standard deviation = 2.31 Hz (F_0 coefficient of variation = 1.06%). Praat analysis parameters: pitch range = 150 to 350 Hz; autocorrelation; voicing threshold = 0.60.

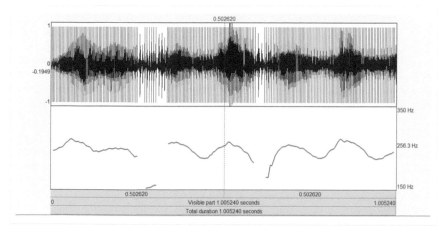

Fig. 4.20 Adult female (47 years old) with severe tremor and intermittent roughness secondary to adductor spasmodic dysphonia producing the sustained vowel /a/ ("ahhh"). Measures from a central portion of the vowel production showed a mean F_0 = 242.96 Hz and the F_0 standard deviation = 21.98 Hz (F_0 coefficient of variation = 9.05%). Praat analysis parameters: pitch range = 150 to 350 Hz; autocorrelation; voicing threshold = 0.60.

increase in vocal pitch and F_0 at the initiation of the vowel followed by a mild tremor.

An increase in the F_0 CV may also be observed in dysphonic voice production even though the perceived vocal pitch is relatively steady. ▶ Fig. 4.19 and **Sample 4.10** demonstrate the sustained vowel sample and F_0 contour for a patient with a moderate breathy voice production. Again, we can see instability in the F_0 contour of the sustained vowel which coincides with an increased F_0 CV (1.06%). In this case, the increased F_0 CV is primarily reflecting the fact that, with increased additive noise in the voice signal during breathiness, the periodicity of the voiced signal becomes disturbed, resulting in increased variation in measurements of period and F_0 during the vowel production.

A more extreme example of combined vocal tremor and dysphonic voice quality is observed in ▶ Fig. 4.20 and **Sample 4.11**. This voice signal was produced by a 47-year-old woman presenting with adductor spasmodic dysphonia (ADSD). We see that tremor produces an obvious "wavelike" rhythmic variation in the F_0 contour. As may be expected, the F_0 CV for this example shows an extreme deviation from our expected less than 1% threshold (F_0 CV = 9.05%). In addition, two intermittent periods of roughness result in extreme variations in the F_0 contour due to frequency jumps and episodes of noise often observed with this form of dysphonic quality.[58]

Total Phonational Frequency Range

Another measure used to document F_0 variation is the *Total Phonational Frequency* (F_0) *Range*. This entails an assessment of the **range between the lowest pitch and frequency in modal register to the highest pitch and frequency in falsetto**. Total phonational range provides an important index of laryngeal health and is often one of the first parameters of vocal capability affected in disordered voice.[15] This measure may be obtained either by using a pitch glide on a sustained sound (e.g., /a/) or in a stepwise fashion.[59] The lowest and highest phonational frequencies should be sustainable (1–2 seconds in duration) and repeatable within the total phonatory range. Because intra- and inter-subject variability on maximum performance tasks may be large and affected by factors such as practice, motivation, or instructions, it is recommended that at least three trials be conducted for both highest and lowest F_0 productions.[60] The total phonational frequency range would then be computed from the highest F_0 and the lowest F_0 productions observed out of the elicited trials.

When assessing the total phonational pitch/frequency range, it is important for the clinician to be aware of the difference between "physiological" range of phonation and the "musical" range.[16,61,62,63,64,65,66] In assessing physiological range, no constraints are placed on quality, pitch, loudness, or duration of the phonation, while the "musical" range entails "controlled" phonations, in which the patient must (**1**) sustain both the lowest and highest frequency for a minimum of 1 to 2 seconds, (**2**) must maintain a relatively steady intensity and frequency level, and (**3**) must produce a "quality" phonation (i.e., no pitch or phonation breaks; no excessive breathiness, harshness, or hoarseness). We suggest that, at the very least, range measures should be repeatable and sustainable, and that extreme vocal attempts (particularly at high pitch levels) be avoided. Case contends that measures of vocal capability are best evaluated during conditions of less than maximum effort, because it may be argued that even an inefficient larynx can produce voice when enough effort is applied.[15] In a similar manner, it may be argued that even inefficient vocal mechanisms may produce extensive vocal ranges if allowed to produce physiological voice, whereas the actual useable range of vocal pitches and frequencies would be much smaller if evaluated under the conditions of "controlled" phonation. *Therefore, we suggest that the total phonational frequency range be assessed in terms of musical range rather than physiological range.*

Within the phonational frequency range, the *highest phonational frequency* has been viewed as having particular importance in voice assessment. Wuyts et al stated that, when extra mass is evenly distributed along the true vocal fold(s), the higher vibratory rates become dampened.[67] The result is a decrease in the upper reaches of the phonational frequency range. Highest phonational F_0 may also be obtained and utilized as part of the **Dysphonia Severity Index** (**DSI**; see discussion on multivariate analysis).

To record the total (musical) phonational range:

1. Use a headset or handheld microphone. Because high pitch levels can be quite loud, it can be useful to hold the microphone by hand for this task and to move the microphone somewhat away from the mouth for the higher pitch productions. Alternatively, the output level of the preamplifier can also be turned down for these productions so as to avoid distorting any recordings.

2. To record the patient's minimum pitch level, provide the following instructions to your patient: "*I am going to ask you to hold the sound "ah" (/a/) at several different notes or pitches. Starting at a comfortable pitch level, I would like you to go down in steps to the lowest note you can hold out without your voice breaking or cracking. It will be similar to singing down a scale, such as...*" (provide an example for your patient here).

3. When the patient gets to the lowest sustainable pitch, have them repeat it at least three times so that (**1**) you can be sure that it is of reasonable quality (do not include vocal fry phonation), (**2**) you can be sure that it is repeatable, and (**3**) you can have the opportunity to cue them to lower productions if you believe that they have not truly reached their minimum pitch limit. When you are confident the patient has reached his or her lower pitch limit, record a brief sample on the computer (1–2 seconds).

4. To record the patient's maximum pitch level, provide the following instructions to your patient: "Starting at a comfortable pitch level, I would like you to go up in steps to the highest note you can hold without your voice breaking or cracking, including falsetto voice—falsetto is a high, thin, reedy voice such as... (provide example). It will be similar to singing up a scale, such as..." (provide an example for your patient here).

5. When the patient gets to his or her highest sustainable pitch, have him or her repeat it at least three times. When you are confident that the patient has reached the highest pitch limit, record a brief sample on the computer (1–2 seconds).

6. To compute the total phonational range in Hz, simply subtract the lowest pitch/frequency level from the highest. To convert the total range in Hz to semitones (STs), consult a chart of musical note/frequency equivalents (▶ Table 4.3) and count the number of semitones between the lowest and highest frequency level (you will probably have to "round" the low- and high-frequency levels to the nearest semitone).

Table 4.3 Table of musical note and frequency equivalents

Note	Frequency (Hz)	Note	Frequency (Hz)	Note	Frequency (Hz)	Note	Frequency (Hz)	Note	Frequency (Hz)	Note	Frequency (Hz)	Note	Frequency (Hz)
C_0	16.35	C_1	32.7	C_2	65.41	C_3	130.81	C_4	261.63	C_5	523.25	C_6	1046.5
$C^{\#}_0/D^b_0$	17.32	$C^{\#}_1/D^b_1$	34.65	$C^{\#}_2/D^b_2$	69.3	$C^{\#}_3/D^b_3$	138.59	$C^{\#}_4/D^b_4$	277.18	$C^{\#}_5/D^b_5$	554.37	$C^{\#}_6/D^b_6$	1108.73
D_0	18.35	D_1	36.71	D_2	73.42	D_3	146.83	D_4	293.66	D_5	587.33	D_6	1174.66
$D^{\#}_0/E^b_0$	19.45	$D^{\#}_1/E^b_1$	38.89	$D^{\#}_2/E^b_2$	77.78	$D^{\#}_3/E^b_3$	155.56	$D^{\#}_4/E^b_4$	311.13	$D^{\#}_5/E^b_5$	622.25	$D^{\#}_6/E^b_6$	1244.51
E_0	20.6	E_1	41.2	E_2	82.41	E_3	164.81	E_4	329.63	E_5	659.25	E_6	1318.51
F_0	21.83	F_1	43.65	F_2	87.31	F_3	174.61	F_4	349.23	F_5	698.46	F_6	1396.91
$F^{\#}_0/G^b_0$	23.12	$F^{\#}_1/G^b_1$	46.25	$F^{\#}_2/G^b_2$	92.5	$F^{\#}_3/G^b_3$	185	$F^{\#}_4/G^b_4$	369.99	$F^{\#}_5/G^b_5$	739.99	$F^{\#}_6/G^b_6$	1479.98
G_0	24.5	G_1	49	G_2	98	G_3	196	G_4	392	G_5	783.99	G_6	1567.98
$G^{\#}_0/A^b_0$	25.96	$G^{\#}_1/A^b_1$	51.91	$G^{\#}_2/A^b_2$	103.83	$G^{\#}_3/A^b_3$	207.65	$G^{\#}_4/A^b_4$	415.3	$G^{\#}_5/A^b_5$	830.61	$G^{\#}_6/A^b_6$	1661.22
A_0	27.5	A_1	55	A_2	110	A_3	220	A_4	440	A_5	880	A_6	1760
$A^{\#}_0/B^b_0$	29.14	$A^{\#}_1/B^b_1$	58.27	$A^{\#}_2/B^b_2$	116.54	$A^{\#}_3/B^b_3$	233.08	$A^{\#}_4/B^b_4$	466.16	$A^{\#}_5/B^b_5$	932.33	$A^{\#}_6/B^b_6$	1864.66
B_0	30.87	B_1	61.74	B_2	123.47	B_3	246.94	B_4	493.88	B_5	987.77	B_6	1975.53

Alternatively, the clinician may use the aforementioned formulas by which the number of semitones (n) between the highest frequency (f2) and the lowest frequency (f1) may be calculated.[68]

Suggested expectations regarding the total phonational range in nondysphonic individuals are as follows:

- **Infants and children**: Phonational range of approximately 1 to 2 octaves (12–24 semitones).
- **Adults**: Phonational range of approximately 2 to 3 octaves (24 to 36 semitones). Adults without singing training or without singing experience may be limited to approximately 20 to 24 semitones.
- **Senescent adults**: Possible decreases in phonational range with increased age.

▶ Table 4.4 provides representative examples of total phonational range in semitones obtained from various literature sources.

4.4.3 Examples of Total Phonational Range Measurements Using Praat

Two examples are provided to illustrate the recording and measurement of total phonational range. In ▶ Fig. 4.21 and **Sample 4.12**, we see the recorded sound wave and F_0 contour for an adult male providing a glide from the lowest phonational pitch and F_0 in modal register to the highest phonational pitch

Table 4.4 Examples of total phonational range from various literature sources

Author	Gender	No. of subjects	Age	Mean and SD	Range
Hollien and Jackson[21]	M	157	17:9–25:8 (M = 20:3)	19.4 T	14.5–27.0
Ramig and Ringel[30, a]	M$_{Y,G}$	8	26–35 (M = 29.5)	32.20 ST (8.77)	N/A
	M$_{Y,P}$	8	25–38 (M = 32.3)	26.65 ST (7.10)	N/A
	M$_{M,G}$	8	46–56 (M = 53.0)	28.29 ST (8.74)	N/A
	M$_{M,P}$	8	42–59 (M = 52.6)	26.84 ST (3.57)	N/A
	M$_{O,G}$	8	62–75 (M = 67.5)	31.37 ST (4.38)	N/A
	M$_{O,P}$	8	64–74 (M = 69.1)	24.30 ST (7.12)	N/A
Pedersen et al[32]	M	19	8.7–12.9	34.4 ST	N/A
	M	15	13.0–15.9	37.5 ST	N/A
	M	14	16.0–19.5	41.4 ST	N/A
Linville[69]	F	24	25–35	33.13 ST (3.43)	28–40
	F	20	45–55	34.00 ST (3.22)	27–38
	F	23	70–80	28.96 ST (4.13)	19–35
Linville et al[51]	F	20	67–86 (M = 76.0; S. D. = 6.09)	36.4 ST (4.1)	29.0–44.0
Awan[61]	M	10	18–30	29.10 ST (5.02)	N/A
	F	10		25.80 ST (4.87)	N/A
Morris et al[37]	M	18	20–35	36.6 ST (4.2)	N/A
	M	14	40–55	36.9 ST (5.0)	N/A
	M	18	>65	29.7 ST (5.2)	N/A
Ma et al[70]	F	35	22–52 (M = 36.03)	40.39 ST (3.73)	N/A
Šiupšinskiene et al[71]	F	76	M = 38.5	30.8 ST (4.3)	N/A
Siupsinskiene and Lycke[72]	M	38	18–67 (M = 33.7)	34.2 ST (3.2)	27.0–41.0
	F	89		29.5 ST (3.3)	22.2–36.7
Hallin et al[73]	M	30	21–50 (M = 30.0)	40.6 ST (4.41)	33.0–51.0

Notes:
a. Young ($_Y$), middle age ($_M$), and old age ($_O$) subjects in good ($_G$) and poor ($_P$) condition. Data are from sustained vowel /a/.

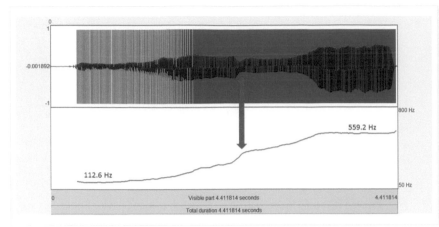

Fig. 4.21 Typical adult male producing a pitch glide from the lowest to the highest phonation pitch and F_0. The total phonational range in Hz is 446.6 Hz (559.2–112.6 Hz), corresponding to 27.74 STs and an approximate range from A2 (110 Hz) to C5 (554 Hz). The transition from modal to falsetto register is indicated with a vertical arrow corresponding to a drop in signal amplitude in the sound wave and a variation in the F_0 contour. Praat analysis parameters: pitch range = 50 to 800 Hz; autocorrelation; voicing threshold = 0.60.

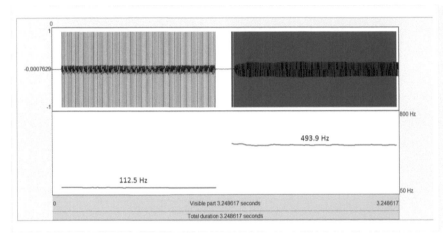

Fig. 4.22 Recordings of the lowest phonation pitch and F_0 in modal register and the highest phonational pitch and F_0 in falsetto register from a typical adult male combined into a single sound file. The total phonational F_0 range is 381.4 Hz (493.9–112.5 Hz), corresponding to 25.61 STs and approximate range from A2 (110 Hz) to B4 (493.9 Hz). Praat analysis parameters: pitch range = 50 to 800 Hz; autocorrelation; voicing threshold = 0.60.

and F_0 in falsetto register. Note that the analysis pitch range has been greatly expanded (50–800 Hz) compared to the more focused analysis ranges we have used for continuous speech and vowel samples in previous examples. In this example, the total phonational range in Hz is 446.6 Hz (559.2–112.6 Hz), corresponding to 27.74 STs and an approximate range from A2 (110 Hz) to C#5 (554 Hz). The transition from modal to falsetto register is indicated in ▶ Fig. 4.21 with a vertical arrow and can clearly be heard in **Sample 4.12** and marked by a sudden drop in signal amplitude and variation in the F_0 contour.

▶ Fig. 4.22 and **Sample 4.13** provide another example of the recording and measurement of the total phonational range, but this time elicited by having the subject going down in steps to the lowest pitch that can be sustained, followed by steps going up to the highest sustainable pitch. In this example, the lowest and highest sustainable pitch and F_0 productions were recorded and have been combined into one sound file. In this example, the total phonational F_0 range is 381.4 Hz (493.9–112.5 Hz), corresponding to 25.61 STs and approximate range from A2 (110 Hz) to B4 (493.9 Hz).

4.4.4 Measures of Vocal F_0 in Normal/ Typical Voice Subjects

Vocal F_0 during Infancy and Childhood

Since we expect there to be variations in habitual pitch as a function of factors such as the typical aging process and sex

differences, we should also expect that these same factors would result in expected variations in mean F_0. The infant voice has been reported to generally have expected F_0s in the range of approximately 400 to 600 Hz, with no observed significant difference between sexes in the F_0.[74,75] A possible tendency for lower F_0s in infants with increased body size has been reported.[76] Pitch and F_0 level gradually lower in both sexes during infancy and through the childhood years, with rapid changes in F_0 occurring during the first 4 months and 1 to 3 years of age.

Increased F_0 variability during vowel-like productions (e.g., cries) in the infant voice has been reported and may reflect a low level of neuromuscular coordination and limited ability to control phonatory parameters such as vocal folds tension.[3] Studies have demonstrated that pitch and F_0 range also develop from infancy through childhood, with the singing range expanding from one to two octaves between the ages of 6 to 11 years.[77,78]

Vocal F_0 during Puberty

F_0 generally becomes distinguishable by sex at about 11 years of age and certainly by 13 years of age. There is a tendency for F_0 variability during vowel productions to decrease with age from infancy to puberty, reflecting increased neuromuscular control during phonation.[79] In females, the fundamental frequency lowers approximately 1 octave from birth to puberty; in males, F_0 lowers approximately 2 octaves, however, because females may mature

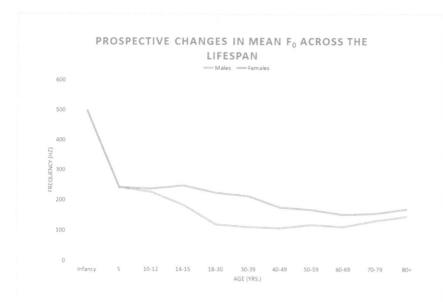

PROSPECTIVE CHANGES IN MEAN F_0 ACROSS THE LIFESPAN

— Males — Females

Fig. 4.23 Prospective changes in mean F_0 across the lifespan. Male versus female differentiation in mean F_0 occurs during puberty. Greatest separation between the sexes occurs postpuberty until the late 40 s/early 50 s. A tendency for a lowering of female F_0 and an increase in male F_0 may result in decreasing differentiation in the mean F_0 of the sexes in older age.

faster than males, they may enter adolescence with slightly lower speaking F_0s.[80] The growth changes in the larynx that occur during puberty (referred to as *mutation*, in which the neck lengthens and the larynx descends and grows in size) are primarily responsible for the observed changes in vocal F_0 in both sexes, with complete mutation occurring within 3 to 6 months.[81] The more drastic pubertal changes in vocal F_0 observed in males are due to increased laryngeal size and increased vocal fold mass and length,[82] but are also consistent with the development of secondary sex characteristics. As an example, Pedersen et al reported on F_0 measures in relation to pubertal development in 48 normal males in three groups (8.7–12.9, 13–15.9, and 16–19.5 years).[32] As expected, mean speaking F_0 dropped considerably between the three groups (273 vs. 184 vs. 125 Hz). In addition, speaking F_0 correlated quite strongly with height ($r = -0.82$), pubic hair stage ($r = -0.87$), testis volume ($r = -0.78$), and total testosterone ($r = -0.73$). The aforementioned laryngeal changes experienced during puberty are also associated with a period of increased pitch instability/variability. Boltezar et al reported that the F_0 CV from sustained vowel /a/ productions was greater in both pubescent males and females than in adult voice, though the pubescent female voice was observed to be somewhat more stable than for pubescent males.[83] The authors attributed this F_0 instability to the inconsistency between gradually developing nervous control of a relatively rapidly growing peripheral speech mechanism. As males and females move through puberty and into adulthood, the range of useable vocal pitches will extend to approximately 2 to 3 octaves.

Vocal F_0 during Adulthood and Senescence

Possible changes in voice characteristics, including pitch and frequency, have been documented as males and females progress through the lifespan toward *senescence* (a state of advanced aging in which a gradual deterioration in bodily function(s) may occur due to biological changes). As females move via adolescence into adulthood, mean F_0 tends to be relatively stable in the vicinity of 180 to 230 Hz until the onset of menopause. Due to factors such as hormonal changes and edema,[25,84] it has been

observed that the pitch and F_0 of the female voice may lower peri- and postmenopause.[35,80,82,85] Awan reported that an 18- to 30-year-old group of females had significantly higher mean F_0 than females in their 40s, 50s, 60s, and 70s.[41] In addition, significant differences in mean speaking F_0 were observed between the 40- to 49- and 50- to 59-year-old groups and the 60- to 69- and 70- to 79-year-old groups. A significant inverse correlation ($r = -0.69$, $p < .001$) observed between mean speaking F_0 and age in the female subjects studied was also reported.[41]

The male vocal pitch and mean F_0 appear to remain relatively stable post-adolescence and throughout adulthood with expected F_0s in the 100 to 150 Hz vicinity. However, there have been studies that indicate that some men may experience a rise in the pitch and F_0 of the voice during senescence.[22,25,34,86,87] It has been hypothesized that pitch and F_0 elevation in the elderly male voice may be due hormonal changes such as decreased secretion of testosterone resulting in a reduction in muscular tissues.[34,82,88] ▶ Fig. 4.23 incorporates data from various studies to illustrate possible changes in mean F_0 with aging for males and females across the lifespan.[19,22,32,35,41,86,89] As in our previous discussion of vocal pitch, substantial variation in vocal F_0 with aging should be expected. However, it is interesting that males and females at both extremes of the lifespan may have a tendency to produce similar pitch and F_0 voices.[1]

In addition to possible changes in mean F_0, evidence exists that increased variability of vocal pitch and F_0 during both continuous speech and sustained vowel production may occur in senescence. In some senescent speakers, a wider range and increased variability of F_0 may be observed during intonation in continuous speech.[35,90] In addition, increased pitch and F_0 variability resulting in a "shaky" or even tremulous-sustained vowel production has been reported in elderly versus younger speakers.[52,91,92] These possible changes in vocal F_0 variability may be due to decrements in sensory feedback, decreased speed and accuracy of motor control, neurochemical changes in the basal ganglia, and structural and physiological changes in the laryngeal mechanism.[93,94] Declinations in pitch/frequency range in elderly persons have also been observed, with senescent persons observed to have reductions in useable pitch and F_0 range, with particular limitations in the production of higher pitch and F_0 levels.[69,95,96]

Possible Effects of Race on Vocal F_0

The possible effect of race on speaking F_0 has been unequivocal. A number of studies have reported significantly lower speaking F_0s for African American speakers compared to that for Caucasians of comparable age.[26,97,98] The possibility of lower F_0s in African American speakers was attributed to possible anatomical differences between racial groups such as increased size of laryngeal structures.[98,99,100,101,102] In contrast to those studies that have speculated on a lower speaking F_0 for African American speakers, several studies have reported no significant difference in the speaking F_0 of African American versus Caucasian subjects.[103,104] Awan and Mueller examined the speaking F_0 characteristics of Caucasian, African American, and Hispanic kindergartners and reported mean speaking F_0 to be significantly lower in African American versus Hispanic children (236.4 vs. 248.5 Hz) but not different from Caucasian children (236.4 vs. 241.7 Hz).[39]

Caution should be exercised when applying the normative speaking F_0 data collected solely from one racial group to decisions regarding the speaking F_0 of other racial groups.[1] Regardless of whether possible anatomical differences in the speech/voice mechanisms of different races exist or not, there may be significant linguistic and societal differences (e.g., differences in pragmatic and interaction styles) between racial and/or dialect groups that influence speaking F_0 characteristics.[1,104]

Effects of Vocal Training on Vocal F_0

Vocal training may result in increased vocal capability and capacity. Persons with vocal training have been reported to learn and use different mechanisms of laryngeal control that may result in an expansion of the phonational F_0 range and, particularly, the ability to produce high F_0s.[105] As an example, a mode of phonation used by trained singers at high frequencies has been described in which only portions of the vibrational length would be used during vocal fold vibration, analogous to shortening the length of a vibrating string to produce a higher pitch tone than the open string by pressing a finger firmly at some intermediate point along the string's length.[106,107] In addition, trained singers may use isometric contractions of the laryngeal musculature to produce wide ranges of acoustic output by varying the tension of the vocal fold independent of changes in vocal fold lengthening that are primarily responsible for vocal fold tension in untrained subjects.[88]

It has been speculated that, unlike untrained vocalists, the trained singer may be able to maintain an acceptable degree of vocal quality and control at even the limits of their vocal capacity and thereby achieve similarity between the "musical" range of phonation and the "physiological" range.[1,61,62,66] In contrast, the "untrained" vocalist often produces a "musical" range of controlled phonation that is distinctly smaller than the "physiological range" that may be available in relatively uncontrolled activities (i.e., no intent to produce or sustain particular target pitch levels) such as screaming, crying, shouting, etc.

4.4.5 Measures of Vocal F_0 in Voice-Disordered Persons

When considering measures of F_0, the possible effects of age, sex, and race must be considered in both normal and voice-disordered persons. With that in mind, the following is a discussion of several disorder types that have been reported to present with changes in the expected F_0 of the voice. Because frequency is a direct correlate of perceived vocal pitch, expectations of changes in vocal frequency will be consistent with expected changes in vocal pitch for various disorders reported in a previous chapter.

4.4.6 Mass Lesions and Distributed Tissue Change

Lesions (e.g., nodules, polyps, and tumors) or added mass (e.g., edema) that develop on or within the vocal fold tissue may have variable effects on vocal pitch and F_0 characteristics.[108] In some cases, mean F_0 may be lowered because of increased vocal fold mass as in cases of edema, benign growths, and erythema.[108,109,110,111] In contrast, vocal pitch and F_0 may increase in these same aforementioned conditions due to increased vocal fold stiffness, or not be substantially effected at all by the presence of laryngeal tissue changes.[108,112,113,114]

The presence of vocal fold lesions or distributed tissue change and associated increased mass and stiffness of the vocal folds may alter the control of vocal fold vibration and therefore result in (1) increased pitch variability during sustained vowel productions and (2) monopitch, limited intonation voice production during continuous speech.[110] Decreased pitch and F_0 range may be observed because the presence of lesion(s) or distributed tissue change results in increased stiffness of the vocal fold(s) and a restricted range of lengthening/tensing motion.[108,109]

Smoking is a form of vocal abuse that is associated with development of mass lesions and distributed tissue change. Several studies have reported changes in vocal F_0 including a decrease in mean F_0, increase in F_0 variability in sustained vowel productions, and limitations in total phonational F_0 range.[84,115,116,117,118,119,120]

Neurological Disorders

Because neurological disorders may affect motor control in a variety of ways, the possible effects of neurological disorders on vocal F_0 are highly varied. Increased mean F_0 has been reported for patients with Parkinson's disease who experience rigidity of the laryngeal musculature[121,122] versus both increased and decreased mean F_0 in certain subjects with amyotrophic lateral sclerosis (ALS)[33] versus a report of no significant differences in mean F_0 in groups of patients with hypo- and hyperkinetic dysarthrias versus normal controls.[123] Flaccidity of the vocal fold musculature may result in increased effective mass resulting in a reduction in mean F_0.

While mean F_0 may be variably effected in dysarthric states, F_0 variability during speaking has been consistently reported to be reduced (monopitch and flattened F_0 contours) in various conditions such as ataxia, right hemisphere lesions, and particularly in patients with Parkinson's disease.[124,125,126,127,128,129]

Increased F_0 SD in sustained vowel productions has also been reported in Huntington's and cerebellar ataxic groups.[123,124]

Muscle Tension Dysphonia/Hyperfunctional Voice

While excessive tension within the vocal musculature may be secondary to neuromotor dysfunction, increased tension in the laryngeal musculature is also observed in many functional voice disorders. In functional cases, the increased tension may occur as a result of factors such as emotional stress, fatigue, use of inappropriate pitch level, or compensatory activity developed in conjunction with organic disturbance (e.g., laryngitis).[1] Muscle tension dysphonia (MTD) is a term used to describe a form of vocal hyperfunction characterized by a presumed overactivation and dysregulation of muscles in and around the laryngeal region in the absence of organic or neurologic laryngeal disorders.[130] When excessive muscular activity occurs in those muscles that affect the lengthening and tensing aspects of vocal fold function, the result may be effort, possible strain, and an increase in pitch and F_0 level.[130,131]

Although increased pitch is most commonly associated with excessive tension, decreased pitch has also been reported in this condition[1,132,133] and may be due to increased tension localized to the thyroarytenoid/vocalis muscle(s) and/or anterior-posterior squeezing of the larynx resulting in vocal fold compression and lower pitch and F_0.[133]

Puberphonia/Mutational Falsetto

As previously stated, a substantial lowering of the pitch and F_0 of the voice is generally observed as males move from childhood to adulthood via puberty. In puberphonia/mutational falsetto, the male subject retains a childlike, higher pitched voice after puberty, resulting in a voice and age mismatch and pitch abnormality (see previous description). Luchsinger and Arnold classified disturbed mutation in boys into three clinical forms: (1) delayed mutation, (2) prolonged mutation, and (3) incomplete mutation. In all three forms, the voice is characterized by high pitch and F_0, highly variable pitch and F_0 production with frequent pitch breaks, and chronic hoarseness.[65] Several studies have described a reduction in mean F_0 as a key outcome of voice therapy for these patients.[134,135,136]

Psychological Disorders

Pitch and F_0 variability has been reported to be substantially reduced in speech contexts (monopitch, flattened intonation) consistent with flat affect in cases of both schizophrenia and severe clinical depression.[110,137,138,139]

Deafness/Hearing Impairment

Patients with congenital or early childhood hearing losses of more than mild severity may be observed to have poor control over vocal F_0 characteristics. Increased mean F_0 in speech contexts has been reported for deaf/severely hearing impaired speakers.[19,140,141] In addition, reduced SD of F_0[19,142] and highly variable speaking F_0[141] (flattened F_0 contours as well as extreme variations in F_0 during speech intonation) have also been reported.

▶ Table 4.5 provides a summary of general expectations for possible changes in vocal F_0 characteristics in the aforementioned disorders.

Table 4.5 A summary of general expectations for vocal F0 characteristics in various disorder types

Disorder	Possible effect on vocal F_0	Comments
Mass lesions and distributed tissue change	Variable	Decreased mean F_0 with conditions resulting in increased vocal fold mass; increased mean F_0 with increased vocal fold stiffness. Increased mass and increased stiffness may counteract to result in minimal change in mean F_0. Increased F_0 variability in sustained voicing; reduced F_0 variability in speech (consistent with monopitch). Decreased F_0 range.
Neurological disorders	Variable	Increased mean F_0 with hypertonia/rigidity (e.g., spasticity; hypokinesias such as Parkinsonism); possibly decreased in flaccidity Increased F_0 variability in sustained vowel productions; reduced F_0 variability in speech (consistent with monopitch; flattened F_0 contours)
Muscle tension dysphonias (MTDs)/hyperfunctional voice	Variable	Increased mean F_0 with increased vocal fold tension and stiffness; mean F_0 may be decreased if tension is focal to the TA/vocalis muscle or results in A-P laryngeal squeezing
Puberphonia/Mutational falsetto	Increased mean F_0; increased F_0 variability in sustained voicing and in speech (consistent with pitch breaks)	Retains childlike, high mean F_0 even though physical development is consistent with transition to adulthood
Psychological disorders	Reduced F_0 variability in speech intonation	Flattened intonation consistent with flat affect in cases of both schizophrenia and severe clinical depression
Deafness/Hearing impairment	Increased mean F_0; F_0 variability in speech may be reduced (consistent with monopitch) or excessive	Patients with congenital or early childhood hearing losses of more than mild severity may be observed to have poor control over vocal F_0 characteristics

4.4.7 Limitations in the Measurement of F_0

Regardless of the computer algorithm that is used for the computation of mean F_0, certain situations will tend to result in miscalculations in estimating vocal frequency.[143] For measures of F_0 to be valid, the acoustic analysis program must be able to identify the fundamental period of the signal. The rapid pitch changes observed during intonation patterns, the effects of voiced-to-voiceless or voiceless-to-voiced transitions, noise within the signal, and (as in various forms of dysphonia) disturbance to the periodicity of voice are all situations in which difficulties in frequency tracking may occur.

Program parameters that dictate how estimates of vocal F_0 are calculated must also be monitored closely by the program user. As an example, most F_0 analysis programs such as those that utilize autocorrelation or waveform matching require the user to provide a frequency range within which the program will search F_0 estimates. For the analysis of the continuous speech of a typical adult male, a range of 80 to 300 Hz would comfortably encompass the mean F_0 of most typical adult males, while also providing an adequate range within which the frequency changes observed within the intonation patterns of the speaker can also be detected. If the range is too wide (e.g., 80–1,000 Hz), the program may produce numerous high-frequency errors in estimating F_0. In contrast, if the range is too limited (e.g., 80–200 Hz), the algorithm may be restricted in its ability to identify F_0 variations observed during normal intonation patterns. In addition, the use of pitch smoothing algorithms will be expected to have an effect on measures of F_0 range and SD (e.g., increased smoothing will reduce measures of F_0 range and average variation for speech samples). The user of a particular program should closely review instructions on how to set these parameters for optimal F_0 processing.

Different software programs with different F_0 analysis algorithms have been reported to have a high degree of correspondence and strong interprogram correlations in estimates of mean speaking F_0, regardless of sex or age of the subject group producing the samples.[54] These results are similar to those reported by Bielamowicz et al for F_0 estimations obtained from sustained vowels. However, poorer correspondence and weaker interprogram correlations have been reported for measures of F_0 SD.[54,144]

4.4.8 Vocal Sound Level (a.k.a. Vocal Intensity)

Sound is the perception of pressure changes in the medium (typically, air).[68] The perceptual attribute that corresponds to the magnitude of the pressure changes is **loudness**, and the magnitude of these pressure changes is reflected in the **amplitude** of the wave. The *sound intensity level (SIL)* of a signal refers to the power of the signal (proportional to the square of the pressure), while the *sound pressure level (SPL)* represents a comparison of the SPL of an observed signal to a reference sound pressure. Because both SIL and SPL give similar result in *decibels (dB)*, it has been suggested that we simply refer to this measurement of sound power/pressure as **sound level** *(SL)*, though the term **vocal intensity** is ubiquitous in the voice literature.[145]

The evaluation of vocal loudness and sound level/intensity provides us with valuable information about the coordination between phonatory and respiratory mechanisms since vocal loudness and intensity relate not only to the degree of respiratory force but also to the amplitude of vocal fold vibration.[146] Specific to phonatory function, Colton and Casper indicated that vocal loudness and intensity is affected by (1) glottal resistance to the expiratory airstream and (2) the rate of airflow change at the moment of closure.[3]

Considerations in Measuring Vocal Intensity

Mouth to Microphone Distance

The measurement of vocal intensity (a.k.a. sound level) is somewhat more complicated than recording the voice for measures of frequency, as the measurement of intensity **is greatly affected by the distance the microphone is from the mouth** (i. e., mouth-to-microphone distance). While the frequency of the vocal signal will be constant regardless of whether the microphone is placed close or relatively distant from the mouth, intensity is effected by the **inverse square law**, which states that, in a free field (i.e., one without reflections), the intensity of sound drops by 6 dB for each doubling of distance from the source. The fact that sound intensity will reduce the farther away from the source should be intuitive in that sound waves spread out in all directions like radiating spheres and, as the radius of the spheres gets larger, the amount of acoustic energy in the disturbance gets distributed over the expanding surface of the sphere. Therefore, the mouth-to-microphone distance substantially affects the intensity of the sound being measured and must be kept as constant as possible if accurate readings of vocal intensity are to be made.

A mouth-to-microphone distance of **30 cm (approximately 12 in)** has been suggested[147] *for handheld or desktop mounted microphones* versus **approximately 4 cm from the lips at a 45-degree angle** *for headset microphones*.[10,11] In practice, the literature on vocal sound level/intensity shows a wide variety of mouth-to-microphone distances being reported. Therefore, it is essential that we know the mouth-to-microphone distance that was used in examples of reported clinical or research data. Headset microphones are strongly recommended because not only do they help considerably in maintaining a consistent mouth-to-microphone distance, but they also provide improved signal-to-noise ratios (due to the short distance from the lips).

Sound Level Meter

While consistent mouth-to-microphone distances help standardize our recordings, the distance by itself does not tell us the actual sound level/intensity of the subject's voice. To actually measure vocal sound level/intensity in dB, we will need a **sound level meter** (SLM). A basic SLM consists of a microphone, an amplifier, a frequency weighting circuit, and a meter (analog or digital) calibrated in decibels.[148] While high-quality SLMs (i.e., Class 1 and Class 2 SLMs which comply with IEC or ANSI standards and provide an accuracy of ±1.5 and ±2 dB, respectively, within the frequency range of 100–1,000 Hz) can be quite expensive, a multitude of low cost SLMs are available (▶ Fig. 4.24) and may be acceptable for clinical purposes.[149,150]

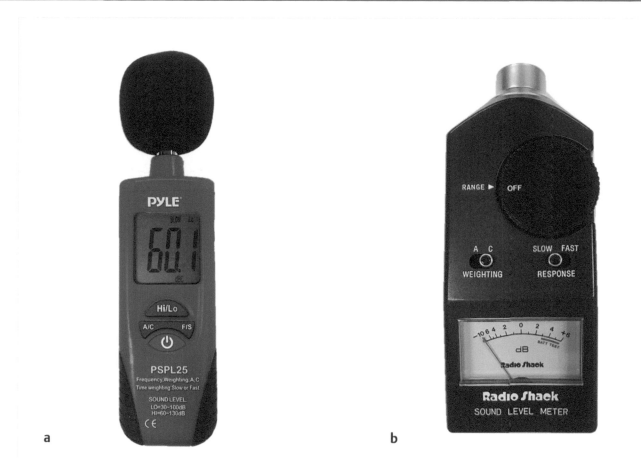

Fig. 4.24 Examples of low-cost sound level meters. **(a)** Pyle PSPL25 sound level meter (https://www.pyleaudio.com/sku/PSPL25/Sound-Level-Meter-with-A-and-C-Frequency-Weighting); **(b)** Analog Sound Level Meter by Radio Shack (Model 33-2050).

Regardless of the SLM being used, it is important to recognize the type of **frequency weighting** being used, as these circuits can have a substantial effect on the sound level measurement provided by the SLM. Two commonly used frequency weighting circuits are A-weighting and C-weighting. The C-weighting circuit (a linear weighted circuit) is preferred for measures of vocal intensity because it (1) measures uniformly over the frequency range (up to approximately 10 kHz) and (2) does not discriminate against low frequencies such as those often found in the F_0s of speech and most singing. In contrast, the A-weighted circuit reduces the influence of low-frequency ambient noise on sound level measurements by attenuating the low-frequency range (i.e., < 500 Hz), resulting in substantially reduced intensity measurements for lower frequency voice productions such as those in the vicinity of the vocal F_0 and other modal register phonations in most subjects.[151]

Although low-cost or free SLM apps are also available for iOS (e.g., iPhone) and Android-based (e.g., Samsung Galaxy) smart phones, these apps do not guarantee sufficient accuracy.[152] In addition, regardless of the quality of the app itself, the characteristics of the microphone or the sound acquisition hardware built into smartphones is often unknown. Because of the potential for poor reliability across various mobile devices, operating systems, and apps, sound level/intensity measures obtained from smartphones should be considered as unclassified SLMs and, therefore, only be used for clinical approximations.[149]

Recording Environment

The environment in which the recording takes place can also have a substantial effect on our measures of sound level/intensity. Ideally, recordings would take place in a soundproofed or treated environment. For measures of sound level, a room should be selected in which the ambient noise level is at least 10 dB lower than the expected lowest sound level/intensity phonation (**optimally, < 38 dB(C) for measurements at 30 cm distance or < 48 dB(C) for measurements with omnidirectional head-mounted microphones**) and reverberations (i.e., echoes) from reflective surfaces are minimized.[153]

4.4.9 Measurement of Modal Vocal Intensity (dB)

The SLM can be used to directly give us a measure of the vocal sound level via its built-in microphone or to calibrate the hand-held or headset microphone that we are using for all of our recordings (including previously mentioned recordings for measures of vocal frequency). The modal vocal sound level/intensity may be obtained from the same continuous speech sample(s) (i.e., portions of the Rainbow Passage—second sentence or second and third sentences; CAPE-V sentences) as used in vocal frequency analyses. Here are a number of methods by which the sound level/intensity of the voice may be measured:

1. The SLM can provide a real-time (i.e., almost "instantaneous") estimate of the *modal sound level/intensity level* (i.e., the most commonly or frequently occurring sound level/intensity). Turn on the SLM, place (e.g., on a tripod) or hold the SLM at a 30 cm (1 ft) mouth-to-microphone distance. Set the range selector to 70 dB—when the range selector is set for 70 dB, the meter will respond to intensity levels between ≈ 60 and 80 dB (70 dB is indicated when the meter points to 0). The 70-dB setting is suggested because **conversational speech levels generally range from ≈ 65 to 70 dB when measured at 30 cm** (1 ft mouth-to-microphone distance). Select C-weighting and slow response. As the patient is reading, closely watch the decibel meter for the most frequently occurring intensity level. The meter will be in a constant state of fluctuation. However, the use of the slow-response setting should allow the meter to "linger" somewhat at the displayed intensity levels, making it easier to identify the most commonly/consistently occurring intensity value (i.e., the modal intensity level). For an approximation of a mean vocal intensity level, record observations of the intensity of speech approximately every 3 seconds during the reading of a standard passage (e.g., the first paragraph of "the Rainbow Passage"). The list of intensity observations can be reviewed for the modal intensity level or averaged to result in an approximately mean intensity level (Appendix 4.1). The clinician should be able to record approximately 9 to 10 intensity observations for a patient reading the first paragraph of "the Rainbow Passage" at a normal speaking rate.

2. The headset microphone may be precalibrated using procedures consistent with Winholtz and Titze[10] and Asplund[154] to indirectly obtain intensity values by converting the microphone signal to a decibel (dB) level. Specifically, to pre-calibrate the headset microphone, a subject is asked to sustain a vowel /a/ at a comfortable pitch and loudness, with a headset microphone placed a fixed distance away from the mouth (e.g., 4 cm) and a SLM placed 30 cm/1 ft away from the mouth (► Fig. 4.25).[154] Recordings of the headset microphone signal can be recorded into a sound acquisition program (e.g., Praat, Audacity) while the SLM is simultaneously monitored for the modal sound level (in dB). The mean amplitude (e.g., root mean squared amplitude) of the recorded signal corresponding to the known SL/intensity level at 30 cm is obtained. For future recordings, the amplitude of the subject's voice production can now be compared to the reference signal amplitude (from 30 cm/1 ft) and be converted to decibels using a standard decibel formula (e.g., $dB = 20Log_{10}(\frac{P_M}{P_R})$, where P_M is equivalent to the RMS amplitude of the signal being measured and P_R is equivalent to the RMS amplitude of the reference signal).

3. Computer programs are also available by which measures of sound level/intensity may be made (e.g., Visi-Pitch; CSL; Praat). These programs are useful for visually depicting the sound level/intensity changes over time for an utterance or for measurements of the sound level/intensity range. However, they do not provide the user with a true measure of vocal sound level/intensity because (1) it is unknown what the reference amplitude/pressure is for the reported intensity level and (2) it is unknown under which conditions the unknown reference was recorded (e.g., mouth-to-microphone distance). Recall that in the calculation of sound level (re: SPL), the reference pressure/amplitude and its equivalent decibel value must be known (e.g., 0.0002 dynes/cm² = 0 dB). Therefore, if the program arbitrarily reports that the mean intensity for an utterance is, for example, 58 dB, the value cannot be regarded as valid because we do not know the reference level used in the reported intensity. However, if a SLM and headset microphone are setup as in no. 2, the difference in reported sound level/intensity between the head-mounted microphone (as measured with the computer and software being used for data analysis) and the SLM at 30 cm distance can then be used as a correction factor to convert software-reported measures to sound levels at 30 cm.

It is essential to note that any changes in equipment setup (e.g., changes in mouth-to-microphone distance; changes in system gain/amplification) will invalidate the measures of sound level/intensity and would require recalibration.

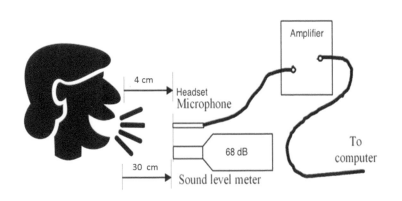

Fig. 4.25 Example procedure by which a headset microphone (e.g., 4 cm mouth-to-microphone distance) may be calibrated in reference to a sound level meter placed at a standard 30 cm mouth-to-microphone distance (see text for full description). The calibration "tone" maybe a steady sustained vowel production or a tone (e.g., 150 Hz triangular wave) produced via a speaker.

General expectations for the sound level/intensity of the speaking voice (30 cm/1 ft mouth-to-microphone distance) are as follows:

- **Children**: 60 to 65 dB.
- **Adults**: 65 to 70 dB.

- **Senescent adults**: Also 65 to 70 dB.

▶ Table 4.6 provides examples of sound level/intensity measures for the speaking voice obtained from various literature sources.

Table 4.6 Examples of speaking sound level/intensity (in dB) from various literature sources

Author	Gender	No. of subjects	Age	Mean and SD	Range
Ryan[155, a]	M	20	40–49	68.1 (2.3)	N/A
	M	20	50–59	68.7 (2.1)	N/A
	M	20	60–69	68.6 (1.6)	N/A
	M	20	70–79	70.7 (2.4)	N/A
Linville et al[51, b]	F	20	67–86 (M = 76.0; S.D. = 6.09)	71.8 (4.0)	64.0–81.6
Awan et al[156, c]	M & F_H	17	5–6 y	61.39 (2.76)	N/A
	M & F_B	17	5–6 y	61.20 (3.07)	N/A
	M & F_W	17	5–6 y	61.77 (3.12)	N/A
Awan[36, d]	M	10	18–30 y	71.36 (2.72)	65.29–75.06
	F	10	18–30 y	67.14 (2.05)	61.80–69.45
Morris and Brown[157, e]	F_Y	25	20–35 (M = 27.2 y)	69.30 (5.57)	56.1–79.7
	F_O	25	70–90 (M = 79.4 y)	70.83 (5.46)	59.8–81.2
Morris et al[37, f]	M	18	20–35	72.8 (4.7)	N/A
	M	14	40–55	70.1 (7.1)	N/A
	M	18	>65	72.4 (4.4)	N/A
Awan[1, g]	M	29	18–30 (mean = 24.24 y)	68.93 (2.60)	64.83–73.50
	M	12	44–58 (mean = 51.69 y)	69.25 (2.80)	65.00–74.33
	F	85	18–30 (mean = 22.57 y)	68.37 (2.17)	65.50–71.93
	F	9	36–41 (mean = 38.99 y)	68.06 (1.78)	65.33–71.00
	F	13	46–80 (Mean = 57.71 y)	67.42 (2.93)	65.60–71.60
Siupsinskiene and Lycke[72, h]	M	38	18–67 (M = 33.7)	62,1	56.7–67.5
	F	89		62.1	55.5–68.6
Hallin et al[73]	M	30	21–50 (M = 30.0)	72.2 (2.14)	67.7–77.6
Goy et al[43, i]	M	55	18–28 (x = 19.4)	69.7 (3.4)	N/A
	M	51	65–86 (x = 73.3)	65.8 (4.9)	N/A
	F	104	18–27 (x = 18.9)	67.8 (4.3)	N/A
	F	82	63–82 (x = 71.1)	66.4 (4.0)	N/A

Notes:
a. Data from impromptu speaking task only (12 mouth-to-microphone distance).
b. Data from sentence reading (6 in. mouth-to-microphone distance).
c. Data for Hispanic ($_H$), Black ($_B$), and White ($_W$) kindergarten age children (9 in. mouth-to-microphone distance).
d. Data for untrained male and female adults only (12 in. [30 cm] mouth-to-microphone distance).
e. Data from young ($_Y$) and old-aged ($_O$) subjects in conversational speech (28.3 cm [11 in.] mouth-to-microphone distance).
f. Data from nonsingers only (25.4 cm [10 in.] mouth-to-microphone distance).
g. Data from oral reading (12 in. mouth-to-microphone distance).
h. dB(A).
i. Data from oral reading (1.5 cm mouth-to-microphone distance; calibrated analogous to 30 cm).

4.4.10 Measurement of Dynamic Range (Sound Level Range in dB)

Because phonation at different intensities assesses the sublaryngeal, laryngeal, and supralaryngeal limits of the phonational system, the dynamic range of the voice would seem to be an important measure in the assessment of vocal function and performance.[151,158] Phonations should be produced with continuous vocal fold vibration and sustained for 2 to 3 seconds (i.e., controlled phonations as with the elicitation of phonational frequency range).

A simple elicitation of the dynamic range of the voice (i.e., lowest to greatest vocal sound level) may be obtained by asking subjects to simply *phonate an /a/ vowel as softly as possible at a comfortable pitch* followed by *phonation of the same vowel as loudly as possible at a self-selected pitch level.*[159] Three trials are generally elicited with the lowest and greatest dB values accepted as the minimum and maximum sound levels, respectively. Because the potential differences between the minimum and maximum sound level/intensity levels may be considerable (40–60 dB in typical speakers), we will have to either (1) adjust the range selector of our SLM to accurately measure the sound level of these extreme phonations or (b) make sure that our amplifier settings are adjusted so that we can capture the entire dynamic range without exceeding the A-to-D clipping.

Within the dynamic range, particular interest has been paid to the **minimum vocal sound level/intensity**. Verdolini speculated that the inability to produce quiet phonation (particularly at higher pitch levels) may be due to the requirement for increased subglottal pressure to put increased mass folds into vibration, thereby negating "quiet" phonation.[160] The inability to produce quiet phonation may also be related to the necessity for increased phonation threshold pressure (PTP) in cases in which the vocal fold mucosal cover has been damaged or dehydrated. PTP is the minimum subglottal pressure required to initiate vocal fold vibration.[161,162] Wuyts et al have stated that structural changes to the true vocal folds, such as distributed or organized mass lesions, may increase glottal resistance such that greater subglottal pressures will be necessary to initiate and maintain vocal fold vibration.[67] Consequently, the lowest phonational intensity will often be increased. Ma has also stated that it is quite common to observe that dysphonic individuals find it difficult to phonate at very low intensity levels compared to vocally healthy individuals.[163] This finding has also been reported in children with voice disorders versus vocally healthy children.[164] It is notable that the lowest vocal sound level/intensity is included as a component of the DSI (see discussion on multivariate analysis methods).

For typical speakers without singing training, the following expectations for dynamic range are suggested:

- **Children:** 30 to 40 dB.
- **Adults:** 40 to 55 dB.
- **Senescent adults:** 30 to 40 dB.

Measures of Vocal Sound Level/Intensity in Normal/Typical Voice Subjects

As was seen with measures of vocal frequency, various factors including age, sex, and vocal training may also have a substantial effect on the sound level/intensity of the voice.

Effects of Aging on Vocal Loudness/Intensity

Vocal Sound Level/Intensity during Infancy and Childhood

Because of their smaller respiratory capacities, it may be expected that the vocal intensity level of the childhood voice would be somewhat lower than that observed in adulthood. Consequentially, children may have to expend more respiratory effort to achieve the same perceptual effect of increased loudness and related sound level/intensity as adults.[165] In terms of overall dynamic range, Böhme and Stuchlik observed that maximum and minimum intensity levels were relatively consistent from ages 7 through 10 years for both males and females.[166] In contrast, Komiyama et al observed increases in dynamic range and associated phonetographic area between the ages of 8 and 9 years in both males and females.[167]

Vocal Sound Level/Intensity during Puberty

During adolescence, dynamic range increases primarily due to by increased respiratory capacity. In a study of 139 male and female subjects between the ages of 6 and 30 years, Komiyama et al observed increases in maximum intensity levels and overall dynamic range between 10 and 14 years and attributed these improvements (particularly observable in male subjects) to increases in physical constitution and vital capacity during this time span encompassing puberty.[167]

Vocal Sound Level/Intensity during Adulthood

The intensity of the speaking voice tends to be in the range of approximately **65 to 70 dB** (mouth-to-microphone distance = 30 cm/1 ft) for both males and females.[36,155,157] However, increased respiratory capacity and expiratory forces, combined with lower fundamental frequencies that may interact with the lower formant frequencies associated with longer vocal tracts, may result in a tendency for increased vocal sound level/intensity in some males.[168-170] These expectations for increased vocal sound level/intensity in males versus females have been reported for both speaking voice and particular levels of the total phonational frequency range.[36,61]

Vocal Sound Level/Intensity during Senescence

Relatively little effect of advanced aging has been observed on the sound level/intensity of the speaking voice, with comparable speaking sound level/intensity values reported for both younger and senescent adults.[155,157,171] However, overall dynamic range may be restricted in senescent adults due to possible decrements in respiratory force and/or laryngeal valving.[157] In particular, minimal intensity productions have been reported to be limited in advanced age (i.e., minimum/low-intensity productions are increased)[172,173] due to respiratory and laryngeal changes. Indeed, as lung compliance decreases, respiratory muscles weaken,[174,175] and vocal folds stiffen,[176] and a greater subglottal pressure may be necessary to initiate and maintain vocal fold vibration,[177] resulting in greater difficulty producing quiet voicing for elderly subjects. Again, it should be kept in mind that the magnitude of aging effects on vocal sound level/intensity may be quite variable person to person and more related to overall physical condition rather than chronological age.[30,157]

Effects of Race on Vocal Sound Level/Intensity

The possible effects of race, dialect, or cultural/linguistic background on vocal intensity have not been studied extensively. It has been speculated that cultural attitudes may be reflected in the use of decreased loudness levels in speech for some individuals.[1,178]

Effects of Vocal Training on Vocal Sound Level/Intensity

Trained subjects have been reported to have the capacity to use a greater storage of air (vital capacity) in conjunction with a greater expiratory force than untrained subjects, and thereby have the capability to produce greater sound level/intensity productions and greater overall dynamic ranges.[64,107,179,180,181] In addition, trained subjects may use less of their capacity in producing similar intensity voice productions as untrained subjects, indicative of more efficient phonatory function.[181,182] At the laryngeal level, increased vocal fold closure time during the vibratory cycle, along with the ability to produce high sound level/intensity productions with relatively small vibration amplitudes, has been reported for trained singers versus untrained subjects. The result is improved efficiency of conversion of airflow to acoustic energy (especially in the higher harmonics) and ability to radiate a greater amount of sound power than the untrained voice.[183,184] Finally, at the supraglottal level, trained singers may learn to "tune" the first formant (i.e., first vocal tract resonance) to the vocal F_0 by adjusting jaw opening, resulting in considerable gains in overall sound level/intensity.[170,185] In light of the aforementioned differences between trained and untrained subjects in terms of vocal sound level/intensity control mechanisms, it has been reported that trained subjects should be able to produce greater maximum intensities and intensity ranges than typical, untrained subjects.[61,105,186]

Measures of Vocal Sound Level/Intensity in Voice-Disordered Subjects

Various disorders that affect the respiratory and/or laryngeal valving capability may adversely affect speaking intensity and/or dynamic range. In addition, abnormalities of vocal loudness/intensity may accompany psychological disorders and disruptions in other components of the speech mechanism. Because sound level/intensity is a direct correlate of perceived vocal loudness, expectations of changes in vocal sound level/intensity will be consistent with expected changes in vocal loudness for various disorders.

Mass Lesions/Distributed Tissue Changes

Speaking loudness/intensity levels may be reduced secondary to mass lesions of the vocal folds.[109,110,178] As an example, Hirano observed that size of glottic gap negatively correlated with maximum SPL level in polyp cases; in carcinoma cases, negative correlations between size of lesion and maximum SPL and SPL range were also observed.[187] However, it should be noted that patients with vocal nodules, other lesions, or irregularities of the vocal fold margins may only be able to sustain phonation while using louder rather than softer voices, and thus may compensate for their disorder with hyperadduction and a louder voice.[110,187]

Neurological Disorders

Several authors have stated that speaking intensity/loudness levels may be reduced in neurological disorders such as Parkinsonism and bulbar palsy (flaccidity).[47,110,122,178] Countryman et al reported decreased vocal loudness/intensity in a patient with Parkinson's disease and subsequent improvement in vocal loudness after voice therapy incorporating the Lee-Silverman Voice Treatment (LSVT).[126] These authors attributed decreased vocal loudness to bowing of the vocal folds or other forms of glottal incompetence in combination with reduced expiratory volumes for speech (resulting from limited thoracic excursion and difficulty coordinating respiratory and laryngeal systems). In a study of 240 patients with unilateral vocal fold paralysis, Hirano et al observed mean speaking intensity to be abnormally low in approximately 70% of the subjects.[188] These authors attributed their findings to glottic incompetence, poor neural control, and asymmetry of vocal fold vibration.

Certain neurological conditions may result in inappropriately high speaking intensity levels. Prater and Swift stated that vocal loudness may be too high in neurological disorders resulting in respiratory and/or vocal hyperfunction.[178] Haynes et al stated that dysarthric patients (particularly those with spasticity or dystonias) may present with a "booming" voice.[189] Inappropriately loud voices have also been reported in patients with multiple sclerosis.[122]

Some patients with neurological conditions may have difficulty in varying sound level/intensity during prosodic patterns used in typical speech. The result will be reduced sound level/intensity variability (consistent with the perception of *monoloudness*) and overall dynamic range.[110,122,178,188,189] In contrast, certain hyperkinetic states (e.g., choreas, dystonias, vocal tremor) may produce excessive variations in sound level/intensity.[110,122]

Muscle Tension Dysphonia/Hyperfunctional Voice

Many hyperfunctional voices initially present with increased vocal sound level/intensity levels during speech followed by periods of reduced vocal intensity/loudness as a result of vocal fatigue.

Psychologically Based Voice Disorders

The sound level/intensity of speech may be reduced in cases of inferiority complex and withdrawal. In addition, monoloudness presenting as a limited sound level variation in speech may be observed in cases of depression.[47,109,110,178,189]

Hearing Impairment/Deafness

Several authors have indicated that hearing impairment may cause speaking loudness/intensity to be too high (e.g., in cases of moderate-to-severe sensorineural losses) or too low (in cases of conductive loss), and overall loudness variability to be reduced.[47,110,111,178]

▶ Table 4.7 provides a summary of general expectations for possible changes in vocal sound level/intensity characteristics in the aforementioned disorders.

Table 4.7 A summary of general expectations for vocal sound level/intensity characteristics in various disorder types

Disorder	Possible effect on vocal sound level/intensity	Comments
Mass lesions/Distributed tissue changes	Variable	Decreased SL in lesions that result in glottal gaps. However, patients may compensate with increased SL
Neurological disorders	Variable	Decreased SL in cases presenting with glottal incompetence (e.g., vocal fold paralysis/paresis; vocal fold bowing in Parkinsonism). Increased SL in cases with vocal hyperfunction/hyperadduction (e.g., spasticity; hyperkinesias). Reduction in SL variability in hypertonic states (e.g., spasticity or rigidity) consistent with monoloudness
Muscle tension dysphonias (MTDs)/hyperfunctional voice	Variable	Many hyperfunctional voices initially present with increased vocal sound level/intensity levels during speech followed by periods of reduced vocal intensity/loudness as a result of vocal fatigue.
Psychologically based voice disorders	Reduced mean SL; reduced SL variability	The sound level/intensity of speech may be reduced in cases of inferiority complex and withdrawal. In addition, monoloudness presenting as a limited sound level variation in speech may be observed in cases of depression
Hearing impairment/deafness	Variable for mean SL; reduced SL variability	Speaking SL may be increased (e.g., in cases of moderate-to-severe sensorineural losses) or decreased (in cases of conductive loss); overall SL variability reduced consistent with monoloudness

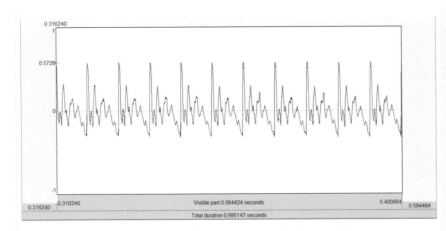

Fig. 4.26 Several cycles of vibration from a typical, nondysphonic adult male speaker. The cycles are highly repetitive with a high degree of cycle-to-cycle similarity in period, amplitude, and profile (i.e., waveform shape).

4.4.11 Correlates of Vocal Quality

Standard English vowels are produced with vocal fold vibration (i.e., voicing), a relatively open vocal tract (i.e., no occlusions or significant constrictions within the supraglottal vocal tract) and, therefore, no purposeful frication or plosive noise. A typical, nondysphonic English sustained vowel produced with a steady pitch and loudness will, therefore, be characterized by a sound wave which is highly periodic in nature, with clearly repetitive cycles of vibration (▶ Fig. 4.26). In addition, if we were to observe the spectrum of this sound wave, we would see that the sound wave is composed of very distinctive evenly spaced **harmonics** (the fundamental frequency [F_0—first harmonic] and integer multiples of the F_0). The amplitude of these harmonics would tend to be substantially greater than any other frequencies (interharmonic or other frequencies) that may be present (▶ Fig. 4.27).

In contrast, in many forms of dysphonia, the highly periodic nature of the voice waveform becomes disturbed by the addition of noise (e.g., turbulent airflow produced in breathiness), irregular vocal fold vibration (e.g., as observed in roughness), or sometimes both characteristics simultaneously (e.g., as in hoarseness). These dysphonic quality voice signals start to deviate from the highly periodic sound wave observed in the typical, nondysphonic voice (▶ Fig. 4.28). In addition, the harmonics in the voice spectrum will now be reduced in amplitude as compared to inharmonic frequencies and, in some cases, will be replaced by noise (▶ Fig. 4.29). Rather than spectral energy concentrated in the harmonics, the spectrum may become dominated by noise that adds energy at *all* frequencies, not just at multiples of the fundamental frequency.[190]

In the next section, we will discuss several methods which may be used to quantify these disturbances in the voice waveform and spectrum.

Measures of Perturbation

The addition of noise to the normal periodic (actually *quasiperiodic*) voice waveform disturbs the repeating pattern of vibration in a number of key ways:

- The period (and thus, the frequency) of vibration is disrupted.
- The amplitude of vibration is disrupted.
- The profile (i.e., shape) of the waveform is disrupted.

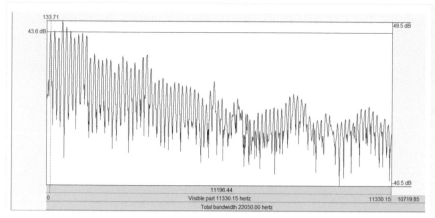

Fig. 4.27 A magnified portion of the sound spectrum for a typical, nondysphonic adult male sustained vowel production. The F₀ (i.e., 1st harmonic) is identified at approximately 133.71 Hz and is followed by a series of distinctive harmonic peaks extending throughout the spectrum at integer multiples of the F₀. Praat analysis parameters: window length = 0.05 s; dynamic range = 90 dB.

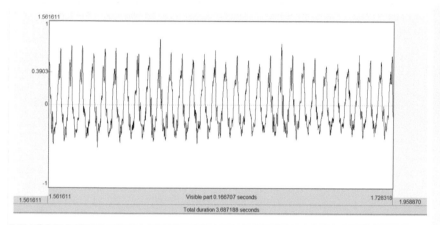

Fig. 4.28 Several cycles of vibration from a moderate breathy female sustained vowel production. Though some degree of repetition is present, obvious cycle-to-cycle variations are created by the addition of additive noise in the voice signal. In this example, cycle-to-cycle variations in amplitude and cycle profile are evident.

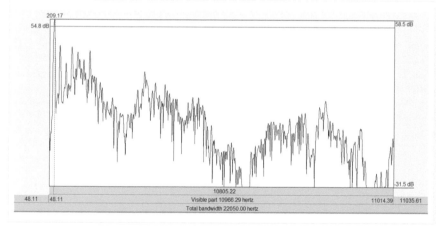

Fig. 4.29 A magnified portion of the sound spectrum for a moderate breathy female sustained vowel production. The F₀ (i.e., first harmonic) is prominent and identified at approximately 209 Hz. However, only a few distinctive harmonics follow the F₀ and most of the spectrum is dominated by inharmonic, unrelated frequencies. Praat analysis parameters: window length = 0.05 s; dynamic range = 90 dB.

The disturbances in frequency, amplitude, and profile are the characteristics we wish to quantify in voice quality evaluation. These disturbances are often referred to as **perturbations**, and measures of perturbation have been used as correlates of dysphonias in which vocal quality is disrupted. Three methods have been regularly used to quantify the voice signal perturbations that are characteristic of voice quality deviations. **Jitter** and **shimmer** are measures of *short-term instability* that quantify *cycle-to-cycle variations* in period/frequency and amplitude, respectively.[46] In addition, **harmonics-to-noise ratio** *(HNR)* is also a method that detects cycle-to-cycle perturbations and

was initially designed as a method for *quantifying spectral noise*. Perturbation measures may be useful in identifying relatively small levels of aperiodicity and, therefore, may be helpful in documenting the severity levels that often present the most difficulty in perceptual judgment (e.g., mild, mild-to-moderate severity dysphonias).[191] Several studies have shown reasonably significant correlations between acoustic perturbation measures and voice quality categories.[192,193,194,195,196]

All of these aforementioned perturbation measures are based on the assumption that the intention of the patient/subject is to produce a sustained vowel at a steady pitch and

loudness, and valid and reliable measures of jitter, shimmer, and HNR may only be obtained from a steady-state vowel production.[68,197,198] Certainly, sustained vowel productions have several key benefits as a voice elicitation task in that sustained vowel production is a nonlinguistic, easily controlled, and standardized task that is easily understood and imitated.[197,199]

Several important points regarding eliciting sustained vowel productions for vocal quality analyses are noted:

1. As stated, use a method of elicitation that provides a pitch/frequency similar to that in continuous speech (we do not want an artificially high/low pitch level that may not correspond well with continuous speech characteristics).

2. Try to obtain a vowel production that reflects the patient's typical voice characteristics. Very importantly, we do not want our instructions to change the natural behavior of the patient. As an example, a hypofunctional patient may present with a quieter, low-intensity voice. If we now ask the patient to produce a vowel at a loudness level that is higher than he or she habitually uses, we may cause the patient to produce a different quality voice with different levels of perturbation than would be found in the habitual voice.

3. We recommend the use of the vowel /a/ since it does not appear to raise the pitch of the voice as with the vowels /i/ and /u/, has a high first formant that tends to not interact with the typical SFF, and may be more beneficial in revealing vocal instability.

4. Obtain multiple repetitions to allow for observation of possible variation in perturbation values but still at a manageable level (three repetitions) for clinical purposes and consistent with the method used in much of the clinical voice literature.

5. Make sure that, if possible, you can obtain at least a **3-second duration** vowel production. In sustained vowel analysis as used for measures of jitter shimmer, etc., we will typically measure the central vowel portion (at least 1 second in duration) and omit vowel onsets and offsets that may artificially inflate perturbation measures. Once we omit the onsets and offsets, we are ideally left with at least a 1-second duration of vowel production to analyze. Though we may not analyze them for perturbation, we should still listen closely to these portions of the patient's vowel productions, since the vowel onsets and offsets may reveal characteristics such as hard onsets, intermittent aphonia, or rough or fry phonation that can be valuable in our perceptual description of the voice.[197]

Jitter

Jitter is a measure of the **cycle-to-cycle perturbations in a vocal period**. Because the reciprocal of period is frequency, there are also methods of computing jitter that report results in Hz. Various methods have been proposed by which jitter may be calculated.[68] One of the more common methods is to calculate *jitter factor* (jitter in %). The mathematical formula for the calculation of jitter factor requires that we (1) sum the cycle-to-cycle absolute differences in frequency (in Hz); (2) divide the sum of the differences by the number of differences (i.e., number of cycles−1); (3) divide the result by the mean frequency; and (4) multiply the final result by 100 to convert to a percentage (%). By expressing the mean cycle-to-cycle perturbation in frequency in relation to the mean overall frequency of the

voice signal, the influence of F_0 (e.g., higher F_0s for adult female vs. male voice) is accounted for:

$$\frac{\frac{1}{n-1}\left[\sum_{i=1}^{i=n-1}\left|F_i - F_{i+1}\right|\right]}{\frac{1}{n}\sum_{i=1}^{n} F_i} \times 100$$

Other methods such as ***jitter ratio*** (the ratio of the average period perturbation to average period reported in ms) and *relative amplitude perturbation jitter* (% RAP—used to remove relatively isolated and/or long-duration fluctuations in cycle-to-cycle perturbation; a smoothed perturbation value) may also be used.

A number of sources have indicated that jitter (%) may be expected to be ≤ 1% in normal subjects,[198,200,201,202] and this expectation may be reasonable depending on the voice analysis program being used (e.g., data from the *Multidimensional Voice Program—MDVP*, KayPentax, Montvale, NJ).[111,203] **However, the combination of improved resolution via high sampling rates (recommended minimum 44 kHz) used in current digital recording methods and improved methods of identifying voice signal cycle boundaries often results in observations of jitter (%) values substantially < 1% and in the vicinity of ≈ 0.4 to 0.6% (or less) in nondysphonic vowel production (e.g., using a program such as Praat).**[1] For absolute jitter (in ms), normative values in the vicinity of 0.04 ms may be expected. ▶ Table 4.8 presents a range of examples of jitter values obtained from normal voice subjects.

Shimmer

Shimmer is a measure of the cycle-to-cycle perturbations in amplitude. Signal amplitude may be measured per cycle in many different ways, including *peak amplitude* (the value of the largest amplitude within each cycle following an a priori decision as to the use of positive or negative peaks), *peak-to-peak amplitude* (the distance between the greatest positive and greatest negative peak amplitudes per cycle), and *root mean squared amplitude* (a form of statistical average amplitude that may be computed per cycle in which all sampled amplitude values are squared and summed, divided by the number of amplitude values per cycle, and the square root computed; ▶ Fig. 4.30).

One of the most commonly used methods of computing shimmer is to report this value in dB. This form of shimmer measurement is an absolute measure of cycle-to-cycle variations in amplitude in which (**1**) the absolute cycle-to-cycle deviations in sound level (dB) are summed, and (**2**) the sum of the differences is divided by the number of differences (i.e., number of cycles−1):

$$\frac{1}{n-1}\left[\sum_{i=1}^{n-1}\left|20 \times LOG\left(\frac{A_i}{Ai+1}\right)\right|\right]$$

As with the measurement of jitter, several methods for carrying out the calculation of shimmer have been proposed, including *percent shimmer* (%) and *relative average perturbation shimmer* (RAP in dB), in which the effects of relatively isolated and/or long-duration fluctuations in cycle-to-cycle perturbation are minimized by smoothing the estimates of cycle-to-cycle amplitude perturbation.[68]

Absolute shimmer (in dB) has been observed to be substantially less than 1 dB in nondysphonic sustain vowel productions, with **typical sustained vowel productions usually observed to have less than 0.5 dB shimmer.**[1,111] Normative percent

Table 4.8 Examples of jitter from various literature sources

Author	Gender	No. of subjects	Age	Mean and SD	Range
Horii[201]	M	31	18–38 (26.6 y)	0.61% (0.20)	N/A
Murry and Doherty[27]	M	5	55–71 (M = 63.8)	0.99%	0.76–1.49
Ramig and Ringel[30, a]	$M_{Y,G}$	8	26–35 (M = 29.5)	0.42% (0.09)	N/A
	$M_{Y,P}$	8	25–38 (M = 32.3)	0.50% (0.09)	N/A
	$M_{M,G}$	8	46–56 (M = 53.0)	0.50% (0.10)	N/A
	$M_{M,P}$	8	42–59 (M = 52.6)	0.70% (0.32)	N/A
	$M_{O,G}$	8	62–75 (M = 67.5)	0.60% (0.15)	N/A
	$M_{O,P}$	8	64–74 (M = 69.1)	0.65% (0.14)	N/A
Horii[48, b]	M	12	24–40	0.085 ms (0.032)	0.035–0.151
				0.87% (0.32)	0.46–1.61
Fisher and Linville[49, c]	F	25	25–35	0.52% (0.18)	0.33–1.02
		25	45–55	0.55% (0.30)	0.31–1.70
		25	70–80	0.91% (1.31)	0.30–6.89
Ludlow et al[204, d]	M	38	M = 42.1 (17.5)	0.047 ms (0.028)	0.011–0.163
	F	61	M = 40.8 (17.9)	0.033 ms (0.013)	0.011–0.074
Linville[50, e]	F	22	18–22 (M = 20.32; S.D. = 0.95)	0.55% (0.36)	0.15–2.30
Linville et al[51]	F	20	67–86 (M = 76.0; S.D. = 6.09)	2.07% (1.56)	0.48–6.10
Deem et al[205]	M	5	26–45	0.56 (0.02)	N/A
	F	7	26–48	0.47 (0.05)	N/A
Orlikoff[52, f]	M_Y	6	26–33 (M = 30.0)	0.042 ms (0.006)	0.034–0.051
				0.46% (0.067)	0.41–0.59
	M_E	6	68–80 (M = 73.3)	0.053 ms (0.015)	0.038–0.081
				0.625% (0.102)	0.468–0.74
Karnell[206]	M	9		0.62 (N/A)	N/A
	F	9		1.128 (N/A)	N/A
Zwirner et al[123]	M & F	12	37–76 (M = 58 y)	0.04 ms (0.02)	0.012–0.07
Kent et al[33]	F	19	65–80 (M = 71.8)	0.073 ms (0.049)	N/A
Walton and Orlikoff[207, g]	M_W	50	M = 30	0.28% (0.12)	0.17–0.89
	M_B	50	M = 29	0.40% (0.36)	0.14–2.33
Dwire and McCauley[208]	M	24	18–25	0.38% (0.17)	N/A
	F	25	18–25	0.89% (0.62)	N/A
Gelfer[209, h]	F	29	20–39 (M = 27:1)	0.333% (0.105)	N/A
Gelfer and Fendel[200, i]	F	30	21–36 (M = 25.5 y)	0.34% (0.11)	N/A
				0.016 ms (0.006)	N/A
Martin et al[194]	M & F	8	23–65	1.18%	N/A
Scherer et al[199]	M & F	24	22–81	0.52% (0.23)	N/A
Stemple et al[131, j]	F	10	22–45 (M = 25.3 y)	0.38% (0.18)	N/A
Wolfe et al[53]	M & F	20	23–65	1.86% (1.89)	0.33–7.52

Table 4.8 continued

Author	Gender	No. of subjects	Age	Mean and SD	Range
Boltezar et al[83]	M & F	8	14.50 y (1.77)	0.81% (0.59)	N/A
Omori et al[210]	M	50	Adult	N/A	0.15–0.53%
	F	50	Adult	N/A	0.07–0.69%
Awan[1]	M	20	18–30	0.43% (0.09)	0.27–0.62
				0.25% RAP (0.06)	0.16–0.36
				0.04 ms (0.01)	0.01–0.06
	F	20	18–30	0.50% (0.15)	0.31–0.82
				0.31% RAP (0.10)	0.16–0.51
				0.02 ms (0.01)	0.02–0.04
	M & F	10	5–6	0.61% (0.21)	0.39–1.08
				0.38% RAP (0.12)	0.26–0.65
				0.02 ms (0.01)	0.01–0.05
Awan[41]	F	10	18–30 (Mean = 23.80 y)	0.36% (0.17)	N/A
	F	10	40–49 (Mean = 43.40 y)	0.47% (0.30)	N/A
	F	10	50–59 (Mean = 54.80 y)	0.82% (0.77)	N/A
	F	10	60–69 (Mean = 65.20 y)	0.51% (0.40)	N/A
	F	10	70–79 (Mean = 72.30 y)	0.46% (0.33)	N/A
Banh et al[211]	M	56	18–27 (Mean = 18.8)	0.37 (0.12)	N/A
	M	11	18–23 (Mean = 18.6)	0.48 (0.19)	N/A
	F	55	65–81 (Mean = 70.7)	0.38 (0.29)	N/A
	F	47	66–78 (Mean = 73.4)	0.45 (0.42)	N/A
Goy et al[43]	M	55	18–28 (x=19.4)	0.38 (0.13)	N/A
	M	51	65–86 (x=73.3)	0.48 (0.20)	N/A
	F	104	18–27 (x=18.9)	0.37 (0.25)	N/A
	F	82	63–82 (x=71.1)	0.47 (0.34)	N/A
Finger et al[212]	F	56	18–40	0.426 (.148)	0.03–0.97

Notes:
a. Young ($_Y$), Middle age ($_M$), and Old age ($_O$) subjects in good ($_G$) and poor ($_P$) condition. Data from vowel /a/ sustained for comfortable duration.
b. Data reported from modal register phonations.
c. Data converted from Jitter Ratio.
d. Jitter converted to ms from microseconds (sec).
e. Data from the vowel /a/ only.
f. Data from healthy young men (M_Y) and healthy elderly men (M_E).
g. Data from White (M_W) and Black (M_B) subjects. Jitter values are based on RAP.
h. Data from vowel /a/ produced at 70 dB (12 in. mouth-to-microphone distance).
i. Data from directly digitized voice samples only.
j. Data from pretest only (pre-laryngeal fatigue).

shimmer is considered to be 5% or less of the voice signal.[111,200,203] ▶ Table 4.9 presents a range of examples of shimmer values obtained from nondysphonic, typical voice subjects.

Harmonics-to-Noise Ratio

We have previously said that the sustained vowel production of a typical, nondysphonic speaker should be highly periodic.

Imagine then that we could somehow separate the highly repetitive, periodic portion of the voice waveform from the aperiodic, random portion of the wave. If we were to compare the amplitude of the periodic portion (i.e., the harmonic) to the aperiodic portion (i.e., the noise) via a ratio (i.e., periodic divided by aperiodic amplitude), we would expect the result to be a large value. In contrast, in dysphonic voices in which the aperiodic contribution to the sound wave is more prominent,

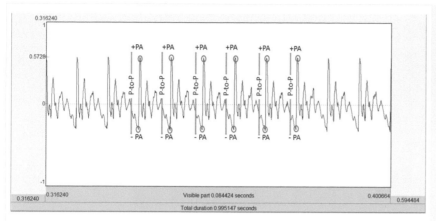

Fig. 4.30 The amplitude per cycle may be measured from the positive peak amplitude (+PA), the negative peak amplitude (–PA), or the peak-to-peak amplitude (P-to-P, the distance between the +PA and the –PA). Cycle amplitude may also be expressed as a form of statistical average referred to as the root mean squared average (see text).

Table 4.9 Examples of shimmer from various literature sources

Author	Gender	No. of subjects	Age	Mean and SD	Range
Horii[201]	M	31	18–38 (26.6 y)	0.47 dB (0.34)	N/A
Ramig and Ringel[30, a]	$M_{Y,G}$	8	26–35 (M = 29.5)	0.27 dB (0.13)	N/A
	$M_{Y,P}$	8	25–38 (M = 32.3)	0.27 dB (0.18)	N/A
	$M_{M,G}$	8	46–56 (M = 53.0)	0.35 dB (0.16)	N/A
	$M_{M,P}$	8	42–59 (M = 52.6)	0.43 dB (0.29)	N/A
	$M_{O,G}$	8	62–75 (M = 67.5)	0.36 dB (0.09)	N/A
	$M_{O,P}$	8	64–74 (M = 69.1)	0.43 dB (0.25)	N/A
Horii[48, b]	M	12	24–40	0.48 dB (0.25)	0.17–1.29
Ludlow et al[204]	M	38	M = 42.1 (17.5)	5.1% (2.9)	1.4–14.3
	F	61	M = 40.8 (17.9)	5.3% (3.9)	1.5–24.1
Deem et al[205]	M	5	26–45	0.56 (0.02)	
	F	7	26–48	0.47 (0.05)	
Orlikoff[52, c]	M_Y	6	26–33 (M = 30.0)	0.257 dB (0.088)	0.154–0.36
				2.93% (1.0)	1.76–4.11
	M_E	6	68–80 (M = 73.3)	0.39% (0.113)	0.269–0.562
				4.42% (1.24)	3.12–6.27
Zwirner et al[123]	M & F	12	37–76 (M = 58 y)	4.1% (3.3)	1.1–12.8
Kent et al[33]	F	19	65–80 (M = 71.8)	2.6% (1.04)	N/A
Walton and Orlikoff[207, d]	M_W	50	M = 30	0.27 dB (0.11)	0.09–0.70
	M_B	50	M = 29	0.33 dB (0.15)	0.11–0.66
Gelfer[209, e]	F	29	20–39 (M = 27:1)	2.53% (0.86)	N/A
Gelfer and Fendel[200, f]	F	30	21–36 (M = 25.5 y)	1.29% (0.34)	N/A
Martin et al[194]	M & F	8	23–65	0.24 dB	N/A
Scherer et al[199]	M & F	18	22–81	1.88% (0.83)	N/A
Wolfe et al[53]	M & F	20	23–65	0.29 dB (0.22)	0.12–1.12
Boltezar et al[83]	M & F	8	14.50 y (1.77)	2.52% (1.40)	N/A
Omori et al[210]	M	50	Adult	N/A	0.45–4.53%

Table 4.9 continued

Author	Gender	No. of subjects	Age	Mean and SD	Range
	F	50	Adult	N/A	0.69–4.52%
Awan[1]	M	20	18–30	0.17 dB (0.05)	0.09–0.27
				0.11 dB RAP (0.02)	0.07–0.15
				1.02% (0.29)	0.54–1.62
	F	20	18–30	0.16 dB (0.06)	0.10–0.33
				0.10 dB RAP (0.03)	0.06–0.20
				1.05% (0.39)	0.61–2.04
	M & F	10	5–6	0.25 dB (0.06)	0.15–0.36
				0.16 dB RAP (0.04)	0.09–0.22
				1.60% (0.37)	0.97–2.35
Awan[41]	F	10	18–30 (Mean = 23.80 y)	4.47% (1.95)	N/A
	F	10	40–49 (Mean = 43.40 y)	4.60% (1.81)	N/A
	F	10	50–59 (Mean = 54.80 y)	7.45% (4.66)	N/A
	F	10	60–69 (Mean = 65.20 y)	6.61% (5.22)	N/A
	F	10	70–79 (Mean = 72.30 y)	6.57% (3.36)	N/A
Banh et al[211]	M	56	18–27 (Mean = 18.8)	2.6 (1.0)	N/A
	M	11	18–23 (Mean = 18.6)	4.4 (2.6)	N/A
	F	55	65–81 (Mean = 70.7)	2.2 (0.8)	N/A
	F	47	66–78 (Mean = 73.4)	26 (1.5)	N/A
Goy et al[43]	M	55	18–28 (x = 19.4)	0.24 (0.09)	N/A
	M	51	65–86 (x = 73.3)	0.37 (0.19)	N/A
	F	104	18–27 (x = 18.9)	0.21 (0.08)	N/A
	F	82	63–82 (x = 71.1)	0.25 (0.16)	N/A
Finger et al[212]	F	56	18–40	0.268 (.197)	0.12–0.69

Notes:
a. Young (y), Middle age (M), and Old age (O) subjects in good (G) and poor (P) condition. Data from vowel /a/ sustained for comfortable duration.
b. Data reported from modal register phonations.
c. Data from healthy young men (M$_Y$) and healthy elderly men (M$_E$).
d. Data from White (M$_W$) and Black (M$_B$) subjects.
e. Data from vowel /a/ produced at 70 dB (12 in. mouth-to-microphone distance).
f. Data from directly digitized voice samples only.

we would expect the HNR to be reduced. In essence, this is what happens in the computation of HNR.

A number of methods have been proposed by which HNR (a.k.a. SNR) may be computed, some of which compute this ratio from the voice waveform and some from the spectrum (e.g., *noise-to-harmonics ratio* [NHR] compares the energy of the nonharmonic components of the spectrum vs. energy of the harmonic components of the spectrum—e.g., the ratio of nonharmonic energy in the range 1,500–4,500 Hz to the harmonic spectral energy in the range 70–4,500 Hz). NHR is most often reported as a nonunit ratio, but could also be reported in dB.[192,213,214,215]

A number of authors have indicated that HNR may be a more comprehensive measure of the voice signal than jitter or shimmer.[199,216,217] This may be because HNR is sensitive to variations in waveform profile/wave shape that occur because of various forms of perturbation and is not restricted to disturbances specific to period and/or focused measures of amplitude (such as measures of peak or peak-to-peak amplitude). Because HNR can account for any type of variation that may occur between cycles, by its nature HNR takes into account the jitter and shimmer in a signal.[216,217]

Expectations for HNR in nondysphonic sustained vowel productions are highly variable dependent on the computer program and specific algorithm used for the analysis. Initial reports of HNR tended to be approximately in the range of 10 to 12 dB.[215] **More recent expectations for normative HNR have been substantially greater, in the vicinity to 15 to 20 dB,[207,216] and most typical voice subjects will have HNRs ≈ 20 dB or higher using the Praat program.**[203] ▶ Table 4.10 presents a range of examples of HNR values obtained from normal voice subjects.

Table 4.10 Examples of HNR from various literature sources

Author	Gender	No. of subjects	Age	Mean and SD	Range
Yumoto et al[192]	M & F	42	19–60	11.9 (2.32)	7.0–17.0
Deem et al[205]	M	5	26–45		
	F	7	26–48		
Zwirner et al[123]	M & F	12	37–76 (M = 58 y)	20.2 (4.1)	12.6–27.9
Kent et al[33]	F	19	65–80 (M–71.8)	21.4 (2.02)	N/A
Awan and Frenkel[216]	M	10	M = 24.2 y	15.63 (1.26)	N/A
	F	10	M = 24.7 y	15.12 (0.85)	N/A
Walton and Orlikoff[207, a]	M_W	50	M = 30	16.32 (2.56)	10.49–21.45
	M_B	50	M = 29	14.77 (3.38)	6.68–20.96
Gelfer[209, b]	F	29	20–39 (M = 27:1)	22.1 (2.9)	N/A
Gelfer and Fendel[200, c]	F	30	21–36 (M = 25.5 y)	27.5 (2.3)	N/A
Scherer et al[199]	M & F	18	22–81	20.26 (2.81)	N/A
Wolfe et al[53]	M & F	20	18–30		
Awan[1]	M	20	18–30	16.25 (2.50)	11.36–21.52
	F	20	18–30	17.89 (2.00)	13.54–21.50
	M & F	10	5–6	13.26 (1.63)	11.09–16.28
Awan[41]	F	10	18–30 (mean = 23.80 y)	16.90 (3.59)	N/A
	F	10	40–49 (mean = 43.40 y)	17.80 (2.73)	N/A
	F	10	50–59 (Mean = 54.80 y)	15.00 (4.62)	N/A
	F	10	60–69 (mean = 65.20 y)	16.42 (3.94)	N/A
	F	10	70–79 (mean = 72.30 y)	16.37 (3.89)	N/A
Banh et al[211]	M	56	18–27 (mean = 18.8)	22.9 (2.8)	N/A
	M	11	18–23 (mean = 18.6)	21.2 (4.6)	N/A
	F	55	65–81 (mean = 70.7)	24.5 (3.0)	N/A
	F	47	66–78 (mean = 73.4)	23.8 (3.7)	N/A
Goy et al[43]	M	55	18–28 (x = 19.4)	22.9 (2.7)	N/A
	M	51	65–86 (x=73.3)	21.9 (3.8)	N/A
	F	104	18–27 (x = 18.9)	25.3 (3.1)	N/A
	F	82	63–82 (x = 71.1)	25.3 (3.8)	N/A
Finger et al[212]	F	56	18–40	19.33 (3.688)	12.6–26.5

Notes:
a. Data from vowel /a/ produced at 70 dB (12 in. mouth-to-microphone distance)
b. Data from vowel /a/ produced at 70 dB (12 in. mouth-to-microphone distance).
c. Data from directly digitized voice samples only.

4.4.12 Examples of Perturbation Measurements Using Praat

We will now examine perturbation measures in several voice samples. All of the samples are sustained vowel productions that have been elicited using the previously described "1, 2, 3, ahhh" method. All examples are analyzed in *Praat* using the cross-correlation method (Pitch | Pitch Settings | Cross-Correlation). To obtain perturbation as well as other voice signal measures, pulses are turned on and a central portion (often 1–2 seconds in duration) is highlighted using the mouse. The selection of **Pulses | Voice Report** will then provide a listing of various measures including F_0 and perturbation statistics.

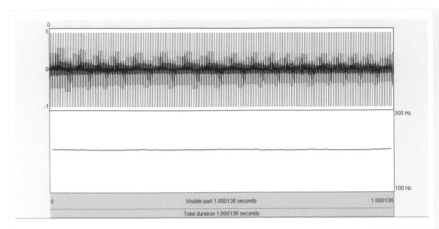

Fig. 4.31 Central 1-second portion of a sustained vowel /a/ produced by a typical, nondysphonic adult female. Jitter = 0.23%; Shimmer = 0.19 dB; HNR = 24.48 dB. Praat analysis parameters: pulses on; Pitch | Pitch Settings | Cross-correlation; voicing threshold = 0.60.

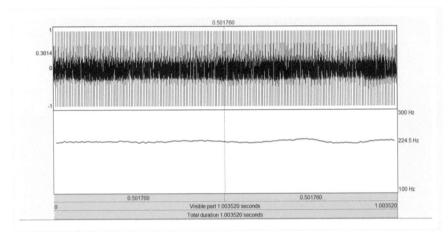

Fig. 4.32 Central 1-second portion of a sustained vowel /a/ produced by an adult female with a mild breathy voice quality. Jitter = 0.59%; Shimmer = 0.34 dB; HNR = 18.36 dB. Praat analysis parameters: pulses on; Pitch | Pitch Settings | Cross-correlation; voicing threshold = 0.60.

▶ Fig. 4.31 and **Sample 4.14** show a central 1-second edit of a sustained vowel /a/ produced by a typical, nondysphonic adult female. The vowel sample is produced at a steady pitch and loudness, and does not have any perceived quality deviation (i.e., no perceived breathiness, roughness, strain, etc.). For this type of nondysphonic sample, we would expect jitter and shimmer to be low and HNR to be high. Results showed jitter = 0.23% (considerably < 1%, and even less than the previously mentioned 0.4–0.6% expectation); shimmer = 0.19 dB (< 0.5 dB expectation threshold); and HNR = 24.48 dB (> 20 dB expectation threshold).

When the voice signal becomes disturbed by factors such as excessive airflow between the vocal folds during vibration (e.g., breathiness) or irregular vocal fold vibration (e.g., roughness), it is expected that measures of perturbation will vary with expected increases in jitter and shimmer and decreases in HNR. ▶ Fig. 4.32 and **Sample 4.15** show the voice signal and F_0 contour for an adult female with a mild breathy quality and mild F_0 instability. Results showed jitter = 0.59% (< 1%, but at the higher limit of the 0.4–0.6% expectation threshold); shimmer = 0.34 dB (< 0.5 dB expectation threshold); and HNR = 18.36 dB (< 20 dB expectation threshold). In very mild cases, we often see that perturbation measures may be near our expected thresholds (i.e., "borderline" atypical) and/or that only one of our measures is sensitive to the mild dysphonia (in this case, HNR is clearly below our expected threshold of > 20 dB for typical, nondysphonic voice). This is one of the reasons why we do not want

to depend on a single measure as a correlate to dysphonic voice quality—depending on the type and severity of the presenting of voice quality, there may be variation in which measures (period/frequency perturbation, amplitude perturbation, HNR) are sensitive to the presenting dysphonia.

In ▶ Fig. 4.33 and **Sample 4.16**, we see the voice signal waveform and F_0 contour for a moderate breathy voice (adult female). Increased disturbance in the F_0 contour is observed due to increased cycle-to-cycle disturbance versus the previously described nondysphonic and mildly dysphonic samples. As the voice signal has increased in the severity of dysphonic voice quality, our measures of perturbation have shown a corresponding increase, with jitter = 1.36% (substantially greater than the 0.4–0.6% expectation); shimmer = 0.62 dB (> the 0.5 dB expectation threshold); and HNR = 13.57 dB (substantially < 20 dB expectation threshold).

The previous examples of breathy voice signals are all examples of relatively periodic signals + additive noise. Breathiness may be described to vary from typical, modal voice via the addition of continuous air escape through the glottis and, while breathiness has been discussed here as a quality that may be associated with disordered voice and possible underlying pathology, it may also be used purposefully to modify communicative intent.[218] We will next examine examples of rough voice quality that may be considered "nonmodal," in that rough voice quality tends to be categorically different from typical, modal voice.[218]

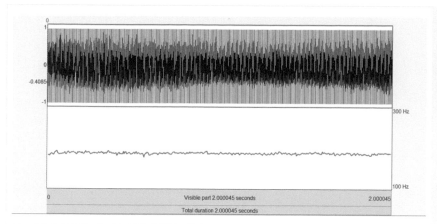

Fig. 4.33 Central portion of a sustained vowel /a/ produced by an adult female with a moderate breathy voice quality. Jitter = 1.36%; Shimmer = 0.62 dB; HNR = 13.57 dB. Praat analysis parameters: pulses on; Pitch | Pitch Settings | Cross-correlation; voicing threshold = 0.60.

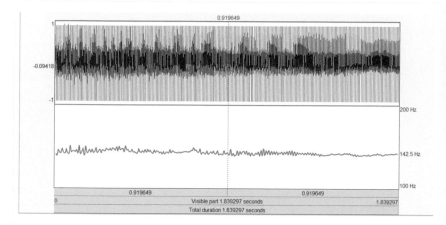

Fig. 4.34 Central portion of a sustained vowel /a/ produced by an adult male with a unilateral vocal fold polyp and rough voice quality. Jitter = 2.05%; Shimmer = 1.11 dB; HNR = 12.99 dB. Praat analysis parameters: pulses on; Pitch | Pitch Settings | Cross-correlation; voicing threshold = 0.60.

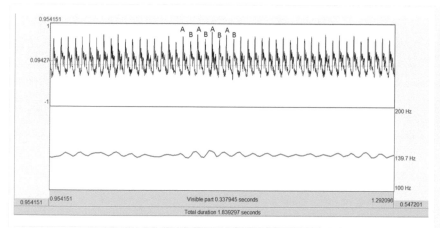

Fig. 4.35 Zoomed portion of the rough voice signal observed in ▶ Fig. 4.34. The sound wave shows alternating large **(a)** versus small **(b)** amplitude cycles. This type of voice waveform pattern has been referred to as an amplitude modulation, and generally coincides with period-doubling and the presence of a subharmonic (i.e., $F_0/2$). Praat analysis parameters: pulses on; Pitch | Pitch Settings | Cross-correlation; voicing threshold = 0.60.

▶ Fig. 4.34 and **Sample 4.17** provide an example of the voice signal and F_0 contour from a sustained vowel /a/ produced by an adult male who presented with a unilateral vocal fold polyp. These types of voice signals are often perceived as low pitched, gravelly, and (unlike some forms of breathy voice) unpleasant. The F_0 contour shows instability, and perturbation measures of jitter and shimmer substantially deviate from expected thresholds (Jitter = 2.05%; Shimmer = 1.11 dB; HNR = 12.99 dB, well below typical expectations). A zoomed-in view of the sound wave (▶ Fig. 4.35) shows that this rough voice sample is characterized by cycles that alternate in terms of amplitude (an *amplitude modulation*). The alternating cycle amplitude pattern also suggests the presence of a subharmonic frequency (i.e., $F_0/2$—also referred to as *period-doubling*), and this type of voice signal has been associated with vocal fold asymmetries and the possible combination of vocal fold and ventricular fold vibration.[218,219,220] The spectrum of a portion of this rough voice waveform (Fig. 4.36) shows the F_0 at approximately 140 Hz and, while there are harmonic multiples of the F_0, there are also visible "interharmonic" spectral peaks. In ▶ Fig. 4.36, the

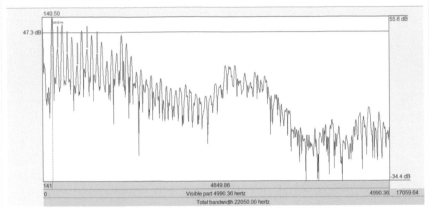

Fig. 4.36 Spectral slice of a portion of the rough voce waveform observed in ▶ Fig. 4.35. Harmonic peaks in the spectrum can be observed at multiples of the F_0 (≈ 140 Hz). However, vertical arrows point to examples of strong interharmonic spectral peaks. The first of these interharmonic peaks occurs at ≈ 210 Hz, and the difference between the F0 and this interharmonic frequency is ≈ 70 Hz (i.e., F_0/2, a subharmonic). Praat analysis parameters: window length = 0.10s; dynamic range = 90 dB; frequency range = 0 to 4,990 Hz.

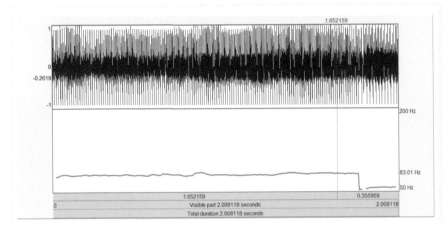

Fig. 4.37 Central portion of a sustained vowel /a/ produced by an adult male presenting with unilateral vocal fold paralysis and rough voice quality. The drastic variation in the F_0 contour near the end of the vowel sample occurs due to a sudden transition in the type/mode of vibration. Jitter = 0.72%; Shimmer = 0.69 dB; HNR = 12.91 dB. Praat analysis parameters: pulses on; Pitch | Pitch Settings | Cross-correlation; voicing threshold = 0.60.

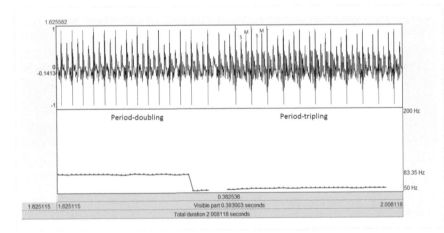

Fig. 4.38 Magnified portion of a section the voice waveform produced by the adult male presenting with unilateral vocal fold paralysis and rough voice quality in ▶ Fig. 4.37. An abrupt transition occurs between period-doubling and period-tripling (two different forms of rough voice signal). The section of period-tripling shows a consistent pattern of large-small-medium (L-S-M) peaks in the waveform produced (in part) by the combination of a F_0 ≈ 169 Hz and a subharmonic at F_0/3 ≈ 56 Hz. Praat analysis parameters: pulses on; Pitch | Pitch Settings | Cross-correlation; voicing threshold = 0.60.

first of these interharmonic peaks occurs at approximately 210 Hz, with the difference between the F_0 (≈ 140 Hz) and this first interharmonic peak ≈ 70 Hz (i.e., F_0/2—a subharmonic).

In ▶ Fig. 4.37, we have another example of a rough voice (adult male; unilateral vocal fold paralysis [UVFP]). This voice waveform is notable in a number of different ways. First, even though we are confident that this voice signal will be perceived a highly dysphonic (see **Sample 4.18**), the jitter (0.72%) and shimmer (0.69 dB) measurements for this voice sample are only slightly above our expectation thresholds and seem disproportionately low as compared to the perceived severity of the voice

sample. Even though rough voice signals may be perceived as dysphonic and are characterized by repeating patterns that extend over more than one apparent cycle, this example shows that the repeating patterns may or may not be excessively perturbed in period/frequency or amplitude. Second, the notable variation in the F_0 contour near the end of the vowel sample occurs due to a sudden transition in the type/mode of vibration, and a zoomed-in view of the voice waveform (▶ Fig. 4.38) shows that this voice signal changes from the *period-doubling* observed in the previous rough example to *period-tripling* with large-small-medium-large-small-medium, etc., amplitude peaks

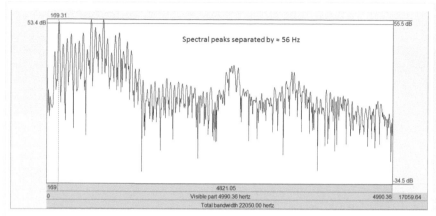

Fig. 4.39 Spectral slice of the period-tripling waveform observed in ▶ Fig. 4.38. The prominent spectral peak at ≈ 169 Hz corresponds to the period (0.005916 s) between medium to large peaks in the period-tripling section of the acoustic waveform. The various harmonic peaks in the spectrum are separated by ≈ 56 Hz, which corresponds to the period (0.0178 s) between large-to-large peaks in the acoustic waveform and is approximately equal to the $F_0/3$. Praat analysis parameters: window length = 0.10s; dynamic range = 90 dB; frequency range = 0 to 4,990 Hz.

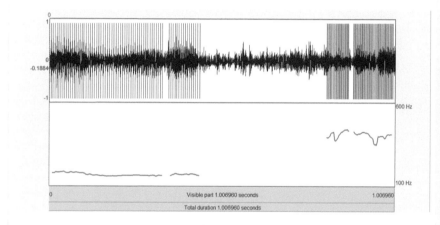

Fig. 4.40 Central portion of a sustained vowel /a/ produced by an adult female presenting with adductor spasmodic dysphonia. The voice is perceived as strained with pitch instability (rising pitch), intermittent roughness, and a period of highly effortful, almost aphonic production near the midpoint of the vowel production. The perturbation measures of jitter (2.03%), shimmer (1.31 dB), and HNR (8.70 dB) are computed from regions of the voice waveform in which possible cycles of vibration are detected. Perturbation data are not applicable to the section of highly aperiodic vibration (region of absent pulses and F_0 contour) that are often perceptually salient. Praat analysis parameters: pulses on; Pitch | Pitch Settings | Cross-correlation; voicing threshold = 0.60.

observed in the waveform. A spectral slice of the zoomed waveform (▶ Fig. 4.39) shows the prominent spectral peak at ≈ 169 Hz to correspond to the period (0.005916 s) between medium to large peaks in the acoustic waveform. The various harmonic peaks in the spectrum are separated by ≈ 56 Hz, which corresponds to the period (0.0178 s) between large to large peaks in the acoustic waveform and is approximately equal to the period × 3 and $F_0/3$. This example shows that there may be several subtypes of the rough voice signal (pitch-doubling, pitch-tripling, etc.) and that these waveforms are not clearly periodic or aperiodic (they have been referred to as "supraperiodic" in nature).[218]

Our final examples show some of the limitations of traditional perturbation with more severe forms of dysphonic voice. ▶ Fig. 4.40 and **Sample 4.19** provide the voice waveform and F_0 contour for an adult female with adductor spasmodic dysphonia (ADSD). The voice is perceived as strained with pitch instability (rising pitch), intermittent roughness, and a period of highly effortful, almost aphonic production near the midpoint of the vowel production. In this example, the perturbation measures computed using the entire sample (jitter = 2.03%; shimmer = 1.31 dB; HNR = 8.70 dB) are certainly well beyond any of the expected thresholds we have discussed and would be consistent with the perception of a severe dysphonia. However, we are actually missing perturbation data from a substantial section of the phonation which is aperiodic with an absence of

detectable cycles of vibration (this is the region of the sound wave in which pulses and an F_0 contour are absent). Therefore, these perturbation measures start to lose their validity with more severe forms of dysphonia which approach aphonia. Because listeners may base their auditory-perceptual judgments and ratings on portions of the voice sample that are more perceptually salient/prominent (regardless of duration) versus F_0 and perturbation measures that will be obtained from portions of the sample that show some degree of periodicity, we may expect poorer correlations between auditory-perceptual ratings and acoustic measures of perturbation in these more severe forms of dysphonic voice.

In ▶ Fig. 4.41, we have dysphonia at its most extreme—aphonia (i.e., a lack of vocal fold vibration). The sound wave is perceived as breathy aphonic and effortful (**Sample 4.20**). Because this signal is completely aperiodic, there are no visible pulses and no visible F_0 contour. In addition, the selections of **Pulses | Voice Report** will simply indicate "undefined" for any measure that is determined by the presence of detectable cycles of vibration in the voice waveform (e.g., F_0, jitter, shimmer, HNR). **This example shows that the acoustic measures we have been using as correlates of the presence and severity of dysphonia completely break down at this most extreme form of dysphonia, leaving us with an absence of objective acoustic data to support our auditory-perceptions.**

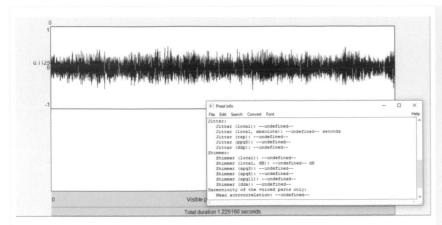

Fig. 4.41 Central portion of a completely aphonic sustained vowel /a/ sample. Pulses (marking cycle boundaries in the waveform) and F_0 contour are absent. The voice report shows "undefined" for any measure that is dependent on the identification of cycles of vibration in the sound wave. Praat analysis parameters: pulses on; Pitch | Pitch Settings | Cross-correlation; voicing threshold = 0.60.

Measures of Perturbation in Normal/Typical Voice Subjects

Measures of Perturbation across the Continuum of Age

In comparison to typical adults, there is some indication that increased perturbation (increased jitter and shimmer; decreased HNR) during sustained vowel productions may be expected in infants and young children, with reductions in vocal perturbation noted as children age.[68,203,221,222,223] Decreased perturbation as children age may be due to factors such as maturity in neuromotor control of phonatory function and membranous vocal fold growth.[224]

It is questionable whether significant differences exist between males versus females on measures of vocal perturbation. Several studies have reported lower amounts of jitter in female voices compared with male voices,[225,226,227] and attributed the lower jitter in female voices to factors such as higher vocal F_0 and possible differences in vocal fold length and vibratory characteristics between women and men.[227,228] In contrast, other studies have reported higher jitter in females versus in males or no difference.[20,67,175,208]

Increased age may produce changes in voice quality due to functional changes in the larynx and general sensorimotor deficits associated with the aging process.[93,94] The possibility of decrement in vocal quality with advanced age may be reflected in measures of perturbation, with higher jitter values observed in older versus young and middle-aged subjects.[49,50,51,52,229,230,231,232] However, as has been previously stated, variability in measures of vocal function (including perturbation) from elderly subjects may be strongly related to physical condition, with other reports indicating no significant difference in perturbation measures between young, middle-aged, and elderly subjects.[175,211,233]

The Possible Effect of Race on Measures of Perturbation

Walton and Orlikoff reported significantly greater jitter and shimmer and lower HNRs in adult African American versus Caucasian men. It was also reported that the perceptual categorization of speakers by race was most successful when substantial differences existed between African American and Caucasian voice pairs in terms of vocal perturbation and additive noise.[207]

Measures of Perturbation in Voice-Disordered Persons

Deviations in voice quality are often the hallmark of abnormal voice production and, as previously mentioned, many of the common dysphonic voice qualities we perceive (e.g., breathiness, hoarseness, roughness) are related to deviations from the highly periodic voice signals produced in sustained vowel contexts by nondysphonic individuals. **The clinician must understand that the numerical results of jitter, shimmer, and HNR analyses may be accounted for by many different perceived voice types and many different underlying physiological conditions. A variety of different underlying causes of vocal dysfunction (e.g., vocal fold paralysis, vocal nodules, and vocal hyperfunction) may all show increases in jitter and shimmer and reduction in HNR.** Similarly, patients with three different voice quality types (breathiness, roughness, and hoarseness) could also show similar increases in the same perturbation measures. *The perturbation measures that we have described simply document the degree of signal disturbance in relation to a perfectly periodic signal that would have 0% jitter, 0 dB shimmer, and an infinitely large HNR—they are not specific to the underlying cause of the voice problem or to the resulting voice quality deviation.* The clinician will have to use other information (e.g., perceptual description of the voice) to understand why increased perturbation is present in the voice signal or not. Clearly, objective acoustic analyses must be a part of a comprehensive voice evaluation that includes detailed case history information, perceptual assessment, other physiological measures (aerodynamics), and laryngeal visualization to achieve a complete understanding and profile of the patient's voice.

Though perturbation measures do not indicate a specific voice quality type, multiple examples are available in which they have been observed to correlate with perceptual ratings of voice quality or show discriminatory ability to separate nondysphonic versus dysphonic voice in a variety of conditions:

- Several studies have reported jitter to significantly correlate with ratings of breathiness,[234] roughness,[196,222] and hoarseness,[192] as well as overall dysphonia severity.[53,193,194,222]
- Shimmer has similarly been reported to correlate significantly with breathiness,[194,235] roughness,[195,236] hoarseness,[237] as well as overall severity.[53]

- Significant correlations between HNR and roughness,[194] as well as overall ratings of dysphonia severity, have also been reported.[53,217]
- Strained voices (i.e., reflective of increased vocal effort) have been reported to be relatively normal in terms of perturbation measures, whereas hoarse voices were substantially abnormal in all parameters.[196,238]
- Various studies have shown that these perturbation measures may have the capability to effectively discriminate between dysphonic and various nondysphonic groups, including laryngeal cancer,[27] vocal nodules,[193,239] vocal polyps,[187] ALS,[33] vocal fold paralysis,[188] and various organic versus hyperfunctional voice-disordered groups.[240] **However, as previously stated, these results should not necessarily be interpreted as indicating that a particular profile of perturbation measures is disorder specific.**

▶ Table 4.11 provides general expectations for commonly used perturbation measures (jitter, shimmer, and HNR) for a number of commonly observed disorder types.

Methodological Considerations in Perturbation Measurement

The clinician should be aware that there are various factors that can have an effect on perturbation measures such as jitter, shimmer, and HNR. In our view, these extraneous variables do not necessarily negate the use of perturbation measures; however, it is important that we have an understanding of how various factors may influence our measurements.

- Differences in the implementation of computer algorithms may result in differences in normative expectations for measures such as jitter, shimmer, and HNR.[144,241] Therefore, normative data should provide a description of the computer program that was used, as well as other key recording parameters (e.g., sampling rate), and inter- and intra-subject comparison must always be conducted using the same computer program and similar parameter settings.
- A number of studies have indicated that vowel type may have an effect on perturbation measurements, with /i/ resulting in

lower jitter and shimmer values than other vowels such as the typically used /a/.[205,209,227] Inter- and intra-subject comparisons on perturbation measures should be conducted on similar vowel productions.

- Even though the computation of percent jitter factor (%) attempts to compensate for the influence of mean F_0, it should be noted that the frequency of phonation can affect measures of perturbation.[52] In particular, higher fundamental frequencies are associated with increased vocal fold tension and increased motor-unit firing rates—both of these factors may result in decreased jitter.[88] The chanted "1, 2, 3" method of elicitation previously described will aid eliciting a more habitual pitch versus higher pitch "sung" productions.
- Short duration phonations should be avoided if at all possible, as they may not provide a representative acoustic profile of the patient's voice. Disordered voice samples may require a larger number of consecutive cycles for analysis than nonpathologic voices, with greater than 100 cycles suggested as a minimum criterion.[199,206] A minimum of a 1-second central portion of the suggested 3-second vowel production should provide a reasonable sample for perturbation analysis for the majority of subjects.
- An inverse relationship between vocal intensity/loudness and measures of jitter and shimmer (i.e., as intensity/loudness increases, perturbation decreases) has been reported.[242] It maybe speculated that increased stability of vibration of the vocal folds at higher intensity phonation may be responsible for this observation.

Limitations of Traditional Acoustic Methods for Voice Analysis

While a number of investigations have reported significant correlations between acoustic perturbation measures and voice quality categories,[194,196,215] key limitations with methods such as jitter, shimmer, and HNR should be noted:

- **Difficulty analyzing more severely dysphonic vowel samples:** Many of the typically used perturbation measures as described here depend on accurately identifying cycle boundaries (i.e., where a cycle of vibration starts and ends).

Table 4.11 A summary of general expectations for vocal perturbation (jitter, shimmer, HNR) characteristics in various disorder types

Disorder	Expectations	Comments
Mass lesions/distributed tissue changes	Increased jitter and shimmer, decreased HNR	May lead to perturbations in the quasi-periodic voice signal. The presence of mass lesions or irregularities to the vocal fold edge(s) may result in additive noise from air escape during phonation (breathiness). Lesions and distributed tissue change may result in irregular vocal fold vibration (roughness), particularly if asymmetric. Combined breathiness + roughness = hoarseness
Neurological disorders	Increased jitter and shimmer, decreased HNR	May lead to hypoadduction (breathiness); irregular vocal fold vibration may be associated with unilateral dysfunction (roughness); combination = hoarseness. Disorders with hypertonia may have harsh voice quality
Muscle tension dysphonias (MTDs)/hyperfunctional voice	Variable	May result in perturbed voice quality. However, effortful, strained voice in the absence of breathy/rough/hoarse quality may be relatively periodic
Psychologically based voice disorders	Typical	Voice dysfunction has been described as primarily pitch/frequency and/or loudness/intensity focused
Hearing impairment/deafness	Variable	Voice quality disturbance and increased perturbation in the voice signal may be present in congenital/prelingual deaf speakers due to poor vocal control. Voice quality in postlingual, acquired hearing impairment is often not effected

However, it is evident that the increased disturbance/perturbation in the voice signal makes it more difficult to accurately locate these cycle onsets/offsets. This problem introduces error in tracking the periodic vibration of the voice signal, and thus contributes to inaccuracy in perturbation measurements.[243] As a result, some researchers have questioned the appropriateness, validity, and clinical usefulness of specific perturbation measures, especially when applied to moderately or severely disordered voices.[144,191] Titze classified acoustic signals into three types: those that were nearly periodic in nature (type I); those that contained modulations or subharmonics (as often observed in rough voice quality; type II); and those that approached random, aperiodic vibration (type III).[220] *While perturbation measures such as jitter and shimmer are applicable to type I voices, these same measures may have difficulty with highly perturbed type II and III signals in which cycles of vibration are not readily discerned.*

- **Excessive variability in the relationship between perturbation measures and perceived vocal quality**: In contrast to the previously cited studies showing significant degrees of relationship between objective measures of quality and perceptual ratings, Ludlow et al concluded that perturbation measures such as jitter and shimmer were not adequate as indices for the detection of laryngeal pathology, and Wolfe et al found no significant correlation between jitter and severity ratings of dysphonia.[53,204] Bielamowicz et al have gone so far as to suggest "abandonment of jitter as a measure of pathological voice" (p. 134).[144]

- **Lack of validity of traditional perturbation measures in the analysis of continuous speech**: In addition to being unreliable with highly perturbed signals, measures such as jitter, shimmer, and HNR are valid only for sustained vowels produced with steady pitch and loudness. Any purposeful changes in vocal pitch or loudness will be measured as increases in vocal perturbation, even though these measurements may not reflect vocal abnormality. Therefore, *the combination of pitch and loudness variations, noise produced via true consonant production (i.e., stop plosives, fricatives, and affricates), and short voicing segments in connected speech may invalidate the results of typically used perturbation measurements from speech segments.*

Because sustained vowels alone may not capture all salient characteristics of a patient's voice, several authors have indicated that *continuous/running speech may (1) provide a more ecologically valid assessment of the patient's control of vocal parameters such as vocal quality, (2) reveal increased degrees of voice impairment, and (3) correlate better with perceptions of dysphonia.*[99,244,245,246,247,248,249,250] In addition, continuous speech incorporates important vocal attributes such as rapid voice onset and termination, and variations in fundamental frequency and amplitude that may have a relatively large impact on short duration signals and, in turn, may be highly relevant to the perception of dysphonia and to clinical decisions regarding the voice quality of the patient.[251,252] It has also been noted that possible differences in dysphonia severity across certain voice contexts may specifically characterize certain voice disorders. As an example, Roy et al reported that the dysphonia associated with sustained vowel production was perceived as less severe

than that observed during connected speech in patients with ADSD.[248] In contrast, the same study reported that patients with MTD did not show variable performance in vowel versus speech contexts. A number of studies have also reported that listeners may rate certain dysphonic qualities (such as breathiness) more severely in sustained vowels than in continuous speech.[53,197,253,254,255]

With these various limitations with traditional perturbation measures such as jitter, shimmer, and HNR stated, the reader may wonder why we have provided some extensive detail in defining these measures and demonstrating their use in voice analysis. As stated, there are some who have urged the abandonment of these measures as indices of dysphonia. However, it is our view that there are a number of valid arguments for voice clinicians to not only have a good understanding of these traditional perturbation measures but to also consider (at least in a limited fashion) the continued use of some of these methods:

- Perturbation measures such as jitter, shimmer, and HNR have a relatively long history of use in the analysis of typical versus disordered voice and are included in most current voice analysis software packages. The ready availability of these measures means that they will continue to be used for both clinical and research purposes and have a level of familiarity among voice clinicians and researchers that may be seen as beneficial.

- Some of these traditional perturbation measures have been included in multivariate (i.e., multiple variables) methods of describing vocal function. The *Acoustic Voice Quality Index* (AVQI)[245] incorporates HNR and shimmer into a measure of estimated dysphonia severity, and the Dysphonia Severity Index (DSI),[67] a general measure of overall vocal function, includes jitter (both the AVQI and the DSI will be discussed in more detail in a later section of this chapter). A thorough understanding of these multivariate measures also requires an understanding of the computation of traditional perturbation measures.

- Traditional perturbation measures may be useful in interpreting *why* changes in more general measures of dysphonia (such as measures obtained from the **cepstrum**—see the following section) are observed (at least for sustained vowel contexts).

While there is certainly reason to have an understanding of traditional perturbation measures from both a historical and a practical standpoints, other methods have been developed in recent years that potentially have a wider range of applicability and address many of the shortcomings of typically used perturbation measures such as jitter, shimmer, and HNR. In particular, the following section will discuss a method of analysis of voice quality for vowels and continuous speech samples that relies upon a technique referred to as *cepstral analysis*.

4.4.13 Cepstral Analysis of Voice

A cepstrum is produced via a Fourier transform of the logarithm power spectrum of an acoustic sound wave. We will remember that the sound wave is a *time × amplitude* waveform. When a Fourier analysis is applied to the sound wave, it produces a *spectrum* which is a *frequency × amplitude* graph. To produce the cepstrum, we will (in a simplified description) repeat the

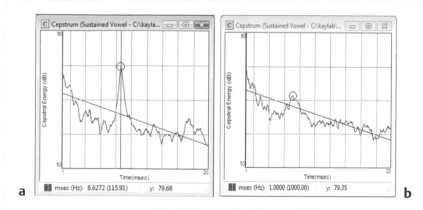

Fig. 4.42 Cepstrum for a typical, nondysphonic voice **(a)** showing a prominent cepstral peak in the region of the fundamental frequency. In contrast, the cepstrum from a moderate breathy voice **(b)** shows a reduced amplitude cepstral peak. The amplitude of the cepstral peak in relation to a linear regression line computed through the cepstrum is referred to as the *cepstral peak prominence (CPP)*. Analyzed using Analysis of Dysphonia in Speech and Voice (ADSV): Default Settings.

Fourier analysis procedure *on the initial Fourier analysis.* **This converts the spectrum back into the *time domain*.** Therefore, when viewing a cepstrum, the *horizontal axis* is a unit of time referred to as **quefrency** (a transposal of the letters in *frequency*) and the *vertical axis* is a unit of **amplitude**. As seen in ▶ Fig. 4.42, the cepstrum of a highly periodic sound wave that has a readily defined fundamental frequency and harmonic structure will show a prominent and relatively high amplitude cepstral peak (▶ Fig. 4.42**a**). The cepstral peak within a predetermined range of quefrencies (i.e., a range of periods) is referred to as the **dominant rahmonic** (an anagram of the word *harmonic*) and generally represents the fundamental period of the voice signal. Of course, the reciprocal of the fundamental period will be the fundamental frequency (F_0), and one of the original applications of cepstral analysis was as a procedure for extracting the fundamental frequency from the spectrum of a sound wave.[253,256]

While the initial interest in the cepstral peak was as a method of computing and tracking the F_0 of the voice, in more recent years, a measure of the amplitude of the cepstral peak in relation to other cepstral coefficients/values has been reported to provide an effective method of quantifying the degree of dysphonia in voices with quality-based disruptions (i.e., breathiness, hoarseness, etc.). As stated, a highly periodic voice signal with strong harmonic/rahmonic energy will be observed to have a relatively high amplitude and dominant cepstral peak, whereas the cepstral peak will be less dominant and decreased in amplitude (due to reduced harmonic energy) in the disturbed periodicity signals often observed in dysphonic voice (▶ Fig. 4.42**b**). *It is this ability of the cepstral peak to provide us information about voice signal characteristics associated with vocal quality (e.g., periodicity of the voice signal; relative amplitude of harmonic energy vs. inharmonic/noise energy) that is of prime value in the evaluation of the dysphonic voice.* In addition, cepstral analysis provides us with a voice evaluation method that addresses key limitations of traditional perturbation analyses of voice (jitter, shimmer, HNR) by providing the following capabilities:

1. Spectral-based acoustic measures such as the cepstrum have shown the ability to characterize the voice signal by extracting characteristics such as the vocal F_0 and the relative amplitude of harmonics versus noise without the necessity of identifying cycle boundaries. Rather than identifying "cycles" of vibration in the voice signal, spectral-based methods obtain acoustic information from "frames" of data (i.e., portions of the sound wave, often described in terms of digital samples or points). Therefore, measures from cepstral analysis have been observed to provide effective indices of dysphonia even in more severe levels of dysphonia in which the voice signal is highly perturbed and distinct cycles of vibration are absent.

2. Measures obtained from the cepstrum have been reported to provide a valid and reliable measure of voice quality, not only in sustained vowel contexts but also in continuous speech samples.

A specific measure of the relative amplitude of the cepstral peak is the **cepstral peak prominence *(CPP)***. While there are several ways by which the relative amplitude may be computed, a frequently used method is to compare the amplitude of the cepstral peak to the expected amplitude of the peak as computed via linear regression analysis (▶ Fig. 4.42). It is this comparison (generally via the difference between the actual cepstral peak amplitude and expected peak amplitude) that was referred to as the CPP in studies by Hillenbrand et al.[257,258] The predictive accuracy of identifying the cepstral peak via automatic signal processing methods is improved by smoothing cepstra across cepstral frames and across quefrency, and most recent reports of computer algorithms used to calculate CPP for voice signals incorporate these smoothing procedures.

A substantial body of evidence exits which supports the use of the CPP in documenting degree of dysphonia in both sustained vowel[233,236,257,259,260,261,262,263] and continuous speech contexts.[99,244,258,264,265,266,267,268,269,270,271,272,273,274] The CPP has also been reported to have strong sensitivity and specificity for the categorization of normal versus dysphonic voice, and also to be a useful measure in documenting change in voice quality secondary to treatment,[233,264,275,276,277,278] and, on the basis of a meta-analysis of acoustic measures of overall voice quality, Maryn et al concluded that a smoothed measure of the CPP was "the most promising and perhaps robust measure of dysphonia severity" (p. 2633).[279]

The CPP has been described as a general measure of dysphonia.[236] Although the measure has been most successful as a measure of dysphonia severity and as a classifier of normal versus disordered voice in cases that have been breathy or hoarse,[236,267,280] the amplitude of the CPP may be effected by various vocal quality deviations. Because voice quality deviations may arise from many different underlying causes, cepstral analysis and measures of the CPP have been used effectively in the description of a variety of diverse disorders including those with hypofunctional voice such as UVFP and presbylaryngis,[265, 270] thyroidectomy,[261,262,264] ADSD,[281] vocal nodules,[260] and ataxia.[280,282] In addition, the CPP has been used as an effective treatment outcomes measure.[262,264,276,283,284]

▶ Table 4.12 provides several examples of published CPP data for typical voice individuals. In addition, ▶ Table 4.13 provides general expectations for changes in the CPP for a number of commonly observed disorder types.

Methodological Considerations in Cepstral Measurement

The ability to compute CPP measurements has become readily available in recent years via software packages that allow for easily computed cepstral calculations from recorded voice signals. Two popular software packages for obtaining CPP measurements are **ADSV** (Analysis of Dysphonia in Speech and Voice; PENTAX Medical, Montvale, NJ) and **Praat** (Paul Boersma and David Weenink, Institute of Phonetic Sciences, University of Amsterdam, the Netherlands; www.praat.org). Both programs provide a smoothed version of the CPP (referred to as CPPs in Praat and simply as the CPP in ADSV) and both programs have been included in a substantial body of clinical voice research. However, there are a number of known differences between the algorithms used in these respective programs that result in differences in reported CPP values[291]:

1. The CPP algorithms used in the ADSV incorporate a simple form of voicing activity detection (VAD) as a means of reducing the potential effect of low amplitude, highly aperiodic signals often associated with breath sounds and/or portions of unvoiced consonants. In contrast, the CPPs algorithm in Praat does not incorporate any form of VAD.

2. Computational differences occur between the programs in which the ADSV program obtains the cepstrum via a forward Fourier transform of the log power spectrum versus taking the inverse Fourier transform of the log power spectrum to obtain the cepstrum in Praat.

3. The programs differ in how they compute the line of best fit by which the relative amplitude of the cepstral peak (i.e., the CPP) is calculated. ADSV uses simple least squares linear regression versus a nonparametric form of linear regression in Praat (the Theil robust fitting method) that is less affected by outlying data points.

4. The regression line is calculated using a lower quefrency value of .0001 s (equivalent to 10 kHz) in ADSV versus 0.001 s (equivalent to 1 kHz) in Praat, tending to result in a greater negative slope to the regression line in ADSV versus Praat.

5. Various minor differences occur between program algorithms such as choice of windowing function (i.e., a Gaussian window in the Praat algorithm vs. a Hamming window in ADSV) and interpolation of the peak value in Praat versus no interpolation in ADSV.

Because of these aforementioned differences, CPP data values obtained via different programs (such as ADSV vs. Praat) may be quite different and, therefore, are not directly comparable. However, in a study examining CPP values from ADSV versus Praat in various elicited (sentence and vowels) and linguistic contexts, Watts et al reported that cepstral measures obtained

with either system are strongly related (e.g., all correlation coefficients were at or greater than r = 0.88) and that CPP values can be converted between programs with relatively small average residual error.[291] Therefore, there appears to be strong parallel-forms reliability between ADSV and Praat for the measurement of CPP in both vowels and connected speech.

In addition to possible differences in computed CPP values between different programs, different CPP values should be expected for different elicited contexts. CPP calculated from continuous speech contexts will tend to be lower in value than those obtained from sustained vowel samples produced at steady pitch and loudness because continuous speech contains both completely voiced (vowel) as well as noise components within consonant sound productions (e.g., stop-plosives, fricatives) and natural and expected variations in pitch and loudness (i.e., prosody). In addition, different sentences and different vowels may also result in different expectations for CPP values.[99,285,289,291] Therefore, *it is essential that both inter- and intra-subject comparisons of measures of the CPP be made using the same elicited sample.*

Examples of Cepstral Measurements in Vowel and Continuous Speech Contexts

The first examples we will discuss are sustained vowel productions analyzed in the *ADSV* program (see Appendix 4.1 for complete instructions for computing cepstral analyses in *ADSV*). ▶ Fig. 4.43 shows acoustic waveforms for sustained vowel productions from a single speaker producing (from L to R) typical/normal voice (**a**), mild breathiness (**b**), moderate breathiness (**c**), and extreme breathiness (aphonia) (**d**). Auditory-perceptual evaluation of the vowel productions (**Sample 4.21**) should confirm that the severity of dysphonia and breathiness increases from example **a** through **d**. Below each vowel production is a representative cepstral frame, and in typical voice production (**a**), the cepstral peak (circled) is prominent and has a relatively high amplitude in comparison to the value of the cepstral regression line immediately below the peak (the relative amplitude of the cepstral peak is referred to as the *CPP*). The value of the mean CPP in the typical voice example (**a**) is 11.86 dB, and decreases with increased voice disturbance (mild (**b**) = 5.90 dB; moderate (**c**) = 3.55 dB, and severe (**d**) = 0.58 dB). *Contrary to perturbation measures such as jitter, shimmer, and HNR, this cepstral-based correlate of vocal quality disturbance is not based on the identification of cycles of vibration in the acoustic waveform. Therefore, we are able to obtain an objective correlate of the presence of quality-based dysphonia and severity even in voice productions that have a tendency toward aphonia and complete aperiodicity.*

In ▶ Fig. 4.44, representative cepstra computed in *Praat* are provided for the same typical/normal voice (**a**), mild breathy (**b**), moderate breathy (**c**), and extreme breathy (aphonic) (**d**) signals in ▶ Fig. 4.43 and **Sample 4.21** (see Appendix 4.1 for complete instructions for computing cepstral analyses in *Praat*). In cepstra **a**, **b**, and **c**, arrows indicate the cepstral peak which reduces in amplitude in relation to the cepstral linear regression line with increasing severity of dysphonia. In cepstrum **d**, the signal was aphonic and aperiodic, and a distinctive cepstral peak is not observed. The mean smoothed CPP (CPP) values computed using Praat are provided for each cepstra. As previously mentioned,

Table 4.12 Examples of CPP, CPP SD, and CSID from various literature sources

Author	Gender	No. of subjects	Age	Sample	CPP	CPP SD	CSID	Software
Awan[275]	M	50	21–45	/a/	13.03 (1.68)	0.63 (0.24)	3.58 (10.37)	ADSV
				Easy onset	6.20 (1.17)	3.75 (0.62)	0.48 (11.33)	
				All voiced	8.04 (1.33)	3.07 (0.60)	−4.48 (7.94)	
				Glottal	5.46 (1.19)	3.24 (0.48)	1.95 (9.87)	
				Plosives	4.75 (1.15)	3.25 (0.51)	10.24 (10.90)	
				Rainbow	6.70 (0.82)	3.82 (0.39)	9.78 (9.75)	
	F	50	21–45	/a/	10.74 (1.61)	0.45 (0.22)	4.43 (8.97)	
				Easy onset	5.45 (0.74)	3.37 (0.45)	11.80 (9.28)	
				All voiced	7.66 (0.95)	3.03 (0.38)	6.44 (7.94)	
				Glottal	4.94 (0.84)	3.27 (0.34)	10.27 (9.30)	
				Plosives	4.66 (0.61)	3.26 (0.35)	21.32 (7.89)	
				Rainbow	6.70 (0.82)	3.82 (0.39)	9.78 (9.75)	
Watts and Awan[270]	M & F	16 (5 M; 11 F)	M = 53	Rainbow	5.42 (1.38)	3.13 (0.52)	N/A	Program developed by Awan (Pre-ADSV)
				/a/	11.08 (1.91)	0.78 (0.54)	N/A	
Awan et al[285]	M & F	92 (42 M; 50 F)	18–30 (M = 21.28)	/a/	7.56 (1.05)	N/A	N/A	ADSV
				/i/	6.53 (0.96)	N/A	N/A	
				/u/	6.78 (1.04)	N/A	N/A	
				/ae/	7.57 (1.12)	N/A	N/A	
Lowell et al[268]	M & F	23 (8 M; 15 F)	26–80 (M = 42.3)	Rainbow	5.96 (0.95)	3.96 (0.45)	15.12 (14.07	ADSV
				/u/	8.70 (2.01)	0.53 (0.21)	11.32 (9.11)	
Barsties et al[286]	F$_{UW}$	9	M = 18.89	/a/	8.00 (1.76)	N/A	N/A	SpeechTool[6]
	F$_{NW}$	13	M = 21.38		8.22 (1.05)	N/A	N/A	
	F$_{OB}$	7	M = 24.57		8.46 (0.69)	N/A	N/A	
Diercks et al[287]	M & F	40	4–17 (M = 9)	/a/	9.82 (2.24)	0.96 (0.69)	21.84 (14.51)	ADSV
		40		Easy onset	5.80 (1.35)	3.16 (0.56)	8.08 (14.68)	
		39		All voiced	7.41 (1.41)	2.60 (0.42)	4.66 (11.70)	
		38		Glottal	4.92 (1.24)	2.88 (0.46)	6.98 (16.82)	
		39		Plosives	4.83 (1.26)	3.08 (0.54)	10.94 (17.07)	
		18		Rainbow	6.03 (1.37)	3.52 (0.42)	N/A	
Heman-Ackah et al[278]	M & F	50	N/A	Marvin Williams passage	4.77 (0.97)	N/A	N/A	Hillenbrand et al[257]; Hillenbrand and Houde[258]
Rosenthal et al[269]	M & F	18 (6 M; 12 F)	18–26 (M = 20.3)	Syllable /pi/ repetitions	6.66 (2.53)	2.55 (0.98)	N/A	ADSV
Carson et al[282]	M & F	20 (10 M; 10 F)	18–25 (M = 20.7)	/a/	11.64 (8.04)	0.98 (0.68)	20.83 (9.85)	ADSV

Table 4.12 continued

Author	Gender	No. of subjects	Age	Sample	CPP	CPP SD	CSID	Software
				/i/	8.04 (1.98)	0.79 (0.26)	38.72 (9.08)	
				/o/	10.33 (1.65)	0.61 (0.36)	20.83 (12.91)	
Vogel et al[124]	M & F	30	M = 36.45	/a/	12.38 (1.85)	0.61 (0.28)	2.71 (10.34)	ADSV
				Grandfather passage	4.69 (0.75)	3.48 (0.42)	11.60 (1.5)	
Watts et al[288]	M	30	20–49 (M = 33.6)	/a/	N/A	N/A	19.32 (13.19)	ADSV
				"We were away a year ago."			-15.62 (10.99)	
		30	50–79 (M = 63.9)	/a/			23.21 (13.08)[290]	
				"We were away a year ago."			-5.24 (10.22)	

Table 4.13 A summary of general expectations for changes in the cepstral peak prominence (CPP) in various disorder types

Disorder	Expectations	Comments
Mass lesions/distributed tissue changes	Decreased CPP	CPP is responsive to breathiness or hoarseness observed in cases of mass lesion(s) or irregularities to the vocal fold edge(s) resulting in additive noise from air escape during phonation. CPP may be less sensitive to rough voice quality secondary to lesions and distributed tissue change that result in irregular vocal fold vibration (roughness), particularly if asymmetric
Neurological disorders		CPP is responsive to breathiness or hoarseness observed in cases of motor dysfunction leading to hypoadduction (e.g., vocal fold paralysis/paresis; iatrogenic effects on laryngeal function). CPP may also be responsible to instability in voice. CPP may not be as responsive to harsh voice quality in hypertonia; not as responsive to rough voice quality
Muscle tension dysphonias (MTDs)/ hyperfunctional voice	Variable	CPP may be responsive to perturbed voice quality. However, CPP may be less responsive to effortful, strained voice in the absence of breathy/rough/hoarse quality (relatively periodic voice signal)
Presbylaryngis		CPP may be responsive to cases in which vocal fold bowing (hypoadduction) is observed. CPP may not detect voice dysfunction that has been described as primarily pitch/frequency and/or loudness/intensity focused
Puberphonia/Mutational falsetto		CPP may not detect voice dysfunction that has been described as primarily pitch/frequency related. May be responsive to possible coexisting voice quality disturbance (e.g., hoarseness)

smoothed CPP values in *ADSV* versus *Praat* are quite different in magnitude (primarily due to differences in how the cepstral linear regression line is calculated), but are based on similar underlying mathematical procedures and correlate very strongly ($r > 0.90$ for sustained vowel productions).[291]

While the mean/average CPP has been reported to be an effective descriptor of disordered voice production, the mean does not provide any information regarding the consistency or steadiness of the CPP over time. However, since cepstral and CPP data are calculated from frames of data over time, it is possible to also calculate a measure of the average variability (i.e., the standard deviation [SD]). Previous studies by Awan and colleagues have shown that the CPP SD can also be an effective discriminator of normal versus disordered voice.[99,264,292] In sustained vowel production, the quality, pitch, and loudness of the voice are expected to be produced with steadiness

and consistency in typical, nondysphonic subjects—the result is that, in vowel production, the CPP SD is expected to be small/low (i.e., very little variability). In contrast, dysphonic voices tend to have reduced steadiness/consistency during sustained voicing, and therefore tend to have increased CPP SDs (i.e., increased variability). ▶ Fig. 4.45 provides examples of CPP data over time for typical versus dysphonic sustained vowel samples.

Let us now look at several examples of cepstral analysis and measures of the CPP in continuous speech samples. These examples will not only show how cepstral measures such as the CPP are able to track voicing characteristics in speech contexts, but will also again demonstrate how these measures are able to provide acoustic correlates of dysphonia even in the most severely dysphonic cases. Let us begin with an example of a typical, nondysphonic female producing the sentence "**We were**

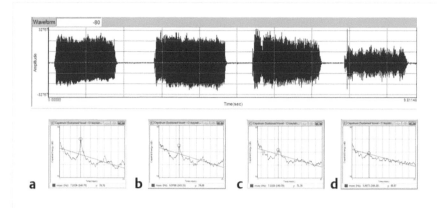

Fig. 4.43 Acoustic waveforms for sustained vowel productions from a single speaker producing (from L to R) typical/normal voice **(a)**, mild breathiness **(b)**, moderate breathiness **(c)**, and extreme breathiness (aphonia) **(d)**. Below each vowel production is a representative cepstral frame. In typical voice production **(a)**, the cepstral peak (circled) is prominent and relatively high amplitude in comparison to the value of the cepstral regression line immediately below the peak. The relative amplitude of the cepstral peak (i.e., the cepstral peak prominence) decreases with increased voice disturbance **(b–d)** and has an amplitude of that approaches 0 dB in the aphonic voice production. Analyzed using Analysis of Dysphonia in Speech and Voice (ADSV): Default Settings (see Appendix 4.1 for analysis instructions).

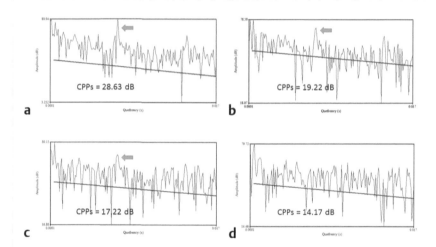

Fig. 4.44 Representative cepstra for typical/normal voice **(a)**, mild breathy **(b)**, moderate breathy **(c)**, and extreme breathy (aphonia) **(d)** sustained vowels (▶ Fig. 4.43) computed in Praat. In **a, b,** and **c**, arrows indicate the cepstral peak which reduces in amplitude in relation to the cepstral linear regression line with increasing severity of dysphonia. In **(d)**, the signal was aphonic, aperiodic, and a distinctive cepstral peak is not observed. Mean cepstral peak prominences (smoothed CPP) values for each cepstra are provided. Analyzed using Praat: see Appendix 4.1 for analysis instructions.

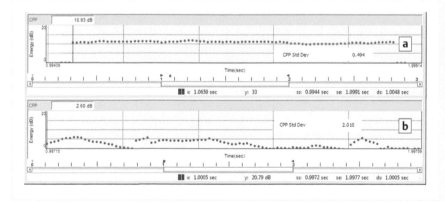

Fig. 4.45 Cepstral peak prominence (CPP) over time showing stability and low variability (CPP SD = 0.494 dB) for a nondysphonic sustained vowel **(a)** versus increased variability (CPP SD = 2.03 dB) in a strained, hoarse vowel sample. Analyzed using Analysis of Dysphonia in Speech and Voice (ADSV): Default Settings (see Appendix 4.1 for analysis instructions).

away a year ago" analyzed in the *ADSV* program (▶ Fig. 4.46 and **Sample 4.22**). While individual cepstra may be visualized (lower right window **f**), window **d** shows the CPP over the duration of the sample. In contrast to sustained vowel production, during continuous speech production, the normal vocal mechanism shows the capability to produce a great deal of variation such as transitions between voiced/voiceless consonants and variations in pitch and loudness observed in normal prosody. The result is that, in continuous speech production, the CPP SD is expected to be increased (i.e., increased variability) in nondysphonic subjects. In contrast, dysphonic voices tend to have reduced variability during continuous speech, and therefore tend to have decreased CPP SDs (i.e., decreased variability). In this sample, the mean CPP = 9.73 dB and the CPP SD = 3.89 dB.

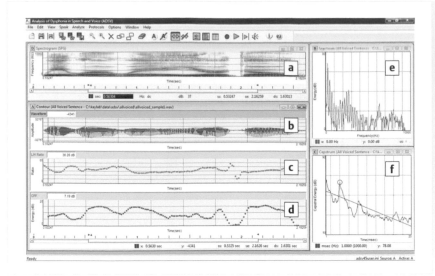

Fig. 4.46 ADSV main screen—spectral/cepstral analyses of a typical, nondysphonic female speech sample ("We were away a year ago"). Analysis windows include **(a)** sound spectrogram; **(b)** sound wave; **(c)** low/high spectral ratio (L/H ratio) over time; **(d)** cepstral peak prominence (CPP) over time; **(e)** focused spectral analysis per data frame; **(f)** focused cepstral analysis per data frame. The mean CPP = 9.73 dB and the CPP shows expected increased variability in speech contexts (CPP SD = 3.89 dB) consistent with natural intonation and vowel-to-consonant and consonant-to-vowel transitions. The Cepstral Spectral Index of Dysphonia (CSID) for this sample is −13.83. Analyzed using Analysis of Dysphonia in Speech and Voice (ADSV): Default Settings (see Appendix 4.1 for analysis instructions).

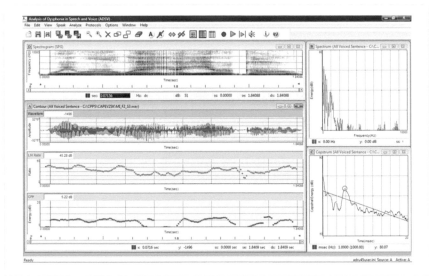

Fig. 4.47 Mild adult female continuous speech sample of "We were away a year ago." This voice sample was perceived as mildly breathy with an intermittent period of roughness in the central part of the sample resulting in an intermittent and substantial drop in the CPP. For example, the mean 4.86 dB and the CPP SD = 1.64 dB (reduced mean CPP and CPP average variation). The Cepstral Spectral Index of Dysphonia (CSID) for this sample is 36.82. Analyzed using Analysis of Dysphonia in Speech and Voice (ADSV): Default Settings (see Appendix 4.1 for analysis instructions).

In ▶ Fig. 4.47, we have an example of a mildly breathy adult female voice sample with an intermittent period of roughness in the central part of the sample (**Sample 4.23**). The brief period of roughness results in a substantial drop in the CPP (window **d**). In this sample, the mean CPP = 4.86 dB and the CPP SD = 1.64 dB (reduced mean CPP and CPP average variation as compared to the typical, nondysphonic sample). ▶ Fig. 4.48 and **Sample 4.24** provide an example of a patient with a moderate and consistent breathy voice. The mean CPP and CPP SD are further reduced (mean CPP = 4.40 dB; CPP SD = 1.30 dB) due to reduced energy in the region of the vocal F_0 and reduced ability to vary voicing parameters with increased dysphonia.

▶ Fig. 4.49 provides an example of a severely dysphonic male speaker. The speech sample is characterized primarily by aphonia and intermittent high pitched, strain (**Sample 4.25**). The CPP approaches 0 dB except for the slight increase in CPP values during a high pitched, strained voice production near the end of the utterance (mean CPP = 0.70 dB; CPP SD = 0.53 dB).

4.4.14 Multivariate Forms of Voice Analysis

It has been recognized that voice (both normal and disordered) varies in a multidimensional manner (i.e., varies in characteristics such as pitch/frequency, loudness/intensity, quality, and/or duration). Because of this, a single (i.e., univariate—single/one variable) measurement procedure may not be able to adequately capture the various distinctive traits of the patient's voice. In response, a variety of multivariate (i.e., multiple variable) approaches that combine the results of several test variables have been developed. Multivariate approaches have the benefit of (**1**) using more information in determining normal/abnormal characteristics than univariate approaches and (**2**) of producing an optimal combination of variables regardless of their individual strength. The hope and expectation is that multivariate approaches may provide a much better reflection of the multidimensional character of the

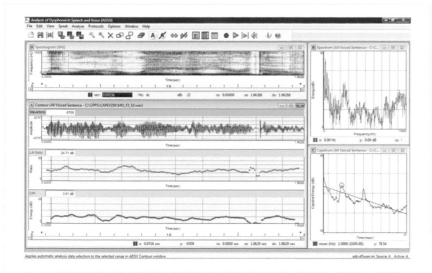

Fig. 4.48 Moderate and continuously breathy adult female continuous speech sample of "We were away a year ago." The mean CPP = 4.39 dB and the CPP SD = 1.30 dB. The Cepstral Spectral Index of Dysphonia (CSID) for this sample is 58.93. Analyzed using Analysis of Dysphonia in Speech and Voice (ADSV): Default Settings (see Appendix 4.1 for analysis instructions).

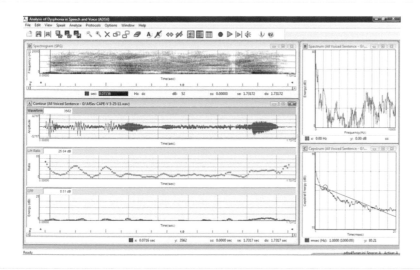

Fig. 4.49 Severe adult male continuous speech sample of "We were away a year ago" characterized by aphonia and occasional high pitch strain. The CPP approaches 0 dB except for the slight increase in CPP values during a high pitched, strained voice production near the end of the utterance. The mean CPP = 0.70 dB and the CPP SD = 0.53 dB. The Cepstral Spectral Index of Dysphonia (CSID) for this sample is 95.08. Analyzed using Analysis of Dysphonia in Speech and Voice (ADSV): Default Settings (see Appendix 4.1 for analysis instructions).

voice signal than individual, isolated voice assessment procedures. We will discuss two multivariate methods of acoustic analysis incorporating some of the aforementioned methods that have been used as correlates of vocal quality (the **CSID** and the **AVQI**). We will also discuss a procedure referred to as the *voice range profile (VRP; a.k.a. phonetogram)* that combines information dealing with the frequency and intensity capabilities of the voice, and finally a multivariate method called the *DSI* that combines measures relating to frequency, sound level/intensity, quality (jitter), and duration of voice production.

The Cepstral Spectral Index of Dysphonia

As stated, the CPP has been observed to be a strong acoustic predictor of dysphonia severity in multiple previous studies of both sustained vowel and continuous speech samples. However, the addition of other measures obtained via the same spectral/cepstral analysis procedures can significantly strengthen these predictions.[99,244] Since these measures can be obtained efficiently via a common core of spectral/cepstral analysis procedures, a multivariate estimate of dysphonia severity which includes

measures in addition to the CPP can be easily computed. Additional spectral and cepstral measures observed to be useful in the characterization of dysphonic voice include the following:

Cepstral Peak Prominence Standard Deviation

As previously mentioned, this is a measure of the *SD* (i.e., *the average variability*) of the *CPP* over time. Previous studies by Awan and colleagues have shown that the *CPP SD* can also be an effective discriminator of normal versus disordered voice.[99,264,292]

General expectations for the CPP SD differ depending on the context in which the CPP SD is elicited. In typical nondysphonic sustained vowel production, we expect the CPP SD to be low (i.e., indicating steadiness with minimal variability—see ▶ Table 4.12) and increased CPP SD in vocal quality-based dysphonia. In contrast, typical nondysphonic continuous speech production generally has an increased CPP SD (consistent with the variations in spectral energy due to consonant/vowel and vowel/consonant transitions and prosodic effects of voice characteristics expected in normal speech production) versus decreased CPP SD in the continuous speech samples of patients with vocal quality-based dysphonia.

Low/High Spectral Ratio

In normal voice signals (particularly during vowel productions), much of the energy found in the voice spectrum is concentrated in the vicinity of the vocal F_0 (i.e., the first harmonic of the periodic spectrum, typically heard as the "pitch" of the voice) and in the first one or two vocal tract resonances/formants. If the spectrum of the voice (computed via the Fourier transform—the precursor the cepstrum) is arbitrarily divided into "low-" versus "high"-frequency regions, a simple **ratio of low/high spectral energy** may be computed (referred to as the *low/high spectral ratio [L/H ratio]*—in the ADSV program the point at which the spectrum is separated into "low-" versus "high"-frequency regions has a default setting of 4 kHz). This ratio is a measure of "**spectral tilt**," and these types of measures have been reported to be particularly important in predicting the severity of breathy voice in which spectral noise is especially noticeable above 2 to 3 kHz.[233,244,258,259,263,293]

Typical, nondysphonic voice signals tend to have a high L/H ratio (i.e., the "low"-frequency energy is substantially greater than the "high"-frequency energy). In contrast, the L/H ratio tends to be reduced (i.e., the "high"-frequency energy begins to compete with the "low"-frequency energy) in dysphonic voices (particularly those that have a breathy component).

L/H Ratio Standard Deviation

The L/H ratio SD provides an indication of the consistency/steadiness of the L/H ratio over time. Expectations for the L/H ratio SD are similar to those mentioned for the CPP SD. Nondysphonic sustained vowel productions are expected to have a low L/H ratio SD value in vowel productions (indicating steadiness and low variability) and an increased value in normal continuous speech with the opposite results expected in dysphonic speakers.

These aforementioned measures provide important information regarding the dysphonic voce signal in their own right, and studies by Awan et al[99,244] showed that the aforementioned individual cepstral (CPP and CPP SD) and spectral (L/H ratio and L/H ratio SD) measures could be combined using mathematical formulae to provide strong multivariate estimates of perceived dysphonia severity (i.e., a rating of dysphonia severity as produced by the listener). When incorporated into the ADSV program, these formulae have been collectively referred to as the *Cepstral Spectral Index of Dysphonia (CSID). The numerical value provided by the CSID is in reference to the 0- to 100-mm scale of the CAPE-V auditory-perceptual rating scale, with nondysphonic voices expected to have very low ratings/scores toward the left end of the scale (i.e., toward "0") and extremely dysphonic voices to have very high ratings/scores toward the right end of the scale (i.e., toward "100").*

Different *CSID* formulas are used for different contexts:

CAPE-V Sentences

For any of the following CAPE-V sentences: (1) easy onset of phonation ("How hard did he hit him?"), (2) all voiced sounds ("We were away a year ago"), (3) hard glottal attack ("We eat eggs every Easter"), and (4) weighted with voiceless plosives ("Peter will keep at the peak"), the predicted CAPE-V severity of sentences ($CSID_{CAPE-V\ Sentences}$) is calculated by the following:

$$CSID_{CAPE-V\ Sentences} = 148.68 - (5.91 \times CPP) - (11.17 \times \sigma_{CPP}) - (1.31 \times \text{L/H Ratio}) - (3.09 \times \sigma_{\text{L/H Ratio}})$$

where CPP is the cepstral peak prominence, σ_{CPP} is the SD of the CPP, L/H ratio is the low/high spectral ratio (using a 4-kHz cutoff), and $\sigma_{\text{L/H Ratio}}$ is the SD of the L/H ratio.[99]

Sustained Vowel

Due to the different expectations for some of the measured variables in vowel samples versus continuous speech samples (as previously described), a different formula is required to estimate dysphonia for vowel samples. The predicted CAPE-V severity of the sustained vowel /a/ is computed by the following:

$$CSID_{Vowel/a/} = 84.20 - (4.40 \times CPP) + (10.62 \times \sigma_{CPP}) - (1.05 \times \text{L/H Ratio}) + (7.61 x \sigma_{\text{L/H Ratio}}) - (10.86 \times G)$$

where G is the gender variable (male = 0; female = 1).[99]

The Rainbow Passage

The following formula was developed by Awan et al[244] for use with samples of the second and third sentences of the Rainbow Passage[16]:

$$CSID_{Rainbow} = 154.59 - (10.39 \times CPP) - (1.08 \times \text{L/H Ratio}) - (3.71 \times \sigma_{\text{L/H Ratio}})$$

▶ Table 4.12 provides several published examples of CSID expectations for typical nondysphonic speakers in various contexts.

4.4.15 Examples of the CSID

We will use the previous examples provided in ▶ Fig. 4.46, ▶ Fig. 4.47, ▶ Fig. 4.48, and ▶ Fig. 4.49 to illustrate the use of the CSID. In ▶ Fig. 4.46, we observed a typical, nondysphonic production of "We were away a year ago." ADSV analyses provided the following results for the measures included in the CSID:

CPP = 9.731; CPP SD = 3.892; L/H ratio = 32.944; L/H ratio SD = 5.945.

When these values are inserted into the $CSID_{CAPE-V\ Sentences}$ formula, we get the following:

$$\begin{aligned} CSID_{CAPE-V\ Sentences} &= 148.68 - (5.91 \times 9.731) - (11.17 \times 3.892) \\ &\quad - (1.31 \times 32.944) - (3.09 \times 5.945) \\ &= 148.68 - 57.51 - 43.47 - 43.16 - 18.37 \\ &= -13.83 (\text{i.e., a very low CSID score}) \end{aligned}$$

When interpreting the CSID, simply remember that (1) like the CAPE-V scale, good-quality nondysphonic voices will be expected to have very low CSID scores and (2) when interpreting the CSID, highly periodic voice signals with strong cepstral peaks and a great deal of spectral energy near the vocal F_0 and lower harmonics may even have negative CSID scores (the lower the better).

Since the CSID has been reported to be a strong direct correlate of the auditory-perceptual rating of dysphonia severity, we will expect the CSID score to increase with increasing severity. ▶ Fig. 4.47 (a mild breathy voice with intermittent roughness) received a CSID score of 36.82, the moderate and continuous breathy voice in ▶ Fig. 4.48 received a CSID score of 58.93, and the primarily aphonic voice in ▶ Fig. 4.49 received a CSID score of 95.08. The reader should listen to the associated speech samples for these various examples to see if their perceived ratings of the dysphonia severity are consistent with the reported CSID values. However, when interpreting the CSID score, the clinician must remember that these formulas provide an acoustic estimate of the overall severity rating on the CAPE-V rating form, and that these estimates should be used with the following caveats in mind:

- The CSID is an acoustic estimate of dysphonia severity that is determined from the entire sample being analyzed via a selected and focused set of acoustic measures (CPP, L/H ratio, and their respective SDs)—this is different from a dysphonia severity rating as provided by a human listener, whose rating/ judgment may be influenced by factors such as listener experience, by articulatory characteristics of the speaker, or by discrete sections of a sample rather than the whole.

- The mathematical formulas used in the CSID estimates have been reported to be very strong correlates of perceived dysphonia severity in patients with vocal quality disturbances. Patients whose disordered voice characteristics deviate from our expectations in some other manner (e.g., a pitch disturbance as may be observed in puberphonia/mutational falsetto) may certainly be perceived as abnormal/atypical but may have a relatively normal/typical CSID score because the voice disturbance is not quality based.

- While the mathematical formulas used in the CSID estimates have been reported to be very strong correlates of perceived dysphonia severity, they are not "perfect" correlates (i.e., correlations equal to 1.0)—as an example, in the study by Awan et al, the best correlation between the acoustic estimates of severity and the listener-perceived severity ratings in a sentence context was for "We were away a year ago" (R = 0.86)—therefore, there is a certain degree of "error variance" unaccounted for in these acoustic estimates of dysphonia severity that may result in differences between acoustic and perceived severity estimates.[99]

- Listener-perceived severity ratings have often been observed to have an "end effect," in which "normal" voices tend to be given very similar low ratings, and "severe" voices tend to be given very similar high ratings.[244] In contrast, the mathematical estimates of dysphonia severity such as the CSID tend to be more "normally" distributed with less of an "end effect."[244] Many "normal" voices that would be scored as 0 by a listener may receive a somewhat higher (though still within normal expectations) CSID score, and severe voices that may be scored as 100 by a listener may have a somewhat lower (though still very high) CSID score. In addition, a mathematical estimate of dysphonia severity such as the CSID is not restricted to the 0 to 100 points severity scale. As an example, normal voices that show strong periodic vocal fold vibration may be observed to have CSID scores less than 0.

Several studies have reported the CSID to be a strong correlate of dysphonia severity[99,244,277,294,295] as well as an effective measure in categorizing normal versus disordered voice.[124,268,288,292] *A study by Awan et al reported that a CSID$_{Rainbow}$ cutoff of ≈ 24 achieved the best balance between sensitivity (i.e., a test's ability to detect a condition or disease when present) and specificity (i.e., an estimate of a test's ability to correctly identify non-cases/non-voice-disordered subjects), whereas a more liberal cutoff score of ≈ 19 may be preferred for screening purposes since this score resulted in higher sensitivity while maintaining respectable specificity. A review of published normative examples for the CSID appears to confirm that CSID scores less than 20 are often observed in continuous speech contexts (▶ Table 4.12).*[277]

The Acoustic Voice Quality Index

An alternative model for the acoustic estimation of dysphonia severity is the *AVQI*.[245] Like the previously described *CSID*, the AVQI was developed to measure dysphonia in both continuous speech and sustained vowel contexts, and also has a primary contribution from a measure of the smoothed CPPs. The *AVQI* uses various measures obtained via the Praat program to provide a numerical index that relates to the perceived overall severity of the dysphonic voice produced via a multivariate regression formula[296]:

$$AVQI_{beta} = 9.072 - (0.2453 \times CPPs) - (0.1613 \times HNR) \\ - (0.4703 \times SL) + (6.1583 \times SLdB) \\ - (0.0713 \times Slope) - (0.1703 \times Tilt).$$

where *CPPs* is the smoothed cepstral peak prominence, *HNR* is the harmonics-to-noise ratio, *SL* is the shimmer local in percent, *SLdB* is the shimmer local in dB, *slope* is the slope of the long-term average spectrum (LTAS), and *tilt* is the tilt of the trend line through the LTAS. *AVQI$_{beta}$* refers to an updated version of the *AVQI* that uses acoustic measures obtained solely via the Praat program. The initial version of the *AVQI* required two separate computer programs to provide the necessary acoustic measures.[245] *The resulting AVQI value falls on a scale with values between 0 and 10, with higher AVQI scores directly related to higher overall dysphonia severity. As examples, Maryn et al reported an AVQI of 2.95 to result in a good balance between sensitivity and specificity, with a positive AVQI score (i.e., > 2.95) very likely to be associated with the presence of dysphonia and a low AVQI score (i.e., < 2.95) very likely to be associated with typical, nondysphonic voice production.[245] Reynolds et al also reported a relatively similar AVQI of 3.46 as a threshold for voice pathology that showed strong sensitivity, specificity, and accuracy.[297]* ▶ Fig. 4.50 and ▶ Fig. 4.51 provide examples of the output of the *AVQI* script run via *Praat* for normal versus disordered voice samples, respectively. A number of studies have indicated that the *AVQI* has strong capability to distinguish voice-disordered from vocally normal participants.[297,298,299,300] Maryn et al also investigated the validity and clinical utility of the *AVQI* as a potential treatment outcome measure.[245]

The *AVQI* and the aforementioned *CSID* certainly have commonalities in that (**1**) they both provide automated, multivariate acoustic estimates of dysphonia severity; (**2**) they are both applicable to sustained vowel and contextual speech analyses; and (**3**) both formulas are heavily weighted toward the value of the CPP. Because the analysis programs used to produce *CSID* and *AVQI* (ADSV and Praat, respectively) produce measures of CPP that are very strongly correlated, it may be expected that the *CSID* and the *AVQI* would also be reasonably correlated.[291] However, the two dysphonia estimates also differ in a number of important ways:

- While both the CSID and the AVQI will analyze both sustained vowel and continuous speech samples, the CSID has completely separate dysphonia severity estimation formula for the two separate contexts which recognize that the potential effects of dysphonia on measures of cepstral and spectral average variability (i.e., the CPP SD and the L/H ratio SD) will be affected in very different ways in sustained vowel versus speech contexts (e.g., in many forms of dysphonia, the CPP SD will be expected to increase in sustained vowel productions, but decrease in continuous speech). In contrast, the AVQI

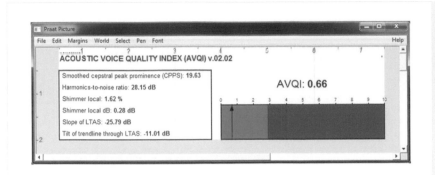

Fig. 4.50 Acoustic Voice Quality Index (AVQI) computed for a normal/typical voice individual. The cepstral peak (CPPs) and harmonics-to-noise ratio values are relatively high, whereas the shimmer values are relatively low. The weighted combination of these measures derived from concatenated vowel + speech samples results in a low AVQI value (0.66) consistent with normal/typical voice production.

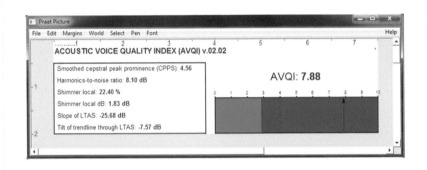

Fig. 4.51 Acoustic Voice Quality Index (AVQI) computed for a severely dysphonic individual. The cepstral peak (CPPs) and harmonics-to-noise ratio values are substantially reduced as compared to the normal/typical example and shimmer values are substantially increased. The weighted combination of these measures derived from concatenated vowel + speech samples results in a high AVQI value (7.88) consistent with a more severe form of dysphonic voice production.

concatenates (i.e., joins) the patient's continuous speech sample to a portion of their sustained vowel production and then analyzes the concatenated sample as a whole to produce a single estimate of dysphonia severity.

- The CSID relies solely on cepstral and spectral measures that do not depend on the identification of prominent cycles of vibration for their measurements. In contrast, like in early studies by Awan and Roy, the AVQI combines cepstral and spectral measures with measures of perturbation (HNR and shimmer).[233,236] As previously stated, the validity of perturbation measures becomes questionable with very severe forms of dysphonia in which the voice signal approaches aperiodicity.

- When analyzing continuous speech samples, CPP values less than 0 dB are removed from further analysis in the ADSV program as a simple form of VAD that was incorporated to reduce the potential effect of low amplitude, highly aperiodic signals often associated with breath sounds and/or portions of unvoiced consonants while still maintaining consonant-to-vowel and vowel-to-consonant transitions.[275] In contrast, the AVQI algorithm very deliberately extracts and concatenates only the voiced segments of the speech sample with a customized script in Praat and then joins them with the medial 3-second portion of the sustained vowel sample prior to further acoustic analyses.

It is expected that studies will be conducted to ascertain the degree of relationship between *CSID* and *AVQI* estimates of dysphonia severity and compare their ability to categorize normal versus dysphonia voice. However, to date, both methods appear to be useful summary measures of overall dysphonia severity that can be useful additions to the acoustic description of voice.

The Voice Range Profile (a.k.a. Phonetogram)

The *VRP (a.k.a. phonetogram)* is a graphical representation of the combined frequency and intensity capabilities of the patient's voice. The contours of the VRP can provide information regarding the ability to control vocal dynamics along the phonational frequency range and within different vocal registers, as well as the ability to coordinate the respiratory, laryngeal, and articulatory subsystems.

In the VRP (▶ Fig. 4.52), frequency (Hz) is displayed from left to right along the *x*-axis, with the lowest phonational frequency levels at the far left. Sound level/intensity (dB SPL) is measured from bottom to top along the *y*-axis, with the lowest intensity, quietest phonations displayed toward the bottom of the graph.

In ▶ Fig. 4.53, regions of different *vocal registers* and the *region of register transition* have been identified. In eliciting the phonations for the VRP, we are interested in modal and falsetto register voice production. In ▶ Fig. 4.53, the lower circled region encompasses the subject's modal register phonations—this region typically contains the greatest dynamic range of the voice (i.e., the difference between maximum and minimum intensity phonations). The higher circled region in ▶ Fig. 4.53 is the region of this subject's falsetto register—dynamic range is typically reduced in falsetto register, though the highest intensity vocalizations within the phonational F_0 range are often produced in falsetto. In many subjects (particularly those who do not have formal singing training), there is a distinctive narrowing of the VRP between the modal and falsetto regions that is representative of the *register transition*—this dynamic range of the voice is not only reduced in in this region but the voice can also be very difficult to control in terms of F_0 and quality. In addition to the

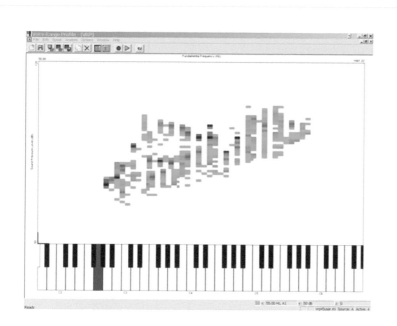

Fig. 4.52 Typical voice range profile (VRP, a.k.a. phonetogram) captured using a real-time VRP program. Analyzed using the Voice Range Profile (KayPentax/Pentax Medical Inc., Montvale, NJ).

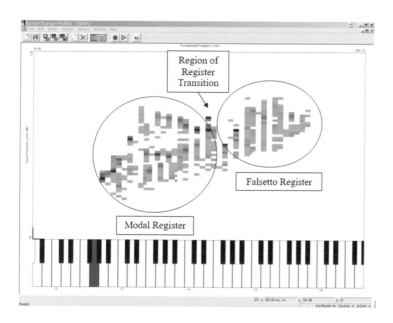

Fig. 4.53 Typical VRP/phonetogram, with regions of modal and falsetto register circled. In addition, the region of register transition has been identified. Analyzed using the Voice Range Profile (KayPentax/Pentax Medical Inc., Montvale, NJ).

aforementioned regions, vocal capability is typically limited in dynamic range when he/she is vocalizing near the extremes of the pitch/frequency range. Awan observed that the mean speaking F_0 was typically in the range of 12 to 16% of the phonational range in semitones, and the speaking F_0 range (i.e., maximum-to-minimum F_0s used in speech) was observed in the lower 25 to 30% region of the VRP.[36]

VRP/Phonetogram Studies

Damsté's description of the VRP/phonetogram was one of the earliest studies to discuss the graphic display of the fundamental frequency range, intensity range, and the area of interaction

between them.[307] The VRP/phonetogram has been used to describe various factors affecting vocal function including the effects of aging,[164,301,302,303] gender,[167,304] and vocal training.[36,61,62,105,151] In addition, the VRP/phonetogram has also been described as a potentially useful "stress test" by which the physiological limitations of the vocal mechanism may be revealed[305] and, once treated, also used as an outcome measure to document the effects of voice therapy.[2,100,306]

VRP/Phonetogram Elicitation Procedures

In creating a VRP/phonetogram, minimal instrumentation can be a simple SLM and a tone generator (pure tone oscillator, pitch

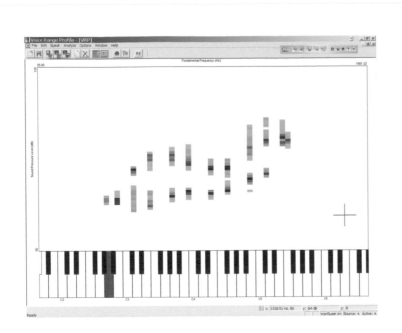

Fig. 4.54 VRP/Phonetogram elicited at approximately 10% intervals of the total phonational F_0 range. In this example, each target frequency has been elicited at maximal and minimal vocal intensities. Analyzed using the Voice Range Profile (KayPentax/Pentax Medical Inc., Montvale, NJ).

pipe, tuned musical instrument).[147] It is important that a constant mouth-to-microphone distance is maintained (e.g., 30 cm if using a SLM). The subject is asked to sustain a vowel (often the vowel /a/, though other vowels have been suggested) at given frequencies within the total phonational F_0 range. Because eliciting and recording a complete VRP/phonetogram at each pitch/F_0 level within the subject's range can be a time-consuming task, shortened versions of VRP elicitation have been used:

- Compute the 10% intervals of the total phonational F_0 range. Vocal intensity levels will be elicited at 11 frequency levels (0, 10, 20 ... 100%; ▶ Fig. 4.54).[61,62,68,305]
- Bless and Hicks suggest a shorter version of the VRP/phonetogram. Phonations are elicited at 10, 50, and 80% levels of the frequency range.[146] Awan suggested the addition of the 30% level (for minimum intensity productions) and 40% level (for maximum intensity productions) to this shortened phonetogram because (1) the 30 to 40% level is often the last frequency in modal register before register transition into falsetto and (2) this level often elicits the greatest dynamic range of the voice.[1]
- Elicit maximum and minimum sound levels at four musical notes (e.g., musical notes E, G, A, C) throughout the subject's entire vocal range.[147,305]

When eliciting voice productions to be used in the VRP, Coleman suggests starting at low-frequency/semitone levels and progressing upward; phonations should be at least 2 to 3 seconds in duration with no excessive breathiness or other quality deviation.[308] The aforementioned pitch/F_0 levels are elicited at the following minimal and maximal vocal sound levels/intensities, with the subject asked to produce minimal levels first. Descriptions of the target sound level/intensity levels are as follows:

- Minimum vocal sound level/intensity ("Pianissimo"): A vowel sustained as quietly as possible without whispering. According

to Gramming and Sundberg, the fundamental frequency (F_0) is the strongest harmonic in soft phonation.[151]
- Maximum Vocal Sound Level/Intensity ("Fortissimo"): A vowel sustained as loudly as possible without pitch breaks. According to Gramming and Sundberg, an overtone of the F_0 is often the strongest partial/harmonic in loud phonation.[151] Therefore, the maximum phonation curve of VRP/phonetogram may reflect an interaction of the voice source fundamental and the resonant characteristics of the supraglottal vocal tract.

In addition to the maximum and minimum intensity levels, target F_0s or musical notes may be elicited at a comfortable sound level/intensity.[61,146]

Evaluating the VRP/Phonetogram

Important information about the subject's use of the singing voice and overall vocal use and control can be observed by a review of the VRP/phonetogram:

- Observation of the subject's habitual or comfortable sound level/intensity within the entire VRP can be useful in assessing whether he or she is consistently using voice near the minimum intensity contour (a form of hypofunctional voice) or habitually using voice in the vicinity of their maximum level (potentially abusive).
- A reduction in total phonational F_0 range may be observed in individuals with laryngeal pathologies. Laryngeal pathologies that produce an increase in vocal fold mass may limit vocal fold vibration at high frequencies. Laryngeal pathologies are also associated with increased vocal fold stiffness which prevents the necessary stretching of the vocal folds for high F_0 phonation.[1,309]
- Individuals with laryngeal pathologies may show a reduction of dynamic intensity range due to increased minimum

phonational intensities.[75] Laryngeal pathologies that result in increases in vocal fold mass and stiffness make phonation at low, quiet levels very difficult. This is because the relatively small subglottal pressure and air flow used for low-intensity phonation is unable to effectively set the vocal folds into vibration in conditions of increased mass and/or stiffness.[160,310]

The Dysphonia Severity Index

Another method for encompassing the multidimensional nature of phonatory function is the *DSI*, developed by Wuyts et al.[67] The DSI makes use of a combination of several voice measures that may be obtained from the VRP/phonetogram, as well as basic aerodynamic and acoustic analyses: the *highest phonational frequency (F₀ high*, in hertz), *lowest intensity (I low*, in decibels), *the maximum phonation time (MPT* in seconds), and *jitter* (in percent).

The DSI was initially described and validated with a large group of 387 subjects (68 normal controls vs. 319 voice-disordered subjects). Each subject provided the aforementioned measures of voice, and each subject's voice was perceptually rated using the GRBAS (grade, roughness, breathiness, asthenia, strain) scale (see section "Auditory-Perceptual Evaluation of Voice" in Chapter 3). The DSI was obtained via multiple regression analysis and is calculated using the following formula:

$$DSI = 0.13 \times MPT(s) + 0.0053 \times F_0 high(Hz) - 0.26 \times I\ low(dB) - 1.18 \times jitter(\%) + 12.4.$$

The results of the study indicated an inverse relationship between the DSI and the grade (G; overall severity) of dysphonia, as well as between the DSI and the Voice Handicap Index.

Evaluating the DSI

In the initial study by Wuyts et al, the DSI was transformed such that a DSI = +5 corresponded to G 0 (i.e., normal voice), and a DSI = –5 corresponded to G 3 (i.e., severe dysphonia).[67] A DSI of +1.6 was determined to be the cutoff point for perceptually normal voices. It was noted by these authors that the DSI is not necessarily restricted to the +5 to –5 range. ▶ Table 4.14 provides expectations for the DSI and the component measures in normal, nondysphonic subjects.

The DSI in Nondysphonic and Dysphonic Voice

In recent years, the DSI has been used to investigate a diverse range of issues dealing with both normal and disordered vocal function, including the following:

- The possible relationship between the DSI and auditory-perceptual ratings of voice.[315,316,317]
- The relationship between the DSI and the Voice Handicap Index.[159,318]
- The possible effects of vocal training on the voice.[312,319,320]
- The possible influence of age and gender on the DSI.[43,175,321,322]
- The effects of smoking on the voice.[313]
- The possible effects of geographical and ethnic background on the DSI.[323]
- The relationship between the DSI and laryngostroboscopic characteristics of the voice.[317]
- The use of the DSI as a treatment outcome measure with thyroidectomy patients and patents with velopharyngeal dysfunction.[324,325]
- The inter-device reliability of DSI measures when obtained using different hardware/software systems.[326]
- The interobserver and test-retest variability of the DSI.[311,314]

Table 4.14 Examples of DSI and component measure data from various literature sources

Author	Gender	No. of subjects	Age	DSI	Jitter (%)	MPT (s)	F0 High (Hz)	I-Low (dB)
Wuyts et al[67]	M	25	18–80	5.22 (0.26)	0.79 (0.10)	16.9 (0.7)	905 (31)	51.3 (0.2)
	F	43	18–80	4.70 (0.40)	0.63 (0.06)	22.2 (1.7)	602 (34)	50.4 (0.5)
Hakkesteegt et al[175]	M	49	Med. = 49.0	4.1 (2.0)	0.77 (0.57)	25 (9.3)	650 (161)	56 (2.9)
	F	69	Med. = 39.0	4.3 (2.01)	0.73 (0.45)	19 (6.7)	943 (243)	57 (3.3)
Hakkesteegt et al[311]	M & F	30 (11 M; 19 F)	20–35 (M = 26.0)	5.60	0.54	23.0	896	54
Awan and Ensslen[312]	M	15	21.66	3.04 (1.98)	0.38 (0.13)	23.42 (8.26)	500.75 (144.47)	56.19 (4.24)
	F	21	22.57	4.69 (1.83)	0.43 (0.24)	20.42 (7.78)	656.94 (187.15)	51.30 (2.94)
Awan[313]	F	30	18–24 (M = 21.46)	5.06 (1.47)	0.37 (0.15)	20.96 (5.11)	756.70 (158.62)	52.43 (3.80)
Awan et al[314]	M & F	49 (21 M; 28 F)	18–25 (21.50)	3.67 (1.56)	0.33 (0.17)	20.83 (6.18)	584.69 (203.71)	54.42 (3.23)
Goy et al[43]	M$_Y$	55	18–28 (19.1)	3.05 (2.19)	0.38 (0.13)	20.2 (8.0)	425 (141)	56.3 (5.1)
	F$_Y$	104		2.34 (1.95)	0.48 (0.20)	18.6 (8.1)	363 (103)	58.6 (6.0)
	M$_O$	51	63–86 (72.0)	1.90 (1.83)	0.37 (0.25)	15.1 (4.4)	517 (124)	58.7 (5.5)
	F$_O$	82		3.72 (2.23)	0.47 (0.34)	18.9 (7.3)	520 (120)	56.5 (6.1)

Abbreviations: DSI, Dysphonia Severity Index; MPT, maximum phonation time.
Note: Young ($_Y$) and old-age ($_O$) subjects.

While Wuyts et al described the DSI as an index of "vocal quality," it is often observed that subjects can have normal perceived voice quality and typical levels of jitter (a correlate of vocal quality dysfunction) in sustained vowel productions, and yet differ in terms of the DSI (e.g., trained singers vs. untrained subjects).[67] This result clearly emphasizes that *the DSI should be interpreted as a measure of vocal function/performance*, and is not necessarily a correlate of perceived or measured vocal quality.[312,313] However, the DSI is unique among the various measures of voice that have been described in this chapter in that it combines measures related to all of the key perceptual characteristics of voice (pitch, loudness, quality, and duration).

4.5 Conclusion

This chapter has summarized acoustic analysis processes for domains of vocal frequency, intensity, and spectral structure which correlate with perceptual domains of vocal pitch, loudness, and quality, respectively. We have provided the reader with rationale, recommendations, and recommended procedures for recording acoustic signals and analyzing those signals to obtain evidence-based acoustic measurements utilized in the diagnostic and treatment process. We have also discussed the expectations for specific acoustic measurements in healthy populations and those with voice impairments. Collectively, these acoustic assessments form (1) part of the larger diagnostic voice profile and (2) one-half of the laryngeal function study procedures.

The process of performing laryngeal function studies includes both acoustic and aerodynamic assessments. The next chapter will focus on the latter. Aerodynamic assessments gather information about the underlying aerodynamic forces which initiate and sustain phonation. We will provide the reader with information associated with the rationale, instrumental options, and procedural requirements for acquiring aerodynamic measurements. We will also provide the reader with knowledge of how physiological impairments resulting in hyperfunctional and hypofunctional voice disorders impact specific aerodynamic measurements. This next chapter will form a bridge to the subsequent instrumental chapter on laryngeal endoscopy, which together with information from Chapters 3, 4, and 5 will form the foundation of a complete voice evaluation and development of a diagnostic voice profile for any patient.

Clinical Case Study

Part 1

Mr. Meine is a 28-year-old man semi-professional rock singer who recently (3 weeks ago) experienced a sudden change in voice. During a recent performance, he noticed a change in his singing voice quality and a noticeable restriction in his upper pitch register. There were no voice symptoms prior to the performance, nor were there any illnesses. In the next few days after the performance, he continued to experience dysphonia and reduced vocal range. He also noticed that his speaking voice became progressively dysphonic in the days after the ini-

tial onset. The problem continued to get worse over the course of a week, at which time he cancelled all future gigs. He consulted an otolaryngologist for an evaluation.

1. Based on the limited information provided above, is your clinical hypothesis leading you to think this impairment is functional, organic, or neurological in etiology? Why?
2. Based on the information above, what would you expect to see when performing video stroboscopy on this patient?

Part 2

Laryngeal videostroboscopy revealed a unilateral hemorrhagic polyp on the right vocal fold with an enlarged vessel feeding into the lesion. The left vocal fold was within normal limits other than mild edema. During phonation, there was a consistent hour-glass closure pattern with reduced mucosal wave and vibratory amplitude at and around the site of the lesion. When prompted to produce voice in his upper frequency range, vibratory dynamics became aperiodic. Both medial compression of the false vocal folds and anterior-posterior compression of the larynx were evidence during all vocalization tasks.

Read the Following Article

de Vasconcelos D, Gomes AO, de Araújo CM. Treatment for vocal polyps: lips and tongue trill. J Voice 2017;31(2):252.e27–252.e36.

1. What elements of history explain why this lesion was a polyp versus vocal nodules?
2. Laryngeal videostroboscopy revealed medial compression of the false vocal folds and anterior-posterior laryngeal compression. What are those signs of?
3. Mr. Meine opted for voice therapy over phonosurgery as an initial treatment for this problem? In singers or professional voice users, what factors might be considered when making this decision?
4. Does the article of de Vasconcelos support voice therapy as an initial intervention for vocal fold polyps? What reasons were given to support this, and how were acoustic measures utilized to determine treatment outcome?

4.6 Review Questions

1. The number of times the amplitude of the sound wave is captured per second is referred to as the _____.
   a) Frequency response.
   b) Nyquist theorem.
   c) Quantization.
   d) Sampling rate.
   e) None of the above.
2. In typical voices, the _____ generally appears as the lowest harmonic frequency in the voice signal and may be observed in the spectrum of the voice signal as the frequency spacing between the harmonics.
   a) Period.
   b) Cycle.
   c) Fundamental frequency (F_0).
   d) Autocorrelation.
   e) a or b.

3. A measure that may be used to describe the average F_0 variability is the _____.
   a) F_0 standard deviation.
   b) F_0 coefficient of variation (a.k.a. vF_0).
   c) SFF.
   d) Total phonational frequency range.
   e) a or b.

4. The term _____ refers to growth changes that occur during puberty in which the neck lengthens and the larynx descends and grows in size.
   a) Flaccidity.
   b) Mutation.
   c) Senescence.
   d) Tremor.
   e) MTD.

5. The following component measure is *not* incorporated into the *Dysphonia Severity Index (DSI):*
   a) Highest phonational frequency (in Hz).
   b) Jitter (%).
   c) Cepstral peak prominence (dB).
   d) MPT (in second).
   e) Lowest vocal intensity (in dB).

6. The following are important considerations in the measurement of vocal sound level/intensity:
   a) Mouth-to-microphone distance.
   b) Weighting circuit.
   c) Ambient noise level.
   d) Type of sound level meter (SLM).
   e) All of the above.

7. _____ is a short-term measure of instability that quantifies cycle-to-cycle variations in frequency.
   a) Shimmer.
   b) HNR.
   c) F_0 standard deviation.
   d) Jitter.
   e) AVQI.

8. Rough voice signals are often characterized by the presence of _____.
   a) Subharmonics.
   b) Amplitude modulations.
   c) Continuous additive noise.
   d) High pitch voice.
   e) a and b.

9. The cepstral peak within a predetermined range of quefrencies (i.e., a range of periods) is referred to as the
   _____.
   a) Spectrum.
   b) HNR.
   c) First harmonic.
   d) Dominant rahmonic.
   e) CSID.

10. The _____ is a graphical representation of the combined frequency and intensity capabilities of the patient's voice.
   a) VRP.
   b) Phonetogram.
   c) Cepstrum.
   d) DSI.
   e) a and b.

4.7 Answers and Explanations

1. Correct: Sampling rate (**d**).
   (**d**) Sampling rate refers to the number of samples (i.e., piece of data) that will be captured per second (in the case of sound waves, multiple measures of the changing amplitude of the sound wave per second will be captured). The higher the sampling rate, the more accurate the digitized reproduction of the sound wave we have recorded will be. A sampling rate of 44.1 kHz is often recommended for detailed voice analyses. (**a**) The term frequency response was used to describe the frequency sensitivity of the microphone used for voice recording. (**b**) The Nyquist theorem states that the sampling rate should be at least two times the highest frequency of interest. (**c**) Quantization refers to the conversion of the continuous amplitude variations of a sound wave into discrete values or increments (related to the number of bits of resolution).

2. Correct: Fundamental frequency (F_0) (**c**).
   (**c**) The fundamental frequency (F_0) is the lowest harmonic in the acoustic spectrum of a voice signal. Because successive harmonics are integer multiples of this frequency, it can be observed in the spectrum of the voice signal as the frequency spacing between the harmonics. (**a**) The period is the time to complete one cycle of vibration and (Hz) = 1/(Period (s)). (**b**) The term cycle refers to a repetitive pattern in the sound wave—sound waves that are periodic will be observed to have a highly repetitive pattern of cyclic vibration. (**d**) Autocorrelation is a mathematical procedure that may be used to identify the period and frequency of a repetitive pattern as may be observed in the voice sound wave.

3. Correct: a or b (**e**).
   (**e**) The F_0 standard deviation is a measure of the average F_0 variability. However, to normalize this value for different voice types (e.g., adult males vs. females), the F_0 standard deviation is often converted to a coefficient of variation: (F_0 standard deviation)/(mean F_0) × 100. Therefore, answers (**a**) or (**b**) may be used to describe the average F_0 variability. (**c**) SFF refers to the speaking fundamental frequency (a.k.a. mean speaking F_0; mean F_0). This measure is related to the habitual pitch of the voice. (**d**) The total phonation frequency range, an assessment of the range between the lowest pitch and frequency in modal register to the highest pitch and frequency in falsetto.

4. Correct: Mutation (**b**).
   (**b**) *Mutation* is a term referring to growth changes that occur during puberty. Specific to the head/neck, during puberty the neck lengthens and the larynx descends and grows in size. (**a**) *Flaccidity* is a state of hypotonia associated with disruptions of the lower motor neuron system. *Senescence* is a state of advanced aging in which a gradual deterioration in bodily function(s) may occur due to biological changes. (**c**) *Tremor* is a rhythmic variation in pitch and/or loudness. (**d**) *MTD* refers to *muscle tension dysphonia*, a form of vocal hyperfunction characterized by a presumed overactivation and dysregulation of muscles in and around the laryngeal region in the absence of organic or neurologic laryngeal disorders.

5. Correct: Cepstral peak prominence (dB) (**c**).

   (**c**) Cepstral peak prominence (dB) is the relative amplitude of the cepstral peak (i.e., the dominant rahmonic). (**a, b, d, e**) As described by Wuyts et al, the Dysphonia Severity Index (DSI) is a multivariate correlate of vocal function which combines measures related to pitch (highest phonational frequency), loudness (lowest vocal intensity), quality (jitter), and duration (MPT—maximum phonation time).

6. Correct: All of the above (**e**).

   (**e**) All answers are important consideration in the measurement of vocal sound level/intensity. (**a**) The mouth-to-microphone distance substantially affects the intensity of the sound being measured since intensity is effected by the *inverse square law*. (**b**) The frequency weighting circuit used (typically, A- vs. C-weighting) may effect measures of vocal sound level/intensity since A-weighting results in substantially reduced intensity measurements for lower frequency voice productions such as those in the vicinity of the vocal F_0 and other modal register phonations in most subjects. Therefore, C-weighting is preferred. (**c**) The environment in which the recording takes place can also have a substantial effect on our measures of sound level/intensity, and recordings should take place in a room in which the ambient noise level is at least 10 dB lower than the expected lowest sound level/intensity phonation. (**d**) Ideally, a high-quality sound level meter (SLM—Class 1 and Class 2 sound level meters which comply with IEC or ANSI standards) is used for measures of vocal sound level/intensity. However, clinical approximations of vocal intensity may be obtained with low costs SLMs or Low-cost or free sound level meter apps.

7. Correct: Jitter (**d**).

   (**d**) Jitter (often reported in % or in ms) is a measure of cycle-to-cycle variations in period or frequency (since 1/period = frequency). (**a**) *Shimmer* is a measure of cycle-to-cycle variations in amplitude. (**b**) The *HNR* detects cycle-to-cycle perturbations and was initially designed as a method for quantifying spectral noise. (**c**) The F_0 standard deviation is a long-term measure of the average variation of the F_0. (**e**) The *AVQI* (Acoustic Voice Quality Index) is a multivariate correlate of dysphonia severity.

8. Correct: a and b (**e**).

   (**e**) Rough voice signals are often observed to contain frequencies found at fractional values (e.g., $F_0/2$, $F_0/3$) referred to as *subharmonics*. In addition, rough voice signals may also be characterized by cycles that alternate in terms of amplitude (e.g., large peak amplitude—small peak amplitude—large peak amplitude, etc., an *amplitude modulation*). (**c**) *Continuous additive noise* is typical of breathy voices, in which a relatively period sound wave produced by vocal fold vibration is combined/added to continuous noise from excessive airflow during phonation. (**d**) In contrast to *high pitch voice*, rough voices are often perceived as low pitched, "gravelly" voices, possibly due to the perception of subharmonics in the voice signal.

9. Correct: Dominant rahmonic (**d**).

   (**d**) The dominant rahmonic (*rahmonic*—an anagram of the word *harmonic*) generally represents the fundamental period of the voice signal. The reciprocal of the fundamental period will be the fundamental frequency (F_0). (**a**) The *spectrum* provides information regarding the frequencies contained within a complex sound wave and their relative amplitudes. (**b**) *HNR* is the harmonics-to-noise ratio, which compares relative amplitude of the periodic versus aperiodic portions of a sound wave—a traditional form of perturbation analysis. (**c**) A *harmonic* is an integer multiple of the fundamental frequency (F_0). Since 1 x the $F_0 = F_0$, the first harmonic (H1) is the same as the F_0. (**e**) The *CSID* is the *Cepstral Spectral Index of Dysphonia*—a multivariate estimate of dysphonia severity that incorporates cepstral and spectral measures.

10. Correct: a and b (**e**)

    (**e**) The terms Voice Range Profile and phonetogram are synonymous. Both refer to a graphical representation of the combined frequency and intensity capabilities of the patient's voice. (**c**) A cepstrum is produced via a Fourier analysis of the log power spectrum of an initial Fourier analysis. (**d**) The DSI is the Dysphonia Severity Index, a multivariate estimate of vocal function which utilizes measures of the highest phonational frequency, the lowest vocal intensity, jitter, and the maximum phonation time (MPT).

Appendix 4.1
Averaging of Decibels[327]

Because decibels are logarithmic units, the appropriate average value is that which corresponds to the average sound intensity, or the average value of p^2 (pressure squared). The average value, L_{AVGE}, of several levels, L_1, L_2, L_3, ... L_N, may be calculated using the formula:

$$L_{AVGE} = 10 Log[(10^{L_1/10} + 10^{L_2/10} + 10^{L_3/10} + ... + 10^{L_N/10}) \times (1/N)]$$

In this formula, the value inside the square brackets [...] corresponds to the average sound intensity.

If one were to calculate the average of four decibel levels (82, 84, 86, and 88 dB) using the logarithmic average formula, the result will be 85.6 dB. This will be different from the arithmetic average of the four levels which is 85.0 dB. While in this case the difference between the logarithmic average and the arithmetic average is very small (0.6 dB), the difference will increase when the range of averaged levels is greater. The logarithmic average will always be greater than the arithmetic average. Examples of decibel calculators are provided at http://www.cesva.com/en/support/db-calculator/.

Cepstral Analysis Instructions for *ADSV* and *Praat*

ADSV

The following commands and parameters will compute the smoothed CPP in ADSV:

1. Select the appropriate protocol for analysis (sustained vowel vs. all voiced sentence) and open the sound file to be analyzed. The selected protocol does not have any effect on how the CPP is computed, but does affect other computations in *ADSV*.

2. If necessary, the user is instructed to place cursors around the section of the sound wave to be analyzed (approx. 50 ms pre- and post-sample is suggested). If samples are pre-edited, cursor selection is not necessary.

3. The "Apply Automatic Data Selection" button is clicked.

4. A graphical display of the CPP over time, as well as other data obtained from the spectral and cepstral analyses (e.g., ratio of low- vs. high-frequency spectral energy (L/H ratio); display of individual cepstral frames), is provided. Default settings that affect CPP analysis found under Options | ADSV Options | Advanced Setup include CPP threshold (dB) = 0; cepstral extraction range (Hz) 60 to 300; spectral window size = 1,024 pts.; maximum frequency for regression line calculation = 10,000 Hz; frame overlap = 75%; cepstral time averaging = 7.

5. Select "Compute/Display New ADSV Results" to provide the mean CPP across the sample being analyzed, as well as other spectral and cepstral statistics.

Praat

The following commands and parameters will generate the smoothed CPP from Praat (v. 6.0.19):

1. After pressing "Analyze Periodicity," choose "To PowerCepstrogram."

2. From the menu proceed with pitch floor (Hz) = 60, time step (s) = 0.002, maximum frequency (Hz) = 5,000, and pre-emphasis from (Hz) = 50.

3. Click on "Query," select "Get CPPS" from the menu, and proceed using the default settings.

The result of this routine is the CPPS measure as described in Maryn and Weenink.[296]

The following commands will draw the cepstrum:

1. After computing the PowerCepstrogram, click on "To Power-Cepstrum (Slice)."

2. Click on "Draw"—this will draw a cepstrum in the Praat Picture window. The quefrency range can be adjusted as necessary (0.0001–0.017 s are used in the examples).

3. Click on "Draw Tilt Line."

References

[1] Awan S. The Voice Diagnostic Protocol: A Practical Guide to the Diagnosis of Voice Disorders. Austin, TX: Pro-Ed Inc.; 2001

[2] Behrman A, Agresti CJ, Blumstein E, Sharma G. Meaningful features of voice range profiles from patients with organic vocal fold pathology: a preliminary study. J Voice. 1996; 10(3):269–283

[3] Colton R, Casper J. Understanding Voice Problems: A Physiological Perspective for Diagnosis and Treatment. Baltimore, MD: Williams & Wilkins; 1996

[4] Behrman A, Orlikoff RF. Instrumentation in voice assessment and treatment: What's the use? Am J Speech Lang Pathol. 1997; 6:9–16

[5] Boersma P, Weenink D. Praat. 2016. Available at: http://www.fon.hum.uva.nl/praat/. Accessed December 1, 2017

[6] Hillenbrand J. SpeechTool. 2008. Available at: http://homepages.wmich.edu/~hillenbr/. Accessed December 1, 2017

[7] Pentax Medical Inc. Multi-Speech, Model 3700. Montvale, NJ: Pentax Medical, Inc. Available at: http://pentaxmedical.com/pentax/en/99/1/Speech. Accessed December 1, 2017

[8] Wevosys. lingWaves. WEVOSYS Medical Technology GmbH; 2016. Available at: https://www.wevosys.com/index.html. Accessed December 1, 2017

[9] Svec JG, Granqvist S. Guidelines for selecting microphones for human voice production research. Am J Speech Lang Pathol. 2010; 19(4):356–368

[10] Winholtz WS, Titze IR. Conversion of a head-mounted microphone signal into calibrated SPL units. J Voice. 1997; 11(4):417–421

[11] Patel R, Awan SN, Barkmeier-Kraemer J, et al. Recommended protocols for instrumental assessment of voice: American Speech-Language-Hearing Association Expert Panel to Develop a Protocol for Instrumental Assessment of Vocal Function. Am J Speech Lang Pathol.

[12] Nyquist H. Certain topics in telegraph transmission theory. Trans Am Inst Electr Eng. 1928; 47(2):617–644

[13] American National Standards Institute. (1973). American national psychoacoustical terminology. S3.20. New York: American Standards Association

[14] Titze IR. Vocal fold mass is not a useful quantity for describing F0 in vocalization. J Speech Lang Hear Res. 2011; 54(2):520–522

[15] Case J. Clinical Management of Voice Disorders. Austin, TX: PRO-ED, Inc.; 1996

[16] Fairbanks G. Voice and Articulation Drillbook. 2nd ed. New York, NY: Harper & Row; 1960

[17] Kempster GB, Gerratt BR, Verdolini Abbott K, Barkmeier-Kraemer J, Hillman RE. Consensus auditory-perceptual evaluation of voice: development of a standardized clinical protocol. Am J Speech Lang Pathol. 2009; 18(2):124–132

[18] Zraick RI, Birdwell KY, Smith-Olinde L. The effect of speaking sample duration on determination of habitual pitch. J Voice. 2005; 19(2):197–201

[19] Horii Y. Some acoustic characteristics of oral reading by ten- to twelve-year-old children. J Commun Disord. 1983; 16(4):257–267

[20] Fitch JL. Consistency of fundamental frequency and perturbation in repeated phonations of sustained vowels, reading, and connected speech. J Speech Hear Disord. 1990; 55(2):360–363

[21] Hollien H, Jackson B. Normative data on the speaking fundamental frequency characteristics of young adult males. J Phonetics. 1973; 1:117–120

[22] Hollien H, Shipp T. Speaking fundamental frequency and chronologic age in males. J Speech Hear Res. 1972; 15(1):155–159

[23] McGlone RE, McGlone J. Speaking fundamental frequency of eight-year-old girls. Folia Phoniatr (Basel). 1972; 24(4):313–317

[24] Horii Y. Some statistical characteristics of voice fundamental frequency. J Speech Hear Res. 1975; 18(1):192–201

[25] Honjo I, Isshiki N. Laryngoscopic and voice characteristics of aged persons. Arch Otolaryngol. 1980; 106(3):149–150

[26] Hudson AI, Holbrook A. A study of the reading fundamental vocal frequency of young black adults. J Speech Hear Res. 1981; 24(2):197–200

[27] Murry T, Doherty ET. Selected acoustic characteristics of pathologic and normal speakers. J Speech Hear Res. 1980; 23(2):361–369

[28] Stoicheff ML. Speaking fundamental frequency characteristics of nonsmoking female adults. J Speech Hear Res. 1981; 24(3):437–441

[29] Bennett S. A 3-year longitudinal study of school-aged children's fundamental frequencies. J Speech Hear Res. 1983; 26(1):137–141

[30] Ramig LA, Ringel RL. Effects of physiological aging on selected acoustic characteristics of voice. J Speech Hear Res. 1983; 26(1):22–30

[31] Moran MJ, Gilbert HR. Relation between voice profile ratings and aerodynamic and acoustic parameters. J Commun Disord. 1984; 17(4):245–260

[32] Pedersen MF, Møller S, Krabbe S, Bennett P. Fundamental voice frequency measured by electroglottography during continuous speech. A new exact secondary sex characteristic in boys in puberty. Int J Pediatr Otorhinolaryngol. 1986; 11(1):21–27

[33] Kent JF, Kent RD, Rosenbek JC, et al. Quantitative description of the dysarthria in women with amyotrophic lateral sclerosis. J Speech Hear Res. 1992; 35 (4):723–733

[34] Shipp T, Qi Y, Huntley R, Hollien H. Acoustic and temporal correlates of perceived age. J Voice. 1992; 6(3):211–216

[35] Awan SN, Mueller PB. Speaking fundamental frequency characteristics of centenarian females. Clin Linguist Phon. 1992; 6(3):249–254

[36] Awan SN. Superimposition of speaking voice characteristics and phonetograms in untrained and trained vocal groups. J Voice. 1993; 7(1):30–37

[37] Morris RJ, Brown WS, Jr, Hicks DM, Howell E. Phonational profiles of male trained singers and nonsingers. J Voice. 1995; 9(2):142–148

[38] Murry T, Brown WS, Jr, Morris RJ. Patterns of fundamental frequency for three types of voice samples. J Voice. 1995; 9(3):282–289

[39] Awan SN, Mueller PB. Speaking fundamental frequency characteristics of white, African American, and Hispanic kindergartners. J Speech Hear Res. 1996; 39(3):573–577

[40] Morris R. Speaking fundamental frequency characteristics of 8- through 10-year-old white- and African-American boys. J Commun Disord. 1997; 30 (2):101–114, quiz 115–116

[41] Awan SN. The aging female voice: acoustic and respiratory data. Clin Linguist Phon. 2006; 20(2–3):171–180

[42] Izadi F, Mohseni R, Daneshi A, Sandughdar N. Determination of fundamental frequency and voice intensity in Iranian men and women aged between 18 and 45 years. J Voice. 2012; 26(3):336–340

[43] Goy H, Fernandes DN, Pichora-Fuller MK, van Lieshout P. Normative voice data for younger and older adults. J Voice. 2013; 27(5):545–555

[44] Gelfer MP, Denor SL. Speaking fundamental frequency and individual variability in Caucasian and African American school-age children. Am J Speech Lang Pathol. 2014; 23(3):395–406

[45] Cox VO, Selent M. Acoustic and respiratory measures as a function of age in the male voice. J Phonet and Audio. 2015; 1(1):1–7

[46] Hartelius L, Buder EH, Strand EA. Long-term phonatory instability in individuals with multiple sclerosis. J Speech Lang Hear Res. 1997; 40(5):1056–1072

[47] Murry T. Phonation: Assessment. In: Lass N, McReynolds L, Northern J, Yoder D, eds. Speech Language, and Hearing. Vol. II. Philadelphia, PA: W.B. Saunders Company; 1982:477–488

[48] Horii Y. Jitter and shimmer in sustained vocal fry phonation. Folia Phoniatr (Basel). 1985; 37(2):81–86

[49] Linville SE, Fisher HB. Acoustic characteristics of women's voices with advancing age. J Gerontol. 1985; 40(3):324–330

[50] Linville SE. Intraspeaker variability in fundamental frequency stability: an age-related phenomenon? J Acoust Soc Am. 1988; 83(2):741–745

[51] Linville SE, Skarin BD, Fornatto E. The interrelationship of measures related to vocal function, speech rate, and laryngeal appearance in elderly women. J Speech Hear Res. 1989; 32(2):323–330

[52] Orlikoff RF. The relationship of age and cardiovascular health to certain acoustic characteristics of male voices. J Speech Hear Res. 1990; 33(3):450–457

[53] Wolfe V, Cornell R, Fitch J. Sentence/vowel correlation in the evaluation of dysphonia. J Voice. 1995; 9(3):297–303

[54] Awan S, Scarpino S. Measures of vocal F0 from continuous speech samples: an interprogram comparison. J Speech Lang Pathol Audiol. 2004; 28(3):122–131

[55] Hema N, Mahesh S, Pushpavathi M. Normative data for Multi-Dimensional Voice Program (MDVP) for adults - a computerized voice analysis system. J All India Inst Speech Hear. 2009; 28:1–7

[56] Petrović-Lazić M, Babac S, Vuković M, Kosanović R, Ivanković Z. Acoustic voice analysis of patients with vocal fold polyp. J Voice. 2011; 25(1):94–97

[57] Aithal VU, Bellur R, John S, Varghese C, Guddattu V. Acoustic analysis of voice in normal and high pitch phonation: a comparative study. Folia Phoniatr Logop. 2012; 64(1):48–53

[58] Herzel H, Berry D, Titze IR, Saleh M. Analysis of vocal disorders with methods from nonlinear dynamics. J Speech Hear Res. 1994; 37(5):1008–1019

[59] Zraick RI, Nelson JL, Montague JC, Monoson PK. The effect of task on determination of maximum phonational frequency range. J Voice. 2000; 14(2):154–160

[60] Kent RD, Kent JF, Rosenbek JC. Maximum performance tests of speech production. J Speech Hear Disord. 1987; 52(4):367–387

[61] Awan S. Phonetographic profiles and F0-SPL characteristics of untrained versus trained vocal groups. J Voice. 1991; 5(1):41–50

[62] Coleman RF, Mott JB. Fundamental frequency and sound pressure level profiles of young female singers. Folia Phoniatr (Basel). 1978; 30(2):94–102

[63] Awan SN, Mueller PB. Comment on "Methodological variables affecting phonational frequency range in adults". J Speech Hear Disord. 1990; 55(4):804–806

[64] Large J. Observations on the vocal capacity of singers. NATS Bulletin. 1971; 28:34–35

[65] Luchsinger R, Arnold G. Physiology and pathology of respiration and phonation. In: Luchsinger R, Arnold G, eds. Voice-Speech-Language. Clinical Communicology: Its Physiology and Pathology. Belmont, CA: Wadsworth Publishing Co.; 1965

[66] Drost HA, VAN OORDTH. Development of the frequency range of the voice in children. Folia Phoniatr (Basel). 1963; 15:289–298

[67] Wuyts FL, De Bodt MS, Molenberghs G, et al. The dysphonia severity index: an objective measure of vocal quality based on a multiparameter approach. J Speech Lang Hear Res. 2000; 43(3):796–809

[68] Baken R, Orlikoff R. Clinical Measurement of Speech and Voice. 2nd ed. San Diego, CA: Singular Publishing Group; 2000

[69] Linville SE. Maximum phonational frequency range capabilities of women's voices with advancing age. Folia Phoniatr (Basel). 1987; 39(6):297–301

[70] Ma E, Robertson J, Radford C, Vagne S, El-Halabi R, Yiu E. Reliability of speaking and maximum voice range measures in screening for dysphonia. J Voice. 2007; 21(4):397–406

[71] Šiupšinskiene N, Adamonis K, Toohill RJ. [Usefulness of assessment of voice capabilities in female patients with reflux-related dysphonia]. Medicina (Kaunas). 2009; 45(12):978–987

[72] Siupsinskiene N, Lycke H. Effects of vocal training on singing and speaking voice characteristics in vocally healthy adults and children based on choral and nonchoral data. J Voice. 2011; 25(4):e177–e189

[73] Hallin AE, Fröst K, Holmberg EB, Södersten M. Voice and speech range profiles and Voice Handicap Index for males-methodological issues and data. Logoped Phoniatr Vocol. 2012; 37(2):47–61

[74] Michelsson K, Eklund K, Leppänen P, Lyytinen H. Cry characteristics of 172 healthy 1-to 7-day-old infants. Folia Phoniatr Logop. 2002; 54(4):190–200

[75] Michelsson K, Michelsson O. Phonation in the newborn, infant cry. Int J Pediatr Otorhinolaryngol. 1999; 49 Suppl 1:S297–S301

[76] Wermke K, Robb MP. Fundamental frequency of neonatal crying: does body size matter? J Voice. 2010; 24(4):388–394

[77] Hedden D. An overview of existing research about children's singing and the implications for teaching children to sing. Update. Applic Res Music Educ. 2012; 30(2):52–62

[78] Wassum S. Elementary school children's vocal range. J Res Music Educ. 1979; 27 4:214–226

[79] Eguchi S, Hirsh IJ. Development of speech sounds in children. Acta Otolaryngol Suppl. 1969; 257 Suppl., 257:1–51

[80] Perkins W. Assessment and treatment of voice disorders: state of the art. In: Costello J, ed. Speech Disorders in Adults. San Diego, CA: College Hill Press; 1985

[81] Aronson AE. Clinical Voice Disorders: An Interdisciplinary Approach. 3rd ed. New York: Thieme Medical Publishers; 1990

[82] Stathopoulos ET, Huber JE, Sussman JE. Changes in acoustic characteristics of the voice across the life span: measures from individuals 4–93 years of age. J Speech Lang Hear Res. 2011; 54(4):1011–1021

[83] Boltezar IH, Burger ZR, Zargi M. Instability of voice in adolescence: pathologic condition or normal developmental variation? J Pediatr. 1997; 130 (2):185–190

[84] Gilbert HR, Weismer GG. The effects of smoking on the fundamental frequency of women. J Linguistic Res. 1974; 3(3):225–231

[85] Xue SA, Deliyski D. Effects of aging on selected acoustic voice parameters: preliminary normative data and educational implications. Educ Gerontol. 2001; 27(2):159–168

[86] Dehqan A, Scherer RC, Dashti G, Ansari-Moghaddam A, Fanaie S. The effects of aging on acoustic parameters of voice. Folia Phoniatr Logop. 2012; 64 (6):265–270

[87] Torre P, III, Barlow JA. Age-related changes in acoustic characteristics of adult speech. J Commun Disord. 2009; 42(5):324–333

[88] Titze I. Principles of Voice Production. Englewood Cliffs, NJ: Prentice-Hall; 1994

[89] Pedersen MF, Møller S, Krabbe S, Bennett P, Svenstrup B. Fundamental voice frequency in female puberty measured with electroglottography during continuous speech as a secondary sex characteristic. A comparison between voice, pubertal stages, oestrogens and androgens. Int J Pediatr Otorhinolaryngol. 1990; 20(1):17–24

[90] Morris RJ, Brown WS, Jr. Age-related differences in speech variability among women. J Commun Disord. 1994; 27(1):49–64

[91] Caruso AJ, Mueller PB, Xue A. Relative contributions of voice and articulation to listener judgements of age and gender: preliminary data and implications. Voice. 1994; 3:1–9

[92] Mueller PB. Voice ageism. Contemp Issues Commun Sci Disord. 1998; 25:62–64

[93] Kahane JC. Age-related changes in the peripheral speech mechanism: Structural and physiological changes. Proceedings of the Research Symposium on Communication Sciences and Disorders and Aging 1990;19:75–87

[94] Liss JM, Weismer G, Rosenbek JC. Selected acoustic characteristics of speech production in very old males. J Gerontol. 1990; 45(2):35–45

[95] Kaplan H. Anatomy and Physiology of Speech. New York: McGraw-Hill; 1960

[96] Ptacek PH, Sander EK, Maloney WH, Jackson C. Phonatory and related changes with advanced age. J Speech, Lang Hear Res. 1966; 9:353–360

[97] Hudson AI, Holbrook A. Fundamental frequency characteristics of young Black adults: spontaneous speaking and oral reading. J Speech Hear Res. 1982; 25(1):25–28

[98] Wheat MC, Hudson AI. Spontaneous speaking fundamental frequency of 6-year-old black children. J Speech Hear Res. 1988; 31(4):723–725

[99] Awan SN, Roy N, Jetté ME, Meltzner GS, Hillman RE. Quantifying dysphonia severity using a spectral/cepstral-based acoustic index: Comparisons with auditory-perceptual judgements from the CAPE-V. Clin Linguist Phon. 2010; 24(9):742–758

[100] DeJonckere PH, van Wijck I, Speyer R. Efficacy of voice therapy assessed with the Voice Range Profile (Phonetogram). Rev Laryngol Otol Rhinol (Bord). 2003; 124(5):285–289

[101] Boshoff P. The anatomy of the South African Negro larynx. S Afr J Med Sci. 1945; 10(2):35–50

[102] Krogman W. Child growth. Ann Arbor, MI: The University of Michigan Press; 1972

[103] Mayo R, Manning WH. Vocal tract characteristics of African-American and European-American adult males. Texas J Audiol Speech Pathol. 1994; 20:33–36

[104] Sapienza CM. Aerodynamic and acoustic characteristics of the adult African American voice. J Voice. 1997; 11(4):410–416

[105] Troup G. The physics of the singing voice. Physics Reports. 1981; 74(5):379–401

[106] Pressman J. Physiology of the vocal cords in phonation and respiration. Archives Otology. 1942; 35:378

[107] Gould W. The effect of voice training on lung volumes in singers and the possible relationship to the damping factor of Pressman. J Res Singing. 1977; 1:3–15

[108] Hirano M, Tanaka S, Fujita M, Terasawa R. Fundamental frequency and sound pressure level of phonation in pathological states. J Voice. 1991; 5 (2):120–127

[109] Boone D, McFarlane S. The Voice and Voice Therapy. 4th ed. Englewood Cliffs, NJ: Prentice Hall; 1988

[110] Andrews M. Manual of Voice Treatment: Pediatrics Through Geriatrics. San Diego, CA: Singular Publishing Group, Inc.; 1995

[111] Dworkin J, Meleca R. Vocal Pathologies: Diagnosis, Treatment, and Case Studies. San Diego, CA: Singular Publishing Group, Inc.; 1997

[112] Baken RJ. The aged voice: a new hypothesis. J Voice. 2005; 19(3):317–325

[113] Murray T. Speaking fundamental frequency characteristics associated with voice pathologies. J Speech Hear Disord. 1978; 43(3):374–379

[114] Hufnagle J, Hufnagle K. An investigation of the relationship between speaking fundamental frequency and vocal quality improvement. J Commun Disord. 1984; 17(2):95–100

[115] Awan SN, Knych CL. Acoustic characteristics of the voice in young adult smokers. In: Windsor F, Kelley L, Hewlett N, eds. Themes in Clinical Phonetics and Linguistics. Mahwah, NJ: Lawrence Erlbaum & Associates; 2002;449–458

[116] Damborenea Tajada J, Fernández Liesa R, Llorente Arenas E, et al. [The effect of tobacco consumption on acoustic voice analysis]. Acta Otorrinolaringol Esp. 1999; 50(6):448–452

[117] Gonzalez J, Carpi A. Early effects of smoking on the voice: a multidimensional study. Med Sci Monit. 2004; 10(12):CR649–CR656

[118] Sorensen D, Horii Y. Cigarette smoking and voice fundamental frequency. J Commun Disord. 1982; 15(2):135–144

[119] Murphy CH, Doyle PC. The effects of cigarette smoking on voice-fundamental frequency. Otolaryngol Head Neck Surg. 1987; 97(4):376–380

[120] Hewlett N, Topham N, McMullen C. The effects of smoking on the female voice. In: Ball MJ, Duckworth M, eds. Advances in Clinical Phonetics. Philadelphia, PA: John Benjamins Publishing Company; 1996:227–235

[121] Canter GJ. Speech characteristics of patients with Parkinson's disease. I. Intensity, pitch and duration. J Speech Hear Disord. 1963; 28:221–229

[122] Darley FL, Aronson AE, Brown JR. Motor Speech Disorders. Philadelphia, PA: W.B. Saunders Company; 1975

[123] Zwirner P, Murry T, Woodson GE. Phonatory function of neurologically impaired patients. J Commun Disord. 1991; 24(4):287–300

[124] Vogel AP, Wardrop MI, Folker JE, et al. Voice in Friedreich ataxia. J Voice. 2017; 31(2):243.e9–243.e19

[125] Kent RD, Rosenbek JC. Prosodic disturbance and neurologic lesion. Brain Lang. 1982; 15(2):259–291

[126] Countryman S, Hicks J, Ramig LO, Smith ME. Supraglottal hyperadduction in an individual with Parkinson disease: a clinical treatment note. Am J Speech Lang Pathol. 1997; 6(4):74–84

[127] Dromey C, Ramig LO, Johnson AB. Phonatory and articulatory changes associated with increased vocal intensity in Parkinson disease: a case study. J Speech Hear Res. 1995; 38(4):751–764

[128] Mori H, Kobayashi Y, Kasuya H, Kobayashi N, Hirose H. Evaluation of fundamental frequency (F0) characteristics of speech in dysarthrias: a comparative study. Acoust Sci Technol. 2005; 26(6):540–543

[129] Bowen LK, Hands GL, Pradhan S, Stepp CE. Effects of Parkinson's disease on fundamental frequency variability in running speech. J Med Speech-Lang Pathol. 2013; 21(3):235–244

[130] Lowell SY, Kelley RT, Colton RH, Smith PB, Portnoy JE. Position of the hyoid and larynx in people with muscle tension dysphonia. Laryngoscope. 2012; 122(2):370–377

[131] Stemple JC, Stanley J, Lee L. Objective measures of voice production in normal subjects following prolonged voice use. J Voice. 1995; 9(2):127–133

[132] Blood GW. Efficacy of a computer-assisted voice treatment protocol. Am J Speech Lang Pathol. 1994; 3(1):57–66

[133] Morrison MD, Rammage LA. Muscle misuse voice disorders: description and classification. Acta Otolaryngol. 1993; 113(3):428–434

[134] Dagli M, Sati I, Acar A, Stone RE, Jr, Dursun G, Eryilmaz A. Mutational falsetto: intervention outcomes in 45 patients. J Laryngol Otol. 2008; 122 (3):277–281

[135] Desai V, Mishra P. Voice therapy outcome in puberphonia. Journal of Laryngology and Voice. 2012; 2(1):26–29

[136] Gama ACC, Mesquita GM, Reis C, Bassi IB. Acoustic and auditory-perceptual analyses of voice before and after speech-language therapy in patients with mutational falsetto. Rev Soc Bras Fonoaudiol. 2012; 17(2):225–229

[137] Cannizzaro M, Harel B, Reilly N, Chappell P, Snyder PJ. Voice acoustical measurement of the severity of major depression. Brain Cogn. 2004; 56(1):30–35

[138] Sobin C, Sackeim HA. Psychomotor symptoms of depression. Am J Psychiatry. 1997; 154(1):4–17

[139] Leff J, Abberton E. Voice pitch measurements in schizophrenia and depression. Psychol Med. 1981; 11(4):849–852

[140] Leder SB, Spitzer JB, Kirchner JC. Speaking fundamental frequency of postlingually profoundly deaf adult men. Ann Otol Rhinol Laryngol. 1987; 96(3, Pt 1):322–324

[141] Monsen RB. Acoustic qualities of phonation in young hearing-impaired children. J Speech Hear Res. 1979; 22(2):270–288

[142] Horii Y. Some voice fundamental frequency characteristics of oral reading and spontaneous speech by hard-of-hearing young women. J Speech Hear Res. 1982b; 25(4):608–610

[143] Papamichalis P. Practical Approaches to Speech Coding. Englewood Cliffs, NJ: Prentice-Hall Inc.; 1987

[144] Bielamowicz S, Kreiman J, Gerratt BR, Dauer MS, Berke GS. Comparison of voice analysis systems for perturbation measurement. J Speech Hear Res. 1996; 39(1):126–134

[145] Titze I. A short tutorial on sound level and loudness for voice. J Sing. 2013; 70(2):191–192

[146] Bless DM, Hicks DM. Diagnosis and measurement: assessing the "whs" of voice function. In: Brown W, Vinson B, Crary M, eds. Organic Voice Disorders Assessment and Treatment. San Diego, CA: Singular Publishing Group, Inc.; 1996:119–170

[147] Schutte HK, Seidner W. Recommendation by the Union of European Phoniatricians (UEP): standardizing voice area measurement/phonetography. Folia Phoniatr (Basel). 1983; 35(6):286–288

[148] Nicolosi L, Harryman E, Kresheck J. Terminology of Communication Disorders Speech-Language-Hearing. 3rd ed. Baltimore, MD: Williams & Williams; 1989

[149] Hunter EJ, Spielman J, Starr A. Acoustic Voice Recording, " I am seeking recommendations for voice recording hardware ....". SIG 3 Perspectives on Voice and Voice Disorders; 2007:66–70

[150] IEC 61672–1. Electroacoustics - Sound Level Meters - Part 1: Specifications. Vol. 2002. Geneva; 2002

[151] Gramming P, Sundberg J. Spectrum factors relevant to phonetogram measurement. J Acoust Soc Am. 1988; 83(6):2352–2360

[152] Kardous CA, Shaw PB. Evaluation of smartphone sound measurement applications. J Acoust Soc Am. 2014; 135(4):EL186–EL192

[153] Šrámková H, Granqvist S, Herbst CT, Švec JG. The softest sound levels of the human voice in normal subjects. The Journal of the Acoustical Society of America. 2015; 137(1):407–418

[154] Asplund A. How loud was it? A Calibration System for Voice Recording in Clinical and Research Applications. In 26th World Congress of the IALP, Brisbane, Australia; 2004:1–5. Available at: http://www.clinsci.umu.se/digital-Assets/50/50362_andersa0902.pdf. Accessed December 1, 2017

[155] Ryan WJ. Acoustic aspects of the aging voice. J Gerontol. 1972; 27 (2):265–268

[156] Awan SN, Mueller PB, Larson G, Summers P. Frequency and intensity measures of Black, White, and Hispanic kindergartners. Paper presented at the Texas Speech-Language-Hearing Association Convention. Houston, TX; 1991

[157] Morris RJ, Brown WS, Jr. Age-related differences in speech intensity among adult females. Folia Phoniatr Logop. 1994; 46(2):64–69

[158] Gauffin J, Sundberg J. Data on the glottal voice source behavior in vowel production. STL-QPSR. 1980; 21(2–3):61–70

[159] Hakkesteegt MM, Brocaar MP, Wieringa MH. The applicability of the dysphonia severity index and the voice handicap index in evaluating effects of voice therapy and phonosurgery. J Voice. 2010; 24(2):199–205

[160] Verdolini K. Voice disorders. In: Toblin J, Morris H, Spriestersbach D, eds. Diagnosis in Speech-Language Pathology. San Diego, CA: Singular Publishing Group; 1994:247–305

[161] Fisher KV, Swank PR. Estimating phonation threshold pressure. J Speech Lang Hear Res. 1997; 40(5):1122–1129

[162] Titze IR. Phonation threshold pressure: a missing link in glottal aerodynamics. J Acoust Soc Am. 1992; 91(5):2926–2935

[163] Ma E. Voice range profile: Phog. In: Ma E, Yui E, eds. Handbook of Voice Assessments. San Diego, CA: Plural Publishing Inc.; 2011

[164] Heylen L, Wuyts FL, Mertens F, et al. Evaluation of the vocal performance of children using a voice range profile index. J Speech Lang Hear Res. 1998; 41 (2):232–238

[165] Sapienza CM, Stathopoulos ET. Respiratory and laryngeal measures of children and women with bilateral vocal fold nodules. J Speech Hear Res. 1994; 37(6):1229–1243

[166] Böhme G, Stuchlik G. Voice profiles and standard voice profile of untrained children. J Voice. 1995; 9(3):304–307

[167] Komiyama S, Watanabe H, Ryu S. Phonographic relationship between pitch and intensity of the human voice. Folia Phoniatr (Basel). 1984; 36(1):1–7

[168] Aronson A. Clinical Voice Disorders. 2nd ed. New York: Thieme Medical Publishers; 1985

[169] Nordstrom PE. Female and infant vocal tracts simulated from male area functions. J Phonetics. 1977; 5:81–92

[170] Sundberg J. The Science of the Singing Voice. Illinois, IL: N. Illinois University Press; 1987

[171] Sapienza CM, Dutka J. Glottal airflow characteristics of women's voice production along an aging continuum. J Speech Hear Res. 1996; 39(2):322–328

[172] Maruthy S, Ravibabu P. Comparison of dysphonia severity index between younger and older Carnatic classical singers and nonsingers. J Voice. 2015; 29(1):65–70

[173] Teles-Magalhães LC, Pegoraro-Krook MI, Pegoraro R. Study of the elderly females' voice by phonetography. J Voice. 2000; 14(3):310–321

[174] Gregory ND, Chandran S, Lurie D, Sataloff RT. Voice disorders in the elderly. J Voice. 2012; 26(2):254–258

[175] Hakkesteegt MM, Brocaar MP, Wieringa MH, Feenstra L. Influence of age and gender on the dysphonia severity index. A study of normative values. Folia Phoniatr Logop. 2006; 58(4):264–273

[176] Ohno T, Hirano S, Rousseau B. Age-associated changes in the expression and deposition of vocal fold collagen and hyaluronan. Ann Otol Rhinol Laryngol. 2009; 118(10):735–741

[177] Huber JE, Spruill J, III. Age-related changes to speech breathing with increased vocal loudness. J Speech Lang Hear Res. 2008; 51(3):651–668

[178] Prater R, Swift R. Manual of Voice Therapy. Boston, MA: Little, Brown and Company; 1984

[179] Gould WJ, Okamura H. Proceedings: respiratory training of the singer. Folia Phoniatr (Basel). 1974; 26(4):275–286

[180] Hixon T, Hoffman C. Chest Wall Shape in Singing. Professional Voice; 1978:9–10

[181] Watson PJ, Hixon TJ. Respiratory kinematics in classical (opera) singers. J Speech Hear Res. 1985; 28(1):104–122

[182] Bouhuys A, Proctor DF, Mead J. Kinetic aspects of singing. J Appl Physiol. 1966; 21(2):483–496

[183] Bell Telephone Laboratories. High Speed Pictures of the Human Vocal Cords. New York: (Motion Picture) Bell Telephone Laboratories Bureau of Publications; 1940

[184] Large J, Baird E, Jenkins T. Studies of male high voice mechanisms. Journal Research Singing. 1980; 3:26–33

[185] Johansson C, Sundberg J, Willbrand H. X-ray study of articulation and formant frequencies in two male singers. Proceedings of the Stockholm Music Acoustics Conference, Stockholm: Royal Swedish Academy of Music; 1983:203–218

[186] Colton RH. Vocal intensity in the modal and falsetto registers. Folia Phoniatr (Basel). 1973; 25(1):62–70

[187] Hirano M. Objective evaluation of the human voice: clinical aspects. Folia Phoniatr (Basel). 1989; 41(2–3):89–144

[188] Hirano M, Mori K, Tanaka S, Fujita M. Vocal function in patients with unilateral vocal fold paralysis before and after silicone injection. Acta Otolaryngol. 1995; 115(4):553–559

[189] Haynes W, Pindzola R, Emerick L. Diagnosis and Evaluation in Speech Pathology. New York, NY: Simon & Schuster; 1992

[190] Denes P, Pinson E. The Speech Chain. New York, NY: Doubleday; 1973

[191] Rabinov CR, Kreiman J, Gerratt BR, Bielamowicz S. Comparing reliability of perceptual ratings of roughness and acoustic measure of jitter. J Speech Hear Res. 1995; 38(1):26–32

[192] Yumoto E, Sasaki Y, Okamura H. Harmonics-to-noise ratio and psychophysical measurement of the degree of hoarseness. J Speech Hear Res. 1984; 27 (1):2–6

[193] Kane M, Wellen CJ. Acoustical measurements and clinical judgments of vocal quality in children with vocal nodules. Folia Phoniatr (Basel). 1985; 37 (2):53–57

[194] Martin D, Fitch J, Wolfe V. Pathologic voice type and the acoustic prediction of severity. J Speech Hear Res. 1995; 38(4):765–771

[195] Takahashi H, Koike Y. Some perceptual dimensions and acoustical correlates of pathologic voices. Acta Otolaryngol Suppl. 1976; 338:1–24

[196] Wolfe VI, Steinfatt TM. Prediction of vocal severity within and across voice types. J Speech Hear Res. 1987; 30(2):230–240

[197] de Krom G. Consistency and reliability of voice quality ratings for different types of speech fragments. J Speech Hear Res. 1994; 37(5):985–1000

[198] Horii Y. Fundamental frequency perturbation observed in sustained phonation. J Speech Hear Res. 1979; 22(1):5–19

[199] Scherer RC, Vail VJ, Guo CG. Required number of tokens to determine representative voice perturbation values. J Speech Hear Res. 1995; 38 (6):1260–1269

[200] Gelfer MP, Fendel DM. Comparisons of jitter, shimmer, and signal-to-noise ratio from directly digitized versus taped voice samples. J Voice. 1995; 9 (4):378–382

[201] Horii Y. Vocal shimmer in sustained phonation. J Speech Hear Res. 1980; 23 (1):202–209

[202] Horii Y. Jitter and shimmer differences among sustained vowel phonations. J Speech Hear Res. 1982a; 25(1):12–14

[203] Glaze LE, Bless DM, Milenkovic P, Susser RD. Acoustic characteristics of children's voice. J Voice. 1988; 2(4):312–319

[204] Ludlow CL, Bassich CJ, Conner NP, Coulter DC, Lee YJ. The validity of using phonatory jitter and shimmer to detect laryngeal pathology. In: Baer T, Sasaki C, Harris K, eds. Laryngeal Function in Phonation and Respiration. Boston, MA: College-Hill Press; 1987:492–507

[205] Deem JF, Manning WH, Knack JV, Matesich JS. The automatic extraction of pitch perturbation using microcomputers: some methodological considerations. J Speech Hear Res. 1989; 32(3):689–697

[206] Karnell MP. Laryngeal perturbation analysis: minimum length of analysis window. J Speech Hear Res. 1991; 34(3):544–548

[207] Walton JH, Orlikoff RF. Speaker race identification from acoustic cues in the vocal signal. J Speech Hear Res. 1994; 37(4):738–745

[208] Dwire A, McCauley R. Repeated measures of vocal fundamental frequency perturbation obtained using the Visi-Pitch. J Voice. 1995; 9(2):156–162

[209] Gelfer MP. Fundamental frequency, intensity, and vowel selection: effects on measures of phonatory stability. J Speech Hear Res. 1995; 38(6):1189–1198

[210] Omori K, Kojima H, Kakani R, Slavit DH, Blaugrund SM. Acoustic characteristics of rough voice: subharmonics. J Voice. 1997; 11(1):40–47

[211] Banh J, Naumenko K, Goy H, Van Lieshout P, Fernandes DN, Pichora-fuller K. Establishing normative voice characteristics of younger and older adults. Can Acoust. 2009; 37(3):190–191

[212] Finger LS, Cielo CA, Schwarz K. Acoustic vocal measures in women without voice complaints and with normal larynxes. Rev Bras Otorrinolaringol (Engl Ed). 2009; 75(3):432–440

[213] Yumoto E. The quantitative evaluation of hoarseness: a new harmonics to noise ratio method. Arch Otolaryngol Head Neck Surg. 1983; 109(1):48–52

[214] Yumoto E. Quantitative assessment of the degree of hoarseness. J Voice. 1988; 1(4):310–313

[215] Yumoto E, Gould WJ, Baer T. Harmonics-to-noise ratio as an index of the degree of hoarseness. J Acoust Soc Am. 1982; 71(6):1544–1549

[216] Awan SN, Frenkel ML. Improvements in estimating the harmonics-to-noise ratio of the voice. J Voice. 1994; 8(3):255–262

[217] Eskenazi L, Childers DG, Hicks DM. Acoustic correlates of vocal quality. J Speech Hear Res. 1990; 33(2):298–306

[218] Gerratt BR, Kreiman J. Toward a taxonomy of nonmodal phonation. J Phonetics. 2001; 29(4):365–381

[219] Bailly L, Henrich N, Pelorson X. Vocal fold and ventricular fold vibration in period-doubling phonation: physiological description and aerodynamic modeling. J Acoust Soc Am. 2010; 127(5):3212–3222

[220] Titze I. Workshop on Acoustic Voice Analysis. Denver, CO: National Center for Voice. 1995:1–36

[221] Ferrand CT. Harmonics-to-noise ratios in normally speaking prepubescent girls and boys. J Voice. 2000; 14(1):17–21

[222] Lopes LW, Cavalcante DP, Costa PO. Severity of voice disorders: integration of perceptual and acoustic data in dysphonic patients. CoDAS. 2014; 26 (5):382–388

[223] Oates JM, Kirkby RJ. An acoustic investigation of voice quality disorders in children with vocal nodules. Australian Journal of Human Communication Disorders. 1980; 8(1):28–39

[224] Dejonckere PH, Wieneke GH, Bloemenkamp D, Lebacq J. Fo-perturbation and Fo/loudness dynamics in voices of normal children, with and without education in singing. Int J Pediatr Otorhinolaryngol. 1996; 35(2):107–115

[225] Milenkovic P. Least mean square measures of voice perturbation. J Speech Hear Res. 1987; 30(4):529–538

[226] Nittrouer S, McGowan RS, Milenkovic PH, Beehler D. Acoustic measurements of men's and women's voices: a study of context effects and covariation. J Speech Hear Res. 1990; 33(4):761–775

[227] Sussman JE, Sapienza C. Articulatory, developmental, and gender effects on measures of fundamental frequency and jitter. J Voice. 1994; 8(2):145–156

[228] Titze IR. Physiologic and acoustic differences between male and female voices. J Acoust Soc Am. 1989; 85(4):1699–1707

[229] Prakup B. Acoustic measures of the voices of older singers and nonsingers. J Voice. 2012; 26(3):341–350

[230] Vipperla R, Renals S, Frankel J. Ageing voices: the effect of changes in voice parameters on ASR performance. EURASIP J Audio Speech Music Process. 2010; 2010:10

[231] Wilcox KA, Horii Y. Age and changes in vocal jitter. J Gerontol. 1980; 35(2):194–198

[232] Winkler R, Sendlmeier W. EGG open quotient in aging voices–changes with increasing chronological age and its perception. Logoped Phoniatr Vocol. 2006; 31(2):51–56

[233] Awan SN, Roy N. Toward the development of an objective index of dysphonia severity: a four-factor acoustic model. Clin Linguist Phon. 2006; 20(1):35–49

[234] Shrivastav R, Sapienza CM. Objective measures of breathy voice quality obtained using an auditory model. J Acoust Soc Am. 2003; 114(4, Pt 1):2217–2224

[235] Hartl DA, Hans S, Vaissière J, Brasnu DA. Objective acoustic and aerodynamic measures of breathiness in paralytic dysphonia. Eur Arch Otorhinolaryngol. 2003; 260(4):175–182

[236] Awan SN, Roy N. Acoustic prediction of voice type in women with functional dysphonia. J Voice. 2005; 19(2):268–282

[237] Wolfe V, Fitch J, Martin D. Acoustic measures of dysphonic severity across and within voice types. Folia Phoniatr Logop. 1997; 49(6):292–299

[238] Wolfe V, Martin D. Acoustic correlates of dysphonia: type and severity. J Commun Disord. 1997; 30(5):403–415, quiz 415–416

[239] Milenkovic PH, Bless DM, Rammage LA. Acoustic and perceptual characterization of vocal nodules. In: Gauffin J, Hammarberg B, eds. Vocal Fold Physiology: acoustic, perceptual, and physiological aspects of voice mechanisms. San Diego, CA: Singular Publishing Group, Inc.; 1991:265–272

[240] Pruszewicz A, Obrebowski A, Swidziński P, Demeńko G, Wika T, Wojciechowska A. Usefulness of acoustic studies on the differential diagnostics of organic and functional dysphonia. Acta Otolaryngol. 1991; 111(2):414–419

[241] Karnell MP, Hall KD, Landahl KL. Comparison of fundamental frequency and perturbation measurements among three analysis systems. J Voice. 1995; 9(4):383–393

[242] Orlikoff RF, Kahane JC. Influence of mean sound pressure level on jitter and shimmer measures. J Voice. 1991; 5(2):113–119

[243] Hillenbrand J. A methodological study of perturbation and additive noise in synthetically generated voice signals. J Speech Hear Res. 1987; 30(4):448–461

[244] Awan SN, Roy N, Dromey C. Estimating dysphonia severity in continuous speech: application of a multi-parameter spectral/cepstral model. Clin Linguist Phon. 2009; 23(11):825–841

[245] Maryn Y, Corthals P, Van Cauwenberge P, Roy N, De Bodt M. Toward improved ecological validity in the acoustic measurement of overall voice quality: combining continuous speech and sustained vowels. J Voice. 2010; 24(5):540–555

[246] Laflen JB, Lazarus CL, Amin MR. Pitch deviation analysis of pathological voice in connected speech. Ann Otol Rhinol Laryngol. 2008; 117(2):90–97

[247] Eadie TL, Doyle PC. Classification of dysphonic voice: acoustic and auditory-perceptual measures. J Voice. 2005; 19(1):1–14

[248] Roy N, Gouse M, Mauszycki SC, Merrill RM, Smith ME. Task specificity in adductor spasmodic dysphonia versus muscle tension dysphonia. Laryngoscope. 2005; 115(2):311–316

[249] Yiu E, Worrall L, Longland J, Mitchell C. Analysing vocal quality of connected speech using Kay's computerized speech lab: a preliminary finding. Clin Linguist Phon. 2000; 14(4):295–305

[250] Qi Y, Hillman RE, Milstein C. The estimation of signal-to-noise ratio in continuous speech for disordered voices. J Acoust Soc Am. 1999; 105(4):2532–2535

[251] Parsa V, Jamieson DG. Acoustic discrimination of pathological voice: sustained vowels versus continuous speech. J Speech Lang Hear Res. 2001; 44(2):327–339

[252] Hammarberg B, Fritzell B, Gauffin J, Sundberg J, Wedin L. Perceptual and acoustic correlates of abnormal voice qualities. Acta Otolaryngol. 1980; 90(5–6):441–451

[253] Maryn Y, Roy N. Sustained vowels and continuous speech in the auditory-perceptual evaluation of dysphonia severity. J Soc Bras Fonoaudiol. 2012; 24(2):107–112

[254] Revis J, Giovanni A, Wuyts F, Triglia J. Comparison of different voice samples for perceptual analysis. Folia Phoniatr Logop. 1999; 51(3):108–116

[255] Zraick RI, Wendel K, Smith-Olinde L. The effect of speaking task on perceptual judgment of the severity of dysphonic voice. J Voice. 2005; 19(4):574–581

[256] Noll AM. Short time spectrum and "cepstrum" techniques for vocal pitch detection. J Acoust Soc Am. 1964; 36(2):296–302

[257] Hillenbrand J, Cleveland RA, Erickson RL. Acoustic correlates of breathy vocal quality. J Speech Hear Res. 1994; 37(4):769–778

[258] Hillenbrand J, Houde RA. Acoustic correlates of breathy vocal quality: dysphonic voices and continuous speech. J Speech Hear Res. 1996; 39(2):311–321

[259] Hartl DM, Hans S, Vaissière J, Riquet M, Brasnu DF. Objective voice quality analysis before and after onset of unilateral vocal fold paralysis. J Voice. 2001; 15(3):351–361

[260] Radish Kumar B, Bhat JS, Prasad N. Cepstral analysis of voice in persons with vocal nodules. J Voice. 2010; 24(6):651–653

[261] Shin YJ, Hong KH. Cepstral analysis of voice in patients with thyroidectomy. Clin Exp Otorhinolaryngol. 2016; 9(2):157–162

[262] Solomon NP, Awan SN, Helou LB, Stojadinovic A. Acoustic analyses of thyroidectomy-related changes in vowel phonation. J Voice. 2012; 26(6):711–720

[263] Wolfe VI, Martin DP, Palmer CI. Perception of dysphonic voice quality by naive listeners. J Speech Lang Hear Res. 2000; 43(3):697–705

[264] Awan SN, Helou LB, Stojadinovic A, Solomon NP. Tracking voice change after thyroidectomy: application of spectral/cepstral analyses. Clin Linguist Phon. 2011; 25(4):302–320

[265] Balasubramanium RK, Bhat JS, Fahim S, III, Raju R, III. Cepstral analysis of voice in unilateral adductor vocal fold palsy. J Voice. 2011; 25(3):326–329

[266] Gaskill CS, Awan JA, Watts CR, Awan SN. Acoustic and perceptual classification of within-sample normal, intermittently dysphonic, and consistently dysphonic voice types. J Voice. 2017; 31(2):218–228

[267] Lowell SY, Colton RH, Kelley RT, Mizia SA. Predictive value and discriminant capacity of cepstral- and spectral-based measures during continuous speech. J Voice. 2013; 27(4):393–400

[268] Lowell SY, Kelley RT, Awan SN, Colton RH, Chan NH. Spectral- and cepstral-based acoustic features of dysphonic, strained voice quality. Ann Otol Rhinol Laryngol. 2012; 121(8):539–548

[269] Rosenthal AL, Lowell SY, Colton RH. Aerodynamic and acoustic features of vocal effort. J Voice. 2014; 28(2):144–153

[270] Watts CR, Awan SN. Use of spectral/cepstral analyses for differentiating normal from hypofunctional voices in sustained vowel and continuous speech contexts. J Speech Lang Hear Res. 2011; 54(6):1525–1537

[271] Halberstam B. Acoustic and perceptual parameters relating to connected speech are more reliable measures of hoarseness than parameters relating to sustained vowels. ORL J Otorhinolaryngol Relat Spec. 2004; 66(2):70–73

[272] Lowell SY, Colton RH, Kelley RT, Hahn YC. Spectral- and cepstral-based measures during continuous speech: capacity to distinguish dysphonia and consistency within a speaker. J Voice. 2011; 25(5):e223–e232

[273] Heman-Ackah Y, Heuer R, Michael D, et al. Cepstral peak prominence: a more reliable measure of dysphonia. Ann Otol Rhinol Laryngol 2003:112(4):324–333

[274] Heman-Ackah YD, Michael DD, Goding GS, Jr. The relationship between cepstral peak prominence and selected parameters of dysphonia. J Voice. 2002; 16(1):20–27

[275] Awan S. Analysis of Dysphonia in Speech and Voice (ADSV): An Application Guide. Montvale, NJ: Pentax Medical, Inc.; 2011

[276] Awan SN, Roy N. Outcomes measurement in voice disorders: application of an acoustic index of dysphonia severity. J Speech Lang Hear Res. 2009; 52(2):482–499

[277] Awan SN, Roy N, Zhang D, Cohen SM. Validation of the Cepstral Spectral Index of Dysphonia (CSID) as a screening tool for voice disorders: development of clinical cutoff scores. J Voice. 2016; 30(2):130–144

[278] Heman-Ackah YD, Sataloff RT, Laureyns G, et al. Quantifying the cepstral peak prominence, a measure of dysphonia. J Voice. 2014; 28(6):783–788

[279] Maryn Y, Roy N, De Bodt M, Van Cauwenberge P, Corthals P. Acoustic measurement of overall voice quality: a meta-analysis. J Acoust Soc Am. 2009; 126(5):2619–2634

[280] Jannetts S, Lowit A. Cepstral analysis of hypokinetic and ataxic voices: correlations with perceptual and other acoustic measures. J Voice. 2014; 28(6):673–680

[281] Roy N, Mazin A, Awan SN. Automated acoustic analysis of task dependency in adductor spasmodic dysphonia versus muscle tension dysphonia. Laryngoscope. 2014; 124(3):718–724

[282] Carson C, Ryalls J, Hardin-Hollingsworth K, Le Normand M-TT, Ruddy B. Acoustic analyses of prolonged vowels in young adults with Friedreich ataxia. J Voice. 2016; 30(3):272–280

[283] Gillespie AI, Dastolfo C, Magid N, Gartner-Schmidt J. Acoustic analysis of four common voice diagnoses: moving toward disorder-specific assessment. J Voice. 2014; 28(5):582–588

[284] Maryn Y, Dick C, Vandenbruaene C, Vauterin T, Jacobs T. Spectral, cepstral, and multivariate exploration of tracheoesophageal voice quality in continuous speech and sustained vowels. Laryngoscope. 2009; 119(12):2384–2394

[285] Awan SN, Giovinco A, Owens J. Effects of vocal intensity and vowel type on cepstral analysis of voice. J Voice. 2012; 26(5):670.e15–670.e20

[286] Barsties B, Verfaillie R, Roy N, Maryn Y. Do body mass index and fat volume influence vocal quality, phonatory range, and aerodynamics in females? CoDAS. 2013; 25(4):310–318

[287] Diercks GR, Ojha S, Infusino S, Maurer R, Hartnick CJ. Consistency of voice frequency and perturbation measures in children using cepstral analyses: a movement toward increased recording stability. JAMA Otolaryngol Head Neck Surg. 2013; 139(8):811–816

[288] Watts CR, Ronshaugen R, Saenz D. The effect of age and vocal task on cepstral/spectral measures of vocal function in adult males. Clin Linguist Phon. 2015; 29(6):415–423

[289] Watts CR. The effect of CAPE-V sentences on cepstral/spectral acoustic measures in dysphonic speakers. Folia Phoniatr Logop. 2015; 67(1):15–20

[290] Shim H, Jung H, Koul R, Ko D. Spectral and cepstral based acoustic features of voices with muscle tension dysphonia. Clin Archives Commun Disord. 2016; 1(1):42–47

[291] Watts CR, Awan SN, Maryn Y. A comparison of cepstral peak prominence measures from two acoustic analysis programs. J Voice. 2017; 31(3):387.e1–387.e10

[292] Watts CR, Awan SN. An examination of variations in the cepstral spectral index of dysphonia across a single breath group in connected speech. J Voice. 2015; 29(1):26–34

[293] Klich RJ. Relationships of vowel characteristics to listener ratings of breathiness. J Speech Hear Res. 1982; 25(4):574–580

[294] Awan SN, Solomon NP, Helou LB, Stojadinovic A. Spectral-cepstral estimation of dysphonia severity: external validation. Ann Otol Rhinol Laryngol. 2013; 122(1):40–48

[295] Peterson EA, Roy N, Awan SN, Merrill RM, Banks R, Tanner K. Toward validation of the cepstral spectral index of dysphonia (CSID) as an objective treatment outcomes measure. J Voice. 2013; 27(4):401–410

[296] Maryn Y, Weenink D. Objective dysphonia measures in the program Praat: smoothed cepstral peak prominence and acoustic voice quality index. J Voice. 2015; 29(1):35–43

[297] Reynolds V, Buckland A, Bailey J, et al. Objective assessment of pediatric voice disorders with the acoustic voice quality index. J Voice. 2012; 26(5):672.e1–672.e7

[298] Barsties B, Maryn Y. The Acoustic Voice Quality Index. Toward expanded measurement of dysphonia severity in German subjects [in German]. HNO. 2012; 60(8):715–720

[299] Maryn Y, De Bodt M, Barsties B, Roy N. The value of the acoustic voice quality index as a measure of dysphonia severity in subjects speaking different languages. Eur Arch Otorhinolaryngol. 2014; 271(6):1609–1619

[300] Ulozaitė N, Petrauskas J, Šaferis V, Uloza V. Correlations between automated dysphonia quantification and perceptual voice evaluation. In: Conference "Biomedical Engineering" Correlations. Lithuanian University of Health Sciences, Kaunas, Lithuania; 2017:147–152

[301] Pedersen M, Alexius Agersted A, Jonsson A. Aspects of adolescence and voice: girls versus boys:a review. J Child Adolesc Behav. 2015; 3(3):3–5

[302] Pedersen M, Moller S, Bennett P. Voice characteristics compared with phonetograms, androgens, oestrogens and puberty stages in 8–19 year old choir girls. J Res Singing Applied Vocal Pedagogy. 1990; 13:1–10

[303] Verdonck-de Leeuw IM, Mahieu HF. Vocal aging and the impact on daily life: a longitudinal study. J Voice. 2004; 18(2):193–202

[304] Coleman RF, Mabis JH, Hinson JK. Fundamental frequency-sound pressure level profiles of adult male and female voices. J Speech Hear Res. 1977; 20(2):197–204

[305] Leborgne WD. Clinical applications and use of the voice range profile. SIG 3 Perspectives on Voice and Voice Disorders 2007;(November):18–24

[306] Speyer R, Wieneke GH, van Wijck-Warnaar I, Dejonckere PH. Effects of voice therapy on the voice range profiles of dysphonic patients. J Voice. 2003; 17(4):544–556

[307] Damsté PH. The phonetogram. Pract Otorhinolaryngol (Basel). 1970; 32(3):185–187

[308] Coleman RF. Sources of variation in phonetograms. J Voice. 1993; 7(1):1–14

[309] Colton RH, Casper JK, Leonard R. Understanding Voice Problems. 3rd ed. Philadelphia, PA: Lippincott Williams & Wilkins; 2006

[310] Andrews M. Manual of Voice Treatment: Pediatrics through Geriatrics. 3rd ed. Clifton Park, NJ: Thompson Delmar Learning; 2006

[311] Hakkesteegt MM, Wieringa MH, Brocaar MP, Mulder PGH, Feenstra L. The interobserver and test-retest variability of the dysphonia severity index. Folia Phoniatr Logop. 2008; 60(2):86–90

[312] Awan SN, Ensslen AJ. A comparison of trained and untrained vocalists on the Dysphonia Severity Index. J Voice. 2010; 24(6):661–666

[313] Awan SN. The effect of smoking on the dysphonia severity index in females. Folia Phoniatr Logop. 2011; 63(2):65–71

[314] Awan SN, Miesemer SA, Nicolia TA. An examination of intrasubject variability on the Dysphonia Severity Index. J Voice. 2012; 26(6):814.e21–814.e25

[315] Hakkesteegt MM, Brocaar MP, Wieringa MH, Feenstra L. The relationship between perceptual evaluation and objective multiparametric evaluation of dysphonia severity. J Voice. 2008; 22(2):138–145

[316] Hussein Gaber AG, Liang F-Y, Yang J-S, Wang Y-J, Zheng Y-Q. Correlation among the dysphonia severity index (DSI), the RBH voice perceptual evaluation, and minimum glottal area in female patients with vocal fold nodules. J Voice. 2014; 28(1):20–23

[317] Uloza V, Vegienė A, Saferis V. Correlation between the basic video laryngostroboscopic parameters and multidimensional voice measurements. J Voice. 2013; 27(6):744–752

[318] Woisard V, Bodin S, Yardeni E, Puech M. The voice handicap index: correlation between subjective patient response and quantitative assessment of voice. J Voice. 2007; 21(5):623–631

[319] Timmermans B, De Bodt MS, Wuyts FL, Van de Heyning PH. Analysis and evaluation of a voice-training program in future professional voice users. J Voice. 2005; 19(2):202–210

[320] Timmermans B, De Bodt M, Wuyts F, Van de Heyning P. Voice quality change in future professional voice users after 9 months of voice training. Eur Arch Otorhinolaryngol. 2004; 261(1):1–5

[321] Boominathan P, Samuel J, Nallamuthu A, Mahalingam S, Dinesh Babu M. Voice characteristics of elderly college teachers: a pilot study. Journal of Laryngology and Voice. 2012; 2(1):21–25

[322] Uchanski RM, Geers AE. Acoustic characteristics of the speech of young cochlear implant users: a comparison with normal-hearing age-mates. Ear Hear. 2003; 24(1) Suppl:90S–105S

[323] Jayakumar T, Savithri SR. Effect of geographical and ethnic variation on Dysphonia Severity Index: a study of Indian population. J Voice. 2012; 26(1):e11–e16

[324] Gnanavel K, Satish HV, Pushpavathi M. Dysphonia Severity Index in children with velopharyngeal dysfunction: a pre-post operative comparison. Innovative J Med Health Sci. 2013; 3:268–273

[325] Henry LR, Helou LB, Solomon NP, et al. . Functional voice outcomes after thyroidectomy: an assessment of the Dysphonia Severity Index (DSI) after thyroidectomy. Surgery. 2010; 147 6:861–870

[326] Aichinger P, Feichter F, Aichstill B, Bigenzahn W, Schneider-Stickler B. Interdevice reliability of DSI measurement. Logoped Phoniatr Vocol. 2012; 37(4):167–173

[327] Peters R, Smith B, Hollins M. Acoustics and Noise Control. 3rd ed. New York: Taylor & Francis; 2013

Suggested Reading

[1] Glaze LE, Bless DM, Milenkovic P, Susser RD. Acoustic characteristics of children's voice. J Voice. 1988; 2(4):312–319

[2] Ma E. Voice range profile: Phog. In: Ma E, Yui E, eds. Handbook of Voice Assessments. San Diego, CA: Plural Publishing Inc.; 2011

[3] Maryn Y, Weenink D. Objective dysphonia measures in the program Praat: smoothed cepstral peak prominence and acoustic voice quality index. J Voice. 2015; 29(1):35–43

[4] Watts CR. The effect of CAPE-V sentences on cepstral/spectral acoustic measures in dysphonic speakers. Folia Phoniatr Logop. 2015; 67(1):15–20

5 Aerodynamic Analyses of Vocal Function

Summary

This chapter describes the processes of aerodynamic analyses as they relate to the clinical evaluation of voice disorders. Aerodynamic properties of subglottal pressure, transglottal airflow, lung capacity, and different measures of phonation efficiency are explained. The physical principles underlying aerodynamic characteristics of phonation are clarified, in addition to the interpretation and clinical application of aerodynamic measurements. The clinical characteristics of aerodynamic measurements in various disordered populations are also explained.

Keywords: subglottal pressure, transglottal airflow, glottal insufficiency, phonation efficiency

5.1 Learning Objectives

At the end of this chapter, readers will be able to
- Compare and contrast clinical aerodynamic measurements of subglottal pressure and transglottal airflow in different clinical populations, including speakers with dysphonia due to hyperfunction or hypofunction.
- Describe measurements of lung capacity and phonation efficiency and their application to the clinical voice evaluation.
- Identify methodological variables which can influence aerodynamic measurements, and different ways to control those variables.
- Describe appropriate reporting methods for clinical aerodynamic measurements.

5.2 Introduction

In Chapter 1, we defined phonation as the aerodynamic and muscular influences acting on the tissue of the vocal folds, setting them into vibration and creating acoustic energy that we call "voice." In the context of clinical voice science, the word "aerodynamic" refers to the physical properties of the air stream which act on the vocal fold tissue to drive phonation. When a voice is perceived as dysphonic, the underlying aerodynamic forces driving phonation are typically altered. Aerodynamic assessments of vocal function have a historic and robust research base supporting their use as a clinical modality and have been recommended as a standard component of voice assessment.[1]

Objective measurement of aerodynamic forces driving phonation, which can include one or more parameters of **volume**, **flow**, **pressure**, and/or **vocal efficiency**. These measures provide valuable clinical evidence which, when combined with the knowledge and skill of the speech–language pathologist, can facilitate important clinical processes including[2]
- Impairment detection.
  - Aerodynamic assessments allow clinicians to measure respiratory function, laryngeal function, respiratory–laryngeal coordination, and whether impairment exists in any of those three domains.

- Objective characterization (measurement) of an impairment.
  - Aerodynamic assessments allow clinicians to objectively quantify physiological substrates of phonation.
- Support the process of differential diagnosis.
  - Aerodynamic assessments can elucidate the underlying physiological causes of dysphonia, providing evidence that informs differential diagnosis.
- Provide a modality for biofeedback during voice treatment.
  - Aerodynamic assessments are simple to employ as part of the clinical process and can serve as a visual biofeedback tool.
- Provide objective measurement of clinical outcome.
  - Aerodynamic assessments can be repeated over time to objectively measure changes in phonation physiology subsequent to voice treatment.

In clinical contexts, *volume and flow* have been measured using direct or indirect estimates of (**1**) vital capacity, (**2**) phonation volume, (**3**) average and peak flow rates, and the ratio of vital capacity to MPT, called (**4**) phonation quotient.[1,3,4,5,6] Estimates of *subglottal pressure* may be measured during habitual pitch and loudness phonation or during soft phonation—when measured during soft/quiet phonation, the measure of subglottal pressure is referred to as phonation threshold pressure.[7,8] Clinical measurement of *vocal efficiency* has included glottal efficiency, laryngeal resistance, maximum phonation time (MPT), and s/z ratio.[1,9,10,11] Advantages and limitations exist for all aerodynamic measures, and to date no individual or set of aerodynamic measures has been demonstrated to be clinically more important or more cost-effective than others. Definitions for the more commonly applied aerodynamic measures are given in ▸ Table 5.1.

5.3 Aerodynamics and Phonation

Voice production is accomplished by converting aerodynamic energy (pressure and flow) into acoustic energy (sound). The aerodynamic energy of voice production originates from differential pressures between the lower vocal tract (lungs and trachea) and upper vocal tract (larynx and supraglottal spaces), resulting in airflow. The larynx acts as a valve that applies varying degrees of resistance to this airflow. Pressure, airflow, and resistance are related to each other. This relationship can be described by applying Ohm's law to fluids (air can be thought of as a type of fluid), as expressed in the formula $U = P/R$, where U = flow, P = pressure, and R = resistance.[7] As you can deduce, increasing or decreasing the value of any one variable on the right side of this equation will influence the result of the equation on the left. As an example, when resistance to the expiratory airstream is low (e.g., in hypofunction), airflow will tend to be increased—we typically perceive a voice produced with increased airflow as breathy. In contrast, if resistance is increased (as in hyperfunctional voice types), airflow will tend to be decreased—we typically perceive this type of voice production as strained. In phonation, airflow may be influenced by modulating pressures below, within, and above the glottis through varying degrees of resistance at the level of the larynx and supraglottal spaces.

Table 5.1 Common clinical aerodynamic measures obtained during the process of voice evaluation

Domain	Measurement	Definition
Pressure	Mean subglottal pressure (Ps)	The average (over time) tracheal air pressure immediately below the vocal folds which initiates and maintains oscillation. Measured in cm H2O
	Peak subglottal pressure (Ps)	The peak subglottal pressure from a narrow (in milliseconds) analysis window within a larger temporal frame (total selected analysis range). Measured in cm H2O
	Phonation threshold pressure (PtP)	The minimum Ps required to oscillate the vocal folds. Measured in cm H2O
Flow	Mean transglottal airflow rate (MTAR)	The average volume of air flowing through the glottis over a specific period of time. Measured in **L/s** or **mL/s**
	Peak transglottal airflow rate (PTAR)	The peak flow rate from a narrow (in milliseconds) analysis window within a larger temporal frame (total selected analysis range). Peak flow is greatest at the release of the plosive preceding onset of the vowel. Measured in **L/s** or **mL/s**
	Phonation quotient (PQ)	An estimate of transglottal airflow. The ratio of vital capacity to maximum phonation time (VC/MPT). Measured in **mL/s**
	Estimated mean flow rate (EMFR)	A regression corrected estimate of mean transglottal airflow rate as derived from phonation quotient, in the formula: $EMFR = 77 + 0.236 \, (PQ)$. Measured in **mL/s**
Volume	Vital capacity (VC)	The quantity of air that can be exhaled from the lungs following as deep an inhalation as possible. Measured in **L or mL**
	Phonation volume	The quantity of air that can be exhaled from the lungs while voicing (e.g., sustained vowel) following as deep an inhalation as possible. Measured in **L or mL**
Efficiency	S/Z ratio	An estimate of aerodynamic efficiency. The ratio of maximum phonation time for /s/ to maximum phonation time for /z/. Measured in **seconds**
	Glottal efficiency	Measured with different formulas depending on published source. One example is the ratio of acoustic power (e.g., in dB) to aerodynamic power (e.g., $P_s \times$ airflow rate)
	Laryngeal resistance	An indicator of the degree of resistance applied to the air supply by the vocal folds. The ratio of P_s to airflow (Ps/flow), measured in **cm H_2O / mL/s**
	Maximum phonation time (MPT)	The maximum duration of sustained vowel production following as deep an inhalation as possible. Measured in **seconds**

In **Table 1.5**, we have listed a number of aerodynamic parameters that drive vocal fold oscillation during phonation. Among these include **subglottal pressure** and **transglottal airflow**, which along with assessments of **lung capacity** and **vocal efficiency** constitute the primary clinical aerodynamic measurements obtained to identify, characterize, and differentially diagnose respiratory and laryngeal impairments underlying voice disorders. A number of physical impairments can cause inefficiencies or ineffectiveness of phonation and the accompanying aerodynamic characteristics. Impairments that result in measurable changes to aerodynamic forces in phonation include, among other things:

- Restricted lung capacity due to disease or muscular weakness.
- Hypokinesia or hyperkinesia of the respiratory and/or intrinsic laryngeal muscles resulting from neurological or functional etiologies.
- Lesions affecting the vocal fold tissue.
- Ineffective posturing of the supraglottal structures and spaces.

These conditions may result in ineffective respiratory support for phonation, altered vibratory dynamics creating irregularities and inefficiencies in vocal fold oscillation, or both. In addition to altered aerodynamic measurements, clinical signs and symptoms related to these impairments include

- Short phrase lengths (few words in one breath).
- Fatigue with prolonged speaking.
- Perceptions of excessive effort when speaking.
- Dysphonia.

5.4 Lung Capacity

Lung capacity refers to **quantities of air exchanged within the lungs during respiration**. The most common lung capacity measurement used in clinical voice practice is **vital capacity** (VC), a measurement used to assess the lung capacity available to support phonation during connected speech. Specifically, VC is defined as the **maximum quantity of air that can be exhaled after a maximum inhalation**—its relationship with other lung capacity measurements is illustrated in ► Fig. 5.1. VC is typically measured using **spirometry** and reported in either liters (L) or milliliters (mL). While high-tech spirometry systems with exceedingly accurate measurement precision are available to measure VC, acceptable measurements of VC are also easily obtained from low-tech and inexpensive hand-held spirometers.

Within the context of phonation, the lungs can be thought of as a gas tank and the air that fills them as the gasoline which drives the engine—the vocal folds. Phonation will occur only as long as air is available to support the process, just as a car engine will only operate as long as gas is available to power it. That is to say, respiratory support is critical for phonation, and measures of VC are one method of quantifying this support.

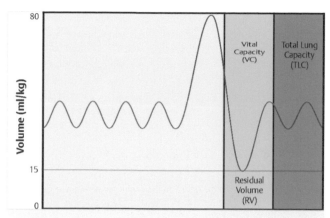

Fig. 5.1 The relationship of vital capacity with other lung capacity measurements. The waveform trace shows four comfortable (tidal) breaths followed by a maximum inhalation and exhalation and return to tidal breaths.

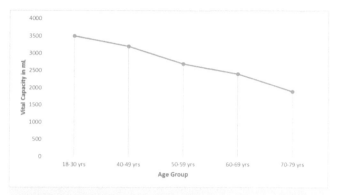

Fig. 5.2 Mean vital capacity of nondysphonic, healthy women between 18 and 79 years old. Significant differences were found between those younger than and older than 50 years, with a strong negative correlation of VC to age. (data from Awan SN. The aging female voice: Acoustic and respiratory data, Clinical Linguistics 2009; 20:2-3, 171-180, DOI: 10.1080/02699200400026918)

While it would be extremely rare that the entire vital capacity would be used during a single sustained vowel or continuous speech utterance, initiating speech/voice with a limited respiratory capacity can lead to undesirable imbalances in phonatory function, vocal effort, and eventual fatigue. As an example, initiating voice with a very low driving capacity often leads to compensatory hyperfunction as a means of conserving air and may lead to fatigue and impaired voice characteristics as the day progresses. Awan has suggested that VC, as a measure of maximum performance, provides evidence that informs the clinician of a speaker's potential ability to produce voice in physically stressful conditions (e.g., extended durations of phonation in connected speech).[6] When combined with measurements of pressure, flow, and phonation efficiency, assessment of VC allows the clinician to rule in or out underlying respiratory etiologies related to a voice disorder. It is typically a good idea to measure VC when dysphonia is present, as respiratory muscle incoordination, weakness, or restricted lung capacity can be contributing factors or underlying causes of voice impairments.

Calculation of VC using commercially available hand-held spirometers is a simple and efficient process. A typical method is described later. This method of eliciting and measuring VC is a form of expiratory vital capacity and has been referred to as **slow vital capacity**, which *does not* require a patient to blow out as forcibly and quickly as possible (forced exhalation is a method of obtaining VC known as "forced vital capacity"—unless a patient suffers from an obstructive lung disease, slow and forced vital capacity are typically very similar).[12]

5.4.1 Measuring Vital Capacity with a Hand-Held Spirometer

- Calibrate the spirometer as per manufacturer's specifications or using a known volume of air.
- Attach a new flow tube onto the spirometer.
- Place a nose clip on the speaker's nares.
- Instruct the speaker as follows: *"Take two comfortable breaths, inhaling and exhaling. On the third breath, inhale as deeply as you can, place your mouth and lips completely around the flow tube, and exhale forcefully into the tube. Keep exhaling until you completely run out of air."*
  - Some speakers will need coaching or encouragement during the performance of this task in order to elicit a true maximum performance.
  - The clinician should make sure the speaker's lips are sealed around the flow tube and that air does not leak around the tube during the task.

A number of factors can influence measures of VC, including the speaker's sex, age, body mass, and height. These factors have been accounted for in equations which can be used to estimate VC in a normal, healthy speaker against which a patient's VC can be compared. Many different reference formulas have been generated based on various population samples. As an example, the following formulas have been used as estimates of predicted VC and referenced in a number of publications associated with voice production[13]:

- **VC (mL) Males**: [27.63 - (0.112 × Age)] × Height (cm).
- **VC (mL) Females**: [27.78 - (0.101 × Age)] × Height (cm).

Why Are Measures of Vital Capacity Sensitive to Respiratory Changes/Impairments?

Respiration requires muscular action to modify lung volumes. Therefore, any condition that causes weakness in the respiratory muscles (e.g., amyotrophic lateral sclerosis, Parkinson's disease) or restricts lung expansion for respiration (e.g., radiation fibrosis) has the potential to affect measures of VC. In all cases, the clinical effect is lowering of VC. Measures of VC also typically decrease with advancing age.[14,15] ▶ Fig. 5.2 illustrates data from an investigation demonstrating that VC in healthy females was significantly greater for those below 50 years compared to those older than 50 years.[15] Thus, clinical measures of VC from dysphonic patients must be considered within the context of biological factors associated with an individual's overall health, age, sex, and height.

It is important to also consider additional sources of variability in clinical measurements of VC. The American Thoracic Society identified at least three sources impacting lung function measurements, including normal biological sources of variation, the presence of disease states, and variability associated with technique or methodology.[16] Within this technical category includes the instrument (spirometer) you will be using and the instructions that you give to a patient. As with methods for acoustic analyses and other aerodynamic measurements; *it is crucial that clinicians develop consistent procedures*, including consistency of equipment used, when measuring and comparing VC within and between patients.

▶ Table 5.2 shows VC measurements from a selection of published studies. Inspection of this table suggests that healthy, young adult male and female speakers typically produce measures of VC within a **range of 3 to 5 L**, with males exhibiting greater measures of VC than females. With advancing age, VC tends to

lower such that measures may be recorded below 3 L for healthy adults older than 65 years. In addition, it should be expected that young children would exhibit much lower VC than adults due to inherently smaller lung structure and available volume.

5.5 Subglottal Pressure

In physics, pressure (P) is defined as the ratio of force applied over a given area, as in the formula: $P = F/A$ (where P = pressure, F = force, and A = area). A common unit of measurement for P is the pascal, although in voice science and clinical voice practice pressure is most often measured in **centimeters of water** (**cm H_2O**; 1 cm H_2O = 98.06 pascals). **Subglottal pressure** can be understood as the tracheal air pressure immediately below the glottis that acts

Table 5.2 Vital capacity from selected published studies reporting data in healthy populations

Authors	Gender	No. of patients	Age range (x)	VC mean (SD)	VC range
[1]Backman et al[17]	M	257	20–84 (47.0)	5.45 (0.94)	N/A
	F	244	20–84 (49.0)	3.73 (0.81)	
[2]Weinrich et al[18]	M	10	6–9 (7.9)	1.82 (0.61)	0.85–3.00
	M	10	10–13 (11.8)	2.25 (0.51)	1.62–3.12
	M	10	14–17 (16.0)	3.60 (1.19)	2.31–6.50
	F	10	6–9 (8.3)	1.57 (0.36)	0.89–1.94
	F	10	10–13 (12.5)	1.98 (0.43)	1.08–2.64
	F	10	14–17 (15.4)	2.77 (0.56)	1.88–3.61
[3]Barsties et al[19]	F	29	17–31 (21.4)	3.30 (0.376)	N/A
[4]Zraick et al[11]	M	32	18–30 (30.6)	4.14 (1.14)	2.10–6.66
	M	19	40–59 (48.6)	4.19 (1.01)	2.11–5.78
	M	18	60–89 (74.1)	3.09 (1.00)	1.15–5.03
	F	47	18–30 (28.8)	2.87 (0.69)	1.02–4.60
	F	22	40–59 (49.6)	2.85 (0.78)	1.33–4.30
	F	20	60–89 (72.9)	2.09 (0.63)	1.14–3.36
[5]Tan et al[20]	M	395	20–44	5.37 (0.77)	N/A
	M	334	40–90	4.82 (0.87)	
	F	417	20–44	3.92 (0.58)	
	F	510	40–90	3.32 (0.71)	
[6]Smolej Narancić et al[21]	M	107	65–86 (71.3)	3.32 (0.64)	2.03–5.14
	F	154	65–86 (71.6)	2.21 (0.46)	1.32–4.03
[7]Piccioni et al[22]	M	509	3–6	1.09 (0.23)	N/A
	F	450	3–6		
[8]Pistelli et al[23]	M	196	8–97 (27.0)	4.78 (1.24)	1.66–7.77
	F	301	8–97 (37.0)	3.48 (0.66)	1.43–5.40
[9]Pistelli et al[24]	M	225	8–64 (18.0)	4.05 (1.28)	N/A
	F	420	8–63 (30.6)	3.36 (0.65)	
[10]Baltopoulos et al[25]	M	38	61–84 (72)	3.24 (0.54)	2.02–4.31
	F	33	61–84 (68)	2.13 (0.33)	1.35–2.64

Notes: All units in liters and from comfortable or forced vital capacity, unless otherwise noted. Standard deviations associated with means and data ranges are noted when reported. For detailed breakdown of VC by age ranges, height, and/or body mass see references studies.
1. **Participants**: Normal Swedish adults; **Spirometer**: Jaeger Masterscope.
2. **Participants**: Normal American children; **Spirometer**: Pentax MEDICAL Phonatory Aerodynamic System.
3. **Participants**: Normal German adult females; **Spirometer**: not reported.
4. **Participants**: Normal American adults; **Spirometer**: Pentax MEDICAL Phonatory Aerodynamic System.
5. **Participants**: Normal Canadian adults; **Spirometer**: Spirotech rolling-seal spirometer.
6. **Participants**: Normal Croatian elderly adults; **Spirometer**: Jager's Pneumoscreen.
7. **Participants**: Normal Italian children; **Spirometer**: Masterscope Rotary Jaeger.
8. **Participants**: Normal Italian adults; **Spirometer**: Biomedin water-sealed spirometer.
9. **Participants**: Normal Italian adults; **Spirometer**: 47804/s Pulmonary System Fleisch pneumotachograph.
10. **Participants**: Normal Greek elderly adults; **Spirometer**: Micro Spiro Hi-298.

as a force distributed over the inferior surface of the vocal folds (▶ Fig. 5.3). This pressure is responsible for initiating oscillation, is the primary determinant of vocal intensity, and plays an important role in sustained oscillation during phonation. It acts on vocal fold tissue during volitional or involuntary voice production, coughing, and other laryngeal behaviors.

During phonation, subglottal pressure (which we will identify by the symbol P_s) is the aerodynamic force that sets vocal folds into motion once they have been approximated or completely adducted by the intrinsic laryngeal muscles. It does this by separating the lower vocal fold edges, allowing a pressurized pulse of air to flow through the glottis at high velocity. As long as respiratory muscles continue to send air from the lungs and the vocal folds are maintained in the adducted position, P_s will continue to build/release during the closed and opening phases of vocal fold vibration, respectively, and continue to modulate

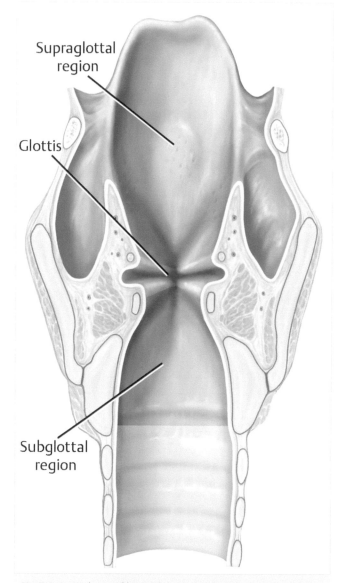

Supraglottal region

Glottis

Subglottal region

Fig. 5.3 Sagittal view of larynx showing location of subglottal pressure forces that act on the vocal fold tissue. (From Schuenke M et al. Thieme Atlas of Anatomy: Head, Neck and Neuroanatomy, Volume 3, 2nd edition. Thieme Publishers: New York, 2016.)

pressure differentials below, above, and within the vocal fold tissue to sustain oscillation.

While P_s can be measured directly by inserting a probe into the trachea below the vocal folds or indirectly by measuring pressure in the esophagus, contemporary clinical applications utilize less invasive and more efficient techniques that provide indirect measures of P_s. **This can be accomplished by measuring intraoral (oral cavity) pressure during the production of unvoiced plosive-vowel syllable trains, such as /pa-pa-pa/ or /pi-pi-pi/.**[26] This is achieved by either inserting a plastic or rubber tube between the lips into the oral cavity connected in line with a pressure transducer (outside the oral cavity), or by routing the intraoral pressure tube through a facemask that is held firmly against the face (examples of masks used in measurement of intraoral pressure are illustrated in ▶ Fig. 5.4).[27] Syllable trains are produced with equal stress, on a single breath, at habitual pitch and loudness. When produced with adequate velopharyngeal and lip seals, it has been demonstrated that peak intraoral pressure measured from the stop-plosive immediately preceding a vowel is a good estimate of the subglottal pressure used during vowel production in speech.[28] This phenomenon can be explained by the fact that, when produced with a sealed supraglottal cavity, the pressure in the vocal tract equalizes from behind the point of articulatory obstruction continuing through the trachea and lungs. Therefore, the peak intraoral pressure measured during /p/ will be the same amount of pressure used to initiate vocal fold oscillation at voicing onset of the subsequent vowel.

Clinical measurements of P_s are typically acquired while a speaker is producing sound at a comfortable or "habitual" F_o and intensity during syllable productions. However, it has also been observed that measuring P_s while a speaker is producing voice at his or her *lowest possible intensity* (e.g., as soft as possible without whispering) is very sensitive to the presence of vocal fold impairments.[29,30] This measurement is called **phonation threshold pressure** (PtP), and can be defined as the **minimum amount of air pressure required to set the vocal**

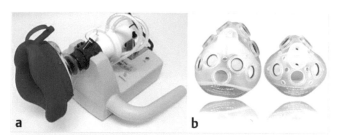

a   b

Fig. 5.4 Two examples of pneumotachograph masks used for measuring air pressure and airflow during voice and speech production. The PENTAX Medical Phonatory Aerodynamic System (PAS—left image) consists of a solid facemask with a wide central tube connected to a flow head, which is attached to a flow transducer. A separate pressure tube can be routed through the flow head and placed between a speaker's lips in the front of the oral cavity for measuring intraoral pressure (the analog of subglottal pressure during plosive production). This tube is connected to a pressure transducer in the main body of the PAS. The Glottal Enterprises Aeroview system (right image) uses a Rothenberg pneumotachograph mask which is circumferentially vented with wire screens, which provide a resistance to flow. Flow and pressure transducers are mounted into the mask and connected to a computer for calculations of airflow and air pressure.

folds into vibration.[31] In healthy speakers, we would expect measures of P_s and PtP to be low, and in speakers with vocal fold impairments we would expect these measurements to be elevated (e.g., speakers with vocal fold impairments require greater pressure to set the vocal folds into vibration, either at their lowest possible intensity or during comfortable speaking intensities). Alternatively, speakers with impaired respiratory support may be unable to generate a sufficient amount of sustained P_s to maintain vocal fold oscillation, and thus exhibit severely breathy voices with marked aphonia during speech.[32]

5.5.1 Why Are Measures of Subglottal Pressure Sensitive to Laryngeal Impairments?

Subglottal pressure is influenced by a number of factors, which include respiratory drive (e.g., activity in the respiratory muscles), glottal configuration (e.g., completely closed vs. posterior gap vs. slightly abducted), medial compression force, and tissue stiffness. Different vocal pathologies can affect these factors and subsequently influence P_s. For example, unilateral vocal fold paralysis (UVFP) results in glottal insufficiency such that many speakers have difficulty closing the glottis completely along the midline. When compared to normal speakers or to posttreatment measures (e.g., when glottal insufficiency has been improved), studies generally find that **P_s is increased in the presence of glottal insufficiency** secondary to UVFP.[33, 34,35] Significant glottal gaps present less surface area at midline against which subglottal pressure can exert force and also result in pressure leaks. While some may expect that glottal gaps would result in low subglottal pressures (due to low resistance), in actual fact this condition requires speakers to increase respiratory drive and residual glottal and supraglottal muscular force to achieve phonation, translating to increased P_s.

Membranous lesions which add mass to the vocal fold tissue can influence P_s because of their influence on vocal fold adduction (e.g., they can cause varying levels of glottal insufficiency along the length of the vocal folds), but in addition can present increased stiffness against the driving pressure. It has been reported that lesions creating higher degrees of stiffness (e.g., polyps and cysts) require greater P_s than those creating less stiffness (e.g., nodules).[36] **Benign mid-membranous lesions** (e.g., nodules, polyps, cysts, and pseudocysts) **typically result in elevated measures of P_s.** In general, speakers with dysphonia typically exhibit measures of Ps **greater than 10 cm H_2O** at comfortable pitch and loudness. In contrast, the literature collectively demonstrates that most healthy speakers without dysphonia exhibit measures of Ps between **5 and 10 cm H_2O** when phonating at comfortable pitch and loudness. ▶ Table 5.3 summarizes P_s data from selected research published since 1988.

It is important for clinicians to consider that patterns of aerodynamic measurements do not always agree across research studies, and do not always move in the direction of "normal" after treatment. This is certainly true for measurements of P_s. For example, while a majority of studies find that surgical improvement of glottal insufficiency lowers P_s, a few studies have reported an opposite pattern or reported that the material/technique used to improve glottal insufficiency influenced the measurements of P_s.[33,35] An important variable to contemplate

when assessing the evidence from clinical studies is the methodology utilized to acquire the aerodynamic measurements, which likely accounts for a large degree of the variability in values across different published investigations. Many methodological factors can influence aerodynamic measurements and P_s measures in particular, and must be accounted for whenever they are obtained in the voice clinic. These will be addressed in the next section.

5.6 Methodological Considerations for Measuring Subglottal Pressure

Among the aerodynamic measurements a clinician might obtain, measurement of P_s requires the most specialized technology. Measurements of P_s will be affected by many methodological factors, among which include

- Equipment.
  - Transducer sensitivity, facemask design, properties of intraoral tubing, and signal processing methods are among the equipment-related factors that will influence measurements of P_s.
- Vocal intensity.
  - P_s is a primary determinant of vocal intensity, which will vary as a function of P_s. In general, the greater the vocal intensity, the greater the P_s.
- Vocal F_0.
  - The influence of P_s on vocal F_0 varies as a function of speaking task. During vowel production increases in P_s will result in increases of F_0—for example, as a speaker moves from modal to falsetto register or chest voice to head voice, P_s will increase. During connected speech, P_s also influences F_0 but in less predictable ways. Speakers often maintain a relatively stable P_s at habitual speaking F_0, even though F_0 will dynamically vary due to intonation. Exceptions to this phenomenon include words or syllables that are stressed during speech, which are characterized by increased F_0, increased vocal intensity, and greater P_s compared to unstressed words and syllables.
- Recording environment.
  - Environmental temperature and humidity can potentially influence the properties of a facemask and tubing when collecting measures of P_s.
- Instructions
  - As previously mentioned, relationships exist between P_s and the intensity and F_0 characteristics of the voice. Both of these factors are modulated in prosody, such that stress patterns of sounds, syllables, and words can also influence P_s. Additionally, lung volume (how deeply a speaker inhales prior to sound production), respiration pattern while speaking (all sounds on one exhalation vs. multiple breaths), speech stimulus, speaking rate, and the degree of coupling (seal) between a facemask and face are all factors that can potentially influence measures of P_s and should be considered when developing a methodology for acquiring clinical measurements.

When developing a clinical voice laboratory for the acquisition of aerodynamic and acoustic analyses, the clinician must decide on what level of control to exert upon the aforementioned factors.

Table 5.3 Ps data from selected published studies

Authors	Gender	No. of patients	Age range (x)	Ps mean (SD)	Ps range
Normal speakers					
[1]Liang et al[37]	F	20	20–45 (x = 31)	6.79	4.93–7.89
[2]Rosenthal et al[38]	M	6	[18–26] (x = 20.3)	7.03 (2.33)	N/A
	F	12			
[3]Awan et al[39]	M	30	[18–31] (x = 23.2)	7.76	N/A
	F	30		6.6	
[4]Zheng et al[40]	M	9	[20–56] (x = 36.9)	5.94 (1.26)	4.31–8.06
	F	18		5.71 (1.49)	3.64–8.14
[5]Zraick et al[11]	M	32	18–30 (30.6)	6.65 (1.98)	3.59–11.43
	M	19	40–59 (48.6)	7.13 (1.50)	4.11–9.63
	M	18	60–89 (74.1)	6.31 (1.94)	2.02–9.46
	F	47	18–30 (28.8)	5.40 (1.37)	2.52–8.68
	F	22	40–59 (49.6)	5.88 (2.06)	2.83–12.99
	F	20	60–89 (72.9)	7.78 (4.23)	3.79–18.39
[6]Cantarella et al[41]	M	20	[20–65] (x = 37.5)	8.31 (2.64)	N/A
	F	19			
[7]Ma et al[42]	M	6	[20–55]	9.75 (1.86)	N/A
	F	35			
[8]Weinrich et al[43]	M and F	5	6	10.05 (2.44)	
	M and F	16	7	9.46 (2.26)	
	M and F	18	8	9.71 (3.47)	
	M and F	19	9	9.08 (2.89)	
	M and F	17	10	8.69 (3.34)	
[9]Yiu et al[44]	F	28	20–50 (33.4)	9.94	N/A
[10]Hartl et al[45]	M	12	49–75 (62)	8.1 (1.9)	N/A
[11]Holmberg et al[46]	M	25	17–30 (22.5)	5.91	N/A
	F	20	18–36 (24.3)	6.09	
Dysphonic speakers					
[12]Fu et al[47]	[a]F	24	[20–54] (37.5)	10.0 (3.08)	N/A
	[b]F	29		11.32 (2.08)	
[13]Dastolfo et al[48]	[a]M and F	13		12.3 (6.5)	N/A
	[b]M and F	17	>18	0.8 (3.4)	
	[c]M and F	32		9.0 (3.4)	
	[d]M and F	8		10.2 (4.4)	
[1]Liang et al[37]	F	21	18–48 (34.0)	10.48	8.45–12.29
[14]Gillespie et al[49]	F	16	18–30	7.27 (3.75)	2.72–18.51 3.87–17.80
	F	13	31–40	8.20 (3.90)	3.04–11.50 5.12–11.39
	F	21	41–50	6.82 (2.07)	3.70–10.90 2.72–14.16
	F	18	51–60	7.58 (1.59)	
	F	10	61–64	7.27 (2.53)	
	F	2	65 +	7.88 (3.58)	
[4]Zheng et al[40]	M	8	[18–56] (38.9)	10.25 (2.69) 10.47 (3.51)	6.53–14.69
	F	18			5.77–17.37
[6]Cantarella et al[41]	M	17	[17–74] (44.4)	12.05 (4.51)	N/A
	F	36			
[7]Ma et al[42]	M	19	[20–55]	16.95 (5.49)	N/A
	F	93			
[8]Yiu et al[44]	F	28	20–50 (33.3)	16.30	N/A
[15]Holmberg et al[50]	F	10	19–35 (24.2)	11.0 (3.70)	N/A

Table 5.3 continued

Authors	Gender	No. of patients	Age range (x)	Ps mean (SD)	Ps range
[9]Hartl et al[45]	M	8	38–78 (61.0)	11.3 (2.1)	N/A
[16]Rosen et al[36]	[a]M	2			
	[a]F	19	(27.4)	6.91	(3.64–10.5)
	[b]M	3	(32.4)	9.00	(1.65–31.9)
	[b]F	61			

Notes: All units of P_s measurement are in cm H_2O. Ages in brackets [ ] indicate data not reported by sex. Standard deviation associated with means and data ranges are noted when reported. All P_s data from comfortable/habitual pitch and loudness productions, unless otherwise noted.
1. **Participants**: Normals and muscle tension dysphonia; **Stimulus**: /pa/; **System**: Pentax Medical Phonatory Aerodynamic System.
2. **Participants**: Normals; **Stimulus**: /pi/; **System**: Glottal Enterprises MS100-A2.
3. **Participants**: Normals: **Stimulus**: /pa/; **System**: Pentax Medical Phonatory Aerodynamic System.
4. **Participants**: Normals and muscle tension dysphonia; **Stimulus**: /pa/; **System**: Pentax Medical Phonatory Aerodynamic System.
5. **Participants**: Normals; **Stimulus**: /pa/; **System**: Pentax Medical Phonatory Aerodynamic System.
6. **Participants**: Normals and benign lesions (nodules, cyst, polyp, Reinke's edema); **Stimulus**: /pa/; **System**: EVA (France).
7. **Participants**: Normals and "dysphonic"; **Stimulus**: /pi/; **System** Kay Elemetrics Aerophone II.
8. **Participants**: Normal children; **Stimulus**: /pa/; **System**: Glottal Enterprises MS100-A2.
9. **Participants**: Normals and "laryngeal pathologies" (Nodules, Polyps, Edema); **Stimulus**: /ipi/; **System**: Kay Elemetrics Aerophone II.
10. **Participants**: Normal smokers and unilateral paralysis; **Stimulus**: /pi/; **System**: Kay Elemetrics Aerophone II.
11. **Participants**: Normals; **Stimulus**: /pae/; **System**: Glottal Enterprises MS100-A2.
12. **Participants**: (a and b): Nodules pretherapy; **Stimulus**: /ipi/; **System**: Kay Elemetrics Aerophone II.
13. **Participants**: (a) Benign lesion (nodule, polyp), (b) unilateral paralysis, (c) muscle tension dysphonia, (d) atrophy; **Stimulus**: /pa/; **System**: Pentax Medical Phonatory Aerodynamic System.
14. **Participants**: Muscle tension dysphonia; **Stimulus**: /pi/; **System**: Kay Elemetrics Aerophone II.
15. **Participants**: Nodules pretherapy; **Stimulus**: /pae/; **System**: Glottal Enterprises MS100-A2.
16. **Participants**: (a) Nodules, (b) polyps and cysts; **Stimulus**: /pi/; **System**: Kay Elemetrics Aerophone II.

Of utmost importance is that equipment choice, environmental factors, and instructions remain consistent within and between patient recordings. The clinician should choose a setup and recording methodology and stick with it. The authors understand that these decisions can be daunting for the novice or inexperienced clinician, and for this reason they provide some recommendations below, which are based on more than six decades of published research evidence and a combined 40 years of clinical experience of the authors.

5.7 Methods for Measuring Subglottal Pressure

Subglottal pressure generation is dependent on the activation of respiratory muscles which cause air to move through the lower respiratory tract to the level of the vocal folds. For this reason, it is very important to remember that clinical measurements of P_s can be influenced by not only laryngeal impairments but also respiratory impairments. Hixon et al developed a very simple, low-cost device that can be used to determine if speakers manifest sufficient respiratory pressure generation for connected speech purposes.[51] This device, illustrated in ▶ Fig. 5.5, utilizes a plastic straw clipped to a glass onto which a ruler is taped. With the straw submerged, the air pressure required to blow a bubble into the water is directly proportional to the depth of the straw. For example, if the end of the straw is at 5 cm, the pressure required to blow a bubble into the water which rises to the surface will be 5 cm H_2O. The authors suggested that speakers with sufficient respiratory function for speech should be able to generate bubbles at 5 cm H_2O for at least 5 seconds. This rule of thumb corresponds well to PtP measures required to initiate and sustain phonation, which range between **2 and 5 cm H_2O** in healthy speakers. This simple low-tech device can be used to assess

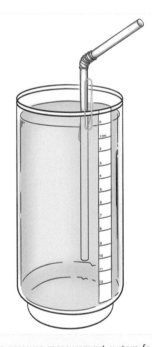

Fig. 5.5 A simple pressure measurement system for determining respiratory support for connected speech purposes. A straw submerged to 5 cm will require an individual to generate 5 cmH_2O to blow a bubble into the water.

respiratory support for phonation, and will further inform your interpretations of subsequent aerodynamic measurements.

A number of commercial equipment applications incorporate pressure tubing into pneumotachograph-based masks (▶ Fig. 5.6) which cover the mouth and nose to allow for simultaneous measurement of pressure and flow. When acquiring pressure

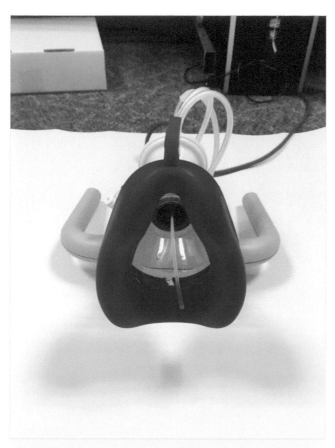

Fig. 5.6 An example of a facemask with intraoral pressure tube routed through it. The tube is placed between the speaker's lips, into the front of the oral cavity, with the facemask held firmly against the face.

measurements using a facemask, it is critical that the patient be instructed to hold the mask "firmly" against their face throughout breathing or speaking trials, and that the intraoral tube be placed between the lips and into the front of the oral cavity above or in front of the tongue. The pressure transducers of commercial applications must also be calibrated on a regular basis.

The literature is consistent in using **/p/** as the bilabial plosive stimulus, but studies vary in their choice of the following vowel and inclusion of other speech sounds. The most commonly used stimuli for measuring P_s include slow (e.g., rate of 1.5 per second) repetitions of either **/pa/** or **/pi/**. It should be noted that the specific vowel and the phonetic environment surrounding the unvoiced plosive may influence measurements of P_s. High vowels following the /p/ release, such as /i/, may result in higher measures of P_s than when using a low vowel such as /a/.[52,53] Some investigations have also attempted to measure P_s during continuous speech samples such as the Rainbow passage, though much less control over the elicited pressure and increased variability may be expected.[54]

The following are methodological recommendations for acquiring measurements of P_s. These are aligned with literature reporting P_s measurements from different commercial systems, with the primary difference being the vowel stimulus used. Current options for equipment capable of measuring P_s are listed in **Appendix 5.1**.
- Ensure system is calibrated to manufacturer's specifications.
- Utilize a new intraoral pressure tube for each patient.

- The tube should be positioned such that it fits between the speaker's lips, with the tip sitting inside the anterior oral cavity in front of or above the tongue.
- A practice recording is recommended to ensure that the intraoral tube is placed correctly (i.e., not loose outside of the lips; not being blocked by the tongue or saliva).
- Instruct the speaker as follows: "*Take a comfortable breath, place the tube between your lips inside the front of your mouth, and repeat the syllables /pa-pa-pa/* [or /pi-pi-pi/] *at a comfortable pitch and loudness, with a slow and steady rate like this* (model a rate of 1.5 syll/sec for the patient). *You will say /pa/* [or /pi/] *five to seven times on a single breath, and I will tell you when to stop.*"
- When the speaker indicates they are ready, begin recording and tell them to "*go.*"

Some clinicians might find that a metronome (easily displayed via a smartphone application) can help a speaker achieve the target syllable rate. When using a facemask (for acquiring synchronous measures of flow), instructions also typically include placing the mask "*firmly*" against the face. Speakers with respiratory impairment and/or significant glottal insufficiency may not be able to produce five to seven repetitions on one breath at the target syllable rate. The authors' clinical experiences suggest that as long as you have a minimum of three repetitions from multiple trials (e.g., x3) which to measure mean data, it will be clinically acceptable. It is important that clinicians monitor the patient's behavior when recording. If they perceive the patient is not producing syllables at a "comfortable" pitch and loudness, they should query the patient on their perception of effort—in the authors' experience, even speakers with typical voice will often push against the mask, resulting in increased intraoral pressures. Re-recording multiple trials will not add significant amounts of time to the clinical process.

Ideally, clinicians should acquire three separate trials (of five to seven syllables each) and use the middle trial or trials which show the best pressure peak characteristics to acquire measurements. The authors' preference is to avoid the first and last syllables (e.g., selection is from the middle syllable trains) when considering from which peaks to measure P_s.

Data from recent studies that have measured P_s using similar methodology as above in normal and dysphonic populations is illustrated in ▶ Table 5.3. This is not an exhaustive listing of the literature but will provide some guidance to the clinicians looking to compare their patients' measures to evidence-based reports using similar methodology.

5.7.1 What to Expect from Normal and Dysphonic Speakers?

Efforts to extract absolute values for what should be expected from normal (nondysphonic) and dysphonic speakers (▶ Table 5.3) can be an exercise in frustration. Published aerodynamic data vary widely from speaker to speaker and study to study, for many different reasons. Among these include (**1**) physiological characteristics and habitual patterns of speakers, (**2**) different instrumentation, (**3**) different speaker instructions, (**4**) different stimuli, and (**5**) different analysis procedures.

Careful analyses of published investigations, in addition to the clinical and laboratory experience of the authors, do allow for some generalizations based on speaker trends for both normal and dysphonic populations. As clinicians consider these "clinical nuggets," we are obliged to again point out that aerodynamic measurements are known to vary widely from speaker to speaker, any mean must be considered along with the associated variability around the mean for a given population (e.g., the typical range of measures in normal speakers or dysphonic speakers), and not all published studies agree with the generalizations below. Clinicians must also accept that some dysphonic speakers will produce P_s within normal ranges, and some normal speakers will produce P_s outside of normal ranges. With this in mind, general trends of P_s measurements in different populations include the following:

- Normal male speakers tend to exhibit greater P_s than normal female speakers (although this trend may not hold for all vowel stimuli or older speakers, e.g., > 60 years of age).[11,39]
- Normal young, middle age, and older speakers do *not* tend to exhibit significantly different measures of P_s.[11]
- Normal speakers tend to produce P_s between 5 and 10 cm H_2O when producing slow repeated /p/ + vowel syllables at comfortable levels.[32,39,40,42,45,46]
- Normal speakers tend to consistently exhibit lower P_s than speakers with dysphonia of various etiologies.[37,40,41,42,44,45,55]
- Speakers with dysphonia due to nonorganic and organic etiologies tend to produce P_s greater than 10 cm H_2O when producing slow repeated /p/ + vowel syllables at comfortable levels.[37,40,41,42,44,47,48,50]
- As vocal intensity increases, measures of P_s will also increase in both normal and dysphonic speakers.[38,50]
- When voice therapy or surgery improves laryngeal physiology (e.g., improves glottal closure), measures of P_s tend to improve in the direction of lowering (exception: rigid Silastic implants used during thyroplasty can add additional stiffness and P_s may not lower).[33,35,37,48]

5.8 Transglottal Airflow

We have previously stated that flow is intimately linked with pressure and resistance as in the formula **U = P/R** (where U = flow, P = pressure, R = resistance).[56] The formula shows that airflow requires a driving pressure. The primary source of driving pressure during phonation is lung pressure, which varies dynamically during breathing and sound production. In accordance with Boyle's law, during expiration, as the volume of air in the lungs decreases, lung pressure will increase, and air will move from the lungs toward the mouth. Vocal fold vibration will occur only when transglottal airflow (i.e., airflow moving between the vocal folds from subglottal to supraglottal regions) is present.

Flow can be defined as the quantity of fluid that moves across a unit of area over a specific unit of time (i.e., volume/time). In voice production, transglottal airflow can then be understood as the volume of air moving through the glottis each second during phonation. It is typically measured in liters per second (**L/s**) or milliliters per second (**mL/s**). The unit of measurement for airflow during phonation reflects a rate of flow, and thus some authors refer to airflow rate as a **volume velocity**.[7] **Fig. 1.20** in Chapter 1 illustrated characteristics of airflow through the glottis during phonation.

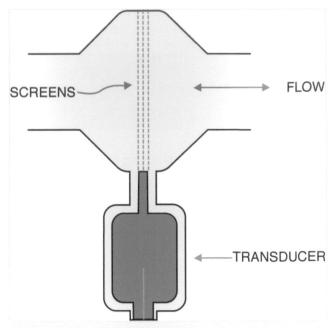

SCREENS — FLOW

← TRANSDUCER

Fig. 5.7 Typical construction of a pneumotachograph.

5.8.1 Measurement of Airflow Using a Differential Pressure Pneumotach

The formula **U = P/R** is a physical phenomenon critical for understanding how airflow is typically measured in clinical voice practice. It can be understood as airflow being the function of pressure and resistance. If the properties of resistance are known, and pressure on either side of the resistance (the pressure differential) can be measured, then airflow rate can be accurately calculated. Most commercial voice analysis systems which measure airflow take advantage of this phenomenon by utilizing a **pneumotach**. As illustrated in ▶ Fig. 5.7, a pneumotach is a device that can measure the drop in air pressure at the point of resistance to airflow (e.g., the change in pressure on each side of the resistance), from which calculations of **transglottal airflow rate** can be obtained using transducers (e.g., a transducer converts one type of energy into another, such as pressure into electrical energy that can be digitized, stored, and analyzed by a computer).[57] As in measures of P_s, transglottal airflow measures acquired with a pneumotach typically place the device in line with a facemask. The mask allows a speaker to produce voice and speech with limited interference on natural articulation and acts as a sealed chamber to capture aerodynamic energy. Together the pneumotach and associated equipment are referred to as a **pneumotachograph**. Different pneumotach-based facemasks are shown in ▶ Fig. 5.4.

5.8.2 The Phonation Quotient: A Low-Cost Estimate of Airflow

Transglottal airflow can also be estimated via low-cost methods. One evidence-based low-cost method of airflow estimation is the calculation of **phonation quotient** (PQ). PQ is derived from the ratio of vital capacity (VC) to MPT, as in the formula **VC/MPT**. MPT can be easily calculated with a stopwatch or temporal measurements from an acoustic waveform (see "**Methodological Considerations for Measuring Phonation Efficiency**" section). PQ was described by Hirano et al as a measure of air consumption during phonation.[3] Hirano et al along with Rau and Beckett found strong correlations between PQ and transglottal flow rates obtained from other instruments.[5] It is important to consider that the total volume of air used during MPT is less than VC, and as a result PQ will typically overestimate measures of transglottal flow rate obtained from pneumotachographs. Rau and Beckett (1984) calculated a regression equation for adjusting measures of PQ as a more accurate predictor of transglottal flow rate. This adjusted measured is referred to as **estimated mean flow rate** (eMFR) and is calculated as follows: **eMFR = 77 + 0.236 PQ**.

5.8.3 Why Are Measures of Transglottal Airflow Sensitive to Laryngeal Impairments?

Transglottal airflow is influenced by many of the same factors as P_s, including the driving pressure from the lungs (respiratory drive), glottal configuration, medial compression force, and tissue stiffness. Different vocal pathologies can affect these factors and subsequently influence airflow. For example, UVFP results in glottal insufficiency such that excess air flows through the glottis during phonation, resulting in increased measures of transglottal airflow (compared to normal speakers) and, typically, breathy voice production. The same is true for other pathologies that result in glottal gaps, including benign midmembranous lesions such as nodules, polyps, and cysts. Alternatively, impairments that add resistance to the air pressure with excessive medial compression of the vocal folds during voicing (e.g., increased medial compression force, as in strained voice and conditions such as muscle tension dysphonia or adductor spasmodic dysphonia) typically result in decreased transglottal airflow. This phenomenon is related to the ratio of opening to closing phases of the vibratory cycle, which are skewed toward increased closed phase duration and faster closing phase in conditions where medial compression is elevated during phonation.[40,48]

5.9 Methodological Considerations for Measuring Transglottal Airflow

Clinical measures of airflow are typically acquired while asking a speaker to produce voice at a "comfortable" pitch and loudness. Measurement of airflow has been reported from sustained vowels and also from the vocalic portion of plosive + syllable repetitions (as in stimuli for measuring air pressure, including /pa/ and /pi/). Peak airflow measures will occur immediately after the burst release of the /p/ (▶ Table 5.1). There are many ways to derive mean airflow from /pa/ or /pi/ repetitions, but a typical measure (sometimes referred to as target airflow) is obtained from a central portion of the steady vocalic portion of the recorded signal. When computed from a sustained vowel,

measures of mean airflow are typically obtained from the steady continuous middle portion of the signal.

As with all aerodynamic (and acoustic) analyses, measurements of transglottal airflow will be affected by many methodological factors, among which include

- Equipment.
  - Transducer sensitivity, pneumotachograph-facemask design, signal processing methods, and spirometer type (for PQ calculations) are among the equipment-related factors that can influence measurements of transglottal airflow.
- Vocal intensity.
  - In general, transglottal airflow tends to increase as vocal intensity increases, although this relationship can be influenced by vocal F_0 (see below).[38,46,58]
- Vocal F_0.
  - Transglottal airflow has been found to vary as a function of vocal F_0 and also in relationship with vocal intensity, Isshiki found that flow rate increased linearly with vocal intensity only in falsetto register (a speaker's highest F_0 range), and increased at comfortable or "modal" F_0 levels only when a speaker produced sound at very high intensities (e.g., above 85 dB).[58] Alternatively, transglottal flow rate did not change as a function of intensity when producing sound at low F_0. This dynamic between vocal intensity, F_0, and flow rate was also reported by Holmberg et al.[59]
- Instructions.
  - Stimulus type can influence some airflow measurements. Higgins et al found that measures of peak airflow were greater when obtained from /pa/ repetitions compared to /pi/, although they did not find a vowel effect on measures of mean transglottal airflow.[52] As previously mentioned, vocal intensity and vocal F_0 can influence measurements of airflow, which must be accounted for when giving instructions to the speaker.

5.10 Methods for Measuring Transglottal Airflow

Transglottal airflow is measured with either pneumotachograph-based system or estimated with calculations of PQ and eMFR. The following are methodological recommendations for acquiring different airflow measurements. These are aligned with the literature reporting airflow measurements from different commercial systems or with low-cost handheld spirometers.

5.10.1 Pneumotachograph-Based System (e.g., Pentax Phonatory Aerodynamic System/Glottal Aeroview system)

- Ensure system is calibrated to manufacturer's specifications.
- If not measuring pressure, make sure pressure tube port is sealed.
- *Measuring from sustained vowel*: Instruct the speaker as follows: "*Take a comfortable breath, place the facemask firmly against your face, and say 'one, two, three ahhhhhh....' at a*

comfortable pitch and loudness, until I tell you to stop. I will tell you to stop after five or six seconds."

- *Measuring from syllable trains:* Instruct the speaker as follows: "*Take a comfortable breath, place the facemask firmly against your face and repeat the syllables /pa-pa-pa/ [or /pi-pi-pi/] at a comfortable pitch and loudness, with a slow and steady rate like this (model a rate of 1.5 syll/sec for the patient). You will say /pa/ [or /pi/] five to seven times on a single breath, and I will tell you when to stop.*"
- When the speaker indicates they are ready, begin recording and tell them to "go."

Ideally, clinicians should acquire three separate trials. For sustained vowels recorded using pneumotachograph-based systems, the authors' preference is to select the middle portion of the vowel (regardless of stimulus type) to calculate mean transglottal airflow rate. As with measures of P_s, it is important to monitor the speaker's behavior during recording. Vocal intensity can influence airflow measures, as can F_o if the speaker is producing sounds at very high frequencies. Data from recent studies that have measured transglottal airflow using pneumotachograph-based instruments in normal and dysphonic populations are provided in ▶ Table 5.4.

Table 5.4 Transglottal airflow data from selected published studies

Authors	Gender	No. of patients	Age range (x)	Flow mean (SD)	Flow range
Normal speakers					
[1]Liang et al[37]	F	20	20–45 (x = 31)	110 (40.0)	N/A
[2]Rosenthal et al[38]	M	6	[18–26] (x = 20.3)	175 (68.1)	N/A
	F	12			
[3]Awan et al[39]	M	30	[18–31] (x = 23.2)	170 (83.0)	N/A
	F	30		130 (49.0)	
[4]Zheng et al[40]	M	9	[20–56] (x = 36.9)	110 (40)	50–170
	F	18		80 (40)	30–150
[5]Zraick et al[11]	M	32	18–30 (30.6)	130 (60)	40–220
	M	19	40–59 (48.6)	170 (100)	30–430
	M	18	60–89 (74.1)	130 (60)	40–200
	F	47	18–30 (28.8)	130 (60)	10–300
	F	22	40–59 (49.6)	150 (70)	40–270
	F	20	60–89 (72.9)	110 (60)	30–270
[6]Cantarella et al[41]	M	20	[20–65] (x = 37.5)	145 (58.36)	N/A
	F	19			
[7]Ma et al[42]	M	6	[20–55]	130 (50)	N/A
	F	35			
[8]Yiu et al[44]	F	28	20–50 (33.4)	100	N/A
[9]Hartl et al[45]	M	12	49–75 (62)	135 (170)	N/A
[10]Holmberg et al[46]	M	25	17–30 (22.5)	185	N/A
	F	20	18–36 (24.3)	139	
Dysphonic speakers					
[11]Fu et al[47]	[a]F	24	[20–54] (37.5)	139 (60.65)	N/A
	[b]F	29		163 (65.07)	
[12]Dastolfo et al[48]	[a]M and F	13	>18	289 (144.0)	N/A
	[b]M and F	17		389 (312.0)	
	[c]M and F	32		192 (117.0)	
	[d]M and F	8		399 (354.0)	
[1]Liang et al[37]	F	21	18–48 (34.0)	110 (40.0)	N/A
[13]Gillespie et al[49]	F	16	18–30	163 (58)	92–278
	F	13	31–40	216 (124)	77–216
	F	21	41–50	166 (93)	74–428
	F	18	51–60	198 (121)	29–553
	F	10	61–64	154 (136)	20–425
	F	2	65 +	107 (42)	51–175
[4]Zheng et al[40]	M	8	[18–56] (38.9)	70 (40.0)	20–120
	F	18		60 (40.0)	10–160
[6]Cantarella et al[41]	M	17	[17–74] (44.4)	214 (156)	N/A
	F	36			

(Continued)

Table 5.4 continued

Authors	Gender	No. of patients	Age range (x)	Flow mean (SD)	Flow range
[7]Ma et al[42]	M F	19 93	[20–55]	170 (90)	N/A
[8]Yiu et al[44]	F	28	20–50 (33.3)	170	N/A
[14]Holmberg et al[46]	F	10	19–35 (24.2)	310 (90)	N/A
[9]Hartl et al[45]	M	8	38–78 (61.0)	463 (125)	N/A

Notes: All units of airflow measurement are in mL/s. Ages in brackets [ ] indicate data not reported by sex. Standard deviation associated with means and data ranges are noted when reported. All airflow data from comfortable/habitual pitch and loudness productions, unless otherwise noted.
1. **Participants**: Normals and muscle tension dysphonia; **Stimulus**: /pa/; **System**: Pentax Medical Phonatory Aerodynamic System.
2. **Participants**: Normals; **Stimulus**: /pi/; **System**: Glottal Enterprises MS100-A2.
3. **Participants**: Normals; **Stimulus**: /pa/; **System**: Pentax Medical Phonatory Aerodynamic System.
4. **Participants**: Normals and muscle tension dysphonia; **Stimulus**: /pa/; **System**: Pentax Medical Phonatory Aerodynamic System.
5. **Participants**: Normals; **Stimulus**: /pa/; **System**: Pentax Medical Phonatory Aerodynamic System.
6. **Participants**: Normals and benign lesions (nodules, cyst, polyp, Reinke's edema); **Stimulus**: /a/; **System**: EVA (France).
7. **Participants**: Normals and "dysphonic"; **Stimulus**: /a/; **System** Kay Elemetrics Aerophone II.
8. **Participants**: Normals and "laryngeal pathologies" (nodules, polyps, edema); **Stimulus**: /a/; **System**: Kay Elemetrics Aerophone II.
9. **Participants**: Normal smokers and unilateral paralysis; **Stimulus**: /a/; **System**: Kay Elemetrics Aerophone II.
10. **Participants**: Normals: **Stimulus**: /pae/; **System**: Glottal Enterprises MS100-A2.
11. **Participants**: (a and b): Nodules pretherapy; **Stimulus**: /ipi/; **System**: Kay Elemetrics Aerophone II.
12. **Participants**: (a) Benign lesion (nodule, polyp), (b) unilateral paralysis, (c) muscle tension dysphonia, (d) atrophy; **Stimulus**: /pa/; **System**: Pentax Medical Phonatory Aerodynamic System.
13. **Participants**: Muscle tension dysphonia; **Stimulus**: /pi/; **System**: Kay Elemetrics Aerophone II.
14. **Participants**: Nodules pretherapy; **Stimulus**: /ae/; **System**: Glottal Enterprises MS100-A2.

5.10.2 What to Expect in Normal and Dysphonic Speakers

As with P_s, extraction of absolute values from ▶ Table 5.4 to use for expected measurements in normal and dysphonic speakers can be challenging. Published airflow data vary widely from speaker to speaker and study to study, for the same reasons as P_s measurements. Among these include (**1**) physiological characteristics and habitual patterns of speakers, (**2**) different instrumentation, (**3**) different speaker instructions, (**4**) different stimuli, and (**5**) different analysis procedures. However, careful analyses of published investigations, in addition to the clinical and laboratory experience of the authors, do allow for some generalizations based on speaker trends for both normal and dysphonic populations. General trends of transglottal airflow measurements in different populations include the following:

- Normal male speakers tend to exhibit greater airflow values than normal female speakers.[11,39,40,46]
- Normal young, middle age, and older speakers do not tend to exhibit significantly different measures of mean transglottal airflow.[11,15]
- Normal speakers tend to produce mean transglottal airflow values **between 100 and 200 mL/s** when measuring airflow from vowels at comfortable levels.[37,38,39,42,46]
- Normal speakers tend to exhibit lower airflow rates than speakers with dysphonia associated with glottal insufficiency —e.g., paralysis, benign mid-membranous lesions.[33,41,42,44,45]
- Normal speakers tend to exhibit higher airflow rates than speakers with dysphonia due to excessive muscle tension.[37,40]
- As vocal intensity increases, measures of transglottal airflow will also increase in normal and dysphonic speakers.[38,46,50]
- As glottal gap size increases, airflow increases. Therefore, when voice therapy or surgery improves glottal closure, measures of airflow tend to decrease.[33,35,37,48]

- When voice therapy reduces laryngeal hyperfunction (e.g., increased medial compression, as in MTD), measures of airflow tend to increase.[37,48]

5.11 Additional Aerodynamic Measures of Voice

Efficiency is a term that reflects a cost-to-benefit ratio. Applied to voice production, phonatory efficiency can be thought of as **the amount of effort or energy (input) required to obtain a desired sound (output)**. In theory, efficient phonation will allow a speaker to meet communication demands in various contexts without excessive phonotraumatic behaviors or effort, and allow them to speak for longer durations without experiencing vocal fatigue. Methods used to assess the degree of efficiency during phonation vary in the literature and in clinical practice, as do the labels given to these measurements. To assess the efficiency of phonation, some authors and clinicians utilize ratios of different aerodynamic measurements to each other, including P_s, transglottal airflow, acoustic power, and aerodynamic power. Others simply use measures of transglottal flow rate, MPT, or other ratios as an indirect assessment of phonation efficiency.

Glottal efficiency is a term representing the efficiency with which a speaker converts aerodynamic energy to acoustic energy during speech production.[60,61] It has traditionally been measured by calculating the ratio of acoustic power to aerodynamic power —e.g., **A_d power/A_c power**, where A_d is the aerodynamic and A_c is the acoustic.[60] **Aerodynamic power** is derived by multiplying P_s by transglottal airflow. **Acoustic power** is the amount of sound energy created over time, as measured in Watts. In speech, acoustic power ranges between 0.01 and 1.0 mW as measured from sound intensities between 70 and 90 dB recorded at a mouth-to-microphone distance of 30 cm.[62] Some authors have used different terms for this same concept. For example, Cantarella et al labeled this ratio "**laryngeal efficiency**," and used the term "glottal efficiency index" in reference to the ratio of sound pressure level (dB) to P_s.[41] Zraick et al used the term "**aerodynamic efficiency**" in their normative study using the Pentax Medical Phonatory Aerodynamic System. Carroll et al and Lundy et al used the term "**glottal efficiency**" in reference to measurements of airflow rate, MPT, and/or phonation quotient.[11,63,64] This variability in defining efficiency related to phonation is important to consider when evaluating published evidence.

Measurements of resistance can also be considered as a construct related to the efficiency of phonation. "**Laryngeal resistance**," "**laryngeal airway resistance**," "**glottal resistance**," and "**translaryngeal resistance**" are similar terms referring to a measurement of the ratio between P_s and transglottal airflow (P_s/flow).[28,38,65] This measurement is reported in cm H_2O/mL and serves as an indicator of the degree of resistance applied to the air supply by the vocal folds (e.g., glottal constriction). Theoretically, this measure can be influenced by muscular activity (e.g., excessive adductor muscle contraction would increase measures of resistance) or glottal closure pattern (e.g., glottal gaps would decrease measures of resistance). For example, in some speakers with diagnosed muscle tension dysphonia, measures of laryngeal resistance are high compared to normal speakers.[11,49] Conversely, in some speakers with UVFP (causing glottal insufficiency), measures of laryngeal resistance are lower compared to normal speakers.[33,45] In both cases, the efficiency of phonation is reduced because the relationship of pressure to flow is unbalanced.

A number of additional measurements have been used to indirectly assess how efficiently a speaker converts aerodynamic energy to acoustic energy. **MPT** has been described as an estimate of "glottal efficiency" which provides information regarding the relationship of glottal closure to respiratory support, or how efficiently the vocal folds valve air during phonation.[66] Kent and Ball also noted the relationship of MPT with glottal closure, citing evidence from published literature in patients with vocal fold paralysis.[67] MPT is assessed by recording the duration of sustained phonation after a maximum inhalation. This measure can be influenced by a number of factors, including lung capacity (and all of the variables that influence those measures—see VC, above), muscle function, and the characteristics of airflow through the glottis. In general, speakers who produce inefficient phonation will exhibit shorter MPT than those who phonate efficiently, and for these reasons MPT is often used as one indicator of the efficiency with which a speaker can valve airflow at the level of the vocal folds.

There have been criticisms of MPT as a valid marker of vocal impairment, for reasons primarily related to intraspeaker and interspeaker performance variability.[68,69,70] The authors of this book have occasionally been surprised by the moderately dysphonic speaker who can sustain a vowel for 30 seconds or more (see typical expected values, below). However, in best practice, MPT is not used as a singular metric for determining phonation efficiency and/or vocal impairment. It is a valuable clinical measurement when used as evidence combined with additional aerodynamic and acoustic information (e.g., the inclusion of MPT in the Dysphonia Severity Index—Wuyts et al[71]), where it helps generate a more complete voice profile of a dysphonic patient. While some patients' MPT will not support your clinical hypotheses, there is abundant research evidence that supports

this measurement lowering in the presence of dysphonia. Clinicians should consider that MPT can be influenced by respiratory impairment, laryngeal impairment, or both—and complementary measurements of vocal function such as those described in this chapter and elsewhere in this book would be needed to differentially diagnose which subsystems of voice are involved.

We previously mentioned the measurement of **phonation quotient** as an indirect assessment of airflow rate during phonation. This measurement has also been conceptualized as a correlate of phonation efficiency, as it can be influenced by the physiology of vocal fold valving and glottal closure pattern. The denominator in the PQ equation is MPT and the same factors influencing that measurement must be considered. Additionally, the numerator in the PQ equation, VC, reflects respiratory function. Thus, measures of PQ can be influenced by respiratory physiology, laryngeal physiology, or both.

PQ is affected by physiological inefficiency and is sensitive to vocal impairment secondary to glottal insufficiency in paralysis and aging in addition to mid-membranous lesions.[4,5,15,72] PQ is also sensitive to improved vocal function and phonation efficiency secondary to treatment, and has been used as a marker of clinical outcomes in a number of research studies.[64,73] Rau and Beckett published normative PQ data based on a sample of 19 young, healthy male and female speakers.[5] While the Rau and Beckett data can be used as a guide for clinical comparison, we previously mentioned that PQ overestimates airflow rate and this must be considered when interpreting the exact values of PQ measurements.

The **s/z ratio** is another measurement associated with the construct of phonation efficiency. Similar in methodology to MPT, this ratio is obtained by measuring the duration of maximum /s/ and /z/ prolongations, and dividing the longest /s/ by the longest /z/. It was originally reported as an indicator of laryngeal pathology and suggested to be influenced by glottal insufficiency due to mid-membranous lesions (e.g., nodules, polyps), which cause the s/z ratio to be elevated.[10] Prolongations of /s/ require valving of airflow only at the point of constriction (the anterior palate), while prolongations of /z/ require valving of air at two points: the vocal folds in addition to the anterior palate. If respiratory physiology is not impaired and also laryngeal function is not impaired, the idea is that sustained duration of each sound should not substantially differ. Conversely, if respiratory physiology is not impaired but laryngeal function is, sustained duration of /s/ should be longer than /z/.

Theoretically, if phonation volume is equivalent, speakers who produce phonation with efficiency should exhibit sustained /s/ and /z/ durations which closely approximate each other, where the s/z ratio approximates a value of 1.0. Eckel and Boone proposed a cutoff value of **1.4** as a predictor of benign mid-membranous lesions, and it would be logical to extend this value as predicting any pathology resulting in glottal insufficiency.[10] That is, a logical clinical hypothesis would be that speakers with glottal insufficiency would be able to sustain the unvoiced /s/ for a longer duration than the voiced /z/, due to the latter sound requiring control of airflow at the vocal folds. Indeed, a body of evidence has found this measure to be elevated (e.g., above 1.4) in speakers with nodules, polyps, cysts, vocal fold paralysis, and glottal gaps due to presbylaryngis.[10,74,75,76]

Since the original reports, some authors have questioned the validity of the s/z ratio's sensitivity to pathology, suggesting that individuals with mid-membranous lesions are able to compensate for laryngeal inefficiency by adjusting control of airflow at the anterior palate during production of /z/ so that its duration is extended to approximate /s/ resulting in ratios near 1.0.[77] The research evidence also shows a large degree of variability in s/z ratio measures across varied clinical populations. In the authors' experience, it is not uncommon to measure s/z ratios under 1.4 in speakers with mid-membranous lesions and speakers with moderate-to-severe dysphonia. It should also be noted that a number of studies of dysphonic children have found that s/z ratios often do not exceed the 1.4 criterion.[78,79,80] Thus, while measures of s/z ratio appear to be sensitive to glottal insufficiency in many speakers, especially adults, interpretation of this measure should be considered along with known inter- and intraspeaker variability. As such, we consider the s/z ratio as a valid and sensitive measurement of phonation efficiency but only when combined within the larger evidence pool (e.g., additional aerodynamic, acoustic, physiological, and history data) of the complete diagnostic profile.

5.11.1 Why Are Measures of Phonation Efficiency Sensitive to Laryngeal Impairments?

Phonation is produced through interaction of coupled subsystems: respiration, phonation, and resonance. Effective and efficient phonation requires a physiological balance between these subsystems.[81] Given unimpaired function in one system, excessive or inadequate function in one or more related systems will result in inefficiencies. Over time these inefficiencies can result in vocal fatigue, hoarseness, and in some cases changes to the vocal fold tissue.

Measures of phonation efficiency are able to indirectly assess the physiological function in the subsystems of respiration and phonation to determine the characteristics of physiological balance. For example, respiratory impairment would be reflected in measures of vital capacity, MPT, and s/z ratio. Laryngeal impairment (e.g., hyperfunction) would be reflected in measures of glottal efficiency, laryngeal resistance, phonation quotient, MPT, and/or s/z ratio. While one measure of efficiency is not adequate to draw diagnostic conclusions, multiple measures of efficiency combined with additional aerodynamic and acoustic measurements facilitate the generation of a complete diagnostic profile which benefits the clinical process during differential diagnosis and treatment planning.

5.12 Methodological Considerations for Measuring Phonation Efficiency

Measurements of glottal efficiency (as defined by Titze[60]—see above) and laryngeal resistance are derived from calculations of P_s and transglottal airflow. They are influenced by the same methodological considerations as mentioned in previous sections. Measurements of acoustic power are acquired from audio signals recorded via a microphone within the context of P_s and airflow measurements (the microphone signal is integrated into the pressure/flow equipment setup). Acoustic power will be affected by those same methodological factors as noted in Chapter 4 ("Acoustic Analysis of Voice").

Measurements of MPT for sustained vowels and the phonemes /s/ and /z/ are influenced by similar methodological phenomena. Instructions for obtaining these measurements are identical except for the prompts given for the specific phoneme. The most common sustained vowel prompt is production of the vowel /a/. For any sound elicited, methodological considerations in calculating MPT include

- **Instructions**: Research has shown that speakers vary their performance when the task is modeled versus unmodeled prior to attempts. Specifically, the longest production was achieved with fewer trials when the task was modeled.[82] The authors of this book and others have also found through clinical experience or research that encouragement (e.g., "coaching") during the speaker's production facilitates maximum performance effort.[83]

- **Equipment:** The most typical method for measuring time during MPT productions is the use of a stopwatch. While this method has been validated based on its ubiquitous use in the research literature and clinical practice, it can be prone to measurement error because it is dependent on manual reaction times of the examiner. One way to limit measurement error is to record the vocal signal and measure the waveform time using acoustic analysis software.

- **Age and sex:** Aggregate research data demonstrates that MPT for adults is longer than that of children. Additionally, younger adults typically exhibit longer MPT than older adults older than 65 years.[6,7] Adult males exhibit longer MPT than females, in theory due to their larger lung capacity.

- **Number of attempts:** A number of studies have found that unmodeled elicitation of MPT is influenced by the number of attempts. Specifically, speakers tend to produce longer MPT when given more attempts—some studies have found that up to 10 trials are needed to elicit a true maximum performance from some speakers.[69,83] The authors of this book and others have been informed by their clinical experience and use the longest production from **three trials** of MPT, where the examiner has modeled the task for them prior to the first production.

5.13 Methods for Measuring Phonation Efficiency

In previous sections and chapters, we have described methods for obtaining VC, P_s, airflow, and acoustics. These variables are used for calculations of PQ, glottal efficiency, and/or laryngeal resistance, and we refer the reader to those sections and chapters for methodological considerations. Commercial systems with integrated pressure and flow transducers, along with proprietary software that computes aerodynamic measurements automatically via custom algorithms, are typically needed to calculate glottal efficiency and laryngeal resistance. The following are the authors' recommendations for measuring MPT and s/z ratio. As a reminder, MPT serves as the denominator for calculations of PQ.

- Instructions for MPT
  - With the speaker sitting or standing (always measure in the same posture), instruct the speaker as follows: "*Take a deep breath and then say the vowel /a/ for as long as you can, until you completely run out of air.*"

- Provide a short model for the speaker, after which you remind them to *"keep going until they have no air left."*
- Ask the speaker if they understand, and then tell them to begin when they are ready. As the speaker nears the end of their breath, verbal encouragement by the examiner is typically helpful to elicit maximum performance.
- Begin and end timer at phonation onset and offset, respectively. Alternatively, record the production using acoustic software and measure the time on a computer.
- Elicit three trials, and **use the longest trial** as your clinical measurement.
- Instructions for s/z ratio
  - S/z ratio is obtained using the same procedures as MPT. The only difference is the sound that the examiner models for

the speaker (/s/ and /z/, respectively). It is common clinical practice to elicit /s/ productions first followed by /z/, although there is no evidence that alternating the order influences resulting measurements.
- Elicit **three productions of each sound**, and use the **longest /s/** and **longest /z/** to calculate the s/z ratio.

5.13.1 What to Expect in Normal and Dysphonic Speakers

▶ Table 5.5, ▶ Fig. 5.6, and ▶ Table 5.7 report selected published data for MPT, s/z ratio, and PQ obtained from healthy, nondysphonic speakers. Some generalizations can be drawn from these tables which can inform clinical interpretation.

Table 5.5 Maximum phonation time

Authors	Gender	No. of patients	Age range (x)	MPT mean (SD)	MPT range
Normal speakers					
Mohseni and Sandoughdar[84]	F	90	30–50	22.5 (5.2)	N/A
Nemr et al[85]	M	17	[20–83]	17.4 (5.4)	N/A
	F	25			
Zhuge et al[86]	M	9	(32.5)	25.7 (6.7)	N/A
	F	22			
Gramuglia et al[79]	M	9	4–6	5.4 (1.4)	
	M	27	7–9	8.1 (2.3)	
	M	23	10–11	9.8 (2.4)	
	F	6	4–6	6.6 (3.2)	N/A
	F	18	7–9	8.4 (2.4)	
	F	17	10–11	8.9 (2.4)	
Goy et al[87]	M	55	18–28 (19.4)	20.2 (8.0)	
	M	51	65–86 (73.3)	18.6 (8.1)	
	F	104	18–27 (18.9)	15.1 (4.4)	N/A
	F	82	63–82 (71.1)	18.9 (7.3)	
Awan et al[39]	M	21	[18–25] (21.5)	20.83 (6.18)	N/A
	F	28			
Maslan et al[88]	M	34	61–70	26.2 (1.2)	16–35
	M	35	71–80	23.1 (1.7)	7–38
	M		81–90	21.7 (1.5)	10–50
	F		61–70	18.8 (2.6)	8–60
	F		71–80	22.8 (1.4)	12–45
	F		81–90	20.6 (1.3)	5–41
Leino et al[89]	M	63	(23.4)	30.0 (10.1)	12–55
	F	189	(25.7)	22.6 (6.0)	10–51
Dysphonic speakers					
Nawka et al[90]	M	6	[19–75] (58.8)	9.5 (5.1)	N/A
	F	30			
Nemr et al[85]	M	7	[20–83]	11.1 (5.5)	N/A
	F	17			
Zhuge et al[86]	M	18	(37.5)	17.1 (3.9)	N/A
	F	48			
Gramuglia et al[79]	M	9	4–6	5.3 (1.4)	N/A
	M	27	7–9	7.9 (2.7)	
	M	23	10–11	7.3 (2.0)	

Table 5.5 continued

Authors	Gender	No. of patients	Age range (x)	MPT mean (SD)	MPT range
	F	6	4–6	4.9 (1.5)	
	F	18	7–9	6.6 (1.9)	
	F	17	10–11	8.6 (2.2)	
Lundy et al[91]	M	13	24–79 (62.5)	5.4 (3.6)	1.5–16
	F	7	39–74 (55.9)		

Mohseni and Sandoughdar: **Participants**: Normal Iranian females; **Stimulus**: /a/.
Nawka: **Participants**: Bilateral vocal fold paralysis (pretreatment); **Stimulus**: /a/.
Nemr: **Participants**: Normal and dysphonic (multiple etiologies); **Stimulus**: /a/.
Zhuge: **Participants**: Normal and vocal polyps; **Stimulus**: /a/.
Gramuglia: **Participants**: Normal children and children with vocal nodules; **Stimulus**: /a/.
Goy: **Participants**: Normal Canadian adults: **Stimulus**: /a/.
Mendes: **Participants**: Normal Brazilian children; **Stimulus**: /a/.
Maslan: **Participants**: Normal older adults; **Stimulus**: /a/.
Leino: **Participants**: Normal young Finnish adults: **Stimulus**: /o:/.
Lundy: **Participants**: Unilateral paralysis; **Stimulus**: /a/.

Table 5.6 Measures of s/z ratio from selected studies

Authors	Gender	No. of patients	Age (x)	Mean s/z (sd)	s/z ratio range
Normal speakers—adults					
Awan[6]	M	53	18–30 (24)	0.95 (0.15)	0.58–1.41
	M	14	41–58 (53)	1.05 (0.16)	0.86–1.54
	M	7	8–13 (10)	0.99 (0.14)	0.82–1.25
	F	206	18–30 (23)	0.98 (0.13)	0.44–1.50
	F	17	32–42 (38)	0.93 (0.12)	0.74–1.86
	F	20	46–80 (55)	1.01 (0.22)	0.79–1.86
Mueller et al[92]	M	20	20–30 (24)	1.10 (0.33)	0.56–1.81
	M	22	65–87 (77)	0.85 (0.33)	0.46–1.78
	F	20	20–30 (24)	1.05 (0.30)	0.66–1.50
	F	22	65–92 (78)	0.89 (0.23)	0.56–1.44
Larson et al[93]	M and F	22	19–41 (25)	1.18 (0.31)	N/A
Eckel and Boone[10,a]	M and F	86	8–88 (28)	0.99 (0.36)	0.41–2.67
Normal speakers—children					
Mendes Tavares et al[94]	M	185	4–6 (N/A)	0.97 (0.17)	N/A
	M	483	7–9 (N/A)	0.95 (0.15)	N/A
	M	156	10–12 (N/A)	0.99 (0.15)	N/A
	F	204	4–6 (N/A)	0.96 (0.15)	N/A
	F	473	7–9 (N/A)	0.99 (0.27)	N/A
	F	159	10–12 (N/A)	1.01 (0.17)	N/A
Sorenson and Parker[95]	M and F	11	5–10 (N/A)	0.97 (N/A)	0.84–1.27
Fendler and Shearer[96]	M	N/A	1st grade	1.42 (0.52)	0.51–2.66
	M	N/A	2nd grade	1.13 (0.33)	0.53–2.13
	F	N/A	1st grade	1.31 (0.38)	0.48–2.02
	F	N/A	2nd grade	1.19 (0.31)	0.52–2.34
Tait et al[97]	M	6	5 (N/A)	0.92 (N/A)	0.82–1.08
	M	9	7(N/A)	0.70 (N/A)	0.52–0.97
	M	6	9 (N/A)	0.92 (N/A)	0.66–1.50
	F	8	5 (N/A)	0.83 (N/A)	0.50–1.14
	F	15	7 (N/A)	0.78 (N/A)	0.51–1.10
	F	8	9 (N/A)	0.91 (N/A)	0.75–1.26

[a]Data include measurements from children and adults.

Table 5.7 Phonation quotient from selected studies (all measurements are in seconds)

Authors	Gender	No. of patients	Normal/Disorder	Age range (x)	PQ (SD)
Normal speakers					
McMullan[98]	M	20	Normal	18–25	189 (77)
	F	20	Normal	18–25	192 (73)
Joshi and Watts[99]	M	20	Normal	25–69	184 (54)
De Virgilio[100]	F	15	Normal	41–49	119
Leino et al[89]	M	63	Normal	(23)	197 (72)
	F	189	Normal	(26)	177 (53)
Lundy et al[64],a	M	15	Normal	18–39	210 (63)
	F	42	Normal	18–39	194 (53)
Carroll et al[63],a	M	7	Normal	(27)	234 (55)
	F	11	Normal	(25)	214 (36)
Rau and Beckett[5]	M	10	Normal	19–28 (21)	137 (19)
	F	9	Normal	21–29 (24)	124 (22)
Hirano et al[3]	M	25	Normal	N/A	145 (44)
	F	25	Normal	N/A	137 (32)
Dysphonic speakers					
Wang et al[73]	M and F	60	UVFP	20–84 (52)	647 (508)
De Virgilio et al[100]	M and F	26	UVFP–RLN	35–76 (50)	550
	F	8	UVFP–RLN and SLN	24–61 (47)	576
Wang et al[101]	M and F	20	UVFP	35–67 (51)	520 (287)
		23	Nodules	N/A–Adult	225 (71)
Iwata and von Leden[4]	M and F	18	Polyps	N/A–Adult	211 (135)
		35	UVFP–Intermediate	N/A–Adult	544 (298)
			UVFP–Paramedian	N/A–Adult	332 (183)
Hirano et al[3]	M	8	Nodules/Polyp	18–56 (41)	278 (105)
	F	10		25–64 (42)	237 (133)
	M and F	6	UVFP	32–71 (45)	584 (364)

Abbreviations: RLN, recurrent laryngeal nerve; UVFP, unilateral vocal fold paralysis.
McMullan 2016: **VC Equipment**: Contec SP10 handheld spirometer.
Joshi and Watts 2016: **VC Equipment**: Contec SP10 handheld spirometer.
Wang et al: **VC Equipment**: Aerophone II.
De Virgilio et al 2014: **VC Equipment**: Aerophone II.
Wang et al: **VC Equipment**: Aerophone II.
Leino et al 2008: **VC Equipment**: VitaloGraph spirometer.
Lundy et al: **VC Equipment**: MultiSPIRO spirometer.
Carroll et al: **VC Equipment**: Tamarac "Presto" spirometer and S&M Instruments spirometer.
Rau and Beckett: **VC Equipment**: Calculair handheld spirometer.
Hirano et al: **VC Equipment**: Collins respirometer.
Iwata and von Leden: **VC Equipment**: Benedict-Roth respirometer.
[a]Participants were singers.

MPT

- Normal healthy children should be able to sustain a vowel for at least **10 seconds**.
- Normal, healthy adult males and females should be able to sustain a vowel for at least **20 seconds**.[6] Some sources have indicated that MPTs may be lower in females (e.g., in the 15–20 seconds range) due to smaller vital capacities in females.

- MPT decreases in older adults (e.g., > 65 years), such that healthy males and females should be able to produce a sustained vowel between **10 and 15 seconds** (expect shorter durations for older speakers).
- Given unimpaired respiratory function, speakers with conditions causing **glottal insufficiency** often (but not always) exhibit MPT below that of healthy, normal speakers.

S/z ratio

- Normal, healthy speakers (males, females, children, and adults) should be able to produce s/z ratios below 1.4 s.
- Given unimpaired respiratory function, speakers with conditions causing glottal insufficiency often (but not always) exhibit s/z ratios at or above 1.4 s.

PQ

- Normal, healthy adult speakers should be able to produce PQ measures between **125 and 225 mL/s**, although measurement system could influence these measures.
- Male speakers tend to produce PQ measures which are larger than those of female speakers.
- Rau and Becket have provided the following means, based on data from their research sample using hand-held spirometers, for use as clinical guides[5]:
  - Males: 135 mL/s (sd = 19.3).
  - Females: 125.8 mL/s (sd = 16.4).
- Speakers with glottal incompetency tend to produce PQ measures **greater than 225 mL/s**.

5.14 Conclusion

Aerodynamic pressures and flows form the foundation for phonation and speech production as a whole. This chapter has reviewed the role of respiratory capacity, subglottal pressure, and transglottal airflow in phonatory function, and has also described both low- and high-cost instrumental methods by which these aerodynamic parameters can be estimated and the efficiency of voice production described. Along with previous chapters dealing with case history, perceptual evaluation of voice, and various objective acoustic measures of voice, the addition of aerodynamic measures gets us closer to a complete voice diagnostic protocol. The last essential component to our protocol (laryngeal visualization via endoscopy and stroboscopy) will be described in our next chapter.

Case Study

Part 1

Mr. Bradshaw is a 64 year-old man who experienced voice change 5 weeks ago, immediately after double coronary bypass surgery. The surgical report detailed some difficulty requiring longer than normal intubation. During the current voice evaluation, the perceptual assessment revealed low volume with a breathy and harsh voice quality. Prior to the initial onset of this problem, he had no history of voice difficulties. Mr. Bradshaw is employed as a foreman in a factory, which requires him to use his voice extensively throughout the day. He is also active in his church and other social groups, where his vocal demands are high. The current problem has caused a handicap or disability in both work and social engagements. He is a non-smoker, drinks one cup of coffee each day, and at least 60 oz of water spaced throughout the day.

1. Based on the short history above, what is your clinical hypothesis regarding the underlying physiological impairment and voice disorder diagnosis?

2. The history provides at least two possible causes for this diagnosis—what are they?

3. Given this diagnosis, what are your hypotheses regarding expected transglottal airflow and maximum phonation time?

Part 2

Read the following article:

Dastolfo C, Gartner-Schmidt J, Yu L, Carnes O, Gillespie AI. Aerodynamic outcomes of four common voice disorders: moving toward disorder-specific assessment. J Voice 2016;30(3):301–307.

1. Explain why patients with unilateral vocal fold paralysis exhibit, in general, greater transglottal airflow than patients with muscle tension dysphonia.

2. Explain why patients with mid-membranous lesions exhibit, in general, greater transglottal airflow than patients with muscle tension dysphonia.

3. What would you expect for measures of MPT in the four groups investigated in the Dastolfo study? Explain your answers.

5.15 Review Questions

1. Which of the following is the most accurate definition of vital capacity?
   a) The maximum quantity of air which can be stored in the lungs.
   b) The maximum quantity of air exhaled after a maximum inhalation.
   c) The lung volume required to sustain life.
   d) The amount of air inhaled after tidal inspiration.
   e) None of the above.

2. In the United States, aerodynamic analyses are often performed along with acoustic analyses as a procedure known as
   a) Behavioral voice analysis.
   b) Laryngeal videostroboscopy.
   c) Laryngeal function studies.
   d) Voice analysis studies.
   e) All of the above.

3. Which if the following is the correct expression of Ohm's law?
   a) $U = P/R$.
   b) $P = 1/F$.
   c) $F = 1/P$.
   d) $P - U = R$.
   e) None of the above.

4. In which of the following populations would we expect the largest measures of vital capacity?
   a) Young adult males.
   b) Young adult females.
   c) Elderly males.
   d) Elderly females.
   e) None of the above.

5. Although measures of vital capacity can vary based on factors including sex, height, and age, in a typical healthy

young adult we would expect measures of vital capacity to be within what range?

a) 2–10 liters.
b) 1–2 liters.
c) 2–8 liters.
d) 3–5 liters.
e) 5–10 liters.

6. Which of the following is an accurate definition of subglottal pressure (Ps)?

a) The tracheal pressure below the vocal folds which maintains lung inflation.
b) The amount of pressure between the lower and upper vocal fold edges during phonation.
c) The air pressure immediately below the glottis that acts as a force distributed over the inferior surface of the vocal folds.
d) All of the above.
e) None of the above.

7. If a patient was diagnosed with glottal incompetency due to unilateral vocal fold paralysis and which also causes a moderate-to-severe breathy voice quality, which of the following would you predict to be the measurement of their subglottal pressure?

a) 2 cm H_2O.
b) 4 cm H_2O.
c) 8 cm H_2O.
d) 15 cm H_2O.
e) All of the above.

8. If a patient was diagnosed with muscle tension dysphonia which also causes a moderate-to-severe rough and strained voice quality, which of the following would you predict to be the measurement of their subglottal pressure (Ps)?

a) 2 cm H_2O.
b) 4 cm H_2O.
c) 8 cm H_2O.
d) 15 cm H_2O.
e) All of the above.

9. When measuring phonation threshold pressure (PtP), what prompt is given to the patient to ensure you are measuring the threshold of phonation pressure and not pressure during some other behavior?

a) Take as deep a breath as possible.
b) Produce sound as soft as possible without whispering.
c) Produce sound as loudly as possible.
d) Sustain a comfortable pitch and loudness.
e) None of the above.

10. Which of the following is an accurate description of a pneumotach?

a) A device which allows for temporal recordings of voice productions.
b) An instrument consisting of a microphone, analog-to-digital converter, and amplifier which allows for the measurement of frequency and amplitude.
c) A device which allows for measurement of the drop in air pressure at the point of resistance to airflow.
d) An instrument placed inside the nasal cavity allowing for measurement of nasal pressures during speech.
e) None of the above.

11. VC/MPT is the formula for which aerodynamic measurement?

a) Vital capacity.
b) Phonation quotient.
c) Estimated mean flow rate.
d) Subglottal pressure.
e) Transglottal airflow.

12. Which of the following statements would be most likely in a clinical context?

a) A patient with muscle tension dysphonia exhibits greater transglottal airflow than a patient with unilateral vocal fold paralysis.
b) A patient with vocal nodules exhibits less transglottal airflow than a patient with muscle tension dysphonia.
c) A patient with unilateral vocal fold paralysis exhibits less subglottal pressure than a normal speaker.
d) A patient with unilateral vocal fold paralysis exhibits greater transglottal airflow than a normal speaker.
e) None of the above.

13. Measurements of transglottal airflow are usually measured from what productions of what stimuli?

a) /pa/ or /pi/.
b) Vowels embedded in sentences.
c) The six CAPE-V sentences.
d) Rainbow passage.
e) None of the above.

14. In a healthy, nondysphonic speaker you would expect measures of transglottal airflow rate to be between what levels when producing speech at comfortable pitch and loudness?

a) 50–100 mL/s.
b) 100–120 mL/s.c. 100–200 mL/s.
c) 200–400 mL/s.
d) 300–600 mL/s.

15. Which of the following would be a transglottal airflow measurement most likely associated with vocal fold bowing secondary to Parkinson's disease causing a moderate-to-severe breathy voice quality with reduced loudness?

a) 75 mL/s.
b) 150 mL/s.
c) 200 mL/s.
d) 300 mL/s.
e) All of the above.

16. Which of the following maximum phonation time (MPT) would you expect from a normal, healthy 30-year-old man?

a) 10 seconds.
b) 12 seconds.
c) 15 seconds.
d) 20 seconds.
e) None of the above.

17. Which of the following s/z ratio measurements would you expect from an individual with unilateral vocal fold paralysis causing significant glottal insufficiency and a severely breathy voice quality?

a) 0.90.
b) 1.00.
c) 1.85.

d) 1.25.

e) None of the above.

18. A healthy, nondysphonic, 10-year-old child would be expected to prolong a vowel for at least what amount of time?
    a) 5 seconds.
    b) 10 seconds.
    c) 20 seconds.
    d) 30 seconds.
    e) All of the above.

19. Which of the following phonation quotient measures would you expect in a patient with significant bowing and glottal insufficiency secondary to presbylaryngis?
    a) 100 mL/s.
    b) 150 mL/s.
    c) 200 mL/s.
    d) 250 mL/s.
    e) All of the above.

20. Which of the following can influence measurements of subglottal pressure and transglottal airflow?
    a) Vocal intensity.
    b) Fundamental frequency.
    c) Vocal fold lesions.
    d) The presence of vocal hyperfunction.
    e) All of the above.

5.16 Answers and Explanations

1. Correct: The maximum quantity of air exhaled after a maximum inhalation (**b**).
   (**b**) Vital capacity (VC) is a measurement used to assess the lung capacity available to support phonation during connected speech. VC is defined as the maximum quantity of air that can be exhaled after a maximum inhalation. It is measured by asking a patient to breathe in as deeply as possible, and then exhale as much air as possible—the amount of air exhaled is measured as VC. (**a**) The maximum amount of air which can be stored in the lungs is referred to as total lung capacity. (**c**) The amount of air needed to sustain life will vary from individual to individual, but is typically not a lung volume measured in a clinical context. (**d**) The amount of air inhaled after a tidal inspiration is referred to as inspiratory reserve volume.

2. Correct: Laryngeal function studies (**c**).
   (**c**) In the United States, aerodynamic and acoustic assessments are typically performed during Laryngeal Function studies (CPT 92520), a procedure that, along with Behavioral and Qualitative Analysis of Voice (CPT 92524) and Laryngeal Endoscopy with Stroboscopy (CPT 31579), constitutes a comprehensive voice evaluation resulting in a complete diagnostic profile of the patient. (**a,b**) Behavioral voice analysis and laryngeal videostroboscopy are labels often given to a behavioral and qualitative analysis of voice and laryngeal endoscopy with stroboscopy, respectively. (**d**) The term "voice analysis studies" is typically not used to refer to acoustic or aerodynamic analyses.

3. Correct: U = P/R (**a**).
   (**a**) Pressure, airflow, and resistance are related to each other. This relationship can be described by applying Ohm's law to fluids (air is a type of fluid), as expressed in the formula U = P/R where U = flow, P = pressure, and R = resistance. (**b, c**) P = 1/F and F = 1/P are formulas used to calculate the period of vibration (P) or the frequency of vibration (F) in the context of voice production. (**d**) P − U = R is an incorrect formula if one wanted to assess the relationship between pressure, flow, and resistance.

4. Correct: Young adult males (**a**).
   (**a**) Young, healthy adult males on average have larger lung capacities than both females and elderly males, due to (**a**) greater physical size and volume of the lungs than females and (**b**) greater physiological capabilities of respiratory musculature and lung tissue than elderly males. (**b**) Females, on average, have smaller lung capacities than males due to smaller physical size and volume of the lungs. (**c, d**) Numerous physiological changes occur with aging, including reduced muscular function and changes to the physiology of lung tissue which can result in decreases in measurements of vital capacity in elderly population.

5. Correct: 3–5 L (**d**).
   (**d**) Healthy, young adult male and female speakers typically produce measures of VC within a range of 3 to 5 liters, with males exhibiting greater measures of VC than females. (**a, b, c, e**) With advancing age, VC tends to lower such that measures may be recorded below 3 L for healthy adults older than 65 years. Young children exhibit much lower VC than adults due to inherently smaller lung structure and available volume.

6. Correct: The air pressure immediately below the glottis that acts as a force distributed over the inferior surface of the vocal folds. (**c**)
   (**c**) Subglottal pressure is the force below the vocal folds which separates the glottis to initiate phonation and helps maintain ongoing vocal fold oscillation. (**a**) Tracheal pressure does help maintain lung inflation but is not the correct definition of Ps. (**b**) The amount of pressure between the lower and upper vocal fold edges is referred to as intraglottal pressure.

7. Correct: 15 cm H_2O (**d**).
   (**d**) Unilateral vocal fold paralysis typically manifests as vocal hypofunction. Subglottal pressure in dysphonia secondary to vocal hypofunction is often measured at levels greater than 10 cm H_2O. (**a, b, c**) During habitual phonation (e.g., comfortable "pitch and loudness"), healthy, nondysphonic speakers typically produce measures of subglottal pressure between 5 and 10 cm H_2O.

8. Correct: 15 cm H_2O (**d**).
   (**d**) Muscle tension dysphonia (MTD) is a form of vocal hyperfunction. As with vocal hypofunction, subglottal pressure in hyperfunctional voices is often measured at levels greater than 10 cm H_2O. (**a, b, c**) During habitual phonation (e.g., comfortable "pitch and loudness"), healthy, nondysphonic speakers typically produce measures of subglottal pressure between 5 and 10 cm H_2O.

9. Correct: Produce sound as soft as possible without whispering (**b**).
   (**b**) Phonation threshold pressure (PtP) is the minimum amount of air pressure required to set the vocal folds into

vibration. It is measured while a speaker produces voice at their lowest possible intensity (e.g., as soft as possible without whispering), and has been found to be very sensitive to the presence of vocal fold. (**a, c, d**) Breathing, producing sound loudly, or producing sound at comfortable levels would not allow the assessment of the threshold pressure required to set the vocal folds into motion.

10. Correct: A device which allows for measurement of the drop in air pressure at the point of resistance to airflow (**c**).
(**a**) A pneumotach contains some internal screen which places a resistance to airflow and is used to measure transglottal airflow rate. A pneumotach is typically used in line with a facemask and together such systems are referred to as a pneumotachograph. (**a**) Temporal or time measurements of voicing are used to measure such variables as maximum phonation time, voice onset time, etc. (**b**) Microphones are most often used when measuring acoustic properties of voice. (**d**) For speech production, nasal cavity pressures are typically not assessed, although measures of nasalance (the ratio of acoustic energy emanating from the nose compared to that emanating from the oral cavity) are of interest in patients with suspected velopharyngeal dysfunction.

11. Correct: Phonation quotient (**b**).
(**b**) VC/MPT represents the formula for phonation quotient (PQ), which is the ratio of vital capacity to maximum phonation time. PQ is typically increased in the presence of voice impairment. (**a**) Vital capacity is the maximum amount of air which can be exhaled after maximum inhalation. (**c**) Estimated mean flow rate can be calculated using a formula derived from an existing measure of phonation quotient. (**d**) Subglottal pressure and transglottal airflow rates do not require calculations of vital capacity or phonation time.

12. Correct: A patient with unilateral vocal fold paralysis exhibits greater transglottal airflow than a normal speaker (**d**).
(**d**) Unilateral vocal paralysis typically causes glottal insufficiency, which translates to excess airflow through the glottis during phonation. This would be measured as increased transglottal airflow. (**a**) Muscle tension dysphonia is often characterized by increased medial compression during adduction, translating to an increased closed phase and rapid closing phase of the vibratory cycle. This can cause decreased transglottal airflow rates. (**b**) Vocal nodules often result in glottal gaps, which can translate to increased transglottal airflow during phonation. (**c**) Normal speakers will typically exhibit lower measures of transglottal airflow compared to speakers with paralysis or other conditions causing glottal insufficiency.

13. Correct: /pa/ or /pi/ (**a**).
(**a**) Measurement of transglottal airflow during speech is most often reported from sustained vowels and also from the consonant release (burst) or vocalic portion of plosive + syllable repetitions (as in stimuli for measuring air pressure, including /pa/ and /pi/). (**b**) Transglottal airflow can be measured from vowels embedded in sentences, but most data available for comparison would come from sustained vowels or vowels from /pa/ or /pi/. (**c, d**) Emerging data exist for transglottal airflow from connected speech

stimuli such as the CAPE-V sentences and Rainbow passage, but to date very few references are available for comparison.

14. Correct: 100–200 mL/s (**c**).
(**c**) Phonation which is not associated with either hyperfunction or hypofunction will usually be measured between 100 and 200 mL/s when produced at comfortable levels. (**a, b, d, e**) Phonation associated with hyperfunction can result in transglottal airflow rates falling near or below 100 mL/s. Phonation associated with hypofunction can result in transglottal airflow rates above 200 mL/s.

15. Correct: 300 mL/s (**d**).
(**d**) Phonation associated with hypofunction such as glottal insufficiency secondary to Parkinson's disease can result in transglottal airflow rates above 200 mL/s. (**a, b, c**) Phonation associated with hyperfunction can result in transglottal airflow rates falling near or below 100 mL/s. The range of normal for nondysphonic phonation produced at comfortable pitch and loudness is 100 to 200 mL/s.

16. Correct: 20 seconds (**d**).
(**d**) Nondysphonic, young, healthy adult males should be able to maximally prolong a vowel for at least 20 seconds. Methodology (e.g., instructions) is important for eliciting a true maximum performance. (**a, b, c**) In healthy young adult males, any MPT measure below 20 seconds would be considered below the range of normal.

17. Correct: 1.85 (**c**).
(**c**) Nondysphonic phonation in speakers with appropriate glottal closure is usually measured below 1.40. Typically normal speakers can prolong the /s/ sound for the approximate duration as the /z/ sound, and resulting s/z ratios will approximate 1.0. (**a, b, d**) S/z ratio measures falling below 1.4 are considered within the range of normal.

18. Correct: 10 seconds (**b**).
(**b**) Young children without dysphonia or other medical conditions should be able to prolong a vowel for at least 10 seconds in duration. Methodology (e.g., instructions) is important for eliciting a true maximum performance. (**a, c, d**) An MPT of 5 seconds in a nondysphonic healthy child would be considered below the range of normal. While MPT measures of 20 or 30 seconds would be impressive for a 10-year-old child, they would be above what would be typically expected.

19. Correct: 250 mL/s (**d**).
(**d**) As with measures of transglottal airflow acquired with a pneumotach, phonation quotient (PQ) will be higher in patients with glottal insufficiency. Measures above 200 mL/s are usually interpreted as falling outside the range of normal. (**a, b, c**) Phonation quotient (PQ) measures at or below 200 mL/s can be viewed as within the range of normal.

20. Correct: All of the above (**e**).
(**e**) All of the variables listed above can influence subglottal pressure and transglottal airflow. It is crucial to establish a consistent measurement method when using to acquire and compare aerodynamic measurements. (**a, b, c, d**) While intensity, frequency, lesions, and hyperfunction alone can influence aerodynamic measurements, collectively they would all affect the resulting calculations of pressure and airflow.

Appendix 5.1 Manufacturers of aerodynamic equipment capable of measuring pressure and/or flow for research and/or clinical applications.

System	Manufacturer	Address/Website
Aeroview	Glottal Enterprises	1201 E. Fayette St, Suite no. 15 Syracuse, NY 13210–1953 United States www.glottal.com
PG-20E and PG-100E (P_s only)	Glottal Enterprises	1201 E. Fayette St, Suite no. 15 Syracuse, NY 13210–1953 United States www.glottal.com
Phonatory Aerodynamic System (PAS)	Pentax Medical	3 Paragon Drive Montvale, NJ 07645–1782, United States www.pentaxmedical.com

References

[1] Dejonckere PH. Assessment of voice and respiratory function. In: Remacle M, Eckel HE, eds. Surgery of Larynx and Trachea. Berlin, Heidelberg: Springer; 2010:11–26

[2] American Medical Association. CPT Assistant. Chicago, IL: AMA; 2006

[3] Hirano M, Koike Y, Von Leden H. Maximum phonation time and air usage during phonation. Clinical study. Folia Phoniatr (Basel). 1968; 20 (4):185–201

[4] Iwata S, von Leden H. Phonation quotient in patients with laryngeal diseases. Folia Phoniatr (Basel). 1970; 22(2):117–128

[5] Rau D, Beckett RL. Aerodynamic assessment of vocal function using handheld spirometers. J Speech Hear Disord. 1984; 49(2):183–188

[6] Awan S. The Voice Diagnostic Protocol: A Practical Guide to the Diagnosis of Voice Disorders. Austin, TX: Pro-Ed Inc.; 2001

[7] Baken RJ, Orkiloff RF. Clinical Measurement of Speech and Voice. San Diego, CA: Singular; 2000

[8] Kostyk BE, Putnam Rochet A. Laryngeal airway resistance in teachers with vocal fatigue: a preliminary study. J Voice. 1998; 12(3):287–299

[9] Dejonckere PH, Bradley P, Clemente P, et al. Committee on Phoniatrics of the European Laryngological Society (ELS). A basic protocol for functional assessment of voice pathology, especially for investigating the efficacy of (phonosurgical) treatments and evaluating new assessment techniques. Guideline elaborated by the Committee on Phoniatrics of the European Laryngological Society (ELS). Eur Arch Otorhinolaryngol. 2001; 258(2):77–82

[10] Eckel FC, Boone DR. The S/Z ratio as an indicator of laryngeal pathology. J Speech Hear Disord. 1981; 46(2):147–149

[11] Zraick RI, Smith-Olinde L, Shotts LL. Adult normative data for the KayPENTAX Phonatory Aerodynamic System Model 6600. J Voice. 2012; 26(2):164–176

[12] Lumb A. Nunn's Applied Respiratory Physiology. 7th ed. Atlanta, GA: Elsevier; 2010

[13] Baldwin ED, Cournand A, Richards DW, Jr. Pulmonary insufficiency; physiological classification, clinical methods of analysis, standard values in normal subjects. Medicine (Baltimore). 1948; 27(3):243–278

[14] Adachi D, Yamada M, Nishiguchi S, et al. Age-related decline in chest wall mobility: a cross-sectional study among community-dwelling elderly women. J Am Osteopath Assoc. 2015; 115(6):384–389

[15] Awan SN. The aging female voice: acoustic and respiratory data. Clin Linguist Phon. 2006; 20(2–3):171–180

[16] American Thoracic Society. Lung function testing: selection of reference values and interpretative strategies. Am Rev Respir Dis. 1991; 144 (5):1202–1218

[17] Backman H, Lindberg A, Od, é, n A, et al. Reference values for spirometry - report from the Obstructive Lung Disease in Northern Sweden studies. Eur Clin Respir J. 2015; 2

[18] Weinrich B, Brehm SB, Knudsen C, McBride S, Hughes M. Pediatric normative data for the KayPENTAX phonatory aerodynamic system model 6600. J Voice. 2013; 27(1):46–56

[19] Barsties B, Verfaillie R, Roy N, Maryn Y. Do body mass index and fat volume influence vocal quality, phonatory range, and aerodynamics in females? Co-DAS. 2013; 25(4):310–318

[20] Tan WC, Bourbeau J, Hernandez P, et al. LHCE study investigators. Canadian prediction equations of spirometric lung function for Caucasian adults 20 to 90 years of age: results from the Canadian Obstructive Lung Disease (COLD) study and the Lung Health Canadian Environment (LHCE) study. Can Respir J. 2011; 18(6):321–326

[21] Smolej Naranci, ć N, Pavlovi, ć M, Zuskin E, et al. New reference equations for forced spirometry in elderly persons. Respir Med. 2009; 103(4):621–628

[22] Piccioni P, Borraccino A, Forneris MP, et al. Reference values of Forced Expiratory Volumes and pulmonary flows in 3–6 year children: a cross-sectional study. Respir Res. 2007; 8:14

[23] Pistelli F, Bottai M, Carrozzi L, et al. Reference equations for spirometry from a general population sample in central Italy. Respir Med. 2007; 101 (4):814–825

[24] Pistelli F, Bottai M, Viegi G, et al. Smooth reference equations for slow vital capacity and flow-volume curve indexes. Am J Respir Crit Care Med. 2000; 161(3, Pt 1):899–905

[25] Baltopoulos G, Fildisis G, Karatzas S, Georgiakodis F, Myrianthefs P. Reference values and prediction equations for FVC and FEV(1) in the Greek elderly. Lung. 2000; 178(4):201–212

[26] Rothenberg M. Interpolating subglottal pressure from oral pressure. J Speech Hear Disord. 1982; 47(2):219–223

[27] Rothenberg M. A new inverse-filtering technique for deriving the glottal air flow waveform during voicing. J Acoust Soc Am. 1973; 53(6):1632–1645

[28] Smitheran JR, Hixon TJ. A clinical method for estimating laryngeal airway resistance during vowel production. J Speech Hear Disord. 1981; 46(2):138–146

[29] Chen SH, Hsiao TY, Hsiao LC, Chung YM, Chiang SC. Outcome of resonant voice therapy for female teachers with voice disorders: perceptual, physiological, acoustic, aerodynamic, and functional measurements. J Voice. 2007; 21(4):415–425

[30] Jiang J, O, ', Mara T, Chen HJ, Stern JI, Vlagos D, Hanson D. Aerodynamic measurements of patients with Parkinson's disease. J Voice. 1999; 13(4):583–591

[31] Titze IR. Phonation threshold pressure measurement with a semi-occluded vocal tract. J Speech Lang Hear Res. 2009; 52(4):1062–1072

[32] Netsell R, Hixon TJ. A noninvasive method for clinically estimating subglottal air pressure. J Speech Hear Disord. 1978; 43(3):326–330

[33] Hartl DM, Hans S, Vaissi, è, re J, Brasnu DF. Laryngeal aerodynamics after vocal fold augmentation with autologous fat vs thyroplasty in the same patient. Arch Otolaryngol Head Neck Surg. 2005; 131(8):696–700

[34] Hartl DM, Hans S, Vaissi, è, re J, Riquet M, Laccourreye O, Brasnu DF. Objective voice analysis after autologous fat injection for unilateral vocal fold paralysis. Ann Otol Rhinol Laryngol. 2001; 110(3):229–235

[35] Shin JE, Nam SY, Yoo SJ, Kim SY. Analysis of voice and quantitative measurement of glottal gap after thyroplasty type I in the treatment of unilateral vocal paralysis. J Voice. 2002; 16(1):136–142

[36] Rosen CA, Lombard LE, Murry T. Acoustic, aerodynamic, and videostroboscopic features of bilateral vocal fold lesions. Ann Otol Rhinol Laryngol. 2000; 109(9):823–828

[37] Liang FY, Yang JS, Mei XS, et al. The vocal aerodynamic change in female patients with muscular tension dysphonia after voice training. J Voice. 2014; 28(3):393.e7–393.e10

[38] Rosenthal AL, Lowell SY, Colton RH. Aerodynamic and acoustic features of vocal effort. J Voice. 2014; 28(2):144–153

[39] Awan SN, Novaleski CK, Yingling JR. Test-retest reliability for aerodynamic measures of voice. J Voice. 2013; 27(6):674–684

[40] Zheng YQ, Zhang BR, Su WY, et al. Laryngeal aerodynamic analysis in assisting with the diagnosis of muscle tension dysphonia. J Voice. 2012; 26 (2):177–181

[41] Cantarella G, Baracca G, Pignataro L, Forti S. Assessment of dysphonia due to benign vocal fold lesions by acoustic and aerodynamic indices: a multivariate analysis. Logoped Phoniatr Vocol. 2011; 36(1):21–27

[42] Ma EP, Yiu EM. Multiparametric evaluation of dysphonic severity. J Voice. 2006; 20(3):380–390

[43] Weinrich B, Salz B, Hughes M. Aerodynamic measurements: normative data for children ages 6:0 to 10:11 years. J Voice. 2005; 19(3):326–339

[44] Yiu EM, Yuen YM, Whitehill T, Winkworth A. Reliability and applicability of aerodynamic measures in dysphonia assessment. Clin Linguist Phon. 2004; 18(6–8):463–478

[45] Hartl DA, Hans S, Vaissi, è, re J, Brasnu DA. Objective acoustic and aerodynamic measures of breathiness in paralytic dysphonia. Eur Arch Otorhinolaryngol. 2003; 260(4):175–182

[46] Holmberg EB, Hillman RE, Perkell JS. Glottal airflow and transglottal air pressure measurements for male and female speakers in soft, normal, and loud voice. J Acoust Soc Am. 1988; 84(2):511–529

[47] Fu S, Theodoros DG, Ward EC. Intensive versus traditional voice therapy for vocal nodules: perceptual, physiological, acoustic and aerodynamic changes. J Voice. 2015; 29(2):260.e31–260.e44

[48] Dastolfo C, Gartner-Schmidt J, Yu L, Carnes O, Gillespie AI. Aerodynamic outcomes of four common voice disorders: moving toward disorder-specific assessment. J Voice. 2016; 30(3):301–307

[49] Gillespie AI, Gartner-Schmidt J, Rubinstein EN, Abbott KV. Aerodynamic profiles of women with muscle tension dysphonia/aphonia. J Speech Lang Hear Res. 2013; 56(2):481–488

[50] Holmberg EB, Doyle P, Perkell JS, Hammarberg B, Hillman RE. Aerodynamic and acoustic voice measurements of patients with vocal nodules: variation in baseline and changes across voice therapy. J Voice. 2003; 17(3):269–282

[51] Hixon TJ, Hawley JL, Wilson KJ. An around-the-house device for the clinical determination of respiratory driving pressure: a note on making simple even simpler. J Speech Hear Disord. 1982; 47(4):413–415

[52] Higgins MB, Netsell R, Schulte L. Vowel-related differences in laryngeal articulatory and phonatory function. J Speech Lang Hear Res. 1998; 41(4):712–724

[53] Netsell R, Lotz WK, DuChane AS, Barlow SM. Vocal tract aerodynamics during syllable productions: normative data and theoretical implications. J Voice. 1991; 5(1):1–9

[54] Gartner-Schmidt JL, Hirai R, Dastolfo C, Rosen CA, Yu L, Gillespie AI. Phonatory aerodynamics in connected speech. Laryngoscope. 2015; 125(12):2764–2771

[55] Zhuang P, Swinarska JT, Robieux CF, Hoffman MR, Lin S, Jiang JJ. Measurement of phonation threshold power in normal and disordered voice production. Ann Otol Rhinol Laryngol. 2013; 122(9):555–560

[56] Titze I. Principles of Voice Production. Upper Saddle River, NJ: Prentice Hall; 2004

[57] Rothenberg M. Measurement of airflow in speech. J Speech Hear Res. 1977; 20(1):155–176

[58] Isshiki N. Regulatory mechanism of voice intensity variation. J Speech Hear Res. 1964; 7:17–29

[59] Holmberg EB, Hillman RE, Perkell JS. Glottal airflow and transglottal air pressure measurements for male and female speakers in low, normal, and high pitch. J Voice. 1989; 3(4):294–305

[60] Titze IR. Physiologic and acoustic differences between male and female voices. J Acoust Soc Am. 1989; 85(4):1699–1707

[61] Titze IR, Maxfield L, Palaparthi A. An oral pressure conversion ratio as a predictor of vocal efficiency. J Voice. 2016; 30(4):398–406

[62] Titze IR. Principles of Voice Production. Englewood Cliffs, NJ: Prentice Hall; 1994

[63] Carroll LM, Sataloff RT, Heuer RJ, Spiegel JR, Radionoff SL, Cohn JR. Respiratory and glottal efficiency measures in normal classically trained singers. J Voice. 1996; 10(2):139–145

[64] Lundy DS, Roy S, Casiano RR, Evans J, Sullivan PA, Xue JW. Relationship between aerodynamic measures of glottal efficiency and stroboscopic findings in asymptomatic singing students. J Voice. 2000; 14(2):178–183

[65] Grillo EU, Verdolini Abbott K, Lee TD. Effects of masking noise on laryngeal resistance for breathy, normal, and pressed voice. J Speech Lang Hear Res. 2010; 53(4):850–861

[66] Deem JF, Miller L. Manual of Voice Therapy. 2nd ed. Austin, TX: PRO-ED; 2000

[67] Kent RD, Ball MJ. Voice Quality Measurement. San Diego, CA: Singular; 2000

[68] Kent RD, Kent JF, Rosenbek JC. Maximum performance tests of speech production. J Speech Hear Disord. 1987; 52(4):367–387

[69] Lewis K, Casteel R, McMahon J. Duration of sustained /a/ related to the number of trials. Folia Phoniatr (Basel). 1982; 34(1):41–48

[70] Solomon NP, Garlitz SJ, Milbrath RL. Respiratory and laryngeal contributions to maximum phonation duration. J Voice. 2000; 14(3):331–340

[71] Wuyts FL, De Bodt MS, Molenberghs G, et al. The dysphonia severity index: an objective measure of vocal quality based on a multiparameter approach. J Speech Lang Hear Res. 2000; 43(3):796–809

[72] Yumoto E. Aerodynamics, voice quality, and laryngeal image analysis of normal and pathologic voices. Curr Opin Otolaryngol Head Neck Surg. 2004; 12(3):166–173

[73] Wang CC, Chang MH, Jiang RS, et al. Laryngeal electromyography-guided hyaluronic acid vocal fold injection for unilateral vocal fold paralysis: a prospective long-term follow-up outcome report. JAMA Otolaryngol Head Neck Surg. 2015; 141(3):264–271

[74] Lodder WL, Dikkers FG. Comparison of voice outcome after vocal fold augmentation with fat or calcium hydroxylapatite. Laryngoscope. 2015; 125(5):1161–1165

[75] Van der Meer G, Ferreira Y, Loock JW. The S/Z ratio: a simple and reliable clinical method of evaluating laryngeal function in patients after intubation. J Crit Care. 2010; 25(3):489–492

[76] Watts CR, Diviney SS, Hamilton A, Toles L, Childs L, Mau T. The effect of stretch-and-flow voice therapy on measures of vocal function and handicap. J Voice. 2015; 29(2):191–199

[77] Trudeau MD, Forrest LA. The contributions of phonatory volume and transglottal airflow to the s/z ratio. Am J Sp Lang Path. 1997; 6:65–69

[78] Farhood Z, Reusser NM, Bender RW, Thekdi AA, Albright JT, Edmonds JL. Pediatric recurrent laryngeal nerve reinnervation: a case series and analysis of postoperative outcomes. Int J Pediatr Otorhinolaryngol. 2015; 79(8):1320–1323

[79] Gramuglia AC, Tavares EL, Rodrigues SA, Martins RH. Perceptual and acoustic parameters of vocal nodules in children. Int J Pediatr Otorhinolaryngol. 2014; 78(2):312–316

[80] Hufnagle J, Hufnagle K. S/z ratio in dysphonic children with and without vocal nodules. Lang Speech Serv Schools. 1988; 19:418–422

[81] Stemple JS, Roy N, Klaben BK. Clinical Voice Pathology Theory and Management, San Diego, CA: Plural; 2014

[82] Neiman GS, Edeson B. Procedural aspects of eliciting maximum phonation time. Folia Phoniatr (Basel). 1981; 33(5):285–293

[83] Finnegan DE. Maximum phonation time for children with normal voices. J Commun Disord. 1984; 17(5):309–317

[84] Mohseni R, Sandoughdar N. Survey of voice acoustic parameters in Iranian female teachers. J Voice. 2016; 30(4):507.e1–507.e5

[85] Nemr K, Sim, õ, es-Zenari M, de Souza GS, Hachiya A, Tsuji DH. Correlation of the Dysphonia Severity Index (DSI), Consensus Auditory-Perceptual Evaluation of Voice (CAPE-V), and gender in Brazilians with and without voice disorders. J Voice. 2016; 30(6):765.e7–765.e11

[86] Zhuge P, You H, Wang H, Zhang Y, Du H. An analysis of the effects of voice therapy on patients with early vocal fold polyps. J Voice. 2016; 30(6):698–704

[87] Goy H, Fernandes DN, Pichora-Fuller MK, van Lieshout P. Normative voice data for younger and older adults. J Voice. 2013; 27(5):545–555

[88] Maslan J, Leng X, Rees C, Blalock D, Butler SG. Maximum phonation time in healthy older adults. J Voice. 2011; 25(6):709–713

[89] Leino T, Laukkanen AM, Ilom, ä, ki I, M, ä, ki E. Assessment of vocal capacity of Finnish university students. Folia Phoniatr Logop. 2008; 60(4):199–209

[90] Nawka T, Sittel C, Arens C, et al. Voice and respiratory outcomes after permanent transoral surgery of bilateral vocal fold paralysis. Laryngoscope. 2015; 125(12):2749–2755

[91] Lundy DS, Casiano RR, Xue JW. Can maximum phonation time predict voice outcome after thyroplasty type I? Laryngoscope. 2004; 114(8):1447–1454

[92] Mueller PB, Larson GW, Summers PA. Letter to the editor. Lang Speech Hear Serv Sch. 1993; 24:177–178

[93] Larson GW, Mueller PB, Summers PA. The effect of procedural variations on the S/Z ratio of adults. J Commun Disord. 1991; 24(2):135–140

[94] Mendes Tavares EL, Brasolotto AG, Rodrigues SA, Benito Pessin AB, Garcia Martins RH. Maximum phonation time and s/z ratio in a large child cohort. J Voice. 2012; 26(5):675.e1–675.e4

[95] Sorenson DN, Parker PA. The voiced/voiceless phonation time in children with and without laryngeal pathology. Lang Speech Hear Serv Sch. 1992; 23:163–168

[96] Fendler M, Shearer WM. Reliability of the S/Z ratio in normal children's voices. Lang Speech Hear Serv Sch. 1988; 19:2–4

[97] Tait NA, Michel JF, Carpenter MA. Maximum duration of sustained /s/ and /z/ in children. J Speech Hear Disord. 1980; 45(2):239–246

[98] McMullan PM. Comparison of acoustic and aerodynamic measurements of laryngeal function using low-cost and high-cost systems. Master's Thesis. Christian University, Texas; 2016

[99] Joshi A, Watts CR. Measurement reliability of phonation quotient derived from three aerodynamic instruments. J Voice. 2016; 30(6):773.e13–773.e19

[100] De Virgilio A, Chang MH, Jiang RS, et al. Influence of superior laryngeal nerve injury on glottal configuration/function of thyroidectomy-induced unilateral vocal fold paralysis. Otolaryngol Head Neck Surg. 2014; 151(6):996–1002

[101] Wang CC, Chang MH, Wang CP, et al. Laryngeal electromyography-guided hyaluronic acid vocal fold injection for unilateral vocal fold paralysis–preliminary results. J Voice. 2012; 26(4):506–514

Suggested Readings

[1] American Thoracic Society. Lung function testing: selection of reference values and interpretative strategies. Am Rev Respir Dis. 1991; 144(5):1202–1218

[2] Holmberg EB, Hillman RE, Perkell JS. Glottal airflow and transglottal air pressure measurements for male and female speakers in soft, normal, and loud voice. J Acoust Soc Am. 1988; 84(2):511–529

[3] Holmberg EB, Hillman RE, Perkell JS. Glottal airflow and transglottal air pressure measurements for male and female speakers in low, normal, and high pitch. J Voice. 1989; 3(4):294–305

[4] Iwata S, von Leden H. Phonation quotient in patients with laryngeal diseases. Folia Phoniatr (Basel). 1970; 22(2):117–128

[5] Rau D, Beckett RL. Aerodynamic assessment of vocal function using hand-held spirometers. J Speech Hear Disord. 1984; 49(2):183–188

[6] Titze I. Principles of Voice Production. Upper Saddle River, NJ: Prentice Hall; 2004

[7] Zraick RI, Smith-Olinde L, Shotts LL. Adult normative data for the KayPEN-TAX Phonatory Aerodynamic System Model 6600. J Voice. 2012; 26 (2):164–176

6 Laryngeal Endoscopy and Stroboscopy

Summary

This chapter describes the roles, responsibilities, and procedures of the speech–language pathologist, as they relate to visualization of the larynx via laryngeal endoscopy with and without strobo- scopy. The use of endoscopy within the professional scope of practice, knowledge and skill requirements, and the interprofes- sional collaborative practices while performing laryngeal endos- copy are defined. Equipment needs and methodological aspects of laryngeal visualization are covered, and interpretation and re- porting guidelines are described. Case study examples and video tutorials are provided to assist the learner.

Keywords: endoscopy, larynx, videostroboscopy, fiberscope

6.1 Learning Objectives

At the end of this chapter, learners will be able to
- Identify the source of validation for laryngeal endoscopy and stroboscopy falling within the scope of practice in speech– language pathology.
- Describe interprofessional collaborative practice patterns of speech–language pathologists and otolaryngologists within the context of performance and interpretation of laryngeal endoscopy and stroboscopy.
- Identify the technology requirements for laryngeal endoscopy and stroboscopy.
- Describe the methodological characteristics of clinical exami- nation using endoscopy and stroboscopy.
- Compare and contrast the visual characteristics of different vocal fold lesions as viewed during laryngeal endoscopy and stroboscopy.

- Describe the clinically relevant characteristics of vocal fold vibratory dynamics as viewed during stroboscopy.
- Develop a model report based on laryngeal endoscopy and stroboscopy evaluation.

6.2 Introduction

Endoscopy (endo—"within"; **oscopy—**"to look at"), in the context of medicine, is a procedure that allows a healthcare professional to look inside the body with the use of an **endoscope**. As illus- trated in ► Fig. 6.1, endoscopes can be made of rigid or flexible material. They contain a fiberoptic system that conveys light from an external source into the body, and a lens system which trans- mits the reflected image of the internal body surfaces. An eye- piece at one end of the scope allows the examiner to see the reflected image or allows for the attachment of a camera for cap- turing and recording of the image. The camera can also be con- nected to a computer or video monitor screen. When the larynx is examined using endoscopy, the process is a type of **laryngo- scopy** (**larynx + oscopy**), although you do not have to have an en- doscope to look at the larynx (it can also be viewed with a mirror). Some professionals prefer the term **phonoscopy** or **pho- noscopic examination** when laryngoscopy is performed by a speech–language pathologist (SLP) for the purposes of evaluating vocal function.[1] This term distinguishes laryngoscopy for voice examination from laryngoscopy for swallowing examination (e.g., fiberoptic endoscopic examination of swallowing [FEES]). Both otolaryngologists and SLPs perform laryngoscopy as a part of standard clinical evaluations. **Stroboscopy** incorporates the use of a stroboscopic (flashing) light or a rapidly shuttered camera to re- sult in the illusion of slow motion. The stroboscopic image allows for the observation and description of vibratory cycles and

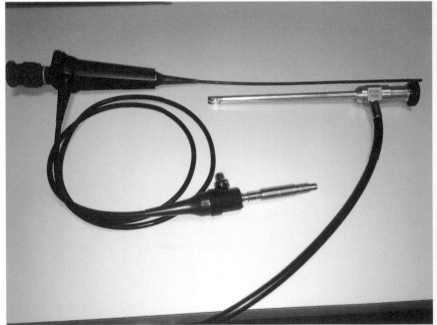

Fig. 6.1 Examples of rigid and flexible endoscopes.

specific characteristics of vibratory dynamics. Stroboscopy has often been referred to as "videostroboscopy," with the "video" prefix referring to the use of a video camera for motion image capture and playback.

6.3 Principles of Stroboscopy

Many of us have been in a club or at a dance where a rapidly flashing strobe light was turned on, making the people in the hall appear as though they were moving in slow motion. This same illusion is used in laryngeal stroboscopy to provide a detailed view of the vibratory characteristics of vocal fold motion. We must remember that, during typical voice production, the vocal folds are vibrating at hundreds of times per second. Like looking at a hummingbird's wing during flight, without some method of slowing down this vibration, our view of the vibrating object would be blurred and indistinct—we know that the structure is moving, but the details of the vibratory movement would be unclear. However, a strobe light (periodically interrupted light) may be used to visualize a rapidly moving object. If the object(s) (e.g., vocal folds) is/are moving in a relatively periodic (repetitive) fashion, the object(s) will appear to move in slow motion if the frequency of the strobe light is slightly different than the frequency of vibration (e.g., vocal frequency = 200 Hz; strobe light frequency = 195 Hz). If the frequency of the strobe light is the same as the frequency of vibration of the moving object(s), then the resulting image will appear to be a still image or "freeze frame." Both of these views are available in most systems used for the stroboscopic evaluation of the larynx, though the key characteristics of vocal fold vibration (e.g., closure pattern, symmetry of vibration, and mucosal wave—see subsequent section) are all observed and described during a "slow-motion" view.

It is important to recognize that we have referred to the slow-motion view observed during stroboscopy as the "illusion" of slow motion. This is because what may appear as a slow-motion view of one cycle of vocal fold vibration is actually made up of different snapshots of multiple cycles of vibration in which the stroboscopic light has illuminated different positions of vocal fold movement during successive vibratory cycles. Just as the individual still frames of a film appear to show continuous movement when viewed rapidly in succession, we see the individual illuminations of successive cycles of vibration as one continuous cycle (i.e., a stroboscopic cycle). This is in contrast to a newer method of laryngeal evaluation referred to as **high-speed video** in which (depending on the system) thousands of images per second are digitized and multiple images are obtained per cycle of vibration.

▸ Fig. 6.2 illustrates how videostroboscopic image perception works. Each row represents a successive vocal fold oscillation. The red dot within an individual circle represents different points within one vibratory cycle, representing a complete cycle (opening-open–closing-closed) moving around a 360-degree circle. Circles in consecutive rows that are highlighted in red represent flashes of a strobe light that will illuminate the visual field. The rate of the strobe light is timed to flash a few milliseconds slower than the actual period of vibration (the amount of time it takes for one vibratory cycle to occur). This results in the vocal folds being illuminated at different points of the vibratory cycle in each successive flash. Although each flash of the strobe creates a separate image that is detected by an examiner's eye,

these discrete images will perceptually blend into a one continuous moving image due to the property of persistence of vision.

Another way to conceptualize visual perception of stroboscopy is shown in ▸ Fig. 6.3. The top waveform symbolizes successive vocal fold oscillations, with the open phase represented by the peak of each oscillation. The lightbulbs underneath represent a flash of the strobe light which illuminates the vocal folds. These flashes occur at different points of the vibratory cycles, but not during the same oscillation. Visually we perceive the motion as a continuous stroboscopic cycle of vocal fold vibration—we do not perceive the fact that different oscillatory cycles are being illuminated. Some may argue that our interpretation of vibratory dynamics in laryngeal videostroboscopy does not represent actual disturbances in any one vibratory cycle—and this is true. However, research evidence shows that the information obtained from videostroboscopy is significant and can add to or change diagnoses in a large percentage of cases.[2,3,4] Evidence strongly supports that visual analysis of vocal fold vibration illuminated with stroboscopic light is highly sensitive to most vibratory disturbances.

6.4 Laryngoscopy/Stroboscopy Frequently Asked Questions

In many graduate SLP programs, basic knowledge of laryngoscopy and stroboscopic examination may be provided, but students often do not get a depth of experience to develop skills in these procedures. Many clinicians develop endoscopic skills and advanced knowledge after graduation through mentored experiences and continuing education. This leaves many new SLPs with questions about their role in the use of endoscopy for clinical evaluation and treatment. To directly address some of the more frequent questions posed by SLPs new to laryngeal endoscopy and stroboscopy, we have organized this introduction into a set of frequently asked questions (FAQ), which will set the stage for the remainder of the chapter.

6.4.1 Does the Use of Endoscopy and Stroboscopy Fall within the Scope of Practice of SLPs?

Yes. And possibly. You are probably confused by this answer. Allow us to explain. According to the American Speech-Language and Hearing Association (ASHA), the clinical services provided by SLPs include "…using instrumentation (e.g., videofluoroscopy, electromyography, nasoendoscopy, **stroboscopy**, **endoscopy**, nasometry, and computer technology) to observe, collect data, and measure parameters of communication and swallowing or other upper aerodigestive functions."[5] ASHA goes further, explicitly stating in a position statement that "It is the position of the American Speech-Language-Hearing Association (ASHA) that vocal tract visualization and imaging for the purpose of diagnosing and treating patients with voice or resonance/aeromechanical disorders is within the scope of practice of the speech–language pathologist."[6] Thus, our national certifying body makes it very clear that visualization of the vocal tract, including the larynx, using endoscopy and stroboscopy is within our scope of practice. As additional supportive evidence, a recent expert panel of ASHA's "Special Interest Group 3: Voice and Voice Disorders" also

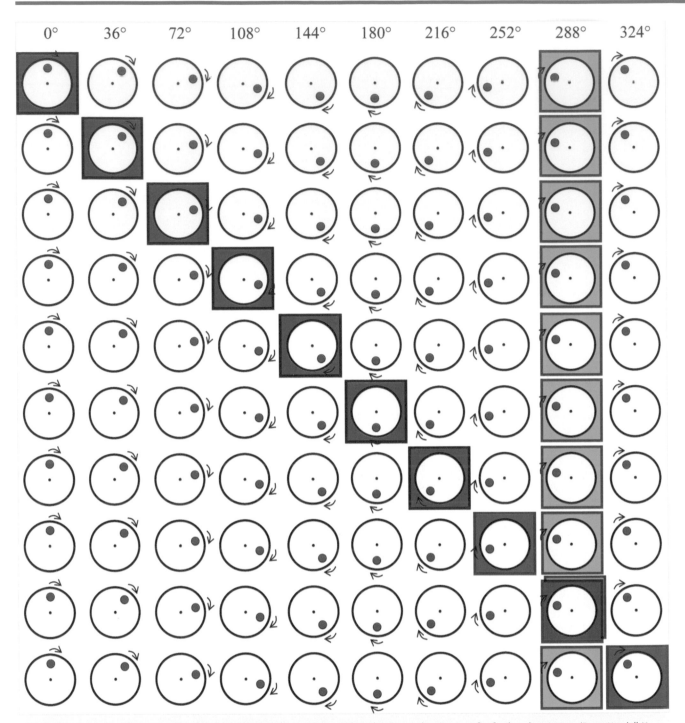

Fig. 6.2 An example of how strobe light flashes different phases of successive vibratory cycles. See text for further description. (From Kendall K, Leonard R. Laryngeal Evaluation, 1st ed. New York: Thieme Publishers, 2010.)

published guidelines for recommended voice evaluation procedures, which included laryngoscopy with stroboscopy.[7]

While ASHA provides certification recognized by the federal government, the right to work as an SLP in any state is regulated by a licensing board. Currently, most state licensing boards allow for laryngoscopy within the SLP scope of practice. However, some states have specific wording in their scope of practice statements that regulates how an SLP might utilize this tool. For example, in California, SLPs are not allowed to diagnose with endoscopy, and must refer any suspected lesion to a physi-

cian for further evaluation. In Michigan and Indiana, an SLP can utilize endoscopy only "…under the authorization and general supervision…" of a physician. In Tennessee, an SLP can use endoscopy but only when they "Obtain written verification from a board-certified otolaryngologist that the SLP is competent in the proper and safe use of an endoscope." It is the SLPs' individual responsibility to be familiar with ASHA's scope of practice (when performing duties as an SLP with a certificate of clinical competence) *and* the scope of practice for the state in which they are licensed.

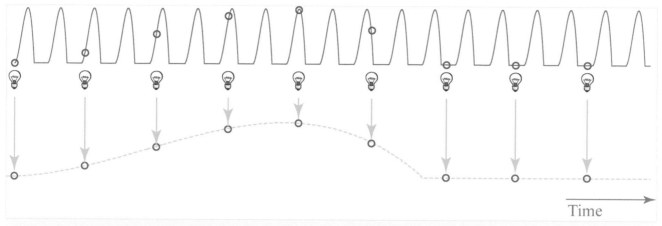

Fig. 6.3 An example of how strobe light flashes different cycles of vibration. Each pulse represents one vibratory cycle. (From Kendall K, Leonard R. Laryngeal Evaluation, 1st ed. New York: Thieme Publishers, 2010.)

6.4.2 Other Than My SLP License/ Certification, Do I Need a Special Certificate or License to Perform Endoscopy and Stroboscopy?

No. But possibly. Sorry to keep doing this to you. According to ASHA's code of ethics, **Principle of Ethics II Rule B**, "Individuals shall engage in only those aspects of the professions that are within the **scope of their competence**, considering their level of education, training, and experience."[7,8] This means that there is no ASHA-required "certificate" or specific training required for utilizing endoscopy and stroboscopy as a certified SLP, but an individual must be certain that they are competent to perform and interpret endoscopic procedures. However, we previously mentioned that each state also publishes a scope of practice which might stipulate requirements for SLP's use of endoscopy, including training requirements. An example was the state of Tennessee, which requires an otolaryngologist to provide written confirmation that an SLP is competent to perform these procedures. It is the responsibility of the SLPs to verify with their state licensing board on educational/training requirements for performing endoscopy.

6.4.3 How Does One Obtain and Demonstrate Endoscopic and Videostroboscopic Competencies?

ASHA gives further guidance on this. The only specific stipulation is that "Some of the training should take place in a clinical setting allowing the SLP to work with more experienced professionals and a number of patients." Otherwise, SLPs can obtain competencies "…by a variety of means," including[9]

- Traditional classroom learning provided in the context of accredited training programs.
- Extended one-on-one work with an SLP or otolaryngologist who has had extensive experience with all aspects of endoscopy in an interdisciplinary environment.
- Extended performance of endoscopy clinical services under the supervision of an SLP and otolaryngologist who has had extensive experience with all aspects of the procedure.

- Organized training provided outside established educational degree programs (continuing education workshops/seminars).
- Review and interpretation of previously recorded endoscopic examination.
- Experience leading to expertise in performing and interpreting endoscopy in the clinical environment.

At the state level, remember that it is the responsibility of the SLPs to verify with their state licensing board regarding any specific educational/training requirements for performing endoscopy. In Appendix 6.1, we provide our recommended guidelines for obtaining and demonstrating competency in performing endoscopic and stroboscopic laryngeal evaluations for voice disorders. We emphasize that these are the recommendations of the authors, and not guidelines endorsed by any state or national agency.

6.4.4 If I See a Lesion, Can I Diagnose It as a Specific Medical Condition Such as Vocal Fold Polyps?

No. ASHA policy is very clear on this, and is stated as follows: "Physicians are the only professionals qualified and licensed to render medical diagnoses related to the identification of laryngeal pathology as it affects voice. Consequently, when used for medical diagnostic purposes, strobovideolaryngoscopy examinations should be viewed and interpreted by an otolaryngologist with training in this procedure."[10] This means that when an SLP uses laryngoscopy with stroboscopy for diagnostic evaluations, the examination needs to be reviewed by an otolaryngologist who will provide a medical diagnosis (if warranted) for the laryngeal condition. SLPs can perform laryngoscopy with stroboscopy independently in the majority of states. However, these examinations should be reviewed collaboratively (preferred) or separately by the otolaryngologist before any final diagnosis is made. How do you know what a medical diagnosis is? You can refer to the International Classification of Diseases, 10th Revision, Clinical Modification (ICD-10) as a guide for diagnostic classifications. ▶ Table 6.1 illustrates the more common ICD-10 codes associated with voice disorders. These are the diagnoses that will be provided by the physician—not the SLP. Some state licensing boards also make this explicit in their scope of practice.

Table 6.1 ICD-10 codes associated with medical diagnoses of voice disorders

ICD-10 code	Description
R49.0	Dysphonia—used for hoarseness
R49.1	Aphonia—used for loss of voice
R49.8	Other voice and resonance disorders—used for vocal hyperfunction
R49.9	Unspecified voice and resonance disorder—used for a general change in voice
J38.01	Paralysis of the vocal cords and larynx, unilateral
J38.02	Paralysis of the vocal cords and larynx, bilateral
J38.1	Polyp of vocal cord and larynx
J38.2	Nodules of vocal cords
J38.3	Other diseases of vocal cords: • Abscess of vocal cords • Cellulitis of vocal cords • Granuloma of vocal cords • Leukokeratosis of vocal cords • Spasmodic dysphonia • Atrophy of vocal cords • Cyst of vocal cords • Pseudocyst of vocal cords
J38.4	Edema of larynx—would be appropriate for Reinke's edema
J37.1	Chronic laryngitis

With that said, as an SLP becomes more knowledgeable and skilled in the evaluation and treatment of voice disorders, they will find that the precision of their diagnostic hypotheses becomes more accurate. In addition to the medical diagnosis provided by an otolaryngologist, our role is to *describe the physiological impairment* that we see on laryngoscopy and stroboscopy. This description should include a report of any visible mass (using non-diagnostic terms such as "lesion"), tissue discoloration, or movement anomaly. It might also include adjectives such as "exophytic," "irregular," "hyperfunction," "erythematous," "plaque-like," "fluid-filled," "immobile," "spasm," and "tremulous" among others, but we leave it to the otolaryngologist to diagnose whether these signs are actually nodules, polyps, cysts, paralysis, spasmodic dysphonia, or primarily hyperfunctional in nature (e.g., muscle tension dysphonia). Thus, the SLP can diagnose impaired physiology, but applying a medical diagnostic label to the disorder is the role of the physician. Ideally, the SLP and otolaryngologist can review these exams together as part of interprofessional collaborative practice, and take advantage of each other's mutual knowledge and skill to guide the process of differential diagnosis.

6.4.5 As an SLP, Can I Use Both Rigid AND Flexible Endoscopes to Perform Endoscopy?

Yes, for ASHA. Possibly, for state licensure regulations. There are more state regulations pertaining to the use of a flexible endoscope during the performance of a FEES than pertaining to the general use of a flexible endoscope for voice examination.

6.4.6 Can I Use an Oral or Nasal Topical Anesthetic to Make the Exam More Comfortable for the Patient?

Possibly. ASHA defers to the state licensing boards on this topic. SLPs routinely use oral and nasal topical anesthetic to decrease oral or nasal sensitivity to endoscopes passed through the mouth or nose. Whether the SLPs can directly administer the anesthetics, if they need another medical professional present during administration, or if they need another medical professional to administer, the decision will be *dictated by state regulations*. Specific wording from ASHA on this topic includes "… speech-language pathologists should address issues of scope of practice as defined by state licensing boards and institutional regulatory committees, professional liability and patient and practitioner safety before engaging in procedures on individuals medicated for sedation or topical anesthesia. These issues should be defined in specific, written protocols that the … speech-language pathologist develop in collaboration with physicians, dentists, and other medical professionals who are responsible for patient care."[11] In this same technical report, ASHA stipulated the requirement to practice collaboratively with medical professionals when administering topical anesthetics, indicating "…collaboration with appropriate medical professionals is required, as topical anesthetics and vasoconstrictors may have undesirable side effects that place patients at risk for adverse medical complications." Many SLPs interpret this to mean that if one is to administer topical anesthesia, they should be in a medical environment with trained health professionals (e.g., nurses, physicians) present (in the facility—not necessarily in the room unless dictated by state regulations) and in communication with the SLP (they are aware that the SLP administers topical anesthesia). ASHA has gone further in their descriptions of the SLP use of topical anesthesia in the context of endoscopic swallowing evaluations, stating that skills needed to perform this procedure include the competence to "Apply topical anesthetic when clinically appropriate and permitted by the licensing regulations of individual states."[12]

ASHA's recommendations justify the SLP practice of topical anesthetic administration in a published guideline, noting "Clinicians may choose to use topical nasal anesthetics alone or in combination with vasoconstrictors to facilitate more comfortable transnasal passage of the flexible endoscope."[13] The administration of nasal vasoconstrictors can increase patient comfort by enlarging the space inside a nostril through constricting small blood vessels and tissue for a brief period. However, ASHA has also published precautions that should be followed by the SLP, which include the following[6]:

- Have available immediate emergency medical assistance when using topical anesthesia or flexible fiberoptic nasoendoscopy.
- Hold a current Basic Life Support Certificate if performing flexible fiberoptic nasoendoscopy or using topical anesthesia.
- Obtain informed consent of the patient and maintain complete and appropriate documentation when performing flexible fiberoptic nasoendoscopy or when using topical anesthesia.

6.5 Rationale for Laryngeal Endoscopy and Stroboscopy

Among the clinical concepts that SLPs might take away from this book, the following are essential: (**a**) functional voice disorders can exhibit perceptual, acoustic, and aerodynamic characteristics that are very similar to organic voice disorders and (**2**) different organic voice disorders can exhibit perceptual, acoustic, and aerodynamic characteristics that are similar to each other. In short, a wide range of voice disorders, including those with a functional origin, those associated with benign lesions, and those associated with more severe organic disorders can all have similar perceptual, acoustic, and aerodynamic characteristics. As examples, the auditory–perceptual features of a speaker with laryngeal cancer can sound exactly like a speaker with primary MTD, with acoustic and aerodynamic measurements also indistinguishable. As another example, an individual with laryngeal papilloma can sound exactly the same as an individual with a vocal fold polyp, where acoustic and aerodynamic measurements also appear similar. However, the treatments for laryngeal cancer, MTD, papilloma, and vocal fold polyp are all very different from each other. These phenomena justify the need to visualize the larynx prior to the development of a treatment plan. Effective treatment plans require accurate diagnoses, and accurate diagnoses of voice disorders require laryngeal visualization.

The question is who performs the laryngoscopy? Here, we present the **Golden Rule of voice therapy**, which all readers should make efforts to memorize and store in long-term memory for the rest of their careers: **Prior to initiating voice therapy, an otolaryngologist must view the larynx (via laryngoscopy) and determine if any medical diagnoses are present**. The SLP can certainly conduct a comprehensive voice evaluation including a behavioral and qualitative assessment, laryngeal function study (acoustics and aerodynamics), and laryngoscopy with videostroboscopy, but before initiating voice therapy the patient must see an otolaryngologist. The laryngeal images viewed by the otolaryngologist might be obtained by their own procedure, or from video obtained by the SLP. In most cases, the physician will obtain the images themselves during their initial clinical examination of the patient. Otolaryngologists can perform laryngoscopy in one of the following three ways: indirectly using a laryngeal mirror (**indirect laryngoscopy**), directly using a flexible endoscope routed through the nose (**flexible laryngoscopy**), or directly using a rigid endoscope routed through the oral cavity (**rigid laryngoscopy**). The most widely used method of laryngeal visualization during initial examinations by otolaryngologists is flexible laryngoscopy.[14]

We have just made the case that laryngoscopy is critical for accurate diagnosis of voice disorders, and that an otolaryngologist must perform laryngoscopy or review laryngoscopic images and provide any medical diagnosis prior to initiation of voice therapy by an SLP (the "Golden Rule"). What about laryngoscopy with videostroboscopy (we will refer to this as **LVS** from this point on)? Unfortunately, most general otolaryngologists do not utilize LVS as part of their initial or follow-up examinations on patients with complaints of voice problems. Fortunately, most laryngologists and most SLPs working in voice clinics do. This is a good thing, because evidence shows that LVS can modify diagnostic decisions, provide additional diagnostic information, and/or change treatment decisions in up to 47% of patients.[4] The reasons for this are multifactorial, but the most important justification for LVS is that it allows you to assess **vocal fold vibratory dynamics** and **glottal closure pattern**, while laryngoscopy without stroboscopy does not. There are many cases in which patients with seemingly normal/typical laryngeal structures show only abnormal/atypical signs when observed during LVS. Vocal fold vibratory dynamics and glottal closure patterns, discussed later in this chapter, inform the otolaryngologist or SLPs about the health of the vocal fold tissue and the extent to which a lesion or tissue change impacts the layered structure of the vocal fold(s) and, in turn, their vibratory characteristics. This information can be the difference between decisions of obtaining a biopsy versus more conservative management, or diagnosing a functional voice disorder instead of a neurological voice disorder.

6.6 Instrumentation

Clinical utilization of laryngoscopy (specifically, phonoscopic examination) with stroboscopy for SLP requires instrumentation that will allow a field of view centered on the larynx and the ability to store and review a recorded image. This requires a specific combination of equipment, illustrated in ▸ Fig. 6.4, including the following:

1. A rigid or flexible **endoscope**.
2. A **light source** to illuminate the field of view and provide an intermittent flash (strobe).

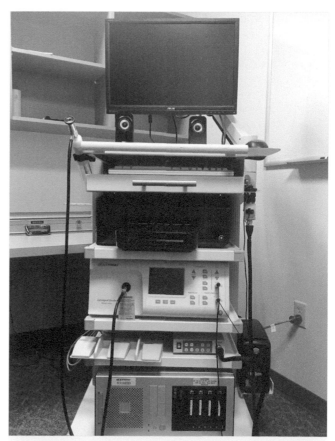

Fig. 6.4 The basic equipment setup for laryngoscopy with stroboscopy.

3. A **microphone** to detect vocal fundamental frequency, which synchronizes the stroboscopic flash and may be used to record the voice signal (depending on the system, this may be achieved via one or two microphones).
4. A **video camera** to capture the image.
5. An analog (e.g., videotape) or digital **recording device** (e.g., computer or DVD recorder) to store the video.
6. Capability to **replay** and/or edit the recording.

Some systems also come with a **foot pedal** to control the characteristics of the light source and to trigger video recording. The endoscope, whether flexible or rigid, allows for an appropriate field of view. There are many endoscope options available commercially in the United States and Europe, and there are many options for the other necessary equipment for LVS. Two of the most important elements of a stroboscopy system are the choice of endoscope and the type of light source used to visualize the larynx. These are described in more detail below.

6.6.1 Endoscopes

Two categories of endoscopes are used during LVS: rigid or flexible, and sometimes both. ▶ Table 6.2 compares and contrasts characteristics of these two options. **Rigid endoscopes** are made of metal and come with a **lens** at the tip that is angled at either 70 or 90 degrees (▶ Fig. 6.5). The lens angle is a matter of preference, but one difference is that the 70-degree lens does not require as deep an insertion into the pharyngeal region to allow visualization of the laryngeal structures versus a 90-degree endoscope. At the opposite end, the lens is an optical **eyepiece** which can be viewed directly or coupled to a camera. Just in front of the eyepiece on the underside of most rigid endoscopes, there is a **fiberoptic cone** to which a light cable can be

attached. Alternatively, the endoscope may be constructed with the light cable fixed to the endoscope. The fiberoptic cable allows light to project internally through the endoscope to illuminate the larynx. Rigid endoscopes are passed through the mouth, with the patient leaned forward, protruding their tongue while sustaining the /i/ vowel. The resolution achieved with rigid endoscopes is much better than standard flexible fiberoptic endoscopes, providing a clear, well-illuminated, and larger view of the larynx and vocal folds. Camera settings can allow for adjustments to brightness, contrast, and color to best visualize tissues.

The typical **flexible endoscope** used for laryngoscopy is made of flexible plastic and rubber and is constructed with mechanical parts not present in a rigid endoscope (▶ Fig. 6.6). One end of the endoscope contains the main **control body** to which a number of components are connected. These include an **eyepiece**, a **fiberoptic cone**, and a **control knob** to control angulation of the endoscope tip, and depending on the endoscope model, **various ports** can be inserted and routed along with the main shaft of the endoscope. The **main shaft** is flexible and contains light-conducting glass fibers (thus, they are sometimes referred to as **fiberoptic endoscopes**). The main shaft can vary in diameter between 2 and 4 mm, with smaller diameter scopes used for pediatric populations. At the end of the shaft is a **bendable tip** whose angulation is manipulated by the control knob on the control body of the endoscope.

Flexible endoscopes are passed through a nostril (they are also referred to as **nasoendoscopes**) so that the tip rests in the pharyngeal space, pointed down toward the larynx. They do not interfere with articulation like a rigid endoscope, so that the patient can produce any type of speech sound the clinician asks of them. However, the image size projected through the lens is smaller than that through a rigid endoscope, and has less resolution. However, recent technological advances have made

Table 6.2 Characteristics of rigid versus flexible laryngeal endoscopes (laryngoscopes) for laryngeal endoscopy with stroboscopy (videostroboscopy)

Characteristics	Rigid laryngoscope	Flexible laryngoscope
	Rigid metal construction	Flexible plastic/rubber construction
	Inserted through oral cavity	Inserted through nasal cavity
	When needed, topical anesthesia to oropharynx	When needed, topical anesthesia to nasal cavity
	70 or 90° angled lens	Different shaft diameters available—angle of tip adjustable
	Can be coupled to standard or high-definition cameras	Chip-in-the-tip high-definition scopes available
	Rigid metal construction	Flexible plastic/rubber construction
Advantages	Larger image with greater resolution	Any vocalization possible
	Greater visible detail of vocal pathology	Less likely to elicit gag reflex
	Requires topical anesthesia less frequently—fewer barriers to use by SLP	Video endoscopes can provide images rivaling HD rigid scopes
	Tolerated by vast majority of patients	Tolerated by vast majority of patients
	Does not require lubricating gel	Patient can be examined in more natural sitting position
Disadvantages	Limited to vowel production	Smaller image with less resolution using standard fiberscopes
	More likely to elicit gag reflex	Requires topical anesthesia more frequently than rigid laryngoscope
	Requires unusual positioning for patient	Video endoscopes very expensive

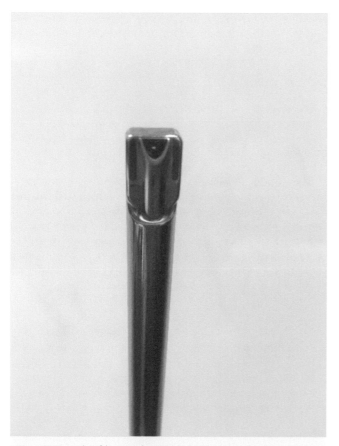

Fig. 6.5 Example of lens angle in a 70-degree laryngoscope.

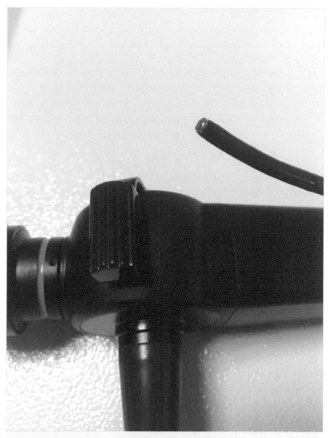

Fig. 6.6 Example of the control knob and flexible tip of a flexible laryngoscope.

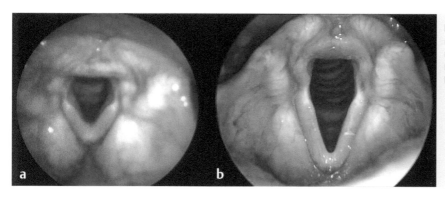

Fig. 6.7 Images taken from the same patient only minutes apart with a flexible endoscope **(a)** and a rigid endoscope **(b)**. (From Kendall K, Leonard R. Laryngeal Evaluation, 1st ed. New York: Thieme Publishers, 2010.)

available **video endoscopes** with a **charged couple device** (CCD) chip and electronics at the distal end of the bendable tip wired back through the shaft and controlled by a video process-or. These are also referred to as "**chip-in-the-tip**" or "**distal chip**" endoscopes, and are equivalent to having a video camera built into the tip. These endoscopes can significantly increase resolution and resulting image clarity even when the image is enlarged on a video screen. Images from current high-definition video endoscope technology rival those from rigid endoscopes, although current flexible video endoscopes have larger diame-ter shafts which can make the examination less comfortable for some patients.

The choice of endoscope used for LVS depends on desired image quality, the type of vocalizations needed for diagnostic purposes, and patient tolerance. Currently, the best image quality can be obtained from rigid endoscopes and chip-in-the-tip flexi-ble endoscopes, especially high-definition versions. Some flexible fiberoptic endoscopes do not illuminate and/or capture sufficient light to thoroughly assess vocal fold vibratory dynamics, which can make accurate interpretation of an LVS examination difficult (▸ Fig. 6.7). Rigid endoscopes, however, limit vocalizations to a sustained vowel-like productions. Flexible endoscopes allow the clinician to assess vocal fold and laryngeal behavior during varied vocal tasks, including connected speech produced with habitual patterns. This can sometimes provide valuable information that would be lost if only a rigid endoscope is used.

Most patients, with the proper procedural technique, can tol-erate rigid endoscopy for LVS. There is a small subset of patients who, no matter how skilled the clinician or how great the amount of topical anesthetic applied, are unable to suppress their gag reflex so that adequate frames of video can be obtained. In these cases, the only option is to switch to a flexible endoscope. And to make things even more interesting for you, there is a small subset of patients who tolerate a rigid endoscope, with or without topical anesthesia, much better than a flexible endoscope due to nasopharyngeal hypersensitivity.

6.6.2 Light Source

Market-leading videostroboscopy systems use either light-emitting diodes (LEDs) or a combination of halogen and xenon bulbs for constant and stroboscopic illumination. LED lighting has the advantage of efficiency, bulb lifespan, low heat output, and economical pricing. However, depending on the quality and construction of the LED array, illumination may not be as good as halogen/xenon light, especially when viewed through a flexible endoscope. Newer LED technology is advancing and overcoming this shortfall. Color temperature will also vary depending on the light source, making the visual perception of tissue color somewhat different depending on the type of light being used.

Most stroboscopy systems allow for manual light adjustment during the exam which, along with camera color balancing technology, can visually approximate true tissue color. Light intensity and color balance must be continually monitored, however, as these factors can alter visual perception of the epithelial surfaces and affect potential diagnostic decisions. Alternatively, color balance can be manipulated by the examiner to better detect specific visual characteristics, such as vascular features of the vocal folds and surrounding laryngeal tissue. Clinicians should become familiar with the light source and camera controls specific to their stroboscopy equipment so that adjustments can be made when needed.

The stroboscopic light flash rate is set at a frequency slightly lower than the actual F_0 being produced to give the visual illusion of slowed vibratory movement. The speaker's F_0 can be **detected via a microphone** placed on the anterior neck (e.g., a contact microphone) or on the endoscope itself, and the signal is fed back into the light source to modulate the strobe flash rate. Other systems can create a stroboscopic effect using a constant light that is shuttered at a high frequency by camera technology. Most stroboscopy systems allow for at least two modes of examination: (**1**) a slow mode which produces the illusion of slow motion and (**2**) a locked mode which produces the illusion of a freeze-frame or still image when the vocal folds are vibrating in a periodic fashion.

6.7 Laryngoscopy and Stroboscopy Procedural Technique

Experience performing laryngoscopy with stroboscopy will lead to clinician's skill and comfort in the procedural aspects of the exam in addition to personal preferences in the examination approach. The following are the authors' recommendations for laryngoscopy with stroboscopy procedure, although it is understood that there may be a wide variation in clinician preference for many dimensions of this protocol. The key to this examination,

regardless of procedural approach, is obtaining a focused and well-lit visualization of the larynx and full view of the vocal folds along their entire horizontal length.

6.7.1 Preevaluation

1. **Exam records**—if the patient has previously been evaluated by an otolaryngologist, those records should be obtained and reviewed prior to the evaluation. Information from these previous laryngeal exams can help guide the subsequent clinical protocol.
2. **Equipment and materials** should be set up so that they are in easy reach of the examiner. In addition to the stroboscopy system, supplies needed for rigid and flexible examinations will include
   a) Personal protective equipment—at minimum, gloves.
   b) Gauze (rigid laryngoscopy)—This will be used to hold the patient's tongue during the examination. We prefer 4 × 4 pads which are then unfolded and then refolded lengthwise.
   c) Cup of warm water (rigid laryngoscopy)—This will be used to warm the tip of the endoscope to prevent fogging once inserted into the patient's mouth.
   d) Lubricant (flexible laryngoscopy)—This may help ease passage of the endoscope through the nasal cavity. Lubricant may be applied to the flexible shaft near the endoscope tip, being careful not to smear any material on the lens.
3. Endoscope preparation.
   a) Endoscopes are coupled to the camera head securely and either placed on top of a sterile pad within easy reach of the examiner or mounted to an equipment rack if purchased for the system.
   b) Once secure in the camera head, the endoscope light cable is connected to the external light source.
   c) The light source is activated while the endoscope is placed over a white surface (for automatic color balancing) and an object with one or more images for focusing. The video monitor will need to be turned on for this step. We use a piece of gauze for automatic white balancing, or a sheet of white paper. If the computer keyboard is white with black letters, we use those to focus the image, or otherwise a sheet of white paper with printed letters.
   d) When using a flexible endoscope, we then apply a thin film of lubricant to the end of the shaft near the tip.
   e) When using a computerized recording system with software that controls the video capture, we use this time to enter patient examination data and prepare the software for recording a new examination. For systems that come with report templates as part of the software, this is a good time to include patient demographic and history information.

6.7.2 Greeting and History

It is customary for the SLP to greet the patient in the waiting room. Some clinics may prefer to have a nurse or aid greet the patient and bring them back to the exam room. In either case, time is taken to say hello, introduce yourself to the patient, and ask the patient how they are doing. This conversation often takes place while walking with the patient to the exam room, or immediately upon entering the room. By careful listening to a patient's responses during these initial greetings, the clinician can get an idea of potential anxiety that can later be mitigated prior to and during the examination.

After initial greetings and once in the examination room, we recommend introducing yourself in a formal manner so that the patient has a clear idea of **your position and role** in the examination about to take place. An example script one might use is as follows (assuming you have already greeted the patient by telling them your name):

"I am a speech-language pathologist by training, and one of my areas of specialty is evaluating and treating voice problems. One of the ways that I evaluate the voice is by looking at the larynx—or voice box—where the vocal folds are located. I can do this with an endoscope—a special camera that allows me to see what is going on inside your neck where your larynx and vocal folds are located. You were referred here today so that we can get some pictures and video of your larynx. This exam is relatively easy for most people and, if we get good images, it should only take 5 or 10 minutes to complete. I will explain to you how we will get these pictures, but first let me know if you have any questions about what I just explained."

The next step is to obtain history information from the patient which would help explain their referral for the examination. When otolaryngology records are available prior to the examination, important history information can be obtained which can be used to devise follow-up questions for the patient's report of history. We typically begin this part of the exam by asking the patient, "*Can you tell me why you were referred here today* (or why you are here today, for those who are self-referrals)?" or "*Tell me what has been going on with your throat and your voice.*" Important follow-up questions are the same as those described in the history section of Chapter 3.

6.7.3 Procedure Explanation

Now that you have a concise history, and the patient understands who you are and what you are about to do, you provide them with further explanation of the examination process. Below are examples of scripts you might use for rigid and flexible examinations, respectively. When showing the patient the rigid or flexible endoscope, it is important not to "threaten" them by pointing it or thrusting it toward them. Hold the endoscope close and in front of your body. The following is an example of what you might say for a rigid laryngoscopic examination:

"To get pictures of your larynx and vocal folds I am going to use this scope (hold the endoscope while standing in front of them but away from their face.) I am going to ask you to sit forward in the exam chair, lean your torso forward and stick out your neck almost like you were trying to sniff something that was in front of you (**give a visual model for the patient**). I will then ask you to open your mouth and stick out your tongue, and I will gently hold your tongue with some gauze. I will gently place the tip of the scope inside your mouth—don't be intimidated by the length of this shaft because only a small portion of the scope will sit in your mouth."

"During the exam I will ask you to take easy breaths and then say the /i/ sound—like this (**give an auditory model of the /i/ vowel, holding it out for about 5 seconds at a comfortable pitch and loudness**). It can be difficult to say the /i/ sound with me holding onto your tongue and the tip of the scope in your

mouth. It is the attempt at /i/ that is important—you might hear me say 'try for more of an /i/ sound' during the exam. This is because some patients start out saying /a/ instead of /i/. The /i/ sound is best because it opens the throat and will give us the best view of your larynx and vocal folds. If you have trouble saying the /i/ sound, sometimes it can help if you smile while saying it, or gently close your teeth around the scope. Remember to take a breath every 4 or 5 seconds, and then just keep saying the /i/ sound until I tell you to do something different. It will also help if you keep your eyes open during the exam so that you can see what is going on—I will remind you to breathe and open your eyes if you forget."

Follow this by having the patient practice sticking out their tongue and prolonging the /i/ vowel for about 4 or 5 seconds, and then take a breath in between productions. When the patient has demonstrated competency in doing this, ask them if they have any questions before you begin.

6.7.4 Positioning and Endoscope Technique

Clinician Position

In the combined experience of the authors, we have found that, for right-handed individuals, positioning oneself on the right side of the patient (as they are facing you) is best. Alternatively, left-handed individuals may find placing themselves on the left side (as they are facing you) is best. However, there is no hard rule and the clinician should determine what configuration will allow them to best handle the endoscope while being able to view and record the video image. Some clinicians also choose to sit in a chair while performing the laryngoscopic exam. When a foot pedal control is used to control the light source and recording, it will be placed within easy reach of the examiner's foot while they are standing or sitting.

Patient Position

For **rigid laryngoscopy**, the patient sits in the examination chair, which might be elevated so that the patient's mouth is at the clinician's eye level. Per previous instructions to the patient, they are asked to sit forward in the chair, lean forward, and protrude their chin as if they were sniffing something in the air, and stick out their tongue (▶ Fig. 6.8). The vast majority of patients will be able to complete the examination in this posture. On occasion, patients may have anatomical differences, whether congenital or acquired (e.g., subsequent to treatment for head/neck cancer), or behavioral reactions to the procedure that necessitate experimentation for the posture that will allow the best visualization of the larynx. In these cases, the examiner needs to be patient and calm, and allow for more time in the process. Having the patient lean farther forward in the chair, sit upright, or even reclined back are just some of the alternative positions that might be attempted to obtain adequate images.

For **flexible laryngoscopy**, the patient can be seated upright with their back resting against the chair. When successfully passed through a nostril, the tip of the endoscope will lie within the oropharynx and point directly downward, and a full view of the larynx is almost always achieved during /i/ productions. If there is difficulty visualizing the entire larynx once the scope

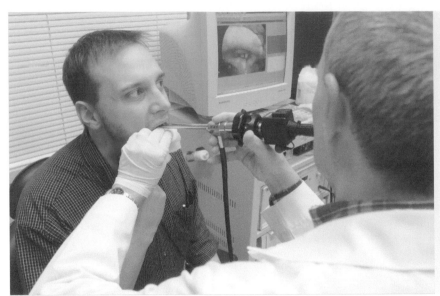

Fig. 6.8 Patient and examiner positioning for rigid endoscopy. (From Kendall K, Leonard R. Laryngeal Evaluation, 1st ed. New York: Thieme Publishers, 2010.)

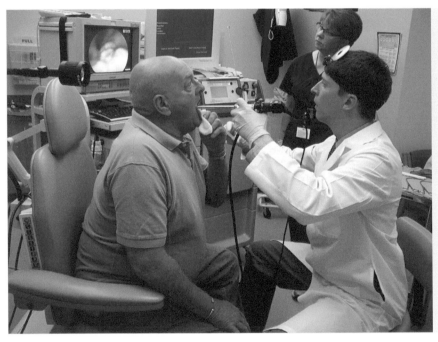

Fig. 6.9 Example of hand position for holding rigid endoscope. (From Kendall K, Leonard R. Laryngeal Evaluation, 1st ed. New York: Thieme Publishers, 2010.)

enters the oropharynx, different positions can be attempted including leaning forward or reclining back.

6.7.5 Handling the Endoscope

There are also no standard rules for how one holds and controls the endoscope. The key is to find a hand position that allows for fine-tuned control of the endoscope in the patient's mouth or nose. For a **rigid endoscope**, we prefer an overhand grip with the index finger resting on the shaft, as illustrated in ▶ Fig. 6.9. Manipulation of the rigid endoscope involves advancing anteriorly in the mouth toward the oropharynx, and then small adjustments with the wrist or fingers to manipulate the scope for the best field of view. Seventy-degree endoscopes may need to

be angled slightly downward to bring the larynx into view. When a clinician first builds competencies in laryngeal imaging, they should experiment to determine which grip and scope position best suits their motor preferences and allows them to manipulate the scope without excessive effort.

For **flexible endoscopes**, an overhand or underhand grip can be used, as illustrated in ▶ Fig. 6.10. In an underhand grip, the thumb is typically used to operate the control knob to manipulate the tip of the endoscope. In an overhand grip, the index or another finger is often used. The free hand will be used to hold and support the endoscope shaft at the nostril entrance. As the scope is passed through a nostril, small adjustments of the tip are made by adjusting the control knob and/or rotating the forearm to direct the shaft at an appropriate angle for advancement.

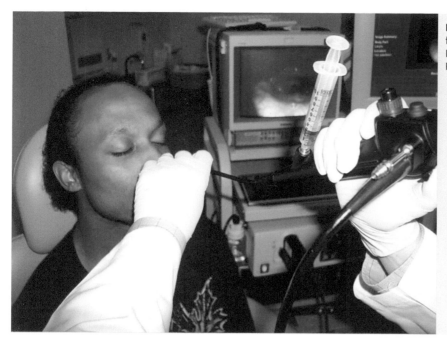

Fig. 6.10 Example of hand position for holding flexible endoscope. (From Kendall K, Leonard R. Laryngeal Evaluation, 1st ed. New York: Thieme Publishers, 2010.)

6.7.6 Inserting the Endoscope—Rigid Laryngoscopy

Before inserting a rigid endoscope, the tip should be placed in a **cup filled with warm water for 5 to 10 seconds** in order to warm the lens and prevent fogging, and then dried with a clean tissue or with the gauze that will hold the patient's tongue. Alternatively, the tip of the endoscope can be placed under warm running water if a sink is near. Some clinicians prefer commercial products such as **dental warming beads** to warm up the endoscope tip or application of an **antifogging gel**.

As the patient leans forward, opens his or her mouth, and sticks out his or her tongue, the clinician should lay the gauze on the tongue and then gently grip the gauze and top of the tongue with their index finger and/or middle finger of their free hand (the one not holding the scope), and grip the bottom of the tongue with their thumb making sure to also wrap the gauze underneath. The scope is then advanced forward into the mouth opening, *paying careful attention not to hit the front teeth*. At this point, the clinician should be looking at the patient's mouth as the endoscope enters and advances inward. The shaft of the endoscope should be braced on the index/middle fingers of the hand holding the tongue to provide a supportive base over which the scope is guided posteriorly and when manipulated during the examination. This also keeps the shaft above the tongue surface and reduces the risk of a gag reflex.

Once the endoscope is inside the mouth, the clinician should now be focusing on the video monitor and continue to use this image as visual guidance for the examination (this is not an oral mechanism examination—looking into the patient's mouth will not help you with visualization of the larynx). Moving eye gaze back-and-forth from the video monitor to the patient's mouth usually results in endoscope drift and disorientation of the endoscope location in the oral cavity. The endoscope is slowly advanced into the mouth until the posterior tongue dorsum and oropharynx become visible. At this point, if the patient is not already doing so, they are prompted to take an easy breath and

say /i/. Another technique for positioning the endoscope at the posterior oropharynx involves rotating the endoscope with the wrist approximately 90 degrees as it enters the oral cavity, so that the buccal cavity (i.e., inside of the cheek) and teeth are visible. When the molars come into view, the endoscope tip is typically at the level of the posterior tongue dorsum. By rotating the endoscope back to a level and straight position as the client produces /i/, the larynx is often immediately revealed and smearing of the lens from saliva/mucus on the tongue is avoided.

Some patients have low vaulted hard palates resulting in a narrow opening within the oral cavity. This can result in the the tongue filling the oral cavity leaving little space for the endoscope. Also, some patients may lift and/or retract the tongue during placement of the endoscope into the mouth. This can sometimes result in the posterior tongue dorsum obstructing advancement of the scope. One technique to overcome this obstacle is to ask the patient to first say /a/ (which requires a low tongue position), get the scope into position with the tip at the posterior tongue dorsum/oropharynx, and then have the patient switch to saying /i/. At this point, the larynx and vocal folds should come into view. Sometimes, it is necessary to apply downward pressure on the tongue dorsum with the shaft of the endoscope if the patient has a highly elevated tongue when producing the /i/ sound. If only a portion of the larynx is visible, a number of additional adjustments can be attempted to bring as much of the larynx and full range of the vocal folds into view as possible:

- Advance endoscope farther posteriorly.
- For 70-degree endoscopes, angle the tip downward with subtle adjustment of the wrist.
- Ask the patient to produce a more /i/-like sound.
- Ask the patient to smile when producing /i/ or gently close their teeth around the endoscope.
- Ask the patient to lean farther forward (you may want to remove and then reinsert the endoscope when they do this).
- Experiment with other postural adjustments.

The clinician should keep in mind that the full horizontal length of the vocal folds, in many patients, can be viewed only when the patient is producing /i/. When breathing, it is typical that the anterior commissure and anterior third of the vocal folds are obscured by the epiglottis. Once the patient produces another /i/, the anterior vocal folds will come back into view. In patients with vocal hyperfunction or who react to the endoscope with vocal strain, increased muscle tension may also obscure the anterior regions of the vocal folds due to a bulging epiglottic petiolus or narrowed laryngeal vestibule. Similarly, the lateral edges of the vocal folds can be obscured due to medial compression of the false vocal folds.

An important concept to remember for rigid laryngoscopy is that when adequate laryngeal and vocal fold visualization is achieved, try to complete as much of the evaluation protocol (see next section) as possible before removing the scope and reinserting. There are times when you may never get as good a view as the last one. With that said, it is common that a number of trial passes are needed to establish patient comfort and familiarity with the scope inside their mouth. The clinician should be a model of serenity during the examination, especially with hypersensitive patients.

A vast majority of patients, given time to accommodate to the examination, can tolerate a rigid endoscope without problems. A small subset of patients will exhibit a gag reflex so strong that, even after several minutes of desensitization (slow, repeated passes of the endoscope into the mouth, moving farther and farther back at each pass), they are not able to tolerate the scope at the back of the oral cavity. These are the cases where topical anesthesia sprayed into the oropharynx can be an option, if the clinician is housed in the appropriate facility and environment (see discussion on FAQs at the beginning of the chapter). Alternatively, the clinician may need to switch to a flexible endoscope to complete the examination.

6.7.7 Inserting the Endoscope—Flexible Laryngoscopy

Before inserting a flexible endoscope, it is wise to ask a patient if he or she can breathe easier through one nostril or the other. This can also be tested by having the patient press against one nostril while inhaling quickly through the other, and then alternate to the other nostril. A restricted nasal passage will result in audible air turbulence, resembling a rustling noise. Alternatively, the clinician can "peek" inside the vestibule (opening) of both nares using the endoscope. The endoscope should always be first passed through the nostril with the greatest space. There is a substantial amount of variability in nasal cavity architecture and available space from patient to patient, and even when no rustling noise is present, finding an adequate pathway through a nostril can be an adventure which even Indiana Jones would be impressed by. Some patients might benefit from application of a topical vasoconstrictor such as Afrin prior to endoscope insertion, which can increase the diameter of the nasal passageway.

The patient can usually be seated upright with their back resting against the exam chair. The clinician raises the flexible endoscope to the level of the nose, holding the tip loosely in the free hand at the edge of a nostril. The entire endoscope is then moved forward, allowing the shaft to slide easily through the fingers of the free hand. The clinician should initially be looking directly at the patient's nose in order to guide the endoscope tip into the nostril entrance, but as soon as the tip enters the nostril, their focus should immediately turn to the video screen for further visual guidance of endoscope passage.

Once inside the nostril, the examiner should use the control knob to manipulate the tip of the scope for inspecting the available space through which the shaft can be advanced. Nasal cavities contain three spaces, the **inferior, middle, and superior meatus**, which provide potential routes through which the endoscope shaft can move (▶ Fig. 6.11). These spaces are separated by three curved bones, the inferior, middle, and superior turbinates (aka conchae), respectively. The largest space, and easiest route for the endoscope, is usually within the inferior meatus. Passage through the middle meatus is sometimes possible and can position the scope higher as it passes the nasopharynx, which can offer a more effective angle for viewing the larynx. Light will reflect off nasal tissues, showing their pink to red color, while the cavities of the nasal meatus will appear as black spaces. The tip of the endoscope should be directed at

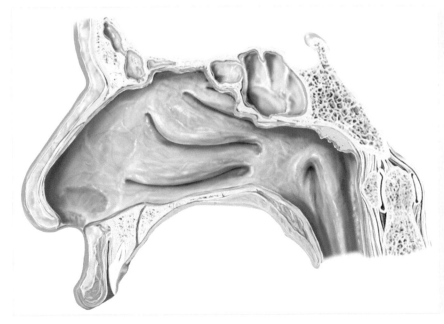

Fig. 6.11 Interior anatomy of nasal cavity. (From Baker E. Anatomy for Dental Medicine, 2nd ed. New York: Thieme Medical Publishers, 2015.)

these spaces while the clinician advances the entire endoscope forward, continually supporting the shaft with the free hand at the edge of the nostril.

As the endoscope enters the nostril, the image on the video screen will show the anterior nose hairs and then, as the shaft advances, the inferior turbinate with inferior and middle meatus below and above, respectively. The clinician should judge which meatus offers the most open route of passage, and direct the tip of the endoscope toward that space while advancing the shaft slowly. It is important to understand that **very small movements of the control knob result in substantial movements of the endoscope tip**, and care should be taken to minimize irritation to the nasal walls and floor. As a general rule, the shaft will follow the direction of the tip. **The tip is used to find open spaces, point toward them, and then guide the shaft as it is advanced further into the nasal cavity**. If, upon entering a turbinate, there is a clear space all the way to the nasopharynx, the control knob can be released as the endoscope advances, leaving the walls of the turbinate to passively straighten out the tip and give a full view of where the endoscope is headed. Some nasal architecture, however, requires fine-tuned manipulation of the tip via the control knob with multiple rotations of the scope using the forearm in order to navigate through the nasal cavity.

As the tip of the endoscope approaches the nasopharynx, the superior surface of the velum will come into view. The velum may move as the patient swallows, sniffs, or speaks while you are advancing the endoscope. Once the tip is at the level of the velum, it can be helpful to ask the patient to breathe through their nose (e.g., a "big sniff"), hum, or produce nasalized syllables such as "mama–mama." This keeps the velum lowered as the tip enters the nasopharynx. As the endoscope slowly advances, the tip should be slowly moved downward using the control knob. The shaft will follow the tip as it abuts the posterior pharyngeal wall and orients the entire front of the shaft downward. Slow advancement of the endoscope will then result in the base of tongue, pharynx, epiglottis, and remainder of larynx coming into view (▶ Fig. 6.12). If the endoscope image is fogged

or smeared by mucus, asking the patient to swallow will usually result in clearing film from the tip of the endoscope.

At this point, the examiner will have an adequate view of the larynx and surrounding spaces. Adequate interpretation of videostroboscopic images requires clear views of the vocal folds. When performing flexible laryngoscopy, this may obligate the examiner to continue advancing the endoscope toward the vocal folds until an adequate visualization is achieved. The image quality will depend on the intensity of light illumination, quality of endoscope and camera, and the patient's anatomical structure. Once adequate visualization is achieved, the examination protocol can begin.

Adverse events: There are very few possible adverse events when using a rigid or flexible laryngoscope. However, risks are present and should be explained to the patient before receiving their permission to proceed with the examination. Of course, in the event of any topical anesthetic use (rigid or flexible) or nasal vasoconstrictor (flexible), the patients must be asked if they have any allergies/reactions to certain medications—whether or not these allergies/reactions may affect the use of topical anesthetic and vasoconstrictor can be confirmed with physician/nursing staff. *Because of the possibility of these adverse events, it is our strong recommendation that rigid or flexible laryngoscopy/stroboscopy* **used in conjunction with topical anesthetic and/or vasoconstrictor** *be conducted in a medical setting with physician/nursing staff readily available.* The following are possible adverse events that can occur during laryngoscopy with stroboscopy:

- Discomfort with rigid scope in mouth or flexible scope in nose.
- Laryngospasm/gag reflex (most likely with rigid endoscope, but possible with either).
- Nasal pain.
- Adverse reaction to anesthetic or vasoconstrictor.
- Nose bleed (not common, but possible).
- Vasovagal response (the patient can pass out—very uncommon, but the authors have heard that it is possible).
- Chipped tooth (from rigid endoscope).

6.8 Evaluation Protocol and Interpretation of Observations

6.8.1 Vocal Tasks

Once the larynx and vocal folds are adequately visualized, a battery of vocal tasks should be elicited from the patient to assess the physiological capabilities of the larynx relative to phonation and, if possible, to assess the prognosis of clinical probes for improving vocal function. The core vocal tasks will be the same whether using a rigid or flexible endoscope, although a flexible endoscope allows for a more extensive investigation because the patient is not restricted to sustained vowel-like productions. For speakers or singers with difficulty in particular voicing contexts, this is also an opportunity to test laryngeal and vocal fold behavior with specificity. Because vocal fold vibratory characteristics change as a function of fundamental frequency and intensity, a range of vocal frequencies and intensities should be tested. We recommend eliciting vocalizations at **comfortable** (e.g., habitual), **soft**, and **loud** intensity and observing vibratory characteristics throughout the patient's physiological frequency range. Sustained vowels should also be

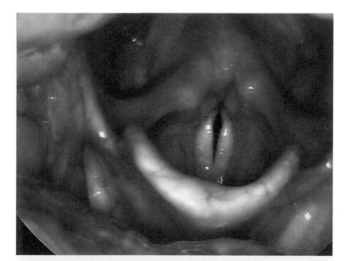

Fig. 6.12 View of the larynx and pharynx via a flexible laryngoscope passed through a nasal cavity. (From Kendall K, Leonard R. Laryngeal Evaluation, 1st ed. New York: Thieme Publishers, 2010.)

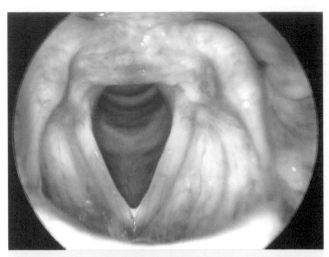

Fig. 6.13 Normal laryngeal appearance under constant light with rigid laryngoscope. (From Kendall K, Leonard R. Laryngeal Evaluation, 1st ed. New York: Thieme Publishers, 2010.)

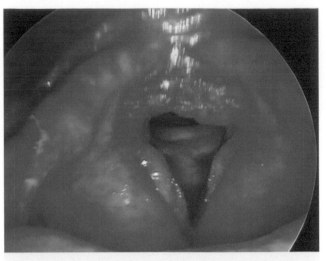

Fig. 6.14 Edema and erythema secondary to chronic laryngitis. (From Kendall K, Leonard R. Laryngeal Evaluation, 1st ed. New York: Thieme Publishers, 2010.)

elicited at comfortable, low, and high fundamental frequencies. The following is a framework for voice tasks elicited during the examination. This framework is similar to that published by ASHA's Committee on Instrumental Voice Assessment Protocols (IVAP—ASHA, 2015). Analysis under stroboscopic light will be most applicable to sustained vowels and pitch glides.

- **Quiet breathing**—ask the patient to breathe quietly while you observe (and record the image).
- **Deep inspiration**—ask the patient to breathe in deeply.
- **Laryngeal diadochokinesis (DDK)**—ask the patient to repeat /hi-hi-hi/ quickly.
- **Quick sniff through the nose followed by /i/**—ask the patient to sniff briskly through the nose, and immediately produce /i/, repeating this gesture rapidly. Provide an example if necessary. This allows for assessment of maximum abduction and adduction movements.
- **Sustained vowels**—ask the patient to produce multiple trials of (**1**) comfortable, (**2**) soft, and (**3**) loud /i/ sounds at (**1**) comfortable, (**2**) low, and (**3**) high frequencies. Model if necessary and repeat each multiple times.
- **Pitch glides**—ask patient to glide up to their highest pitch, and then down to their lowest pitch on the /i/ vowel. Model if necessary, and repeat multiple times.
- **Dynamic voicing**—when using a flexible endoscope, the patient can be asked to produce connected speech and/or sing so that dynamic laryngeal and vocal fold behaviors can be observed. Dynamic voicing can also be elicited using a rigid scope by having the patient sing a well-known tune (e.g., "Happy Birthday") while using an /i/ or a humming sound (often easier to elicit).

6.8.2 Domains of Observation

A complete laryngoscopy with stroboscopy examination by the SLP, regardless of endoscope used, should include three domains of observation: (1) laryngeal and pharyngeal **color**; (2) laryngeal and pharyngeal **structure**; and (3) laryngeal **movement**, including vocal fold **vibratory dynamics**. The first two and part of the third domains do not require a stroboscopic

light, but observation and analysis of vibratory dynamics must occur under stroboscopic light (or using a high-speed camera). **Tissue color** of the larynx and pharynx can be observed with the patient breathing comfortably. When healthy, laryngeal tissue appears *pink with a glistening surface* reflecting an invisible blanket of thin, clear mucous (▶ Fig. 6.13). Healthy vocal folds appear as a *pearly white color* with *minimal vascularity* present along their horizontal surfaces. When vascularity is present, there should not be abundant vessels and those that are visible should be thin. Color balance and the intensity of illumination can greatly influence visual perception of tissue color—it is important to keep this in mind when evaluating this domain and adjust as needed. The following are descriptors of common visual signs of color impairment during laryngoscopy, typically observed during quiet breathing or sustained vowel production:

- **Erythema/Hypervascularity**—reddened tissues or prominent blood vessels on the vocal fold surface ("bloodshot" appearance). For example, signs of reflux or recent phonotrauma can include erythema/hypervascularity at the vocal processes of the arytenoids and the interarytenoid space during the acute wound healing stages or as a sign of chronic irritation (▶ Fig. 6.14; ▶ Fig. 6.15).
- **Edema**—fullness or puffy epithelium. For example, the vocal folds may appear enlarged and somewhat grayish or translucent secondary to phonotrauma or irritation. Signs of laryngopharyngeal reflux can also include edematous or irregular tissue (interarytenoid dysplasia) at the interarytenoid space that appears translucent, grayish, or white (not the normal pink color—**Fig. 2.13**).
- **Excessive mucous (white or opaque mucous)**—a blanket of translucent mucous normally coats the epithelium of the larynx and pharynx, serving to lubricate the surface and protect from foreign particles. When the larynx is irritated or when a person is dehydrated, mucous often becomes thick, opaque, or sometimes white. It can be cleared by swallowing, clearing the throat, or coughing but will return after a few seconds of voicing. If this mucous pools on the vocal fold surface or medical edges, it can disrupt phonation (**Fig. 2.8**).

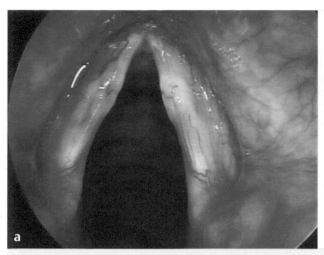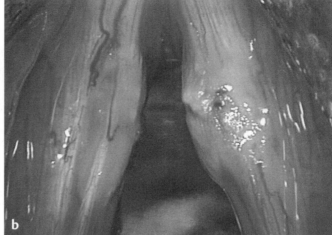

Fig. 6.15 Hypervascularity characterized by bilateral prominent vasculature.

- **Discolored plaques**—Any discoloration that is excessively red, white, or patchy should be noted. These plaques are sometimes just thick, sticky mucous which are difficult for the patient to clear. However, discolored plaques can be anything from mucous to cancer, which is why we always have an otolaryngologist evaluate and diagnose before initiating voice therapy (**Fig. 2.22**).

Structural observations include inspection of the *shape*, *size*, and *position* of the laryngeal cartilages and vocal folds. It is important to remember that there can be great variability in normal shape and size of laryngeal structures, especially the epiglottis and arytenoids, as illustrated in ► Fig. 6.16 and ► Fig. 6.17, respectively. Important structural characteristics to assess are the position of the arytenoids during rest and adduction, and the shape, size, and position of the vocal folds. Impairments in either region can significantly affect phonation. Arytenoid shape may be asymmetrical even in nondysphonic speakers, but their shape during adduction should not alter significantly from their resting shape. The vocal fold tissue should be **smooth** on the surface, free of any exophytic masses, with a **straight** medial edge. The following are descriptors of common visual signs of structural impairment during laryngoscopy, typically observed during quiet breathing, sustained vowel production, and pitch glides:

- **Prolapsed arytenoid**—one or both arytenoids are positioned tilted inward toward the glottis at rest or during adduction. This is a sign of potential paresis/paralysis (**Fig. 2.19**).
- **Overrotation of one arytenoid**—during adduction, one arytenoid is positioned past midline while it is in contact with its counterpart. This can be a sign of dysmotility in the opposite arytenoid.
- **Reduced vocal fold elongation**—the vocal folds do not sufficiently stretch anteriorly during pitch glides. This can be a sign of superior laryngeal nerve (SLN) disruption and cricothyroid paresis/paralysis.
- **Atrophy and bowing**—atrophy is characterized by visible thinning of one or both vocal folds. This is often accompanied by a prominent vocal process on the affected side, where the membranous vocal fold curves laterally at its posterior attachment. Bowing can occur with or without atrophy, and is characterized by a concave shape to the vocal fold along its medial edge (► Fig. 6.18).
- **Exophytic mass**—various possible masses which protrude from the surface or medial edge of the vocal folds or laryngeal tissue. "Exophytic" is an adjective (it means "protruding from the surface") used to describe a noun, while "excrescence" is often used as a general noun referring to a raised structural abnormality. For example, descriptions might be, "*There was an exophytic mass on the right vocal fold*" or "*There was an excrescence on the right vocal fold*" (► Fig. 6.19).
- **Irregular medial edge**—different lesions can impair the normally smooth, straight shape of the vocal fold medial edge (► Fig. 6.19).

Movement observations include adduction and abduction actions of the vocal processes, in addition to longitudinal stretching of the vocal folds. This will require the patient to vocalize or breathe in different ways (see previous vocal tasks). On inspiration, the vocal processes should move laterally (abduct) and on expiration return toward their resting position. This abduction movement should be brisk if asked to sniff quickly and forcibly. During vocalization, the arytenoids should move medially with symmetry, and remain adducted throughout the production of voiced sounds. As the patient produces different pitches, there should be noticeable elongation of the vocal folds in the anterior direction. The following are descriptors of visual signs of movement impairment during laryngoscopy, typically observed during deep inspiration, laryngeal DDK, sustained vowels, and pitch glides:

- **Paresis/Paralysis** (**Video 6.1**)—failure of the arytenoids and vocal folds to move medially (adduct) or laterally (abduct) during voicing attempts or inspiration. If the impairment affects the SLN, the visual sign can also be failure to elongate anteriorly. These signs can be observed during laryngeal DDK, sustained vowels, or pitch glides.
- **Paradoxical movement**—lateral movement (abduction) of the arytenoids and vocal folds during voicing attempts, when those structures should normally move medially (adduct).

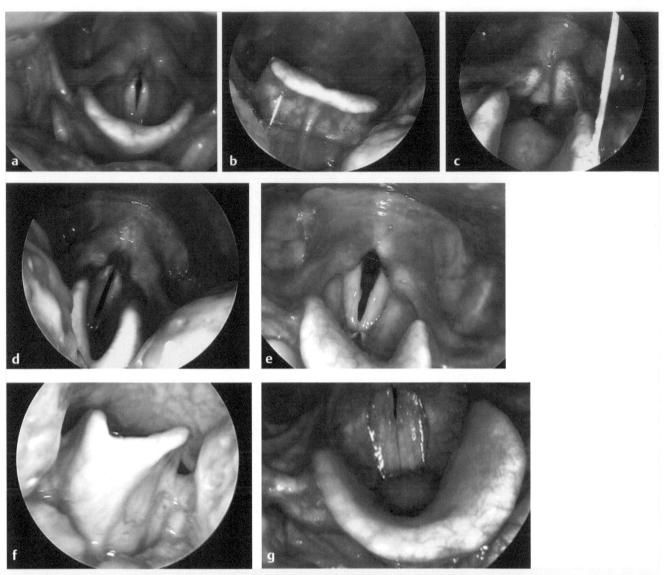

Fig. 6.16 (a) Typical appearance of the epiglottis from above during laryngeal imaging. **(b)** In this image, the epiglottis has less curvature as seen from the lingual surface of the structure. The vallecula is open and easily visualized in this example. **(c)** This is an example of an omega-shaped epiglottis. The rim is **U**-shaped, and the petiole is quite prominent. **(d)** Asymmetry of the epiglottis is within the range of normal variation. This example demonstrates an asymmetric and very curved epiglottis. **(e)** This epiglottis has a "normal" amount of curvature but is asymmetric, with an **L**-shape. **(f)** This lingual surface view of the epiglottis reveals the asymmetry in the shape of the epiglottic cartilage. **(g)** The petiole of the epiglottis is quite prominent in this example. (From Kendall K, Leonard R. Laryngeal Evaluation, 1st ed. New York: Thieme Publishers, 2010.)

- **Tremor** (**Video 6.2**)—rhythmic oscillations of the arytenoids, entire larynx, and sometimes pharynx when at rest or during phonation.
- **Dystonic movements**—irregular spasm-like contractions characterized by quick, transient, but involuntary hyperadduction or abduction of the arytenoids and vocal folds. These occur during phonation attempts.
- **Medial compression of ventricular folds** (**Video 6.3**)—when present, typically characterized by both ventricular (false) folds compressed toward each other. This can obscure portions of the true vocal folds below. This is a sign of hyperfunction, such as in primary or secondary MTD.

- **Anteroposterior laryngeal compression**—the anterior portion of the vocal folds can be obscured by bulging of the epiglottic petiolus or posterior tilting of the entire epiglottis. This is a sign of hyperfunction.

6.8.3 Definition and Interpretation of Vibratory Dynamics

The primary role of videostroboscopy as part of the laryngoscopic examination is to enable the assessment of vibratory dynamics during phonation. **Vibratory dynamics refer to the visual characteristics of vocal fold tissue physiology within**

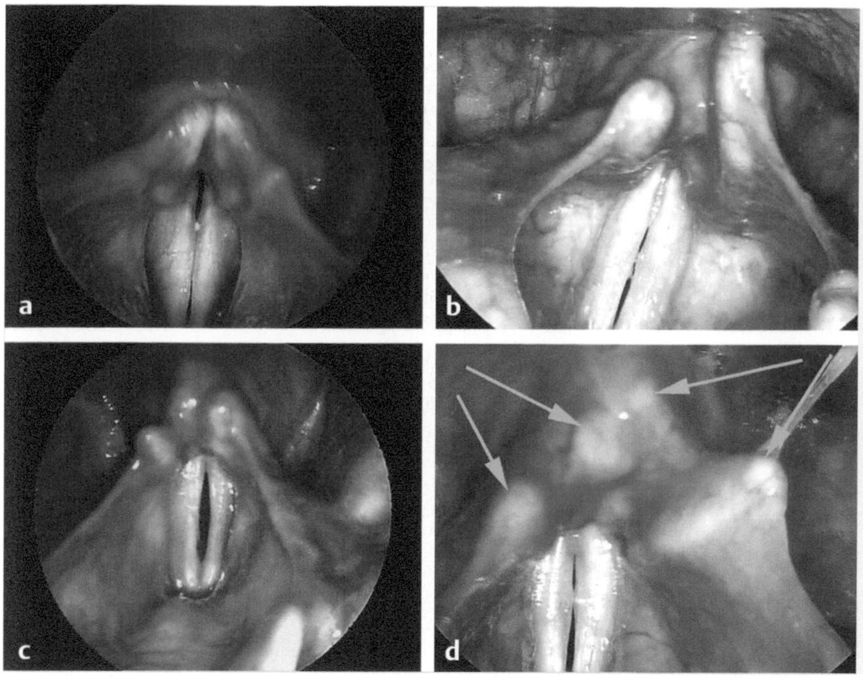

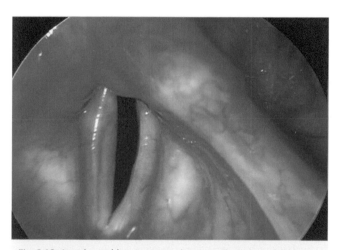

Fig. 6.17 **(a)** In this example, the arytenoid cartilages, with the smaller corniculate and cuneiform cartilages composing their most superior portions, appear quite symmetric in size, shape, and relative location. **(b)** The arytenoid cartilages can be significantly asymmetric. This example shows the left side posterior to the right side. **(c)** Another example of arytenoid asymmetry with the left arytenoid posterior to the right arytenoid. **(d)** In this example, the arytenoid cartilages may be symmetric relative to each other, but the corniculate and cuneiform cartilages (*green arrows*) are asymmetric in their position giving an overall appearance of significant asymmetry. (From Kendall K, Leonard R. Laryngeal Evaluation, 1st ed. New York: Thieme Publishers, 2010.)

Fig. 6.18 Atrophy and bowing secondary to unilateral vocal fold paralysis. (From Kendall K, Leonard R. Laryngeal Evaluation, 1st ed. New York: Thieme Publishers, 2010.)

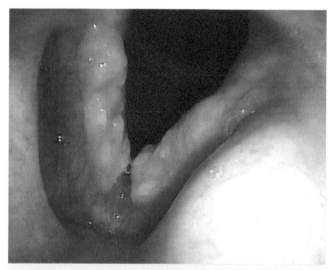

Fig. 6.19 Fungal laryngitis causing bilateral exophytic and irregular vocal fold edges.

and between individual cycles of vibration. These characteristics fall under the domain of movement but require a separate discussion due to the specialized knowledge required to interpret their features. Vibratory dynamics can only be visualized with a strobed image or with high-speed videography. When viewed under constant light, the vibration rate of the vocal folds is too fast for cycles of vibration to be visually perceived. Instead of separate cycles, the medial edges of the vocal folds appear blurred. High-speed video is emerging as a potential clinical modality, but, at the time of this publication, remains more of a research tool due to its high cost and issues with efficiency of implementation. In almost all voice clinics today, vibratory dynamics are assessed as a patient phonates while the larynx is illuminated with stroboscopic light (or the camera shutter is operated to give a stroboscopic effect, depending on the system used). The perceived vocal fold image appears as slow cycles of vibration. As previously mentioned, this is actually a **visual illusion**, and the actual stroboscopic cycle observed represents a composite of vocal fold images from multiple cycles of vibration at different points along the vibratory cycle.

Attempts should be made to observe the following dynamic characteristics under stroboscopic light. **Video 6.4** provides an example of laryngoscopy where all parameters were judged to be within normal limits. *At the very least, the following vibratory dynamic characteristics will be described from phonation during a relatively long duration (at least 2–3 seconds) sustained /i/ at comfortable pitch and loudness.* This is because a number of these characteristics will naturally change or differ from typical comfortable pitch and loudness voice production when voice is produced at high pitch levels (e.g., falsetto voice) or at differing loudness levels. As examples, partial or incomplete vocal fold closure, increased vocal fold stiffness, and decreased or restricted mucosal wave are commonly observed during high pitch/falsetto voice production, while these observations during comfortable pitch and loudness productions would be abnormal/atypical.

- **Symmetry**—the degree to which the vocal folds appear as mirror images of each other during a glottal cycle in the timing of opening, closing, and maximum lateral-medial excursion.[7] Vocal fold vibration symmetry can be viewed and described in two ways: (**1**) as the **phase relationship** (i.e., timing characteristics) between left and right vocal folds, in both the medial-lateral dimension (closing and opening movements) and anteroposterior dimension (front to back); and (**2**) in terms of the **amplitude** of vocal fold vibration. Amplitude refers to the extent of lateral movement of the vocal fold edges and can be observed as the degree to which a vocal fold moves laterally during the opening-to-open phase of vibration.[7]

Varying degrees of asymmetry occur in nondysphonic voices which should be considered when interpreting this vibratory parameter. Asymmetry of vibration typically indicates some difference (visible or nonvisible) in vibratory or tissue characteristics between the vocal folds. Structural changes to the vocal fold tissue, such as segments of tissue with increased stiffness or additional mass, can alter the vibratory characteristics of one or both vocal folds causing them to oscillate at different phases or amplitudes during the vibratory cycle. Excessive muscle tension can also influence vibratory symmetry. At comfortable, high, or low pitch and loudness levels, the vocal folds should move with symmetry where the phases of vibration occur at the same time and the extent of amplitude of vibration is similar. When phase symmetry is impaired, it can appear as a *side-to-side wavelike motion* of the vocal folds (e.g., **left-to-right asymmetry**) or *teeter-totter appearance* (e.g., **front-to-back asymmetry**)—the glottal opening will appear to wobble. Asymmetry of amplitude will appear as an asymmetric glottal opening as the vocal folds move from the closed to the open phase of vibration. The Stroboscopy Evaluation Rating Form published provides a scale that allows for documentation of the percentage of time asymmetry occurs in 20% temporal increments.[15] **Video 6.5** provides an example of phase asymmetry characterized by the left vocal fold "chasing" the right.

- **Stiffness**—Stiffness/tension within vocal fold tissue greatly affects the amplitude of vibration. When stiff segments or excessive tension occur in the vocal fold cover (e.g., due to mass lesion or hyperfunction, respectively), it can reduce the lateral displacement of a vocal fold. Impairments to vibratory amplitude characteristics due to changes in stiffness are typically labeled as reduced or increased. A *normal benchmark* at comfortable pitch and loudness is a **vibratory amplitude of one-third of the equivalent visible vocal fold width**.[16]

It is also important to note that vocal F_0 and intensity will influence stiffness and amplitude of vibration. The higher the F_0, the greater the stiffness and the smaller the vibratory amplitude. When vocal intensity increases, there will generally be some increase in vocal fold stiffness, but vibratory amplitude will increase. The F_0 and vocal intensity is often calculated and displayed on a digital videostroboscopy system.

Video 6.6 provides an example of reduced vibratory amplitude in the right vocal fold (asymmetry of amplitude).

- **Regularity**—the degree to which one videostroboscopic glottal cycle is consistent with successive videostroboscopic glottal cycles.[7] Regularity is also known as "**periodicity**" and can be thought of as the regularity of vocal fold oscillation from one stroboscopic cycle to the next. Impairments affecting the stiffness and tension of the vocal folds can alter vibration regularity, causing consistent or inconsistent irregularity or aperiodicity of vibration (quite common in rough voice quality). Under stroboscopic light, vibration irregularity (as observed in rough voice) causes the image to be perturbed or "jump" for very brief periods of time such that other dimensions of vibratory dynamics are difficult to judge. These perturbations can be validated not only by visual judgment but also by (**1**) the F_0 tracking display (the displayed F_0 will vary across a wide range of frequencies during the perturbations) and (**2**) the inability to "freeze" vocal fold motion when using the locked mode available on most stroboscopic systems.

Complete or near-complete irregularity will impede the ability of the strobe light flash rate to align with vocal F_0, so that the visual display is consistently blurred. In normal speakers producing comfortable, high, or low pitch and loudness phonation, attempts should always be regular (periodic). **Video 6.7** provides an example of phonation irregularity causing a blurred image due to the inability of the microphone to detect a stable fundamental frequency.

- **Mucosal wave**—the independent movement of the mucosa (i.e., epithelial cover) over the body of the vocal fold.[7] The mucosal wave is a wave-like displacement of the vocal fold cover during vibratory cycles. In healthy, nondysphonic voices producing sound at comfortable pitch and loudness, the vocal fold cover is pliable and becomes displaced during vibration somewhat independently of the body. This wave-like displacement can be seen moving from the bottom vocal fold edge superiorly toward the top edge and then across the surface of a vocal fold.

As with amplitude, mucosal wave is influenced by vocal F_0 and intensity in the following ways: (**1**) **the higher the F_0, the smaller the mucosal wave**; (**2**) **the greater the vocal intensity, the larger the mucosal wave**. Stiff vocal fold segments will typically decrease the mucosal wave on a vocal fold, either at the site of the lesion or across the entire vocal fold. Impairments to mucosal wave characteristics are typically labeled as reduced or increased. A normal benchmark at comfortable pitch and loudness is a **mucosal wave which travels at least one-half of the equivalent visible vocal fold width**.[16] As with vibratory amplitude, the corresponding F_0 should be notated for reference. **Video 6.8** demonstrates reduced mucosal wave on the left vocal fold due to the presence of a cyst, with normal mucosal wave properties on the right vocal fold.

- **Closure Pattern**—the glottal configuration during maximum closure.[10] This can be thought of as the degree of vocal fold closure at midline along the length of their horizontal (front-to-back) dimension. In healthy, nondysphonic comfortable pitch and loudness phonation, the left and right vocal folds should completely approximate each other in the vibratory portion of the vocal fold(s) (the anterior two-thirds portion) during the closed phase of vibration. In the majority of females and in a relatively smaller percentage of males, it is acceptable to observe a small posterior gap limited to the cartilaginous glottis.

Irregularities caused by lesions on the medial edge of one or both vocal folds, structural alterations such as atrophy or sulcus, and excessive muscle tension and stiffness can all compromise glottal closure.

- **Complete**—this is what should be expected in healthy, non-dysphonic speakers allowing for a small posterior gap in some patients (majority of females; smaller percentage of males).
- **Hourglass**—this is typical of unilateral or bilateral midfold swelling or mid-membranous lesions such as edema, nodules, polyps, and cysts. The exophytic nature of the lesion(s) does not allow tissue on either side to fully approximate.
- **Incomplete**—can be associated with a range of impaired physiology including paresis/paralysis to muscle tension dysphonia.
- **Irregular**—this can be associated with a range of structural lesions at any point along the vocal fold edge where varying segments of the vocal fold are exophytic and/or concave.
- **Posterior gap**—this may be normal in the majority of females and in some males when it is limited to the cartilaginous glottis (i.e., the posterior one-third of the length of the vocal fold comprising the vocal process region). In males or females, posterior gaps that include the membranous glottis (anterior two-third vibratory portion of the vocal folds) are considered abnormal and may be a sign of excessive muscle tension. Alternatively exophytic lesions located in the posterior glottis could cause a gap in that region.
- **Anterior gap**—this is most commonly associated with excessive muscle tension, and is an abnormal sign in both males and females. May also be observed in patients with SLN disruption or in patients who have swelling of the mid-to-posterior edges of the vocal folds.
- **Spindle (elliptical) gap**—this pattern occurs when the middle section of the membranous glottis does not approximate, while the anterior and posterior glottal regions do. It is most commonly associated with vocal fold bowing (e.g., as in Parkinson's disease) and/or bilateral vocal fold atrophy (e.g., as in presbylaryngis).
- **Closure duration**—the relative portion of each glottal cycle that the glottis is closed.[7] This can be observed and judged as the amount of time the vocal folds are in the closed phase of vibration relative to the open phase. In hyperfunctional kinetic voicing behaviors, it is not uncommon for the closed phase to take up a greater portion of the vibratory cycle than the other phases. Alternatively, in hypofunctional disorders where a glottal gap is present, it is not uncommon for the opening or open phases to dominate.
- Laryngeal videostroboscopy allows for additional assessment of vocal fold characteristics that can provide valuable clinical information. This would include the presence of a **vertical level difference**, which refers to the relative vertical level of the two vocal folds as they meet at midline. This is typically judged as either on-plane (e.g., "level") or off-plane, and when the level is noted as off-plane the clinician should note which vocal fold is above or below the other.[7] The presence and location of **nonvibrating segments** can also add valuable information to the diagnostic process (see **Video 6.8**, where there

is marked reduction of mucosal wave due to the presence of a cyst). Small and/or soft lesions may only impact vibratory amplitude and mucosal wave at the site of lesion, resulting in a limited region of stiffness along a vocal fold. This is typical of early vocal fold nodules or edematous lesions. Larger and stiffer lesions, especially those which anchor the vocal fold cover to the vocal ligament, can impact stiffness to a greater degree and is visually characterized by a larger affected region across the vocal fold.[16]

6.9 Billing and Reimbursement Issues

Speech–language pathology services can be provided on a pro-bono (free) basis or fee for service. The fees charged for services can be billed to the patient directly (e.g., "private pay") or billed through a third-party insurer that covers the patient. In the United States, health care services that are billed to insurance companies are required to identify the specific procedure with the use of codes. The most common coding scheme used in the United States is the **Current Procedural Terminology** coding system (CPT; American Medical Association). Specific CPT codes are established and revised by an expert panel of 17 individuals (the majority are physicians) authorized by the American Medical Association.

▶ Table 6.3 illustrates the three most common procedures that are conducted as part of a comprehensive voice evaluation protocol. As of the year 2017, laryngoscopy with stroboscopy (whether conducted with a rigid or flexible endoscope) is identified by CPT code **31579**. Since this is a medical code, 31579 must be co-signed by a physician for some insurance policies. This procedure can be conducted with other voice diagnostic

Table 6.3 Current Procedural Terminology (CPT American Medical Association) codes for procedures specific to voice evaluation.[a]

Billing code	Descriptor	Medicare Part B rate
31579	Laryngoscopy, flexible or rigid fiberoptic, with stroboscopy	$178.01
92520	Laryngeal function studies (i.e., aerodynamic testing and acoustic testing)	$77.16
92524	Behavioral and qualitative analysis of voice and resonance	$90.08

Procedure 1	Procedure 2	Modifier
31579	92520	-59
31579	92524[b]	N/A
92520	92524[b]	N/A

[a]These three codes constitute procedures that complete a comprehensive voice diagnostic protocol. Medicare Part B reimbursement rates correspond to the 2017 Medicare Physician Fee Schedule used by the Centers for Medicare and Medicaid Services of the United States. For Medicare billing, all claims should be accompanied by the **–GN** modifier to indicate services provided under speech–language pathology plan of care.

[b]When only completing one component of 92524 (e.g., only acoustic, or only aerodynamic), a **-54** modifier onto the code is required to indicate a partial procedure.

procedures including Laryngeal Function Studies (92520—acoustic and aerodynamic procedures) and the Behavioral and Qualitative Analysis of Voice (92524). When 31579 is conducted on the same day as 92520, it must include an extension, called a "modifier," of **-59** which indicates that it is a separate and distinct procedure.

The Centers for Medicare and Medicaid Services publishes an annual schedule of fees (the "Physician Fee Schedule") which indicates the amount Medicare will reimburse a provider (e.g., the SLP) for specific procedures identified by CPT codes. As ▶ Table 6.3 shows, these amounts vary widely among the three diagnostic codes listed, although currently the reimbursement rate for videostroboscopy is more than double the rate for other diagnostic procedures.

Third-party insurance companies often base their reimbursement rates on the Physician Fee Schedule, which means it is important that clinicians who are billing for services be familiar with the current published guidelines. It is also important to understand that what an insurance company will reimburse for a procedure and what a clinician or practice charges for the procedure are different. In most cases, the fee for service is greater than the amount the insurance entity will pay, and the patient will be responsible for the difference in the form of a co-pay or an amount that includes but also exceeds the co-pay. The specific fee schedules set by different clinical practices vary greatly from region to region.

6.10 Conclusion

This chapter has summarized the essential role of laryngeal endoscopy and stroboscopy as a key method for laryngeal visualization necessary to complete our voice diagnostic protocol. The laryngeal visualization tasks and procedures described in this chapter provide not only a detailed description of the laryngeal and associated structures used in phonation but also an in-depth analysis of subtle vibratory characteristics that underlie dysphonic voice in the many cases in which obvious structural impairments (e.g., the observation of vocal fold lesion(s) of demonstrated paralysis/paresis) are absent.

The order of the chapters that we have led the reader through has been quite purposeful, as a detailed and appropriate diagnostic methodology provides the necessary direction for treatment (i.e., a thorough and accurate diagnosis is essential for successful treatment). Now that our detailed voice diagnostic protocol (composed of information obtained from case history, perceptual, acoustic, aerodynamic, and laryngeal visualization) is complete, we are ready to move on to descriptions of various behavioral, surgical, and pharmaceutical voice treatment methods.

Clinical Case Study

Mrs. Granger is a 31-year-old woman who has experienced dysphonia for 8 months. Her current symptoms began to form gradually after spending the summer as a vocal coach at a singing camp. The camp required heavy vocal demands on a daily basis including singing and loud speaking. Over the last 2 weeks of the camp, she noticed a sudden onset of a change in her voice (it started one morning and then got worse over the next 2 weeks), which she characterized as a lower speaking pitch,

a loss of her upper frequency range when singing, and vocal fatigue when speaking or singing for an extended amount of time. The problem has affected her job as a high-school voice (singing) teacher, which requires her to work with individuals and small groups throughout the day. She reports that her voice quality is beginning to further deteriorate when speaking and singing, and that she is no longer able to hold notes in the upper part of her register. She was evaluated by an otolaryngologist 3 weeks ago who diagnosed her with vocal nodules.

Mrs. Granger has a college degree in voice and she continued professional voice lessons after college for 3 years. Prior to the onset of the current problem, she participated in an amateur band on weekends performing contemporary music (pop, soft rock). Due to her problems she has stopped performing. She has no history of voice problems prior to the current issues, is a non-smoker, and drinks at least five glasses of water per day, two cups of green tea during the day, but no other caffeinated beverages. She is not taking any medications currently and has no priory history of surgeries.

Laryngeal videostroboscopy revealed a large unilateral polyp at the mid-membranous (anterior one-third to posterior two-thirds juncture) portion of the true vocal fold, with a contralateral reactive lesion. The polyp is broad based with prominent blood vessels surrounding it. The contralateral lesion appears edematous and translucent.

Questions to Consider
1. For purposes of differential diagnoses, what other questions would be informative to ask this patient?
2. Based on the patient's age, gender, and vocal use history, what clinical hypotheses would you develop with regard to the potential diagnosis (e.g., functional vs. organic) and why?
3. Describe a theory which explains why polyps form.
4. What does it mean that a polyp is a "benign" laryngeal lesion?
5. Does the patient's description of the onset of her voice problem fit with the description of time-course for onset of polyps described on voicemedicine.com?
6. What is the recommended initial form of treatment for this lesion and why?

6.11 Review Questions

1. Another word used for laryngoscopy when it is performed by a speech–language pathologist is?
   a) Mirror evaluation.
   b) Phonoscopic exam.
   c) Laryngeal palpation.
   d) Endoscopy.
   e) None of the above.
2. Which credential demonstrates the obtainment of knowledge and skill necessary to perform laryngoscopy with stroboscopy for speech–language pathologists?
   a) Certificate of clinical competence (CCC-SLP).
   b) State license.
   c) Both a and b.

d) All of the above.

e) None of the above.

3. The medial edge of the vocal fold (the "vibratory edge," where one fold contacts the other) should, in normal healthy tissue, be characterized by
   a) Smooth and straight.
   b) Concave at cartilaginous portion and convex at membranous portion.
   c) Yellowish in appearance.
   d) Thin and hypotonic.
   e) All of the above.

4. What flexible endoscope technology can produce images that rival those from rigid endoscopes?
   a) Flexible laryngoscopes.
   b) Nasoendoscopes.
   c) Video endoscopes.
   d) Stroboscopes.
   e) Both a & c

5. Which of the following is *not* a material/equipment needed when performing laryngoscopy with stroboscopy?
   a) Gloves.
   b) Gauze.
   c) Light source.
   d) All of the above.
   e) None of the above.

6. What information controls the flash rate of stroboscopic light for laryngoscopy with stroboscopy?
   a) The patient's F_o.
   b) The patient's vocal intensity.
   c) The size of the patient's vocal folds.
   d) The patient's gender.
   e) Both b and c.

7. Which of the following is an advantage of a flexible endoscope over a rigid endoscope?
   a) Larger image with greater resolution.
   b) Less likely to elicit a gag reflex.
   c) Allows for production of /i/ vowel.
   d) Tolerated by most patients.
   e) None of the above.

8. A recommended patient position for rigid laryngoscopy includes
   a) Leaning back with chin up.
   b) Standing with shoulders in line with the torso.
   c) Sitting forward with chin out as when sniffing.
   d) Sitting straight in the chair with good posture.
   e) All of the above.

9. When passing a flexible endoscope through a nostril, what visual characteristic does the examiner look for to guide where to direct the shaft?
   a) Dark regions indicating space.
   b) The location of the superior turbinate.
   c) The Eustachian tube.
   d) None of the above.
   e) All of the above.

10. Why would you dip the end of a rigid endoscope into warm water?
    a) To clean it.
    b) To prevent fogging.

c) To lubricate it.

d) To ease insertion into the oral cavity.

e) Both c and d.

11. Which of the following are *not* possible adverse effects of either rigid or flexible laryngoscopy?
    a) Nose bleed.
    b) Chest pain.
    c) Gag.
    d) Discomfort.
    e) None of the above.

12. Which of the following would most likely cause the greatest disruption in the mucosal wave?
    a) Vocal fold nodules.
    b) Vocal process granuloma.
    c) Vocal fold cyst.
    d) Vocal fold edema.
    e) All of the above.

13. Which of the following disorders would likely cause closure duration of the vibratory cycle to be much greater than the open-opening duration?
    a) Vocal fold paralysis.
    b) Muscle tension dysphonia.
    c) Laryngeal cancer.
    d) Presbylaryngis.
    e) None of the above.

14. Healthy vocal folds are characterized by what color?
    a) Pink.
    b) Pearly white.
    c) Translucent red.
    d) Deep red.
    e) Both c and d.

15. In what way would fundamental frequency affect vibratory amplitude and mucosal wave?
    a) Higher F_o = less amplitude and smaller mucosal wave.
    b) Higher F_o = more amplitude and greater mucosal wave.
    c) Lower F_o = less amplitude and greater mucosal wave.
    d) Lower F_o = more amplitude and smaller mucosal wave.
    e) None of the above.

6.12 Answers and Explanations

1. Correct: Phonoscopic exam (**b**).
   (**b**) Laryngoscopy is sometimes referred to as "phonoscopy" or a "phonoscopic exam" to differentiate it from the laryngoscopy performed by a physician or an endoscopic examination conducted during FEES. (**a**) The term "mirror evaluation" is not used in the context of laryngoscopy. Some otolaryngologists might utilize a laryngeal mirror when visualizing the larynx, which is called indirect laryngoscopy. (**c**) Laryngeal palpation involves manipulation of the laryngeal cartilages using the hands on the outside of the neck. (**d**) Endoscopy is a general term and can be performed by medical professionals in addition to the SLP.

2. Correct: None of the above (**e**).
   (**e**) There is no credential that certifies or licenses an SLP to perform stroboscopy. However, the ability to conduct stroboscopic examinations is included in the SLP scope of practice of ASHA and most state licensure boards. (**a**) The Certificate

of Clinical Competence does not specifically certify an SLP to perform stroboscopic procedures. However, they are included within the scope of practice. (**b**) State license to work as an SLP Competence does not specifically certify an SLP to perform stroboscopic procedures. However, they are included within most state boards' scope of practice.

3. Correct: Smooth and straight (**a**).

(**a**) Healthy vocal fold medial edges appear smooth and straight, allowing for complete glottal closure when the vocal folds are adducted. (**b**) Concave medial edges typically result in elliptical glottal closure patterns. (**c**) Healthy vocal folds appear white all along their length, not yellowish. (**d**) Thin, hypotonic medial edges of vocal fold are often a sign of atrophy and/or paralysis.

4. Correct: Video endoscopes (**c**).

(**c**) Recent technological advances have made available video endoscopes with a charged couple device chip and electronics at the distal end of the bendable tip wired back through the shaft and controlled by a video processor. These are also referred to as "chip-in-the-tip" or "distal chip" endoscopes, and are equivalent to having a video camera built into the tip. (**a**) Flexible laryngoscopes typically result in smaller images with less resolution than standard rigid laryngoscopes. (**b**) Nasoendoscopes are a type of flexible laryngoscope, and typically result in smaller images with less resolution than standard rigid laryngoscopes. (**d**) The term "stroboscope" is a general term that can refer to any endoscope utilizing a stroboscopic light.

5. Correct: None of the above (**e**).

(**e**) Gloves, gauze, and a light source are three of the important materials and equipment needed to perform laryngoscopy with or without stroboscopy. (**a**) Gloves are an important piece of personal protective equipment used during laryngoscopy. (**b**) Gauze is an important piece of material used during laryngoscopy. (**c**). A light source is needed to illuminate the larynx during laryngoscopy.

6. Correct: The patient's F_0 (**a**).

(**a**) The stroboscopic light flash rate is set at a frequency slightly lower than the actual Fo being produced to give the visual illusion of slowed vibratory movement. (**b**) Vocal intensity is detected via a microphone with most stroboscopy systems, but does not influence the strobe flash rate. (**c**) The size of a patient's vocal folds can be visualized with endoscopy or stroboscopy, but do not influence the flash rate of the strobe. (**d**) Gender will have an influence on a patient's F_0, but it is the F_0 that influences flash rate, not gender (e.g., some females speak at F_0s near some males).

7. Correct: Less likely to elicit a gag reflex (**b**).

(**b**) Because flexible endoscopes bypass the region near the faucial arches in the oropharynx, they are less likely to elicit a gag reflex compared to rigid endoscopes. (**a**) Rigid endoscopes produce larger images with greater resolution compared to standard flexible endoscopes. (**c**) While a patient can produce /i/ when being examined with a flexible endoscope, they can produce any vowel when being examined with a rigid endoscope. (**d**) Both rigid and flexible endoscopes are tolerated by most patients.

8. Correct: Sitting forward with chin out as when sniffing (**c**).

(**c**) Having the patient sit forward with his or her chin out will help best expose the larynx to the field of view as the patient produces an /i/ sound during rigid endoscopy. (**a**) Leaning back, and especially with the chin up, may tilt the epiglottis posteriorly which would obscure views of the larynx. (**b**) Endoscopic examinations are almost always performed with the patient sitting in a chair. (**d**) Sitting straight in a chair is the preferred position for flexible endoscopy, but not for rigid endoscopy.

9. Correct: Dark regions indicating space (**a**).

(**a**) During flexible endoscopy, dark regions indicate space through which the endoscope can pass freely. (**b**) The superior turbinate is located high in the nasal cavity and can be difficult to reach with a flexible endoscope in many patients. (**c**) The eustachian tube is located in the posterior oral cavity, at the anterior portion of the oropharynx—not in the nasal cavity.

10. Correct: To prevent fogging (**b**).

(**b**) Dipping the tip of an endoscope into warm water will warm it, so that when it encounters the warm breath of a patient the lens does not fog. (**a**) Endoscopes should be cleaned with high-level disinfectants after each use, not water. (**c**) Gel is used to lubricate the shafts of flexible endoscopes, not water. (**d**) Rigid endoscopes do not need lubricant or water to place within the oral cavity.

11. Correct: Chest pain (**b**).

(**b**) Because endoscopes do not put pressure or impinge upon sensory nerves of the chest, chest pain is not a typical adverse effect associated with endoscopy. (**a**) Nose bleed during flexible endoscopy is rare, but one of the possible adverse effects. (**c**) Gag reflex is a common adverse effect related to rigid endoscopy. (**d**) Nasal discomfort and general discomfort in the oral cavity are possible adverse effects of flexible endoscopy and rigid endoscopy, respectively.

12. Correct: Vocal fold cyst (**c**).

(**c**) Vocal fold cysts can anchor to the vocal fold ligament, which can cause significant stiffness and great disruption to the mucosal wave. (**a**) Vocal nodules affect epithelium but generally result in less mucosal wave disruption than cysts. (**c**) Vocal process granulomas occur posteriorly and generally do not have a substantial impact on mucosal wave. If they do, the disruption will be confined to the posterior vocal fold region. (**d**) Compared to vocal fold cysts, mucosal wave disruptions from edema are typically less.

13. Correct: Muscle tension dysphonia (**b**).

(**b**) Muscle tension dysphonia is characterized by excessive contraction of the adductor muscles. This tends to increase the duration of the closed phase of the vibratory cycle compared to the open phase. (**a**) Vocal fold paralysis is characterized by greater open phase than closed phase of the vibratory cycle. (**c**) Laryngeal cancer, when it is at the level of the glottis, would result in greater open phase durations due to the excrescence and glottal gap. (**d**) Presbylaryngis is typically characterized by vocal fold bowing and glottal insufficiency, resulting in a greater open phase duration.

14. Correct: Pearly white (**b**).

(**b**) Healthy vocal folds are typically pearly white with minimal vascularity visible on the surface. (**a**) Vocal folds with a pink color may indicate recent phonotrauma. (**c**) Translucent vocal folds indicate edema, while redness (erythema) indicates irritation. (**d**) Deep red color on the vocal folds indicates hypervascularity and recent phonotrauma.

15. Correct: Higher F_0 = less amplitude and smaller mucosal wave (**a**).

(**a**) Higher F_0 results from increased vocal fold tension, which has the effect to reduce vibratory amplitude and mucosal wave. (**b**) Higher F_0 would result in reduced amplitude and reduced mucosal wave due to the added stiffness in the vocal fold. (**c**) Lower F_0 would result from decreased vocal fold stiffness, which has the effect of reducing increasing mucosal wave. (**d**) Lower F_0 tends to increase the mucosal wave dynamics compared to higher F_0.

Videos

Video 6.1 Vocal fold paralysis. (From Kendall K, Leonard R. Laryngeal Evaluation, 1st ed. New York: Thieme Publishers, 2010.)

Video 6.2 Vocal tremor. (From Kendall K, Leonard R. Laryngeal Evaluation, 1st ed. New York: Thieme Publishers, 2010.)

Video 6.3 Medial compression of false vocal folds. (From Kendall K, Leonard R. Laryngeal Evaluation, 1st ed. New York: Thieme Publishers, 2010.)

Video 6.4 Normal vibratory parameters

Video 6.5 Phase asymmetry. (From Kendall K, Leonard R. Laryngeal Evaluation, 1st ed. New York: Thieme Publishers, 2010.)

Video 6.6 Reduced amplitude of vibration. (From Kendall K, Leonard R. Laryngeal Evaluation, 1st ed. New York: Thieme Publishers, 2010.)

Video 6.7 Vibration irregularity. (From Kendall K, Leonard R. Laryngeal Evaluation, 1st edition. New York: Thieme Publishers, 2010.)

Video 6.8 Reduced mucosal wave. (From Kendall K, Leonard R. Laryngeal Evaluation, 1st ed. New York: Thieme Publishers, 2010.)

Appendix 6.1 An example of competency guidelines for laryngeal endoscopy with stroboscopy

Skills   Mentors' initials

These competencies are a condensed representation of the American Speech-Language-Hearing Association policy statement (2004). *Knowledge and Skills for Speech-Language Pathologists with Respect to Vocal Tract Visualization and Imaging [Knowledge and Skills]*

Recognition of voice and resonance disorders and identification of patient qualifications for specific procedures

Proficient in discussing all aspects of videoendostroboscopy with the patient and/or significant others as that procedure relates to voice disorders

Proficient in using various tools and procedures that are needed to perform videoendostroboscopy

Proficient in interpretation of the effects of vocal behavior on the laryngeal anatomy as well as the laryngeal anatomy effects on laryngeal physiology in conjunction with medical colleagues and concisely describe videoendostroboscopic findings and interpretations for professional communication purposes

Proficient in the management of voice disorders with the use of visual feedback from obtained laryngeal images

Must complete one of the following: _____
1. Completion/Attendance of continuing education   _____
course on methodology and use of endoscopy/   _____
stroboscopy (e.g., Pentax-Kay Elemetrics Strobo-   _____
scopy Course, Vanderbilt Stroboscopy Course, Doug   _____
Hicks Stroboscopy course, etc.)............................   _____
....
2. Participation in a mentorship program with an experienced speech–language pathologist to develop skills related to trouble-shooting, interpretation, and report writing of endoscopic/stroboscopic examinations...
Must complete two of the following:
1. Obtaining a score of at least 85% on a written examination covering specific knowledge and application of vocal tract visualization procedures...
2. Establishing at least 90% reliability of judgments on rigid and flexible laryngeal videostroboscopic findings with two clinicians competent in these procedures..
3. Complete *Perspectives* quarterly continuing education associated with ASHA Special Interest Division 3...
4. Must read chapters 5 and 6 of *Videostroboscopic Examination of the Larynx* by Hirano and Bless..

Completion of the following with the number of   _____
hours listed under the supervision of an   _____
experienced/trained mentoring clinician or otolar-   _____
yngologist.   _____
Observation of 10 endoscopic and/or stroboscopic   _____
examinations..   _____
10 examinations on normal individuals without suspected problem utilizing rigid endoscope...
10 examinations on normal individuals without suspected problem using flexible endoscope...
15 examinations on patients utilizing rigid endoscope...
15 examinations on patients utilizing a flexible endoscope...
Less than 15 patient examinations based on demonstrated competency
Once the mandatory number of hours under trained clinician procedure is completed, the evaluator will determine if further supervision is necessary (i.e., comfort level; skills; techniques)

_____ has satisfactorily demonstrated competency in completing advanced graduate training in Laryngeal Stroboscopy Diagnostic Examination and is prepared to perform this procedure under further supervision as a SLP clinical fellow/intern

_____ has **NOT** satisfactorily demonstrated competency in completing advanced graduate training in Laryngeal Stroboscopy Diagnostic Examination and will require further supervision prior to independent practice. Guidelines of supervision will be posted in employee file.

Mentoring plan has been established and a new assessment will be completed by:_____ (date)

_____

Mentor Signature Date

_____ _____

Clinician Signature Date

Note: These guidelines were adapted from recommendations by Kimberly Chachere-Coker, MS, CCC-SLP.

References

[1] Leonard RJ. Flexible laryngoscopy in speech-language pathology evaluation. In: Kendall KA, Leonard RJ. eds. Laryngeal Evaluation: Indirect Laryngoscopy to High-Speed Digital Imaging. New York: Thieme Medical Publishers; 2010

[2] Mehlum CS, Rosenberg T, Groentved AM, Dyrvig AK, Godballe C. Can videostroboscopy predict early glottic cancer? A systematic review and meta-analysis. Laryngoscope. 2016; 126(9):2079–2084

[3] Paul BC, Chen S, Sridharan S, Fang Y, Amin MR, Branski RC. Diagnostic accuracy of history, laryngoscopy, and stroboscopy. Laryngoscope. 2013; 123(1):215–219

[4] Sataloff RT, Spiegel JR, Hawkshaw MJ. Strobovideolaryngoscopy: results and clinical value. Ann Otol Rhinol Laryngol. 1991; 100(9, Pt 1):725–727

[5] American Speech-Language-Hearing Association. Scope of practice in speech-language pathology [Scope of Practice]. 2007, Available at: www.asha.org/policy. Accessed December 4, 2017

[6] American Speech-Language-Hearing Association. Vocal tract visualization and imaging: position statement [Position Statement]. 2004a, Available at: www.asha.org/policy. Accessed December 4, 2017

[7] ASHA Committee on Instrumental Voice Assessment Protocols (IVAP). Recommended Protocols for Instrumental Assessment of Voice: Draft Summary of Recommendations. January 24, 2015

[8] American Speech-Language-Hearing Association. Code of ethics [Ethics]. 2010, Available at: www.asha.org/policy. Accessed December 4, 2017

[9] American Speech-Language-Hearing Association. Knowledge and skills for speech-language pathologists with respect to vocal tract visualization and imaging [Knowledge and Skills]. 2004, Available at: www.asha.org/policy. Accessed December 4, 2017

[10] American Speech-Language-Hearing Association. The roles of otolaryngologists and speech-language pathologists in the performance and interpretation of strobovideolaryngoscopy [Relevant Paper]. 1998, Available at: www.asha.org/policy. Accessed December 4, 2017

[11] American Speech-Language-Hearing Association. Sedation and topical anesthesia in audiology and speech-language pathology. 1992. ASHA Suppl. 1992; 34 7:41–42

[12] American Speech-Language-Hearing Association. Knowledge and skills for speech-language pathologists performing endoscopic assessment of swallowing functions [Knowledge and Skills]. 2002, Available at: www.asha.org/policy. Accessed December 4, 2017

[13] American Speech-Language-Hearing Association. Role of the speech-language pathologist in the performance and interpretation of endoscopic evaluation of swallowing: guidelines [Guidelines]. 2004, Available at: www.asha.org/policy. Accessed December 4, 2017

[14] Thomas JP. Why Is There a Frog In My Throat? Portland, OR: James P. Thomas; 2012

[15] Poburka BJ. A new stroboscopy rating form. J Voice. 1999; 13(3):403–413

[16] Hirano M, Bless DM. Videostroboscopic Examination of the Larynx. San Diego, CA: Singular; 1993

Suggested Readings

[1] Hirano M, Bless DM. Videostroboscopic Examination of the Larynx. San Diego, CA: Singular; 1993

[2] Kelkar AS, Cox KT, Hough M, Ball L, O, ', Brien K. Participant anxiety and presence of hyperfunction in stroboscopy. Folia Phoniatr Logop. 2013; 65 (6):275–279

[3] Kendall KA, Leonard RJ. Laryngeal Evaluation: Indirect Laryngoscopy to High-Speed Digital Imaging. New York: Thieme Medical Publishers; 2010

[4] Woo P. Stroboscopy. San Diego, CA: Plural Publishing; 1999

7 Medical Treatment of Voice Disorders

Summary

This chapter describes the roles and practices of the otolaryngologist specific to evaluation and treatment of patients with voice impairments. The framework of the office examination is described along with the procedures used by the otolaryngologist for differential diagnosis. Surgical management options are described and associated with targeted voice impairments. The role of voice rest as part of the postsurgical voice recovery phase is detailed, along with pharmacological management for various conditions associated with voice disorders.

Keywords: laryngology, laryngeal framework surgery, injection laryngoplasty, botulinum toxin

7.1 Learning Objectives

At the end of this chapter, readers will be able to
- Compare and contrast the otolaryngologist's clinical evaluation compared to the clinical evaluation of voice performed by the speech–language pathologist.
- Describe the framework of the otolaryngology office evaluation.
- Identify surgical procedures used by otolaryngologists for specific voice disorder etiologies.
- Identify the rationale for administration of specific medications for voice disorders, and the potential side effects of those medications.

7.2 Introduction

Speech–language pathologists (SLPs) who evaluate and treat populations with voice disorders work collaboratively with other medical professionals as part of a **voice care team**. In most situations, the primary members of the voice care team will be the voice therapist and otolaryngologist. Additional members may include but are not be limited to neurologists, gastroenterologists, singing voice teachers, psychologists, pulmonologists, allergy specialists, and endocrinologists. Members of the team may be physically located near each other (e.g., in an otolaryngology private practice or medical center), in the same community, or sometimes spread across different cities and states. Regardless of team member locations, it is key that they communicate effectively and efficiently with each other to maximize care and management of the patient.

Otolaryngologists who specialize in laryngeal disorders affecting voice, swallowing, and airway are known in the United States as "**laryngologists.**" There is no formal degree or credential which certifies one as a laryngologist, although many complete a postresidency laryngology fellowship where they learn the specialty under the mentorship of an experienced physician (who will also be a laryngologist). Training guidelines for laryngology fellowships have been developed by the American Laryngological Association (ALA). According to the ALA, there were at least 23 laryngology fellowship programs participating in the National Resident Matching Program as of 2017. Other laryngology fellowship programs are also offered which do not participate in this program. Otolaryngologists who complete a fellowship are often referred to as a "Fellowship trained Laryngologist." According to

www.voicedoctor.net, as of the year 2017, there were a total of 212 laryngologists in the United States, and 368 practicing worldwide.

When one practices as a voice therapist, it is important that the "*golden rule of voice therapy*" is always considered. It is as follows: **before developing and implementing a voice treatment program, a patient must be evaluated by an otolaryngologist for the determination of an existing medical diagnosis**. This does not mean that the voice therapist must wait to conduct a voice evaluation—in fact, that information can be of great value to the otolaryngologist's subsequent examination. However, although knowledge and skill domains of the voice therapist and otolaryngologist overlap, and both may perform laryngeal endoscopy, it is only the otolaryngologist who will determine the final medical diagnosis regarding organic disorders affecting the larynx. The otolaryngologist possesses advanced knowledge of systems and structures and are the only medical/health professional qualified to diagnose specific organic vocal fold impairments. These pathologies must be ruled in or out before initiating behavioral voice treatment.

7.3 The Otolaryngology Office Examination

n treatment-seeking populations, the clinical otolaryngologic exam is either the first or last stage of assessment prior to the initiation of treatment. When voice therapy is warranted, the patient might come to the voice therapist via otolaryngology referral, or it may be the voice therapist who refers to the physician before initiating treatment if that patient has not yet been evaluated by an otolaryngologist. The otolaryngology office examination will consist of a series of steps which facilitate the process of differential diagnosis. Typically, these steps will follow the order outlined below.

7.3.1 Patient Questionnaires

As with the voice evaluation performed by the voice therapist, the otolaryngologist may ask the patient to complete questionnaires or ratings of self-perception prior to the office examination. These indices will be used to evaluate self-perceived handicap, quality of life, and/or reflux-associated symptoms. Examples include the following:
- Voice Handicap Index.[1]
- Singing Voice Handicap Index.[2]
- Voice Related Quality of Life.[3]
- Voice Symptom Scale.[4]
- Glottal Function Index.[5]
- Voice Activity and Participation Profile.[6]
- Reflux Symptom Index.[7]

7.3.2 Patient History

After greeting in the office, the otolaryngologist will ask the patient a series of questions regarding domains of voice use and problem history. The questions presented to the patient are designed to elicit information which will elucidate (1) the patient's perception (description) of the current voice difficulties; (2) the temporal (time) development of the current voice problem; (3) potential behavioral, medical, environmental, and psychological etiologies associated with the problem; and (d) the patient's personality, motivation, occupational, and social activities which may contribute to the current problem and which may influence subsequent treatment decisions.

7.3.3 Physical Examination

The otolaryngologist will complete a general evaluation of systems and structures associated with the head and neck. The goal of the physical examination is to rule in or out conditions which may be causing the current voice problem(s), and to further characterize the nature of an existing problem. Among the domains assessed during this part of the clinical examination are

- Otoscopic view of ears.
- Oral and nasal cavity exam.
- Palpation of nodes and glands within the neck.
- Perceptual evaluation of voice quality and function.

7.3.4 Laryngeal Visualization

The penultimate step in the otolaryngology office examination is visual observation of laryngeal structure and function (**laryngoscopy**). There are three primary methods with which the otolaryngologist can visualize the larynx: (**1**) indirect mirror laryngoscopy, (**2**) direct laryngoscopy using a flexible fiberscope (nasoendoscopy) routed through the nose, and (**3**) direct laryngoscopy using a rigid endoscope routed through the mouth. A majority of general otolaryngology practices will utilize a flexible endoscope routed through the nose to complete laryngeal visualization. In laryngology practices, the physician may use a standard flexible fiberscope, a distal chip nasoendoscope, or a rigid endoscope, all of which may be used with a steady light source or with stroboscopy for examination of vibratory dynamics. ▶ Fig. 7.1 shows the three tools (laryngeal mirror, flexible endoscope, and rigid endoscope) with which an otolaryngologist can visualize the larynx and vocal folds.

7.3.5 Debriefing, Diagnosis, and Referral Pathways

The office examination concludes with the otolaryngologist considering all the evidence collected from the procedures described earlier. The physician will describe to the patient which findings were suggestive of physiological impairment and indicate what options might be available to rehabilitate or improve those impairments. The collective evidence may lead to the determination of a medical diagnosis from which the appropriate treatment recommendations can be made. In some cases, the otolaryngologist will need more detailed information of internal structure as well as neurological and systemic function that requires referral to another medical professional or subsequent otolaryngologic procedure. Examples include

- *X-ray, computed tomography or computed axial tomography (CT or CAT), magnetic resonance imaging (MRI) scan*: these examinations are completed to better visualize internal bony structures and spaces (X-ray), or soft tissues such as the brain,

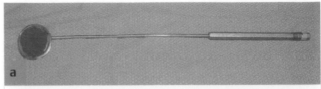
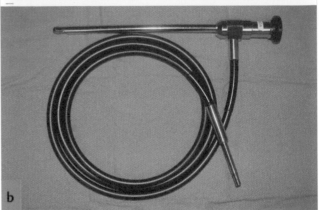
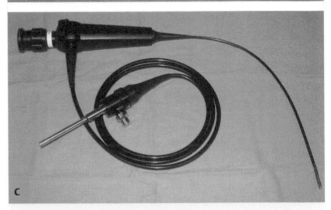

Fig. 7.1 Instrumentation used for laryngoscopy: **(a)** laryngeal mirror, **(b)** rigid endoscope, and **(c)** flexible endoscope. (From Aronson A, Bless D. Clinical Voice Disorders. 4th ed. New York: Thieme Publishers, 2009.)

nerve pathways, and blood vessels (CT and MRI). These referrals are often made to rule out tumors or structural irregularities which cannot be visualized using laryngoscopy.

- *Gastroenterology examination*: referral to the gastroenterologist is sometimes made when the otolaryngologist suspects laryngopharyngeal reflux. The current gold-standard assessment for reflux is **24-hour dual-channel pH monitoring**.[8] In this examination, probes are placed above and below the upper esophageal sphincter. The probes are attached to a monitor which records the pH levels of the probes. The patient wears the monitor with probes in place for 24 hours, and the pH levels are recorded across this time frame.

- *Oncologist*: when laryngeal cancer is diagnosed, the multidisciplinary medical management will typically include referral to an oncologist when recommended treatment will include irradiation and/or chemotherapy. Oncologists are medical doctors with specialty training in the prevention, diagnosis, and treatment of cancers. To practice as an oncologist, the educational requirements necessitate completion of a postresidency fellowship in oncology. The oncologist may remove large or complex head/neck tumors (these are referred to as "surgical oncologists"), they may administer chemotherapy (these are referred to as "medical oncologists"), or they may administer radiotherapy (these are referred to as "radiation oncologists").

- *Allergist/Immunologist*: the otolaryngologist may need to rule in or out allergic or immunologic conditions associated with the current voice problems. When this need exists, the physician may refer to an allergist (or allergist/immunologist). These medical professionals are physicians with specialty training in the form of a fellowship in allergy/immunology, and in the United States are certified by the American Board of Allergy and Immunology. The allergist/immunologist can conduct specialized testing to investigate the presence of allergic reactions to various substances, asthma, and immune system disorders.

- *Endocrinologist*: referral to the endocrinologist might be needed when the otolaryngologist needs to rule out impairments to the endocrine system. The endocrine system controls hormone levels in the body, and the endocrinologist is the medical specialist who diagnoses diseases to this system. Of importance to the otolaryngologist is the status of the thyroid gland, as voice quality change such as hoarseness can be a clinical manifestation of a hypoactive thyroid.[9]

- *Neurologist*: the otolaryngologist can diagnose certain neurological disorders—among these include vocal fold paralysis, spasmodic dysphonia, and voice tremor. However, additional and more specific neurological information may be needed and in these cases assessment by a neurologist can be warranted. Voice disorders can be associated with degenerative or acute neurological disease processes, which the neurologist is specially trained to assess and diagnose.

- *Electromyographic testing*: when vocal fold paralysis is suspected, the otolaryngologist may need to perform electromyography (EMG) to test the function of peripheral nerves innervating the laryngeal muscles. Fellowship-trained laryngologists may have the knowledge and skills to perform this procedure, otherwise the otolaryngologist can refer the patient to a neurologist. Laryngeal EMG can provide important information for the differential diagnosis of paresis/paralysis based on the electrical activity of laryngeal muscles (needles connected to electrical sensors are inserted into the muscles), and possibly provide information that can inform prognosis for recovery. However, it has been suggested that information obtained from laryngeal EMG is most useful within 6 months from problem onset, and assessments after that time frame may provide misleading information.[10]

7.4 Surgical Management Options

Once an accurate medical diagnosis is established, the otolaryngologist will recommend the appropriate options for treatment. Ultimately, the patient is responsible for choosing the option that best meets their goals for health, function, and quality of life. Depending on the specific diagnosis, these options can include (**1**) temporal observation of the problem and subsequent follow-up appointment with the otolaryngologist, (**2**) referral to the voice therapist for further evaluation and behavioral treatment of the disordered voice, (**3**) pharmaceutical

management, (**4**) surgical management, and/or (**5**) referral to another medical specialist. Kirtane et al have developed an algorithm (▶ Fig. 7.2) to assist the otolaryngologist in determining the appropriate course of referral when pathological tissue is detected during the examination.[8] A significant factor affecting the decision pathway in this model is the suspicion of laryngeal cancer. The algorithm leads to three possible pathways: (**1**) multidisciplinary management for confirmed malignancy, as described earlier; (**2**) observation, pharmaceutical and/or behavioral voice therapy with subsequent follow-up; or (**3**) surgery.

Some diagnoses will most effectively be treated with surgical procedures. Surgeries performed by otolaryngologists for the purposes of sustaining, restoring, or improving vocal function are known collectively as **phonosurgery**. Phonosurgical procedures can be organized into three general categories: (**1**) phonomicrosurgery via microlaryngoscopy, (**2**) laryngeal framework surgery, and (**3**) office-based phonosurgery (OBP).

Phonomicrosurgery is performed in an operating room using a microscope to visualize the vocal folds and surrounding regions (**microlaryngoscopy**). An example of the operational setup is illustrated in ▶ Fig. 7.3. The primary purpose of phonomicrosurgery is to *remove abnormal tissue*. Abnormal tissue may be malignant or benign, and surgery will be chosen when there is a strong possibility for cure or improved vocal function upon removal of the tissue. Microlaryngoscopy provides a detailed, close-up view of the vocal folds, pathological tissue, and surrounding structures as demonstrated in ▶ Fig. 7.4. Once an otolaryngologist has visualized the vocal folds, they can remove pathological tissue using different surgical options, which include the following:

- **Microflap dissection:** epithelial microflaps are a preferred technique for removing submucosal (below the outer epithelium) vocal fold lesions. This option is used for lesions such as cysts, polypoid degeneration, scar, and sometimes polyps.[11,12] Microflap procedures require microdissection of the epithelium to create a flap, which is then raised and moved laterally to expose the superficial layer of the lamina propria (SLLP). Lesions are then removed while maintaining as much integrity to the SLLP as possible, and the epithelial flap is then laid back in place to support the healing process. This technique preserves epithelium and minimizes disruption to the vocal fold cover to facilitate mucosal wave function after surgery.

- Another type of microsurgical dissection has been used in selected cases of spasmodic dysphonia. **Selective laryngeal adductor denervation–reinnervation surgery** has been used to improve vocal function in patients with Adductor Spasmodic Dysphonia (ADSD).[13] This surgery dissects the adductor branches of the recurrent laryngeal nerve innervating the thyroarytenoid (TA) and lateral cricoarytenoid (LCA) muscles. These branches are severed and treated in a manner which prevents their resprouting toward their former muscle targets.[14] The distal axons of the recurrent laryngeal nerve which enter the TA muscle (the tips which are left after the remainder of the nerve has been dissected away) are then reanimated by connection to the sternohyoid branch of the ansa cervicalis nerve (formed by portions of spinal nerves C1–C3).[15]

- **Mass resection with cold instruments:** lesions which occur on the epithelial surface or superior to the SLLP may be

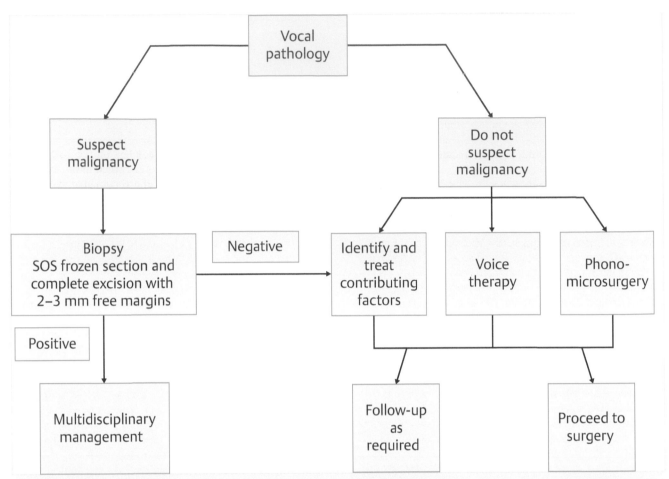

Fig. 7.2 Decision-making algorithm outlining the key steps in the management of vocal pathology. (From Bhattacharyya A. Laryngology: Otorhinolaryngology—Head and Neck Surgery Series. 1st ed. New York: Thieme Publishers, 2014.)

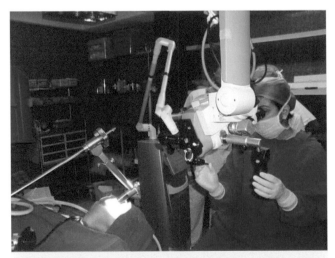

Fig. 7.3 Operation theatre setup for phonomicrosurgery. (From Bhattacharyya A. Laryngology: Otorhinolaryngology—Head and Neck Surgery Series. 1st ed. New York: Thieme Publishers, 2014.)

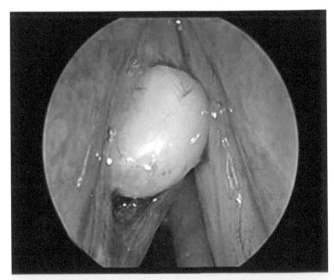

Fig. 7.4 Example of laryngeal visualization during microlaryngoscopy. Here a subepithelial cyst is being removed. (From Bhattacharyya A. Laryngology: Otorhinolaryngology—Head and Neck Surgery Series. 1st ed. New York: Thieme Publishers, 2014.)

resected using various microinstruments including scissors, forceps, and microdebriders. These devices are made of medical grade metals and are also referred to as "cold steel instruments." This option is used for lesions such as vocal fold nodules, polyps, premalignant lesions, cancer, granulomas, vascular lesions, and papilloma. These lesions are literally cut off from the vocal fold surface, which results in an obligatory injury to the vocal fold epithelium. Surgeons attempt to spare as much epithelium and deeper tissue as possible, and may further trim the epithelium to create a smooth vocal fold vibratory edge.[16]

- **Laser resection:** Some surgeons prefer to use laser technology to remove abnormal tissues from the vocal folds and surrounding laryngeal regions. These have been used in place of cold instruments or as the primary choice for a wide variety of impairments, including premalignant lesions and vocal fold cancers, papilloma, vascular lesions, hemorrhagic polyps, cysts, nodules, polypoid degeneration, and granulomas.[10] While CO_2-type lasers are the most commonly employed, other laser technologies are preferred by certain surgeons and include pulse dye lasers, yttrium aluminum garnet lasers, and potassium titanyl phosphate lasers.[10] Laser technology can be advantageous for lesion removal because the beams can be directed to small focal regions of tissue. They have also been preferred for removing vascular injuries and disrupting the vascular supply to papilloma.[17] Lasers produce heat, however, and the settings of the instrument must be monitored closely by the surgeon to prevent thermal injury to surrounding vocal fold regions.

Laryngeal framework surgery is designed to alter or improve vocal fold position, shape, and tension or to reconstruct the larynx. Another name for this type of phonosurgery is **laryngoplasty**. Laryngoplasty techniques manipulate the cartilaginous framework of the larynx to achieve targeted results. The laryngeal framework can be modified using various methods, which include (**1**) medialization laryngoplasty (ML) using implants, (**2**) arytenoid repositioning (arytenoid adduction or arytenopexy), or (**2**) cricothyroid repositioning (approximation or subluxation).

Laryngoplasty performed as an open procedure in the operating room (as opposed to injection laryngoplasty, described later) creates permanent changes to the laryngeal framework. Because the vagus nerve can spontaneously recover in many cases of vocal fold paresis/paralysis, it is recommended that many forms of laryngoplasty, and especially thyroplasty (see later), be delayed for at least 6 months post-onset, and possibly up to 1 year to allow for recovery to take place. As the patient is observed by the otolaryngologist over this time, behavioral voice therapy can be applied and has shown to be effective for rehabilitation of vocal function secondary to vocal fold paralysis, especially when the vocal fold is positioned closer to midline (as opposed to a more abducted position) and has some residual adductor movement.

- **Medialization laryngoplasty** was first described by Isshiki et al in the 1970s as "thyroplasty," and also goes by the name "medialization thyroplasty." Isshiki et al originally described four types of thyroplasty techniques which require augmentation of the thyroid cartilage to achieve different results:
  (**1**) **Type 1 thyroplasty**, designed to medialize the vocal fold;
  (**2**) **Type 2 thyroplasty**, designed to lateralize the vocal fold;

(**3**) **Type 3 thyroplasty**, designed to shorten and relax the vocal fold to lower fundamental frequency; and (4) **Type 4 thyroplasty**, designed to lengthen and tense the vocal fold to increase fundamental frequency.[18] Type 1, the most commonly employed thyroplasty technique, is used to correct glottal insufficiency secondary to vocal fold paralysis, presbylaryngis, and in some cases of bowing secondary to Parkinson's disease.[19,20]

ML (Type 1 thyroplasty) has evolved over time such that various materials can be used to medialize one or both immobile vocal folds. The procedure is performed in the operating room and requires the creation of a rectangular window in the thyroid cartilage at the level of the vocal fold (▶ Fig. 7.5 and ▶ Fig. 7.6). The window is marked and cut out using various instruments. Silicone or Silastic blocs can be placed through the window to press against the paralyzed vocal fold, pushing it toward midline (▶ Fig. 7.7). Sutures hold the implant in place, and the healing process will further secure the implant within the cartilaginous framework.

The anesthesia level provided to the patient can be adjusted so that they are able to follow directions and vocalize on instruction from the surgeon. This allows for testing the effectiveness of the implant placement prior to completion of the surgical procedure. The silicone bloc can be modified during the operation to create a customized shape which will be most effective for the patient. Some otolaryngologists prefer to use materials other than silicone blocks, with one popular option being GORE-TEX. This is a flexible material manufactured by W. L. Gore & Associates (*www.gore.com*), which allows the surgeon to modify the location of the GORE-TEX ribbon within the excised window of the thyroid to produce desired outcomes.

- **Arytenoid repositioning** techniques include arytenoid adduction and arytenopexy. **Arytenoid adduction**, when performed, is typically used in conjunction with ML *to facilitate improved closure of the posterior glottis*. The technique re-creates the physiological adduction properties of the LCA muscle, although it results in a fixed adducted vocal fold position.[10] The arytenoid is repositioned using monofilament sutures, which are routed through the muscular process and thyroid cartilage. Tension is applied to physically rotate the arytenoid such that the vocal process and vocal fold tissue moves medially, and the suture is fixed.[21]

Arytenopexy is a procedure designed to improve upon the arytenoid adduction technique. The arytenopexy procedure is accomplished by the surgeon manually manipulating the arytenoid cartilage on the surface of the cricoarytenoid joint (e.g., it is dislocated from the joint). A unique suture technique routes monofilament through the cricoid cartilage and muscular process of the arytenoid, tension is added, and then the suture is fixed. The orientation of the arytenopexy suture is thought to not only improve posterior glottal closure but also increase the length of the paralyzed vocal fold, improve the horizontal plane of the paralyzed vocal fold so that it is better aligned with the opposite fold, and also improve the vertical orientation of the targeted arytenoid cartilage (e.g., it sits higher and in a more vertical position, as opposed to a prolapsed position).[22,23] It is thought to accomplish this by re-creating the adductor action of the LCA, TA, and interarytenoid muscles in addition to the antagonistic abductor action of the posterior cricoarytenoid (PCA) muscle.[24]

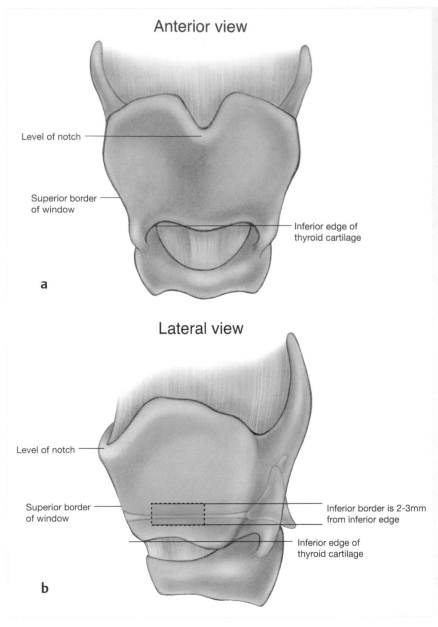

Anterior view

Level of notch

Superior border
of window

Inferior edge of
thyroid cartilage

a

Lateral view

Level of notch

Superior border
of window

Inferior border is 2-3mm
from inferior edge

Inferior edge of
thyroid cartilage

b

Fig. 7.5 (a,b) Landmarks of the thyroid cartilage showing location of the window within the thyroid cartilage created for medialization laryngoplasty (Type 1 thyroplasty). (From Fried M, Tan M. Clinical Laryngology. 1st ed. New York: Thieme Publishers, 2014.)

- **Cricothyroid repositioning** is used to adjust the relationship of the cricoid and thyroid cartilage to the remaining framework of the larynx. One procedure, **cricothyroid subluxation**, can be utilized in conjunction with ML or be combined with ML and arytenopexy as a triple laryngoplastic procedure.[25] Cricothyroid subluxation is designed to add length and tension to the paralyzed vocal fold, restoring substantial range to the patient's physiological frequency abilities. It is accomplished by the surgeon tying a suture to the inferior cornu of the thyroid cartilage on the affected side, routing the suture underneath and around the cricoid so that it returns to the inferior cornu, as illustrated in ▶ Fig. 7.8a,b. Tension is added which creates a traction on the thyroid and cricoid so that the distance between the anterior commissure of the thyroid and the vocal process of the arytenoid is increased. This has the effect of elongating and tensing the vocal fold, allowing for higher vibration frequencies.[25]

Thyroplasty Types 3 and 4 also alter the relationships of the cricoid and thyroid cartilages. **Type 3 thyroplasty** shortens the vocal fold (and thus "relaxes" the cover, lowering vibration frequency) by dissecting the thyroid cartilage in half, and then suturing the paralyzed side in a position that more closely approximates the arytenoid cartilage (e.g., this is an anteroposterior shortening on one side of the thyroid cartilage).[26] **Thyroplasty Type 4** results in a cricothyroid approximation, which has the effect of lengthening the vocal fold to add tension (increasing vibration frequency). Other procedures to reposition the cricoid and/or thyroid cartilage include **anterior commissure advancement** (to increase vibration frequency, such as for a male-to-female transgender) and **thyroid cartilage advancement** (also to increase vibration frequency).

Office-based phonosurgery allows the otolaryngologist to perform surgical procedures on an outpatient basis in the offices of their medical practice. There are numerous advantages to

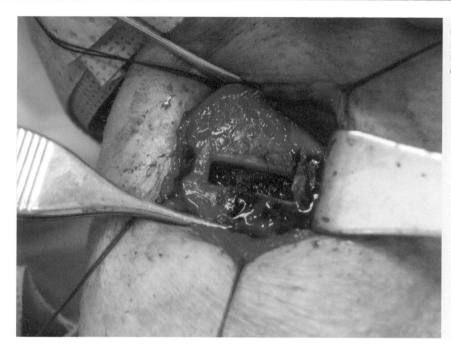

Fig. 7.6 Thyroplasty window excised from the left thyroid lamina. (From Fried M, Tan M. Clinical Laryngology. 1st ed. New York: Thieme Publishers, 2014.)

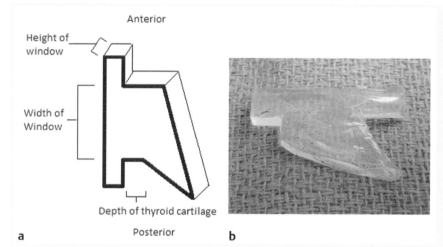

Anterior

Height of window

Width of Window

Depth of thyroid cartilage

Posterior

a

b

Fig. 7.7 Example of a Silastic implant used for medialization laryngoplasty (Type 1 thyroplasty). This bloc can be customized to the patient. (From Fried M, Tan M. Clinical Laryngology. 1st ed. New York: Thieme Publishers, 2014.)

OBP, among which include time, cost, and materials savings (which benefit both the patient and surgeon). OBP procedures utilize endoscopes to provide a visual guide for the surgeon. Endoscopes with side ports can also be used to thread surgical instrumentation through. OBP is performed using local anesthesia applied to the mucosa of the regions through which instruments will pass and tissue that will be worked on, which include the nasal cavity, oral cavity, and larynx. The patient is awake and positioned in an exam chair while the surgeon operates.

A large percentage of OBP procedures are **vocal fold injections** (see later) to correct glottal insufficiency.[27] **Lasers** can also be used in OBP for tissue resection in cases of papilloma, premalignant lesions, and dysplasia.[12] Some surgeons have also used OBP laser techniques for the removal of benign mid-membranous lesions, such as polyps.[28]

- **Injection augmentation** is used to correct glottal incompetence (via medialization) or to improve vocal fold shape, most notably the contour of the vibrating edge. Conditions for which

this may be appropriate include vocal fold paresis/paralysis, atrophy (such as in presbylaryngis), bowing, sulcus, scar, and tissue defects of the membranous vocal folds.[10] Various substances have been used to inject into the vocal folds, including autologous fat (fat harvested from the patient), collagen-based substances, and hyaluronic acid-based substances. ▶ Table 7.1 provides an overview of some of the more common injectable substances and their reported duration of action. As this table illustrates, most injectable substances are temporary because they are reabsorbed by the body. Because of this, they are often used in the acute stage after the onset of vocal fold paralysis. In these cases, injection augmentation can provide restoration of adequate vocal function while the patient waits for spontaneous recovery and/or voice therapy to facilitate the return of physiological adductor function. After 6 months to a year, if adequate function does not return, the patient may choose for a more permanent solution, such as medialization thyroplasty.

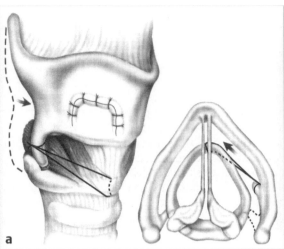
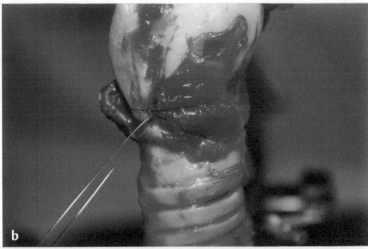

Fig. 7.8 (a) Cricothyroid subluxation: a suture is first tied to the inferior cornu of the thyroid cartilage and the routed under and around the anterior rim of the cricoid cartilage. **(b)** Cricothyroid subluxation: the suture is routed back to the inferior cornu and the appropriate tension is added. This orientation increases the distance between the vocal process of the arytenoid and anterior commissure of the thyroid, resulting in increased length and tension of the vocal fold. (From Dailey S, Verma S. Laryngeal Dissection and Surgery Guide. 1st ed. New York: Thieme Publishers, 2013.)

Table 7.1 Injectable materials

Material	Ease of use	Duration	Comments
Gelfoam	++	1–2 mo	Large bore needle
Collagen—bovine	+++	1–6 mo	Requires pretesting
Collagen—human	++	4–6 mo	Short shelf life, cross-infection risk
Collagen—human autologous	+	Variable	Perfect biocompatibility, requires skin harvest, expensive
Fat	+	6 + mo	GA, donor site, superficial or deep use
Radiesse voice gel	+++	2–3 mo	Inert, low allergy risk, supplied ready to use
Hyaluronic acid	+++	6–12 mo	Good rheology, superficial or deep use
Glycerine	++	2–6 wk	Safe, short-term use only
Calcium hydroxylapatite	+++	Up to 2 y	Bony defects, nonvibratory, overinjection required
Silicone—polydimethylsiloxane	+++	Permanent	Long-term studies awaited, extrusion
Teflon	+++	Permanent	Granuloma, extrusion, rarely used

Source: From Bhattacharyya A. Laryngology. 1st ed. New York: Thieme Publishers, 2013.

While injection augmentation can be performed under general anesthetic in the operating room, in the office setting this can be performed using a number of different approaches which place the injection needle into the vocal fold. **Peroral** approaches utilize a curved injection needle routed through the oral cavity, under visual guidance from a flexible nasoendoscope. **Percutaneous** approaches utilize needles inserted through the cricothyroid membrane (**transcricothyroid**), the thyrohyoid membrane (**transthyrohyoid**), or directly through the thyroid cartilage (**transthyroid**).[8] Injections designed to medialize the vocal fold tissue will typically be placed deep within the vocal fold layers, while injections designed to correct defects, such as scar or minor defects of the vocal fold edge, will be placed more superficially, closer to the epithelium.[10]

- **Botulinum toxin (BTX) injections** are used to treat spasmodic dysphonia and organic (essential) voice tremor. BTX is a neurotoxin which inhibits the release of acetylcholine into the neuromuscular junction, inhibiting muscle contraction. BTX injection levels are measured in "mouse units" (mu or U; mouse units are based on the amount of neurotoxin required to kill a mouse of a specific size). There are varied injection approaches which may be used to deliver the BTX into the vocal fold musculature, including an **EMG-guided percutaneous method**, an **endoscopically guided percutaneous method**, and an **endoscopically guided peroral method** which has been used for BTX injection into the false vocal folds.[8,10,29]

The specific dose level will be individualized for each patient over time, and is largely dependent on the patient's response. Typically, initial doses for ADSD are around 2.5 U, divided into two for bilateral injection.[8,10] Subsequent dose levels may be adjusted up or down. In ADSD, injections are targeted into the TA muscle and sometimes the LCA. Larger doses are used for ABSD, and are usually applied unilaterally during the initial stages of treatment. Of course, for ABSD, the target muscle is the PCA.

The overall response pattern to BTX injections for spasmodic dysphonia is generally similar, but the duration of the stages making up this pattern can vary widely across patients. One to 2 days postinjection, the patient will experience the onset of a breathy voice. The duration of this **breathy stage** might last anywhere from 3 or 4 days to upwards of a week (and in some patients longer).[8,30] Patients may also experience swallowing difficulties during this stage (e.g., potential laryngeal penetration and aspiration).[30]

Following the breathy stage, the patient will enter a stage of **acute voice recovery** lasting anywhere from a few days to a week. The voice will eventually reach a stage of **peak function**, which on average will last around 15 weeks (although this can vary widely, from 8 to 24 weeks in duration).[31] Toward the end of this stage, the voice will begin to **decline toward baseline**, and it will be during this period that the patient is seen for reinjection.

Response to BTX injections into the PCA for ABSD follows a similar pattern, although on average the stage of peak function takes longer to develop after injection, is shorter in duration, and the degree of voice improvement is not as great as in ADSD.[8,31] Dosage can be modified based on the temporal pattern of these stages, the degree of impairment during the breathy stage, and the degree of improvement during the peak function stage.

BTX has also been used for **voice tremor**, which can occur in isolation (e.g., organic voice tremor) or in conjunction with spasmodic dysphonia or Parkinson's disease.[31,32] Injections are typically bilateral into the LCA and TA, but in lower doses than used for spasmodic dysphonia. While BTX can improve vocal function in up to 80% of patients with tremor, many will experience a prolonged breathy stage and the degree of improvement may not be as significant as when BTX is used to treat ADSD or ABSD.[10,32]

7.5 Post–Phonomicrosurgical Voice Recovery

Phonomicrosurgical techniques which remove tissue from the surface or underneath the vocal fold epithelium have the potential to induce scar formation. As mentioned previously in this book, scar is fibrous, stiff, interferes with vibratory dynamics, and is currently irreversible. For this reason, it is common practice for the otolaryngologist and voice therapist to recommend a period of voice rest in the acute period after phonomicrosurgery. It is believed that preventing the vocal folds from vibrating during this period will facilitate normal wound healing and/or reepithelization, and inhibit the formation of scar. Among otolaryngologists and voice therapists, there is a great variety in preferences for postsurgical voice rest recommendations, including those who recommend no voice rest at all.[33]

For those recommending some degree of postsurgical voice rest, the specific regime may include **modified voice rest** (low intensity vocalization only during instances requiring the need for voicing) or **total voice rest** (no voicing at all). The most important period of healing likely occurs within the first 3 days after surgery, which has been verified in animal models of vocal fold wound healing.[34] This is often stressed to the patient as the most critical period of adherence to the voice rest recommendations. The rapid proliferation of cells into the vocal fold tissue tapers off after the first 3 days, and a more stable process of cellular activity ensues to complete the wound healing process.

After a period of modified or total voice rest, the patient will then be instructed to follow a tapered schedule of gradual voice use and structured voice building exercises, a period which might last 3 to 4 weeks or more before presurgical voice use patterns are reestablished.[35] The voice building techniques employed for professional voice users should be customized to their abilities and performance needs. This process of voice building most commonly occurs 1 week after surgery. Across a large section of otolaryngology practices, the average length of modified or total voice rest was reported as 7 days.[33] A recent randomized clinical trial compared patients undergoing 5 days of rest to those undergoing 10 days of rest, finding that the only significant difference in vocal function between the two groups was in measures of maximum phonation time (longer in those resting for 10 days).[36]

Ossoff and Cleveland have published guidelines on a postoperative voice treatment plan tailored to singers.[37] This plan recommends a four-stage progressive hierarchy of voice building over a 3-month period. In **stage 1**, the patient adheres to total voice rest. In **stage 2**, the patient begins to gradually increase the amount of time they vocalize in the morning and in the afternoon over a 4-week period. They will also work with the voice therapist during this stage. In **stage 3**, from week 4 to 12, the patient will work with the voice therapist and singing voice professional on healthy and balanced speaking and singing technique. In **stage 4**, which begins after week 12, the singer is able to resume his or her rehearsal and performance schedule, though care is taken to utilize the voice therapy and singing techniques learned in the previous stages. The patient will gradually increase the number of minutes and hours they vocalize each day. Details of the recommended voice building plan are given in ▶ Table 7.2, where voice loads (in minutes) represent the maximum recommended amount of voice use.

Table 7.2 Example of a voice rest and recovery schedule postphonosurgery

Time period	AM	PM
One wk postsurgery	Total rest	Total rest
Day of post-op visit	5 min	5 min
2nd day post-op visit	10 min	10 min
3rd day post-op visit	20 min	20 min
4th day post-op visit	45 min	45 min
5th day post-op visit	1 h	1 h
6th day post-op visit	2–4 h throughout the day	
7th day post-op visit	4–6 h throughout the day	
8th day onward	Add half hour each day	

Please note that none of the aforementioned guidelines mention *whispering*. **Whispered voice is to be avoided since it will inevitably lead to the development of hyperfunctional behaviors, excessive extralaryngeal muscle tension, and strain in the attempt to compensate for this ineffective form of communication.** In addition, the inefficient and ineffective consequences of whispering may become habituated by the patient and contribute to the maintenance of dysphonia.

7.6 Pharmaceutical Management

In addition to surgery, otolaryngologists can treat voice disorders by prescribing medications. Patients may also choose to treat symptoms and causes of voice problems using self-administered over-the-counter (OTC) medicines. There are many medical conditions associated with voice problems that respond favorably to pharmaceutical treatment. At the same time, many pharmaceutical medications can have adverse effects on the subsystems of voice, and it is important that the voice care team be familiar with both positive and negative effects of medications on voice. Sataloff et al have suggested that most medications will have some effect on laryngeal function, though in most cases the impact is not substantial.[38] However, this also means that some medicines can have a significant impact on laryngeal function, and it is these classes of drugs which will be the focus for the remainder of this section.

▶ Table 7.3 lists major groups of drugs based on their biological actions. Many of these are available in prescription strength (acquired through a written prescription from a physician) or in lower strength formulas available in OTC forms. A number of these medications will have benefits for patients with voice disorders which far outweigh possible negative side effects. However, some can produce systemic changes which can put the tissue of the vocal folds at risk for irritation and/or trauma, potentially causing a voice problem or making an existing problem more severe. SLPs should be familiar with the more commonly encountered drug groups prescribed or self-administered in treatment-seeking populations, and the risk of these medications causing adverse laryngeal reactions. Copious web-based resources are available to quickly check on the side-effects of administered medications reported by patients during the history portion of the voice diagnostic.

7.6.1 Medications with Potential Adverse Laryngeal Effects

Medications That Can Dry Mucosa

In healthy laryngeal function, the vocal fold tissues are coated with a blanket of thin mucous. This mucous serves to lubricate the vocal folds and, in theory, reduce vibratory friction and thus prevent irritation, edema, and inflammation. In Chapter 8, we will describe appropriate hydration levels as a target within a vocal hygiene program. Therefore, the clinician and patient must consider medications which could disrupt systemic hydration levels. Unfortunately, there exists a large number of medications across different drug classes which can dry mucosa.

Table 7.3 Medications commonly prescribed or self-administered (over-the-counter) in treatment-seeking populations with voice disorders

Drug Group	Purpose / Actions	Examples
Antihistamine	Reduces systemic allergic reactions (edema, inflammation, itching) by blocking histamine release from histamine-1 receptors	Fexofenadine (Allegra); diphenhydramine (Benadryl); Desloratadine (Clarinex)
Anti-inflammatory (non-steroid)	Reduces inflammation by blocking cyclooxygenase. Non-steroid anti-inflammatories may also result in pain relief and fever reduction	Ibuprofen (Advil, Motrin); Naproxen (Aleve)
Antibiotic	Kills or controls bacterial infections by destroying bacterial cells	Amoxicillin; Doxycycline; Ciprofloxacin
Antireflux	Inhibits gastroesophageal and laryngopharyngeal reflux through various mechanisms of action, including antacids, H2 antagonists, and proton pump inhibitors, among others	Aluminum/Magnesium/Simethicone (Mylanta); Esomeprazole (Nexium); Omeprazole (Prilosec); Ranitidine, Lansoprazole (Prevacid)
Antitremor	Inhibits involuntary tremor in skeletal muscles.	Beta-blockers (Propranolol); antiseizure (Primidone)
Antitussive	Also known as cough suppressants. Thought to depress activity in the brainstem cough centers to reduce cough frequency	Dextromethorphan; Codeine
Cholinesterase inhibitor	Facilitates acetylcholine action at the neuromuscular junction by inhibiting the enzyme responsible for the reuptake of acetylcholine. Used for myasthenia gravis	Pyridostigmine (Mestinon)
Decongestant	Reduces swelling in tissues—for voice, this can target the nasal cavities to improve breathing and resonance	Oxymetazoline (Afrin); Phenylephrine (Sudafed); Pseudoephedrine
Expectorant	Increases and thins airway secretions, loosening mucous and making it easier to cough it out of the airways	Guaifenesin (Mucinex, Robitussin)
Steroids	Controls inflammation in the lower airway (e.g., for asthma) and upper airway (e.g., vocal folds, nasal cavity)	Prednisone; Prednisolone; Mometasone (Nasonex); Fluticasone (Flonase; Advair; Flovent); Budesonide (Pulmicort)

Some of the more commonly administered medications which can potentially dry the vocal fold mucosa include

- Antihistamines.
- Antihypertensive medications (e.g., beta-blockers, angiotensin-converting enzyme inhibitors).
- Antipsychotic medications (e.g., Quetiapine [Seroquel], Asenapine [Saphris]).
- Antidepressants (e.g., Bupropion [Wellbutrin], Fluoxetine [Prozac]).
- Antibiotics.
- Antireflux medications (H2 blockers and proton pump inhibitors—not all are associated with dryness, but the clinician and patient should check).
- Central nervous system stimulants (e.g., Adderall, Focalin).
- Diuretics (e.g., Furosemide [Lasix]).
- Opioid pain medications (e.g., Oxycodone [OxyContin, Percocet], Hydrocodone [Lortab]).

Medications That Can Cause Cough

Cough is necessary to clear adverse stimuli from the lower airway, but may also result in phonotrauma. Some medications are administered specifically to control cough, but other medications used to treat certain medical conditions can produce cough as a side effect. Some of these include

- Angiotensin-converting enzyme inhibitors.
- Steroid-based inhalers (only some with reported side effect of cough, e.g., Fluticasone; others may actually be used to help treat cough).
- Antidepressants (e.g., Citalopram, Escitalopram [Lexapro]).

Medications That Can Alter Laryngeal Tissue (e.g., Edema, Infection, Atrophy)

Some medications can cause acute or chronic changes in the vocal fold tissue. Two examples of these changes are edema and vocal fold atrophy. Cessation of these medicines often results in reversal of the local effects on the vocal fold tissues. Examples of medications with side effects of edema or atrophy include

- Inhaled corticosteroids (some have been associated with hoarseness thought to be related to tissue irritation, candidiasis, and/or vocal fold atrophy. Some of these changes may be due to the devices used to administer the steroid).
- Antibiotics (associated with laryngeal candidiasis).

7.7 Conclusion

This chapter has reviewed the essential role and practices of the laryngologist in both the diagnosis and treatment of voice disorders. Because the speech pathologist (as a behavioral voice therapist) works collaboratively with the laryngologist as part of the voice team, it is important that he or she has knowledge of the various surgical and pharmaceutical options which may be used as primary treatment methods or in combination with the behavioral voice therapy methods that will be described in the subsequent chapter.

Case Study

Part 1

Mr. Nunez is a 65-year-old man who recently (3 weeks ago) underwent cardiac surgery to repair a heart valve. After a 5.5-hour surgery, he awoke with a hoarse voice which he described as "a whisper." After 2 weeks with minimal improvement, he was referred to you by his general otolaryngologist. During the voice evaluation, Mr. Nunez indicated that he had never experienced voice problems prior to the onset of the current issue, and that up until the time of surgery he sung tenor in his church choir—evidence that he had a strong voice. He related that he is unable to produce sustained voice for a substantial amount of time, he is unable to produce high pitched sounds, and he describes his voice as very weak in volume. He also indicated that he hears a "sound" when he breathes in.

1. Based on the limited information provided above, is your clinical hypothesis leading you to think this impairment is functional, organic, or neurological in etiology? Why?
2. Identify three clinical measurements (e.g., diagnostic measures which may or may not require instrumentation) which might provide valuable information to help in differential diagnosis and better characterize the impairment—what do you expect these measures to show (i.e., identify a measure and then indicate what you expect this patient's data to be).
3. Based on the information above, what would you expect to see when performing video stroboscopy on this patient?

Part 2

Laryngeal videostroboscopy revealed a left unilateral vocal fold paralysis/paresis (some residual adductor and abductor movements of the vocal fold), with the vocal fold positioned in an intermediate position at rest. The left vocal fold appeared thinner than the right. During attempted phonation, there was a consistent elliptical glottal gap. When prompted to produce a very loud voice, he was able to achieve near-complete adduction and sustained phonation for 4 seconds. During maximal loudness attempts, the right vocal fold appeared to cross the midline as it approximated the left vocal fold.

  Watch the following video:
  http://voicedoctor.net/videos/laryngology-vocal-cord-paralysis

1. List two possible reasons why this patient developed unilateral vocal fold paralysis during surgery.
2. What explains why the left vocal fold is thinner than the right?
3. Other than surgery, what two other etiologies that can cause vocal fold paralysis?

Part 3

Read the following article and answer the questions:
  Young VN, Smith LJ, Rosen C. Voice outcome following acute unilateral vocal fold paralysis. Ann Otol Rhinol Laryngol 2013;122(3):197–204.

1. Based on ▶ Table 7.1, is it likely that patients experiencing vocal fold paralysis due to surgical procedures other than thyroidectomy will have a return of vocal fold motion? Explain your answer.

2. What are two *positive* prognostic indicators for Mrs. Nunez, based on the information in Part 2?
3. Why would temporary vocal fold injections for vocal fold paralysis be a beneficial option for a patient?

7.8 Review Questions

1. What two health care professionals typically serve as the primary members of a voice care team?
   a) Otolaryngologist and singing voice teacher.
   b) Otolaryngologist and speech–language pathologist.
   c) Speech–language pathologist and neurologist.
   d) Speech–language pathologist and singing voice teacher.
   e) None of the above.
2. An otolaryngologist who completes a postresidency specialty training focusing on voice and swallowing impairments is referred to as what title?
   a) Surgeon.
   b) Ear, nose, and throat doctor.
   c) Laryngologist.
   d) Physician.
   e) None of the above.
3. Which of the following best matches the *"golden rule of voice therapy"*?
   a) A patient must be evaluated by an otolaryngologist before initiating voice therapy.
   b) A patient must be evaluated by a speech–language pathologist before he or she is referred to the otolaryngologist.
   c) A patient must be evaluated by an otolaryngologist before he or she is evaluated by the speech–language pathologist.
   d) A patient must receive at least six sessions of voice therapy for it to be effective.
4. Which of the following surgical techniques utilizes a laryngoscope which is connected to a microscope within in the operative room?
   a) Laryngectomy.
   b) Phonomicrosurgery.
   c) Laryngeal framework surgery.
   d) Office-based phonosurgery.
   e) All of the above.
5. Which surgical procedure raises the epithelium to expose the lamina propria, from which lesions will be removed?
   a) Injection augmentation.
   b) Type 3 thyroplasty.
   c) Arytenopexy.
   d) Microflap dissection.
   e) None of the above.
6. Which of the following best describes the purpose of Type 1 thyroplasty?
   a) To elongate a vocal fold.
   b) To shorten a vocal fold.
   c) To medialize a vocal fold.
   d) To lateralize a vocal fold.
7. Which of the following vocal fold lesions would be an appropriate choice to use laser surgery for removal?
   a) Glottic cancer and papilloma.
   b) Vocal fold cysts.

c) Vocal fold nodules and any type of polyp.
   d) None of the above.
   e) All of the above.
8. Which of the following is *not* an approach for injection augmentation?
   a) Peroral.
   b) Transcricothyroid.
   c) Transthyrohyoid.
   d) Transepiglottis.
   e) Percutaneous.
9. Which category of phonosurgery would arytenoid adduction belong to?
   a) Phonomicrosurgery.
   b) Laryngeal framework surgery.
   c) Office-based phonosurgery.
   d) Laser resection.
   e) None of the above.
10. What is a major reason why otolaryngologists and voice therapists recommend some form of voice rest after phonosurgery?
    a) To prevent the formation of a cyst.
    b) To prevent the formation of polyps.
    c) To prevent the formation of nodules.
    d) To prevent the formation of scar.
    e) None of the above.
11. Which of the following medications have been associated with potential drying of the vocal fold mucosa?
    a) Antihistamines.
    b) Steroid-based inhalers.
    c) Aspirin.
    d) Vitamin C.
    e) All of the above.
12. Which of the following medications have been associated with coughing?
    a) Steroid-based inhalers.
    b) Angiotensin-converting enzyme inhibitors.
    c) Some antidepressants.
    d) None of the above.
    e) All of the above.

7.9 Answers and Explanations

1. Correct: Otolaryngologist and speech–language pathologist (**b**).
   (**b**) The primary members of the voice care team in most situations will be the voice therapist and otolaryngologist. Their respective knowledge and skills related to anatomy, physiology, and impairment complement each other. (**a, c, d**) Although the otolaryngologist and the speech–language pathologist are typically the primary members of a voice team, additional members may include but are not be limited to neurologists, gastroenterologists, singing voice teachers, psychologists, pulmonologists, allergy specialists, and endocrinologists.
2. Correct: Laryngologist (**c**).
   (**c**) Otolaryngologists who specialize in laryngeal disorders affecting voice, swallowing, and airway are known in the United States as "laryngologists." There is no formal degree or credential which certifies one as a laryngologist, although many complete a postresidency laryngology fellowship where they learn the specialty under the mentorship of an experienced physician (who will also be a laryngologist). (**a**) The title "Surgeon"

is used for any medical doctor who is trained and qualified to perform surgeries. Not all doctors are surgeons. (**b**) The title "ear, nose, and throat" doctor (ENT) is simply another name for "otolaryngologist." (**d**) The title "Physician" refers to someone who is qualified to practice medicine—it is a synonym of "doctor."

3. Correct: A patient must be evaluated by an otolaryngologist before initiating voice therapy (**a**).

   (**a**) The otolaryngologist possesses advanced knowledge of systems and structures and are the only medical/health professional qualified to diagnose specific organic vocal fold impairments. Before an SLP initiates a voice treatment plan, the medical diagnosis must be established or ruled out by the otolaryngologist. (**a, b**) A patient can be evaluated by an SLP at any time—either before or after they are seen by an otolaryngologist. (**d**) The duration of voice therapy is completely dependent on the patient's response. Some voice problems can be resolved in one therapy session. Others can take multiple sessions over many months.

4. Correct: Phonomicrosurgery (**b**).

   (**b**) Phonomicrosurgery is performed in an operating room using a microscope to visualize the vocal folds and surrounding regions (microlaryngoscopy). (**a**) Laryngectomy is an "open procedure," where they cut through the external skin. A microscope is not needed. (**c**) Laryngeal framework surgery is performed in the operative room, and also involves "open" approaches where incisions are made through the external skin. (**d**) Office-based phonosurgery is not performed in the operating room and does not utilize a microscope.

5. Correct: Microflap dissection (**d**).

   (**d**) Microflap dissection is a type of phonosurgery where epithelial microflaps are raised and separated from the lamina propria, from which lesions such as cysts are removed. This is the preferred technique for removing submucosal (below the outer epithelium) vocal fold lesions. (**a**) Injection augmentation involves the injection of substances into the vocal folds to medialize or correct abnormalities. (**b**) Type 3 thyroplasty uses an open approach to surgery where the vocal fold is shortened, or "relaxed." (**c**) Arytenopexy is a type of surgical procedure which repositions the arytenoid cartilage to better align it when another medialization procedure is performed.

6. Correct: To medialize a vocal fold (**c**).

   (**c**) Type 1 thyroplasty involves the creation of window in the thyroid cartilage, through which material is placed to medialize a vocal fold. (**a, b, d**) Type 4 thyroplasty elongates a vocal fold. Type 3 thyroplasty shortens a vocal fold. Type 2 thyroplasty lateralizes a vocal fold.

7. Correct: Glottic cancer and papilloma (**a**).

   (**a**) Lasers have been used in place of cold instruments or as the primary choice for a wide variety of impairments, including premalignant lesions and vocal fold cancers, papilloma, vascular lesions, hemorrhagic polyps, cysts, nodules, polypoid degeneration, and granulomas. (**b, c**) Lesions which occur on the epithelial surface, such as nodules, or superior to the SLLP, such as polyps, may be resected using various

microinstruments including scissors, forceps, and microdebriders. Cysts are typically removed using microlaryngoscopic Microflap dissection.

8. Correct: Transepiglottis (**d**).

   (**d**) Injections for vocal fold augmentation must be directed toward the vocal folds. The epiglottis lies superior to the vocal folds, which would not make it a logical choice through which to place the needle. (**a, b, c, e**) Vocal fold augmentation injections are placed using a peroral or percutaneous approaches. The percutaneous approach might utilize a transcricothyroid, transthyrohyoid, or transthyroid location to place the needed.

9. Correct: Laryngeal framework surgery (**b**).

   (**b**) Laryngeal framework surgery is designed to alter or improve vocal fold position, shape, and tension or to reconstruct the larynx. The laryngeal framework can be modified using various methods, which include (**1**) medialization laryngoplasty using implants, (**2**) arytenoid repositioning (arytenoid adduction or arytenopexy), or (**3**) cricothyroid repositioning (approximation or subluxation). (**a**) Phonomicrosurgery is performed in an operating room using a microscope to visualize the vocal folds and surrounding regions (microlaryngoscopy). (**c, d**) Office-based phonosurgery is performed in a physician's office and can include injection augmentation or injections of botulinum toxin.

10. Correct: To prevent the formation of scar (**d**).

    (**d**) Phonomicrosurgical techniques which remove tissue from the surface or underneath the vocal fold epithelium have the potential to induce scar formation. Scar is fibrous, stiff, interferes with vibratory dynamics, and is currently irreversible. (**a**) Cysts are caused by blocked mucous gland ducts or epithelial entrapment and are often related to heavy voice use, but are not caused by phonosurgery. (**b**) Polyps are caused by phonotrauma, not phonosurgery. (**c**) Vocal fold nodules are caused by phonotrauma, not phonosurgery.

11. Correct: Antihistamines (**a**).

    (**a**) Antihistamines work by histamine receptors. One side effect is mucosal drying. (**b**) Steroid-based inhalers have been associated with laryngeal irritation and tissue atrophy, but not drying. (**c**) Aspirin is an analgesic and has not been associated with vocal fold drying. (**d**) Vitamin C is a supplement which is thought to support the immune system, but has not been associated with laryngeal drying.

12. Correct: All of the above (**e**).

    (**e**) Steroid-based inhalers, angiotensin-converting enzyme inhibitors, and antidepressants have all been associated with triggering abnormal cough. (**a, b, c, d**) Steroid-based inhalers, angiotensin-converting enzyme inhibitors, and antidepressants have all been associated with triggering abnormal cough.

References

[1] Jacobson BH, Johnson A, Grywalski C, et al. The Voice Handicap Index (VHI): development and validation. Am J Sp Lang Path. 1997; 6:66–70

[2] Cohen SM, Jacobson BH, Garrett CG, et al. Creation and validation of the Singing Voice Handicap Index. Ann Otol Rhinol Laryngol. 2007; 116(6):402–406

[3] Hogikyan ND, Sethuraman G. Validation of an instrument to measure voice-related quality of life (V-RQOL). J Voice. 1999; 13(4):557–569

[4] Deary IJ, Wilson JA, Carding PN, MacKenzie K. VoiSS: a patient-derived Voice Symptom Scale. J Psychosom Res. 2003; 54(5):483–489

[5] Bach KK, Belafsky PC, Wasylik K, Postma GN, Koufman JA. Validity and reliability of the glottal function index. Arch Otolaryngol Head Neck Surg. 2005; 131(11):961–964

[6] Ma EP, Yiu EM. Voice activity and participation profile: assessing the impact of voice disorders on daily activities. J Speech Lang Hear Res. 2001; 44(3):511–524

[7] Belafsky PC, Postma GN, Koufman JA. Validity and reliability of the reflux symptom index (RSI). J Voice. 2002; 16(2):274–277

[8] Kirtane MV, de Souza CE, Bhattacharyya AK, Nerurkar NK. Laryngology. New York: Thieme Medical Publishers; 2014

[9] Hari Kumar KV, Garg A, Ajai Chandra NS, Singh SP, Datta R. Voice and endocrinology. Indian J Endocrinol Metab. 2016; 20(5):590–594

[10] Rosen CA, Simpson CB. Operative Techniques in Laryngology. Berlin: Springer-Verlag; 2008

[11] Courey MS, Gardner GM, Stone RE, Ossoff RH. Endoscopic vocal fold microflap: a three-year experience. Ann Otol Rhinol Laryngol. 1995; 104(4, Pt 1):267–273

[12] Halum SL, Moberly AC. Patient tolerance of the flexible CO2 laser for office-based laryngeal surgery. J Voice. 2010; 24(6):750–754

[13] Chhetri DK, Mendelsohn AH, Blumin JH, Berke GS. Long-term follow-up results of selective laryngeal adductor denervation-reinnervation surgery for adductor spasmodic dysphonia. Laryngoscope. 2006; 116(4):635–642

[14] DeConde AS, Long JL, Armin BB, Berke GS. Functional reinnervation of vocal folds after selective laryngeal adductor denervation-reinnervation surgery for spasmodic dysphonia. J Voice. 2012; 26(5):602–603

[15] Blumin JH, Berke GS. Spasmodic dysphonia. In: Merati AL, Bielamowicz SA, eds. Textbook of Voice Disorders. San Diego, CA: Plural Publishing; 2007

[16] Jamal N, Berke GS. Principles of phonosurgery. In Fried MP, Tan M, eds. Clinical Laryngology. New York: Thieme Medical Publishers; 2015

[17] Burns JA, Zeitels SM, Akst LM, Broadhurst MS, Hillman RE, Anderson R. 532 nm pulsed potassium-titanyl-phosphate laser treatment of laryngeal papillomatosis under general anesthesia. Laryngoscope. 2007; 117(8):1500–1504

[18] Isshiki N, Morita H, Okamura H, Hiramoto M. Thyroplasty as a new phonosurgical technique. Acta Otolaryngol. 1974; 78(5–6):451–457

[19] Isshiki N. Mechanical and dynamic aspects of voice production as related to voice therapy and phonosurgery. J Voice. 1998; 12(2):125–137

[20] Roubeau B, Bruel M, de Crouy Chanel O, Périé S. Reduction of Parkinson's-related dysphonia by thyroplasty. Eur Ann Otorhinolaryngol Head Neck Dis. 2016; 133(6):437–439

[21] Fried MP, Tan M. Clinical Laryngology: The Essentials. New York: Thieme Medical Publishers; 2014

[22] Hochman II, Zeitels SM. Phonomicrosurgical management of vocal fold polyps: the subepithelial microflap resection technique. J Voice. 2000; 14(1):112–118

[23] Zeitels SM, Hochman I, Hillman RE. Adduction arytenopexy: a new procedure for paralytic dysphonia with implications for implant medialization. Ann Otol Rhinol Laryngol Suppl. 1998; 173:2–24

[24] Zeitels SM. Adduction arytenopexy and cricothyroid subluxation. In: Dailey SH, Verma S, eds. Laryngeal Dissection and Surgery Guide. New York: Thieme Medical Publishers; 2013

[25] Zeitels SM. New procedures for paralytic dysphonia: adduction arytenopexy, Goretex medialization laryngoplasty, and cricothyroid subluxation. Otolaryngol Clin North Am. 2000; 33(4):841–854

[26] Isshiki N. Progress in laryngeal framework surgery. Acta Otolaryngol. 2000; 120(2):120–127

[27] Verma SP, Dailey SH. Overcoming nasal discomfort–a novel method for office-based laser surgery. Laryngoscope. 2011; 121(11):2396–2398

[28] Kim HT, Auo HJ. Office-based 585 nm pulsed dye laser treatment for vocal polyps. Acta Otolaryngol. 2008; 128(9):1043–1047

[29] Rosen CA, Murry T. Botox for hyperadduction of the false vocal folds: a case report. J Voice. 1999; 13(2):234–239

[30] Kim JW, Park JH, Park KN, Lee SW. Treatment efficacy of electromyography versus fiberscopy-guided botulinum toxin injection in adductor spasmodic dysphonia patients: a prospective comparative study. Sci World J. 2014; 2014:327928

[31] Blitzer A, Brin MF, Stewart CF. Botulinum toxin management of spasmodic dysphonia (laryngeal dystonia): a 12-year experience in more than 900 patients. Laryngoscope. 1998; 108(10):1435–1441

[32] Sulica L, Louis E. Essential voice tremor. In: Merati AL, Bielamowicz SA, eds. Textbook of Voice Disorders. San Diego, CA: Plural Publishing; 2007

[33] Behrman A, Sulica L. Voice rest after microlaryngoscopy: current opinion and practice. Laryngoscope. 2003; 113(12):2182–2186

[34] Mitchell JR, Kojima T, Wu H, Garrett CG, Rousseau B. Biochemical basis of vocal fold mobilization after microflap surgery in a rabbit model. Laryngoscope. 2014; 124(2):487–493

[35] Bhattacharyya AK, Nerurkar NK, Ifeacho SN. Principles of Phonomicrosurgery. In: Kirtane MV, de Souza CE, Bhattacharyya AK, Nerurkar NK, eds. Laryngology. New York: Thieme Medical Publishers; 2014

[36] Kiagiadaki D, Remacle M, Lawson G, Bachy V, Van der Vorst S. The effect of voice rest on the outcome of phonosurgery for benign laryngeal lesions: preliminary results of a prospective randomized study. Ann Otol Rhinol Laryngol. 2015; 124(5):407–412

[37] Ossoff RH, Cleveland TF. Postoperative voice care of the singer. In: Benninger MS, Murry T, Johns MJ, eds. The Performer's Voice. San Diego, CA: Plural Publishing; 2015

[38] Sataloff RT, Lawrence VL, Hawkshaw MJ, Rosen DC. Medications and their effects on voice. In: Benninger MS, Jacobson BH, Johnson, AF, eds. Vocal Arts Medicine: The Care and Prevention of Professional Voice Disorders. New York: Thieme Medical Publishers; 1994

Suggested Reading

[1] Behrman A, Sulica L. Voice rest after microlaryngoscopy: current opinion and practice. Laryngoscope. 2003; 113(12):2182–2186

[2] Kirtane MV, de Souza CE, Bhattacharyya AK, Nerurkar NK. Laryngology. New York: Thieme Medical Publishers; 2014

[3] Dailey SH, Verma S. Laryngeal Dissection and Surgery Guide. New York: Thieme Medical Publishers; 2013

[4] In Fried MP, Tan M. Clinical Laryngology. New York: Thieme Medical Publishers; 2015

8 Voice Treatment: Orientations, Framework, and Interventions

Summary

This chapter introduces the reader to classifications and orientations for different voice treatment approaches. Recent literature is utilized to present a new organizational framework into which different voice treatment approaches can be conceptualized. Examples of long-term and short-term goals that align with this organizational framework and which guide the treatment process are provided. Finally, a description of the rationale, characteristics, and processes of indirect and direct interventions for voice disorders are detailed. Direct treatments are organized into approaches which address kinetic hyperfunction and those which address kinetic hypofunction. The major focus of the chapter centers on treatments which have been supported with scientific evidence. Where possible, the framework and steps of specific interventions are detailed.

Keywords: vocologist, voice therapy, dysphonia, vocal function exercises, stretch-and-flow, resonant voice therapy

8.1 Learning Objectives

At the end of this chapter, learners will be able to
- Differentiate the goals of voice habilitation and rehabilitation.
- Describe the characteristics of measureable long-term and short-term goals specific to voice treatment.
- Compare and contrast treatments in different domains of the voice treatment taxonomic model.
- Describe the factors influencing the choice of treatment approach.
- Describe the frameworks and list the procedural steps for indirect voice treatment approaches.
- Compare and contrast treatments utilized for vocal hyperfunction and vocal hypofunction.
- Identify the rationale for selecting one treatment approach over another.
- Describe the frameworks and list the procedural steps for multiple voice treatment approaches.
- Describe age-related issues associated with treating children compared to adults.
- Identify the special needs of professional voice users which might impact treatment plans.

8.2 Introduction

Habilitation is the processes of helping an individual with an impairment or limitation realize their maximum potential—its purpose is to enable and enhance. **Rehabilitation** is the process of helping an individual recover function after an injury or illness—its purpose is to repair and restore. Speech–language pathologists (SLPs) who administer voice treatments are involved in both voice habilitation (e.g., facilitating skills to produce a desired voice in a healthy way for professional or performance voice needs) and voice rehabilitation (e.g., restoring phonation abilities

secondary to vocal fold paralysis). The SLP who provides voice therapy is often involved in both habilitation and rehabilitation simultaneously. That is, while we attempt to restore vocal function secondary to disorder or disease, we must recognize that, depending on factors such as the severity of the disorder, we may never be able to restore a typical or "normal" voice. Instead, we focus on the patient achieving their maximum potential to produce the best voice possible. SLPs who practice this subspecialty (voice impairments) are sometimes referred to as **vocologists** ("vocology" refers to the science and practice of voice habilitation) **or voice therapists**. A smaller subset of voice therapists also have a background in singing voice pedagogy and are able to work with singers on not only voice production and vocal health but also *singing technique*, and are referred to as **singing voice specialists**.

The profession of SLP has provided services to patients with vocal impairments since it was first officially organized. Over time, our knowledge of vocal anatomy and physiology, the interaction of voice production and the psychological state of the patient, and the effectiveness of specific treatments has advanced our understanding of how the larynx responds to various habilitation and rehabilitation processes. Today voice therapists base treatment selection on (**1**) the patient's needs and goals, (**2**) the underlying impaired physiology, (**3**) the research evidence that supports a specific treatment, and (**4**) the competency (knowledge and skill) of the clinician. Selected treatments then rehabilitate or habilitate vocal function by targeting the underlying physiological impairments and/or improving physiological function to advance the patient's ability to vocalize or communicate via phonation.

In this chapter, we will use rehabilitation terminology with specific meanings that you should commit to memory to best understand the material. The words "rehabilitation," "treatment," and "therapy" have been used in different contexts by different authorities. For the purposes of this book, we will define these terms as follows:
- **Voice habilitation/rehabilitation**—the *process* of enhancing or restoring vocal abilities to a desirable (habilitation) or previous (rehabilitation) level of function. This process is conducted via patient and clinician collaboration (including, where necessary, affiliated health professionals) and typically includes pedagogy (education), counseling, and the administration of one or more specific voice treatments through extrinsic or intrinsic delivery methods. We will use the word "rehabilitation" throughout the remainder of this chapter to refer to both habilitation and rehabilitation processes.
- **Voice therapy**—synonymous with voice rehabilitation.
- **Voice treatment**—a specific method (technique) of care provided to a patient, focused on one or more of the following voice production domains: musculoskeletal, respiratory, vocal function, auditory, or somatosensory. Alternatively, a voice treatment can be administered indirectly in the context of pedagogy, counseling, or vocal hygiene treatments. Voice treatments, when used to achieve clinical goals, will include a specified framework, duration, frequency, and expected level of outcome.

- **Voice tool**—synonymous with voice treatment.
- **Voice treatment program**—an organized group of treatments, typically structured in sequence with each other, and administered using one or more delivery methods. Traditionally, these have been referred to as "eclectic voice therapy."
- **Voice disorder**—The presence of a deviation in voice quality, pitch, loudness, flexibility, and/or stamina from expectations related to factors such as age, sex, body type, speaking community, communication needs, and/or performance needs.
- **Vocal impairment**—synonymous with voice disorder.

When we administer a treatment as part of the rehabilitation process, we do so with the goal of alleviating an impairment to reduce or eliminate a handicap or disability. The selection of specific treatments is dependent on the diagnosis and the associated etiology. This means that **treatment decisions should only be determined after (accurate) diagnosis has been prescribed and a firm hypothesis regarding the underlying physiological impairment has been determined.** The rationale for this is clear: **certain voice treatments are inappropriate, and can be contraindicated, for certain diagnoses and etiologies.** For example, you would not use circumlaryngeal massage as the primary treatment for a case of laryngeal cancer or choose treatments that would encourage increased muscular effort for cases of phonotrauma such as vocal nodules.

8.3 Voice Treatment Orientations

Through the years, there have been a number of philosophies and principles that have provided a basis for the goals of voice therapy as a whole, and for support underlying voice therapy techniques. The following provides several examples[1]:

8.3.1 Symptomatic Voice Therapy

This treatment orientation focuses on targeting the functional misuse(s) or abuse(s) of the voice that are responsible for perceived atypical vocal characteristics such as breathiness or atypical low pitch. Once identified, misuses (behaviors that result in inefficient/ineffective technical use of the voice) and/or abuses (inefficient/ineffective forms of vocalization that have a greater tendency to damage the vocal fold mucosa via **phonotrauma**) are eliminated or reduced through various voice therapy–facilitating techniques. A voice therapy–facilitating technique is a technique which, when used by a patient, enables him/her to easily produce an improved voice. The facilitating technique and the resulting improvement in voice characteristic(s) become the symptomatic focus for voice therapy.[2] Many of these facilitating techniques attempt to elicit improved vocalization by eliciting nonlinguistic or nonpurposeful forms of phonation. As an example, **vegetative vocalization** (cough, throat clear, and/or humming that is shaped into connected speech) has been used effectively as a treatment for patients with mutational falsetto and has been implemented by these authors to elicit improved voice function in severely hyperfunctional cases of aphonia.[3] In summary, the main focus of symptomatic therapy is the direct modification of the vocal "symptoms" (i.e., atypical voice characteristics) to minimize phonotrauma and inefficient vocal technique through the application of facilitative techniques.

8.3.2 Hygienic Voice Therapy

This treatment orientation focuses on the improvement of the health of the vocal fold cover and surrounding laryngeal tissues via modifying or improving vocal hygiene. Some examples of behaviors representative of poor vocal hygiene include excessive loud voice (e.g., shouting, talking loudly over noise, and vocal noises during play), excessive loud coughing and throat clearing, and poor hydration. When the inappropriate behaviors are identified, treatments and recommendations are provided that will modify or eliminate the condition and result in improved laryngeal health and environment. Once modified, voice production has the opportunity to improve or return to normal. Inappropriate voice use may also be a factor in poor vocal hygiene.

8.3.3 Etiologic Voice Therapy

This type of treatment philosophy is based on the view that the primary focus of voice therapy is on the identification and subsequent modification and/or elimination of the underlying physiological cause(s) (i.e., the etiology) of the presenting voice disorder. This orientation is aligned with the biomedical model, which assumes that physiological impairment is related to a finite number of etiologies. When these causes are removed or reduced, the disability resulting from the physiological impairment will be modified or eliminated.[4] Furthermore, when the initial cause is no longer present but changes in function persist, those factors responsible for maintaining the impairment can be identified and subsequently eliminated or modified. Once all etiologic factors are treated, the expectation is that disordered voice characteristics will improve.

8.3.4 Psychogenic Voice Therapy

This type of therapy orientation views emotional and psychosocial disturbances as key factors in the initiation and maintenance of the presenting voice disorder.[5] The relationship(s) between factors such as stress, anxiety, and the presenting voice characteristics are key elements that are brought to the attention of the patient during treatment. The expectation is that once identification of and reduction/elimination of these factors is achieved, voice production will improve.

8.3.5 Physiologic Voice Therapy

Voice treatment programs targeting more than one direct physiological domain have been referred to as **physiological voice treatment** approaches.[1] Since phonation is produced when respiratory pressures and airflow interact with laryngeal structures capable of vibration, this treatment approach focuses on modifying and improving the balance between respiratory and laryngeal systems. In particular, the primary focus is on (**1**) directly modifying and improving the balance of laryngeal muscle effort to the supportive airflow and (**2**) on effectively resonating and focusing the phonatory vibration for improved vocal quality. The physiologic voice therapy approach attempts to directly modify ineffective or inefficient respiratory/laryngeal physiologic activity through direct therapy techniques.

8.3.6 Eclectic Voice Therapy

This treatment orientation incorporates various views and techniques from the aforementioned philosophies into a comprehensive approach to voice treatment.[1,6] As an example, the therapist may have key goals of (**1**) improving vocal hygiene (hygienic voice therapy); (**2**) identifying and relieving causes of phonotrauma and inefficient vocal technique (etiologic voice therapy); (**3**) emphasizing relaxed, easy onset phonation via a yawn/sigh technique (symptomatic voice therapy); and (**4**) improving vocal efficiency and effectiveness via the use of vocal function exercises (physiologic voice). This orientation allows for a flexible selection of voice treatment approaches customized to the individual patient.

8.3.7 Dysphonic Physiology Reversal

Our orientation to effective voice therapy and the selection of voice therapy techniques is based on a very simple but, in our experience, highly effective tenet: **dysphonic physiology reversal (DPR)**. Each word in the name of this approach to voice treatment has importance.

Dysphonic

Dysphonic refers to disrupted phonation. You will see that this philosophy or approach to treatment, as with all potentially successful forms of treatment, is inseparable and dependent on accurate and detailed diagnosis. Diagnosis refers to the detection and description of the cause and features of a disease.[7] To prescribe an effective treatment, it is essential that we can accurately describe the cause and disruption affecting the patient's ability to produce phonation/voice. This description may be based on individual history, perceptual, acoustic, aerodynamic, and laryngeal imaging observations, or ideally from a multidimensional combination of these forms of voice assessment.

Physiology

Once we have clearly defined the cause and described the dysphonia, we must develop a viable hypothesis regarding the underlying physiology of the impairment. *Physiology* is the study of how structures such as cells, muscles, organs, or systems interact to produce a particular outcome. In the case of dysphonia, we must develop a hypothesis regarding the underlying physiological impairment associated with the voice disorder (i.e., how structures are or are not working, or are or are not working together to produce the observed dysphonia) and potential behaviors/factors which may be maintaining disability associated with that impairment.

Reversal

With the development of a strong and logical hypothesis regarding the underlying physiological impairment associated with the observed dysphonia, the last step in this treatment philosophy/approach is very simple: reverse the underlying physiological disruption. There may be several therapy techniques that may be applicable to treat and reverse the underlying physiological deficit, and we may choose a particular technique/method based on

factors such as the severity of the presenting disorder, the duration of the dysphonia, patient health status, clinician familiarity, and expertise with certain treatment techniques. Regardless of the method selected, if (**1**) our hypothesis regarding the underlying physiological deficit is correct and (**2**) our selected treatment technique logically aids in reversal of the physiological deficit, some degree of success in voice therapy will be probable.

Here are a few examples to illustrate the DPR approach to voice therapy:

1. Perception of dysphonia characterized by breathy voice → underlying physiological deficit is hypothesized and confirmed via observation to be hypoadduction → selection of treatment method(s) that reverse hypoadduction (i.e., increase vocal fold adduction). These options may include behavioral (e.g., exercises facilitating increased muscle activation to achieve glottal adduction) or medical options (e.g., vocal fold augmentation).
2. Perception of dysphonia characterized by strained voice and fatigue → underlying physiological deficit is hypothesized and confirmed via observation to be hyperfunction and increased muscle tension → selection of treatment method (s) that reverse hyperfunction and decrease muscle tension. These options may include behavioral (e.g., laryngeal massage) or medical options (e.g., use of Botox in adductor spasmodic dysphonia cases).
3. Perception of dysphonia characterized by low pitched, rough voice → underlying physiological deficit is hypothesized and confirmed via observation to be increased mass (swelling) and accompanying irregular vocal fold vibration → selection of treatment method(s) that reverse (i.e., decrease) vocal fold swelling. These options may include behavioral (e.g., vocal hygiene techniques, techniques to reduce phonotrauma, focus on reduction in vocal loudness) or medical options (e.g., use of prednisone to reduce swelling).

Key underlying physiological deficits that we may attempt to "reverse" in DPR are *excessive laryngeal motor activation* in the form of **vocal hyperfunction** and/or *reduced laryngeal motor activation* in the form of **vocal hypofunction**. Vocal hyperfunction is exemplified by muscle tension dysphonia (MTD), where the impaired physiological balance usually includes excessive activation of intrinsic and extrinsic laryngeal, supralaryngeal, and respiratory muscles. Voice disorders associated with phonotraumatic behaviors would also fall into this category. Vocal hypofunction is exemplified by vocal fold paresis/paralysis, where reduced activation of intrinsic laryngeal muscles causes glottal incompetency. Vocal fold bowing and/or atrophy associated with presbylaryngis and the physiological changes to the respiratory, laryngeal, and articulatory systems subsequent to Parkinson's disease would also fit into this category. It is important to remember that glottal insufficiency does not always relate to hypofunction, as some forms of MTD result in hyperfunctional activation of both adductor and abductor muscles (which are antagonistic to each other) resulting in an excessive posterior glottal gap.

It is critical to the DPR orientation that the clinician also assesses and identifies any psychological processes tied to the onset, development, and/or maintenance of the voice disorder. As noted in Chapter 2, psychological processes are intimately linked to and constantly influence phonation. A comprehensive understanding of the patient's personality characteristics, their specific needs, and how they react to their environment will help the clinician understand the multidimensional nature of a voice disorder. This information can then be used to develop a comprehensive DPR treatment approach, which in some cases may include counseling and/or referral to appropriate mental health professionals.

8.4 An Organizational Framework for Voice Treatments

Depending on which orientation of voice therapy we ascribe to, we will next have to determine the specific voice treatment technique(s)/method(s) that we will use to achieve the overarching goal of the selected voice treatment approach. In the following sections of this chapter, we will organize voice treatments into a taxonomy structured around **direct interventions** and **indirect interventions**. We will also identify those treatments which are effective for specific underlying physiological disruptions common to many vocal impairments, including vocal hyperfunction and vocal hypofunction. It will be emphasized that many treatments *cross categorical boundaries* and can be applied to both hyperfunctional and hypofunctional impairments. In addition, mitigating barriers to treatment participation and compliance and taking advantage of opportunities that will facilitate treatment success will be discussed.

Numerous models for classifying voice treatments have been proposed, although no consistent model has been universally accepted. Van Stan et al published a comprehensive and detailed taxonomic model which can be used as a classification scheme for most voice treatments supported with published research evidence. In this model, specific voice treatments are referred to as "**tools.**"[8] As illustrated in ► Fig. 8.1 and ► Fig. 8.2, the taxonomy consists of two levels. At the first-order level, voice treatments are organized into two intervention approaches: indirect interventions and direct interventions. ***Indirect interventions*** include treatments that modify the cognitive, behavioral, psychological, and physical *environment* in which voicing occurs. These environmental characteristics are modified through two possible domains, **pedagogy** and **counseling**, which are defined as follows:

- **Pedagogy**: rehabilitating or enhancing vocal function by providing knowledge and strategies to modify vocal health.
- **Counseling**: rehabilitating or enhancing vocal function by identifying and modifying psychosocial factors that negatively impact vocal health.

In contrast, ***direct interventions*** include treatments that *modify vocal behavior* through one or more physiological domains including musculoskeletal, respiratory, vocal function, auditory, and somatosensory modification. These five domains can be defined as follows:

- **Musculoskeletal modification**: rehabilitating or enhancing motor execution by modifying muscular, skeletal, and/or connective tissue structures and systems.

- **Respiratory modification**: rehabilitating or enhancing motor execution by modifying respiratory function.
- **Vocal function modification**: rehabilitating or enhancing motor execution by modifying phonation.
- **Auditory modification**: rehabilitating or enhancing auditory-perception by modifying the auditory input.
- **Somatosensory modification**: rehabilitating or enhancing somatosensory perception by modifying somatic and visual input.

The administration of any specific tool within a domain requires the application of a specific *method of delivery*. Extrinsic treatments are those administered and overseen solely by a clinician, whereas intrinsic treatments are those administered and overseen by the patient (under clinician guidance).

Intervention Approach	
Direct	**Target**
Musculoskeletal modification	Rehabilitating or enhancing motor execution by modifying muscular, skeletal, and/or connective tissue structures and systems.
Respiratory modification	Rehabilitating or enhancing motor execution by modifying respiratory function.
Vocal Function modification	Rehabilitating or enhancing motor execution by modifying phonation.
Auditory modification	Rehabilitating or enhancing auditory perception by modifying the auditory input.
Somatosensory modification	Rehabilitating or enhancing somatosensory perception by modifying somatic and visual input.
Indirect	**Target**
Pedagogy	Knowledge and strategies to modify vocal health.
Counseling	Identification and modification of psychosocial factors that negatively impact vocal health.

Fig. 8.1 Taxonomy of voice treatments. The first-order level organizes treatments into categories of direct and indirect intervention approaches, and identifies the delivery methods with which those treatments can be administered. Within the direct intervention category, voice treatments are organized into five different domains of modification: auditory, somatosensory, musculoskeletal, respiratory, and vocal function. Examples of these treatments are shown within these domains. Within the indirect intervention category, voice treatments are organized into two different domains of modification—pedagogy and counseling. The domains of modification in either intervention category can be delivered using extrinsic or intrinsic methods. (Used with permission from Van Stan JH, Roy N, Awan S, Stemple J, Hillman RE. A taxonomy of voice therapy. Am J Speech Lang Pathol 2015; 24(2): 101–125.)

Direct Treatment Approaches	

Musculoskeletal modification	• **Neck Modification**
	  ○ Digital manipulation
	  ○ Myofascial release
	• **Orofacial Modification**
	  ○ Tongue position
	  ○ Chewing
	  ○ Yawn-Sigh
	• **Postural Alignment**
	  ○ Head/Neck position
	  ○ Body posture
	• **Stretching**

Respiratory modification	• **Respiratory Support**
	  ○ Incentive Spirometry
	  ○ Abdominal breathing
	  ○ Expiratory Muscle Training
	• **Loudness Modification**
	  ○ Loud Vocalization
	  ○ MPT Exercises
	  ○ Messa di Voce
	• **Respiratory Coordination**
	  ○ Easy Onsets
	  ○ Flow phonation

Vocal Function modification	• **Glottal Contact**
	  ○ Push/Pull Exercises
	  ○ Flow Phonation
	  ○ Half Swallow Boom
	• **Pitch Modification**
	  ○ Pitch Range Exercises
	  ○ Lip Trills
	  ○ Tongue Trills
	• **Vegetative Vocalization**
	  ○ Throat Clear
	  ○ Cough
	  ○ Hum

Auditory modification	• **Sensorineural**
	  ○ Pitch Monitoring
	  ○ Loudness Monitoring
	  ○ Voice Quality Monitoring
	• **Conduction**
	  ○ Ear Occlusion
	  ○ Delayed Auditory Feedback

Somatosensory modification	• **Nociception**
	  ○ Pain/Discomfort Monitoring
	  ○ Thermal Stimulation
	• **Discrimination**
	  ○ Frontal Focus
	  ○ Semi-Occluded Vocal Tract Exercises
	• **Visual Processing**
	  ○ Mirror Use
	  ○ Video Endoscopy Feedback

Fig. 8.2 The second-order level more thoroughly organizes treatments into the domains of modification for the direct intervention category. Each treatment is administered by focusing the patient's attention to the domain in which it resides. Some treatments overlap domains of modification. This allows the clinician to refocus the patient's attention to another domain while utilizing the same treatment. (Used with permission from Van Stan JH, Roy N, Awan S, Stemple J, Hillman RE. A taxonomy of voice therapy. Am J Speech Lang Pathol 2015; 24(2): 101–125.)

8.5 Indirect Interventions: Pedagogy, Vocal Hygiene, and Counseling

8.5.1 Pedagogy

Vocal pedagogy entails imparting knowledge to the patient by explaining the anatomical and physiological processes of phonation in terms they can understand, and teaching them behaviors which will promote vocal health over time. Pedagogical intervention is a characteristic of most comprehensive voice treatment programs. One important reason for the application of pedagogy and counseling during the initial stages of voice rehabilitation is to shape the patient's perspective regarding the acceptance and adherence of treatment. Both knowledge and perspective can impact a patient's acceptance of treatment, which in turn is a major factor influencing his/her adherence to a treatment program.[9] Patients who do not understand why you are asking them to perform a behavior or how that behavior

relates to vocal improvement are likely to lose motivation, and those who are less motivated are less likely to comply with treatment recommendations.

Pedagogy includes knowledge enhancement (education) and implementation of vocal hygiene programs. **Knowledge enhancement** is designed to increase the patient's understanding of how they create sound through phonation, and how behaviors or conditions can negatively influence that process. When explaining these concepts to a patient, a recommended core set of topics includes the following (described in language familiar to the patient):

• Basic structure of the larynx.
• Relationship between respiratory, laryngeal, and articulatory systems.
• Process of phonation in healthy, nondysphonic production.
• Effect of phonotrauma on vocal fold tissue and voice quality.
• Effect of hydration, irritants (including reflux) on vocal fold tissue and voice quality.
• Effect of lesions, paralysis (if applicable to the patient) on phonation and voice quality.
• The role of treatment in rehabilitating vocal impairments.

It is useful to utilize visual aids when educating the patient, which are readily available from images in this book or via download from the Internet. Additionally, the laryngeal examination video (endoscopic and/or stroboscopic) can itself be a powerful tool for learning.[1]

8.5.2 Vocal Hygiene

The purpose of a vocal hygiene program is to establish knowledge and behaviors which will expose the larynx to an environment where internal and external irritants are minimized. Although vocal hygiene alone is often not sufficient for rehabilitating most vocal impairments, this form of treatment can help reinforce the clinical effects of other direct and indirect interventions. Interprofessional collaboration with the otolaryngologist is important when initiating vocal hygiene treatment as certain recommendations (e.g., hydration through increased fluid intake) need to be made in the context of the patient's larger medical management plan and ensure that recommendations/treatments do not conflict. ▶ Table 8.1 illustrates an example of a vocal hygiene program which includes four domains. This can be used as a guide for treatment, and a version of ▶ Table 8.1 can be provided to the patient as additional learning material. The four domains described in this table include

• **Hydration**: The influence of internal and external hydration on phonation physiology is explained during the process of education. In vocal hygiene, specific recommendations are provided to the patient that will establish behaviors to promote sufficient hydration.
• **Respiratory health**: The heat and chemicals in cigarette smoke can both irritate and damage vocal fold tissue. An emphasis on exposure to smoke is an important domain relative to hygiene. Smokers are encouraged to stop or reduce the frequency of smoking in order to minimize vocal fold exposure. Patients who are frequently exposed to second-hand smoke are encouraged to change lifestyle behaviors to limit that exposure.
• **Vocal habits**: Phonotraumatic behaviors impacting the tissue of the vocal folds are explained during education. Here, the

Table 8.1 Vocal hygiene guidelines

Domain	Recommendations
Hydration	64 oz of water per day
	Limit caffeine intake
	Limit alcohol
	Offset drying medications with extra water
	Use steam inhalation if beneficial
	Avoid menthol products
Respiratory health	Avoid smoking
	Limit exposure to 2nd hand smoke
Vocal habits	Instead of clearing throat, dry swallow or wet swallow; use hard swallow if those do not work alone
	Instead of shouting, use noise device to call attention
	Limit vocal loudness when speaking in the presence of loud background noise
	Do not sing out of your range
	Try to limit overall amount of talking time
	Take frequent voice rests
Vocal irritants (including reflux and postnasal drainage)	Know your reflux and allergy triggers and use medications as prescribed
	Limit intake of spicy, acidic, and fatty foods
	Try not to eat or drink within 3–4 h of going to bed
	Elevate head of bed

clinician provides specific recommendations to reduce or eliminate phonotrauma, individualized to the patient based on their reported vocal habits.

- **Vocal irritants (including reflux and postnasal drainage precautions)**: Laryngopharyngeal reflux (LPR) and postnasal drainage are associated organic etiologies in many patients with voice disorders. If a patient has a history of LPR or postnasal drainage, it is crucial that steps are taken to minimize laryngeal exposure, as indicated in ▶ Table 8.1. Although not listed in the table, an emphasis on adhering to prescribed medication schedules should be provided, as failure to consistently take reflux medication or use prescribed nasal sprays impacts their clinical effectiveness.

8.5.3 Counseling

The process of **counseling** in the context of voice rehabilitation involves rehabilitating or enhancing vocal function by identifying and modifying psychosocial factors that negatively impact vocal health. Some information related to these factors will be obtained during the diagnostic interview (case history). During the initial phase of treatment, counseling can help the patient further understand how psychosocial factors may contribute to their voice impairment. This process is best accomplished with

an open and honest discussion regarding how the patient's personality, life situations, and reactions to stress manifest in laryngeal signs and symptoms. Many patients do not make a connection between stressful life events or their personality characteristics and the onset or maintenance of voice problems. Counseling brings these relationships to light and can help the person better understand how the physiological problem they are experiencing is connected to their own cognitive processing. Referral for professional psychological counseling that goes beyond explaining the relationship between voice and factors such as stress and anxiety should be a necessary consideration.

8.6 Direct Interventions: Facilitative Approaches for Vocal Hyperfunction

Direct interventions include treatments that modify vocal behavior through one or more physiological domains (including musculoskeletal, respiratory, vocal function, auditory, and somatosensory modification). These behavioral treatments allow the clinician and patient to directly target, reverse, and thus rehabilitate underlying impairments in which the disruption occurs in one or more of those physiological domains. Some of these treatments target a singular component of physiology rather than multiple sources of impaired physiology. Treatments which target singular components of voice have been referred to as **facilitative or symptomatic approaches**.[2,10] Many of these treatments have a long history of use in SLP, and several have been precisely described in other publications.[2] We will summarize a sample of facilitative approaches which, in our own clinical experiences, have proven effective for selected patients with voice disorders associated with both hyperfunction and hypofunction.

8.6.1 Resonant Focus

As a facilitative technique, resonant focus can be used dynamically in conjunction with other techniques to "unload" laryngeal muscular hyperfunction. This is accomplished by establishing an **awareness of oronasal vibratory sensations during vocalization**. These sensations arise when voice energy resonated in the facial region is associated with vocal folds that are not excessively compressed together.[11] Resonant or frontal focus is also a fundamental target of a frontal resonance treatment (FRT) approach (see subsequent section).

A useful tool for establishing resonant focus is **humming**. This gesture facilitates vibrotactile sensory awareness due to the sound energy being concentrated in the nasal cavity and along the palate. This effectively moves the placement of sound energy perception from the larynx to the facial region. Patients with severe hyperfunctional dysphonia may need to produce a hum in different postures to achieve an appropriate degree of sensory awareness. This might include gently tucking the chin toward the chest or leaning over with the head facing the floor and the forearms resting on the knees while producing repeated hums. Humming is typically best elicited by modeling the behavior for the patient, prompting them to also take in a comfortable, supportive breath each time.

To monitor performance accuracy, the clinician can assess (**1**) his/her own perception of the patient's voice quality, which should improve when a voice with resonant focus is produced correctly; (**2**) the patient's perception of the sound quality; and (**3**) the patient's perception of vocal effort. Accurate productions of resonant voice when humming should result in improved voice quality perceived by the clinician and patient, in addition to a sense of minimal effort by the patient. In the authors' experience, some patients may require ear training to establish a perceptual anchor for what improved voice quality sounds like.

Once improvements in voice quality are established with humming, the goal is to shape the resonant production into speech. This can be accomplished using a traditional hierarchy of a nasal + vowel (e.g., hum, followed by "ma-ma-ma"), single syllable words starting with nasals (e.g., "hum, followed by "mom," "mum," and "non"), single-syllable words with and without nasals (e.g., numbers—hum followed by "one," then "two"), multisyllabic words, **phrases**, sentences, and conversation.

8.6.2 Tongue Advancement

The goal for patients with vocal hyperfunction is to change the maladaptive motor pattern into one that is more efficient and effective for communication. However, some patients have difficulty consciously monitoring their own internal sensations, monitoring their own voice quality, or experience severe degrees of hyperfunctional muscle contraction such that achievement of initial therapeutic goals is difficult. In these cases, tongue advancement (e.g., "protrusion") may be attempted as a facilitating technique. Because the tongue is attached directly to the hyoid bone, which is itself attached to the larynx, forward movement of the tongue dorsum applies traction to the larynx, altering the degree of muscular tension in the laryngeal muscles. This muscular response often has the effect of changing the patient's hyperfunctional pattern so that vocal fold vibration becomes more periodic and voice quality improves. Tongue advancement also opens the pharynx, which may lead to less laryngeal compression. In contrast, tongue retraction (as in back focus) compresses the pharynx, larynx, and results in increased muscular tension in the laryngeal region.

Tongue advancement is best accomplished by utilizing a high front vowel, such as /i/,[2] as follows:

1. The clinician prompts the patients to slightly open their mouth and stick out their tongue so that it is past the lips (but not as far as they can protrude it—the posture should be comfortable for the patients).
2. They are then asked to take an easy breath in and sustain the /i/ vowel for a few seconds, with attention paid to voice quality and level of effort. This is repeated multiple times, and different degrees of protrusion and mouth opening can be explored in attempts to achieve a target voice quality.
3. When voice quality improves and the patient indicates that voice production is not effortful, they are asked to retract the tongue to the level of the lips and produce /mi-mi-mi/ with the tongue staying between the lips on each repetition.
4. The goals continue to remain as a perception of improved voice quality and reduced level of perceived effort. With continued accuracy, the patient is asked to move the tongue inside the mouth to the natural /i/ position while repeating the

syllable. With continued mastery, the clinician can introduce the traditional hierarchy of stimuli with the goal of progressing to conversational speech while maintaining the improved voice quality and ease of effort.

8.6.3 Vegetative and/or Automatic Voicing

Vegetative voicing includes non-speech vocalizations such as throat clearing, grunting, phonating on inhalation, coughing, and the common form of automatic voicing resulting in the production of "uh-huh" as a conversational response. These types of voicing can be useful starting points in the treatment of patients with severe MTD in the form of aphonia (sometimes referred to as non-adducted hyperfunction and traditionally as a form of psychogenic aphonia). In these cases, an initial goal of treatment is to achieve vocal fold adduction which allows for phonation of any type. This can be accomplished with numerous techniques, including the use of vegetative/automatic voicing tasks that provides the patient with a physical and auditory cue that vocal fold adduction and voicing is possible.

Attempts to elicit voicing often require the clinician to move quickly from one technique to another. The clinician will elicit productions by choosing an initial vegetative or automatic gesture and model it for the patient. If the patient fails to produce voice after multiple attempts, the clinician models a different gesture and asks the patient to repeat. Experimentation is often necessary in the form of prompting the patient to produce the gestures at different pitches and loudness levels. It can also be useful to cycle through the techniques, coming back to the first or second vegetative/automatic voice type after attempting the oher forms.

Once achieved, it is crucial that the clinician brings the occurrence of phonation to the conscious awareness of the patient and has them repeat the gesture. With repeated success on one type of vocalization, the clinician should then prompt the patient to vary the production by changing pitch, changing loudness, and changing duration. With continued success, the vegetative/automatic vocalization should be shaped into a vowel (e.g., vocalization + vowel), followed by a traditional stimulus hierarchy. Implementation of vegetative/automatic voicing, especially in patients with long-standing aphonia, requires persistence and perseverance from the clinician. Typically, maladaptive hyperfunctional patterns of phonation do not improve in seconds or a few minutes. However, for the patient without significant psychological comorbidity, these techniques can be very successful in eliciting an improved or even normal voice quality in the first treatment session.

8.6.4 Chewing

The chewing method was first described by Emil Fröschels as a treatment for vocal hyperfunction.[12] The theoretical basis for the application of this approach centers on the shared neuromuscular pathways employed during the act of speaking and mastication. Froeschels reasoned that voiced speech sounds were a natural evolution from noises produced during chewing while eating food.[12] He generated a clinical hypothesis which suggested that if the neuromuscular pathways producing these chewing noises were the same as those for laryngeal function during speech, one behavior could be used to influence the other. This was supported by the observation that chewing movements and chewing noises remain unaffected in many patients with hyperfunctional voice disorders, even though similar muscles are being used for voice production during speech.[13] Based on this rationale, he developed a treatment approach which utilizes exaggerated chewing movements of the tongue, facial, and mandibular muscles in concert with voice production to counteract the hyperfunctional contraction of laryngeal muscles associated with voice impairment and dysphonia. The steps in utilizing the chewing method are as follows:

1. The clinician introduces the concept of chewing to the patient as a method of removing excessive laryngeal tension during speaking. It is emphasized that vocal noises can be produced while chewing, which is what the clinician and patient will explore together. The clinician should emphasize that once an improved voice quality is achieved, chewing movements will be reduced.

2. The clinician prompts the patient to produce exaggerated movements of the jaw as if chewing a large bolus. In prompting the patient, the clinician first provides a model and asks the patient to replicate. Key concepts of instruction include the following:

   a) The jaw position for a majority of the movements should be lowered so that the mouth is open. Closing movements of the mouth will correspond to adduction of the lips during chewing motions. Jaw movements are vigorous and should include up-down and side-to-side actions. The patient can be given a cue to chew as if they had a large piece of meat or bread in their mouth.

   b) Lip movements are exaggerated by wide opening, closing, pursing, and retraction (e.g., smiling) gestures.

   c) Tongue movement includes large excursions throughout the oral cavity in all directions.

3. As the patient replicates the exaggerated chewing, the clinician introduces visual feedback utilizing a mirror. The patient is asked to continue exploring random chewing movements while being reminded to move the lips and tongue extensively. The clinician continues to monitor the patient to ensure that range of movements are substantial, especially those of the tongue.

4. The patient is asked to add voicing during the act of chewing. The resulting sound is monitored by the clinician for two characteristics:

   a) The resulting speech sounds should perceptually resemble variegated babbling and include a range of phonemes due to the numerous positions of the articulators during chewing actions. If a patient produces a monotonous "yam yam" it is a cue that the tongue is not moving throughout a wide range of motion.

   b) If laryngeal tension is in fact decreased, the quality of the voiced sounds should improve. This is noted by the clinician and brought to the attention of the patient so that their perception is acutely aware of the voice change.

5. Once an improved voice quality is established consistently, the patient is then asked to continue the chewing actions while chanting the numbers one through ten, as if counting slowly. It is not important that articulation of these numbers is precise—the focus is on voice quality rather than articulatory precision.

6. Once improved voice quality during counting is consistent, the patient is prompted to chant **phrases** while chewing in the same manner. Initial phrase stimuli can be structured with many nasal consonants to promote a frontal resonance but should transition to stimuli with a wide variety of sounds.

7. Once improved voice quality during phrase production is consistent, the patient is then prompted to decrease the large chewing movements into a more natural oral posture during speech, with an emphasis on flexibility of the jaw, tongue, and lips. The **phrases** are repeated in this manner while chanting, and perceptual focus remains on the maintenance of an improved voice quality.

8. Once consistency is established, the patient is asked to transition the **phrases** from chanting to a more natural speech prosody. Finally, the patient is asked to read **passages** and then engage in conversation while maintaining the improved voice quality.

8.7 Direct Interventions: Facilitative Approaches for Vocal Hypofunction

8.7.1 Glottal Adduction Exercises

Exercises requiring maximum concentric contraction of intrinsic vocal fold muscles have been utilized in combination with other techniques to rehabilitate adductor muscles when physiological impairments cause vocal hypofunction. The theory behind these exercises is that **vocal fold adduction performed with maximum residual motor unit recruitment during muscular contraction will facilitate neuromotor adaptation in the target muscles and neuromotor pathways**, particularly when completed in sets of numerous repetitions and with high frequency across a day or week. These exercises will be most beneficial when combined with phonation attempts in a hierarchy of voicing difficulty (moving from sustained vowel productions to syllables and toward actual speech contexts). Two examples of glottal adduction exercises include push/pull and glottal attack exercises.

Push/pull exercises can be performed in diverse ways, such as in the following methodology:

1. The clinician prompts the patient to press or pull against a surface, as if holding their breath as tightly as possible.[14] This exercise promotes maximal adduction of the vocal folds by simulating the glottal closure reflex.

2. The patient is instructed to hold the contraction for 3 or 4 seconds, and then release. This is repeated multiple times to complete a set, with multiple sets completed numerous times each day.

3. The technique can be performed while seated, where the patient presses with both hands against the surface of their chair or the desk in front of them, or also be performed while standing where the patient presses against a wall or table or presses both hands against one another. In addition, these exercises may also be carried out using an isometric contraction in which the patient links the fingers of each hand together and pulls to initiate glottal closure.

4. The exercises can be combined with phonation by asking the patient to perform the push/pull maneuver while attempting to phonate a sound. It is essential that the clinician help the patient to time the contraction to occur along with phonation attempts. With this technique, the goal will be to shape away the push/pull gesture while maintaining the improved glottal closure and sound quality.

While push/pull exercises are not typically used as the only technique for glottal insufficiency, their use in combination with other techniques has been supported by a number of published investigations.[15,16,17,18] It should also be remembered that there may be patients who, due to physical health, may not be candidates for this treatment, such as those with high blood pressure.[19]

Glottal attack exercises attempt to achieve a similar effect as the push/pull exercises with the exception that the patient will hold the contraction for only a few seconds and then release it into a sustained vocalized vowel. This can be prompted with instructions such as: *"Take a deep breath, hold your breath by squeezing tightly with your vocal folds, and then say "ahhhh" with a loud volume."* With mastery, the technique can be modified to initiate phonation immediately after maximum glottal adduction without holding the breath. Glottal attack exercises have been utilized for glottal incompetence that affects both voice production and swallowing.[10,17,20] For those who manifest slower progress, another exercise, the "**pseudo-supraglottic swallow**," can be added to the sets. This exercise requires the patient to take a breath and hold it as in the initial part of the supraglottic swallow, but instead of swallowing the patient is asked to cough forcefully after a few seconds of breath hold. This is repeated, along with the other exercises, in multiple repetitions over 5 minutes, and performed numerous times each day. A similar exercise to the pseudo-supraglottic swallow is the "**half-swallow boom**," which requires the patient to take a breath, swallow, and attempt to produce a sharp "boom!" in the middle of the swallow while the vocal folds are maximally adducted. Evidence for the effectiveness of this exercise when combined with other treatments has been reported in multiple studies.[21,22]

8.7.2 Digital Manipulation

Using the hands for applying pressure to the thyroid cartilage on the affected side in unilateral vocal fold paralysis is another technique which has been utilized to facilitate and improve glottal closure.[15,17,22] One approach to digital manipulation is as follows:

1. The fingers of a free hand (the other hand can be used to support the patient's head) are placed on the thyroid lamina of the weak/paretic side, near the middle of the vertical dimension of the thyroid. The thumb can be placed on the opposite thyroid lamina to fixate the unaffected side so that it can serve as a base against which the opposite side approximates.
2. Using the fingers, the clinician applies inward (medial) pressure to the thyroid, pushing the affected side toward the midline. The patient is asked to vocalize by sustaining a vowel as the clinician applies the pressure.
3. As the patient produces a vowel, the clinician and patient should listen for a change in voice quality. Varying degrees of pressure can be applied to elicit improved voice, monitoring and querying the patient about his or her level of comfort.

4. When a positive voice change is elicited, the clinician brings this to the conscious awareness of the patient. When both clinician and patient can perceive the change and it can be consistently elicited on multiple trials (e.g., 8-10 consecutive trials), the clinician then begins to eliminate the manipulation by releasing pressure during vocalization on successive attempts.
5. The patient is asked to maintain the improved voice as pressure is released. This requires greater muscular effort on the part of the patient, which is the motor behavior this exercise is designed to elicit. With mastery, the clinician prompts the patient to produce the vocalization without digital manipulation, and then voice production is moved through a hierarchy of stimulus contexts terminating in conversational speech with the improved voice.

8.8 Direct Interventions: Comprehensive Voice Treatment Programs for Vocal Hyperfunction

Voice treatment programs are organized collections of different treatments representing varied direct and indirect domains. Most voice treatment programs are delivered with some extrinsic structure (clinician led), but may also include intrinsic delivery structures as part of the program. Seven different voice treatment programs were recently described within the context of the voice treatment taxonomy.[8] Voice treatment programs targeting more than one direct physiological domain have been referred to as **physiological voice treatment** approaches, and when incorporating both direct and indirect approaches have been referred to as **eclectic voice treatment**.[1,23]

We will focus our subsequent discussion of voice rehabilitation on the characteristics of voice treatment programs supported by at least a minimal level of published research evidence (i.e., evidence for the program's effectiveness exists in the peer-reviewed literature).

8.8.1 Stretch-and-Flow

Stretch-and-flow (SnF) is a voice treatment program designed to rehabilitate vocal function in the presence of a physiological imbalance within the vocal subsystems, usually when the imbalance is related to functional hyperkinetic motor execution.[24] It can be adapted for patients with vocal hypofunction, especially in speakers who have developed compensatory maladaptive hyperfunctional vocalization patterns to overcome glottal insufficiency. SnF has also been referred to as **flow phonation**, and was first described in the early 1980s as a program for children with functional voice disorders.[25,26] Evidence for the clinical effectiveness of SnF has been demonstrated in populations with voice impairments ranging from nodules, polyps, and MTD, and has recently been investigated within the context of a randomized controlled trial.[24,27]

The program of SnF targets multiple direct and indirect domains. Direct domains include **musculoskeletal** (orofacial modification and postural alignment), **respiratory** (coordination and support), **vocal function** (glottal contact and pitch modification), **auditory** (sensorineural), and **somatosensory** (discrimination). The SnF program is typically administered along with an indirect approach focusing on the domain of **pedagogy** (knowledge enhancement and vocal hygiene). The delivery method is primarily extrinsic and characterized by a **hierarchical** structure, which is illustrated in ▶ Fig. 8.3.

A fundamental goal of SnF is to *facilitate volitional neuromotor control of the vocal subsystems while maintaining a perception of minimal effort*. To accomplish this, the patient moves through a hierarchy of progressively challenging vocal tasks. SnF structure initially focuses on the respiratory domain with voiceless airflow control techniques. As the patient demonstrates mastery, airflow is combined with the vocal function domain of glottal contact by progressively increasing the degree of vocal fold adduction onto the stream of airflow, first with a breathy voice and then with a more engaged glottal contact pattern. The program culminates with mastery of coordinated neuromuscular control characterized by phonation in connected speech produced with equilibrium between respiration, phonation, and resonance.

The SnF hierarchy presents a progressive structure along the continua of muscle activity levels (*x*-axis of ▶ Fig. 8.3) and motor complexity stages (*y*-axis of ▶ Fig. 8.3). Each muscle activity level of the hierarchy is referred to as a skill, and the patient is required to progress horizontally through each skill level while working vertically through the hierarchy of motor complexity stages. The motor complexity hierarchy begins with unvoiced airflow and culminates with connected speech. When a patient masters all motor complexity stages within a skill level, they move to the next skill in the horizontal muscle activity hierarchy.

The muscle activity skill levels are as follows (as defined in the study of Watts et al[24,27]):

- **Level 1: Flow.** The goal for this skill level is for the speaker to gain control over airflow. The speaker's task is to produce a *steady flow of unvoiced air without effort* through rounded lips, as in a slow, comfortable exhalation. A piece of soft-tissue paper held at the front of the mouth is used for visual feedback, with successful productions resulting in forward movement of the tissue along with patient perceptions of relaxed exhalation. The patient's hand placed in front of the mouth can be used in lieu of the tissue, as a form of tactile biofeedback (airflow emanating from the mouth stimulates sensory receptors on the hand). When mastery is established for voiceless airflow, the clinician may choose to progress to the next skill level or another stage in level 1 (stage 1B on the *y*-axis of ▶ Fig. 8.3) by modeling and eliciting a breathy voiced vowel (e.g., /u/) with emphasis on the perception of effortless flow. The goal for level 1 stage B is a steady flow of air and minimally engaged vocal folds to produce breathy voice quality with minimal effort. For patients who may have difficulty comprehending the sequence of SnF, this preliminary stage can help build understanding of how airflow will be combined with voicing as the treatment progresses.
- **Level 2: Stretch-and-flow.** The goal for this skill level is for the speaker to produce minimal effort, **voiceless** airflow through the glottis along with slow (stretched out) movements of the

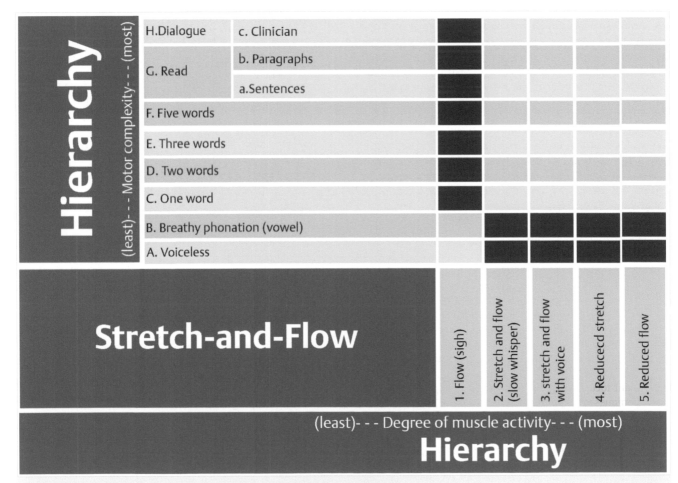

Fig. 8.3 The hierarchical structure of stretch-and-flow (SnF) voice treatment program.

articulators. Accurate productions should be perceived as effortless, whispered connected speech at a slow rate. Tissue can also be used for visual feedback. Stages in the vertical hierarchy (*y*-axis) begin with one-word and then progress to multiple-word stimuli as the patient masters each stage. Stimuli in stages C to E in this skill level and subsequent skill levels have included numbers (e.g., "one," "one-two," "one-two-three"), or words beginning with /h/ or /w/ + /u/ to facilitate airflow in the context of semiocclusion.[24,25,27]

- **Level 3**: **Stretch and voiced flow**. The goal for this skill level is for the speaker to produce **voiced** airflow through the glottis along with slow (stretched out) movements of the articulators, while using minimal effort. Accurate productions should be perceived as breathy, effortless voice quality in connected speech at a slow rate of speech. Tissue can also be used for visual feedback.
- **Level 4**: **Reduced stretch with increased flow**. The goal for this skill level is for the speaker to produce voiced airflow through the glottis with a faster speech rate, while maintaining minimal effort. Accurate productions should be perceived as effortless voiced but breathy speech with a normal rate of speech.
- **Level 5**: **Reduced air flow (target voice)**. The goal for this skill level is for the speaker to produce a normal voice quality with an appropriate rate of speech, while maintaining minimal effort. Accurate productions should be perceived as appropriate conversational loudness with normal (nonbreathy) air flow, normal speech rate, and modal (natural for that person) pitch.

The development of treatment goals for individual patients receiving SnF can be structured with percent correct benchmarks dependent on factors such as the patient's response to diagnostic probes and their initial response to the treatment techniques. Published research has set mastery criteria at 90% accuracy at each stage within a skill level.[24] It is possible that initial criteria for a particular stage can be set lower, and the goal adjusted as the patient attains increasing degrees of mastery. For example, an initial goal of the program might be "*Patient XX will produce level 1 flow productions with continuous voiceless exhalations (stage A) on 7 of 10 (70%) consecutive trials.*" When the patient reaches that level of mastery, the criterion can be increased and the goal modified to 9 of 10 consecutive trials or 90% accuracy. When mastery at 90% is reached, the patient moves on to the next stage within that skill level.

8.8.2 Frontal Resonance Treatment (FRT)

The concept of directing conscious awareness to resonant sensations in the oral and nasal cavities to facilitate vocal flexibility and target voice quality has been used in singing pedagogy for centuries. Many treatment concepts utilized in vocal rehabilitation emerged from early singing voice instructors, and it is not surprising that techniques used to improve vocal control such as resonant focus are shared among SLPs and teachers of singing. Techniques which attempt to exchange muscular tension at the larynx for increased oral cavity movement, airflow, and vibratory sensations have existed in the profession of SLP since at least the early 1940s as a means of reducing or eliminating vocal hyperfunction.[28] Resonant focus is understood as **the conscious perception of vibrotactile sensations in the oral and nasal cavities** (e.g., frontal regions of the face) **during sound production**. These sensations are related to actual tissue and bone vibrations in the facial region which are elicited by vocal tract shaping during resonant voice production.[29] Clinical theory suggests that transferring a patient's attention of effort away from the larynx and toward the resonant cavities of the upper airway has the effect of reducing excessive laryngeal motor execution, or hyperfunction.[2] This theory has been supported by published evidence which has demonstrated that glottal adduction during resonant voice production allows for normal voice quality and function with minimal tissue contact that is beneficial for patients with voice disorders related to hyperkinetic muscular control and/or phonotraumatic behaviors.[11]

The framework of many physiologically based resonant voice programs is built on modifications of the work of Arthur Lessac, a renowned voice teacher who developed the "Kinesensic" approach.[30] One of the foundational components of his method is awareness of movement and energy throughout the body. **The perception of oral vibratory sensations in the context of perceived easy or effortless phonation is a fundamental target of contemporary resonant voice therapy programs**.[1] Two evidence-based resonant approaches used widely by SLPs include the Lessac-Madsen Resonant Voice Therapy (LMRVT) program developed by Kathrine Verdolini and the associated program of Resonant Voice Therapy (RVT) developed by Joseph Stemple and colleagues.[10,31,32,33] These treatments or other associated adaptions of resonant focus have been used successfully in patients with vocal hyperfunction and vocal hypofunction, especially when the glottal incompetence of hypofunction is accompanied by compensatory maladaptive strain and effort.

Measurable effects of Stemple's RVT approach and adaptions of the program have been supported by numerous published investigations.[9,32,34,35] The physiological domains and treatment characteristics of RVT have also been applied to the previously described taxonomy of voice treatment by Van Stan et al.[8] A video example illustrating administration of the RVT approach is provided in **Video 8.1** and is further detailed by Roy et al.[32] The following methodology for FRT (related but distinct from LMRVT and RVT), is derived from the authors' clinical experiences, and is built upon decades of advancing knowledge of the physiological effects that resonant focus imparts upon the vocal subsystems. Authors and voice therapists who have advanced this knowledge include but are not limited to Emil Froeschels, Friedrich Brodnitz, Ed Stone, Thomas Cleveland, Daniel Boone, Katherine Verdolini, Joseph Stemple, and Kimberly Coker, among others.[36] Additionally, clinicians can use the process described below in a flexible and dynamic manner to fit the needs of the patient.

Fundamental Characteristics of FRT

The perceptual target of FRT is the **conscious awareness of focused, oral vibratory sensations in the context of minimal effort**. Although the perceptual focus of FRT is on resonance, the physiological requirements for accurate resonant productions require coordination of respiratory, laryngeal, and supralaryngeal muscles. FRT facilitates rehabilitation or enhancement of motor patterns and requires the implementation of motor learning strategies, of which copious repetition of target resonant voice production in varying speech contexts is crucial.

- Stage 1: Establishing frontal resonance
  - *Teaching the foundations of voice*: The process of FRT begins with education. The clinician will introduce the patient to the anatomy and physiology of phonation in terms that the patient can understand. An emphasis on the connection between the three subsystems of voice should be provided. This emphasis will help the patient better understand how shaping the supraglottal vocal tract can influence laryngeal muscle function and subsequent phonation.
  - *Exploring current function*: The purpose of this step is to increase the patient's conscious awareness of current vocal technique. The clinician begins by asking the patient to inhale slowly and deeply, and then exhale. Close attention is paid to diaphragmatic and rib cage expansion in relation to the upper torso tension. This process is repeated. Inefficient motor patterns for respiration can be identified and brought to the patient's attention at this point, and subsequently corrected.

The patient is then asked to produce a vowel at comfortable pitch and loudness. The clinician guides the patient through the process of perceptually identifying (**1**) levels of effort, (**2**) anatomical regions of muscular tension, and (**3**) perceptual impressions of voice quality. The patient is also asked to describe the location at which they feel voice effort is focused—such as at the level of the chest, the throat, or higher in the oral cavity.

- *Locating vibrotactile energy*: This step is designed to establish a kinesthetic sense of vibration in the facial region. Establishing a physical sensation of orofacial vibrations is a key to this step. The clinician begins by leading the patient through different voice gestures to find one or more strategies which lead to orofacial vibratory awareness *and* improved voice quality. Successful attempts will be characterized by improvements of voice quality *within the context of reduced effort* (*note*: it should not be harder for the patient to produce these gestures … it should be easier). Among the prompts that can be attempted to establish frontal resonance, all of which are preceded by an easy inhalation to support voicing, include the following:
  - A gentle, sustained hum at a constant pitch lasting 3 to 5 seconds—the head should be in a neutral, relaxed position.
  - Gently humming with descending pitch, as in a sigh.[1]
  - Gently humming while tucking the chin to the chest.
  - While seated, leaning over with hands on knees, head toward the floor, while gently humming.
  - Turning the head to the left or right while gently humming.
  - Rounding the lips (as if whistling) while gently humming.

It is important to realize that the perceptual responses to these attempts can be variable from patient to patient. Some patients will report a strong sense of vibrotactile energy, while others may feel none. Others may report the sense of vibration within the nose, while others may report the sense at the lips, palate, or somewhere general within the oral cavity. The perception of vibrotactile energy anywhere in the oral and nasal regions is a positive predictor, and subsequent repetitions of the gesture(s) should prompt the patient to consciously focus on the feeling of energy at those regions. Mastery at this stage of the FRT protocol occurs when the patient can *consistently* produce repeated gestures with the following treatment targets: (**1**) a physical perception of

vibrotactile energy in the oral or nasal region, (**2**) an auditory-perceptual improvement in sound quality, and (**3**) the perception of minimal effort when producing the voice gesture.

This stage of FRT can last as little as 10 minutes, or may require multiple treatment sessions with subsequent home practice to achieve mastery. Some patients will have more difficulty establishing the physical sense of vibrotactile energy and progress more slowly during the treatment process. Some modifications for facilitative gestures which might aid those patients can include the following[36]:

- Ask the patient to place a finger on the side of the nose while prompting them to monitor touch sense for nasal vibrations.
- Ask the patient to gently hum through a straw held between the lips.
- Ask the patient to produce a comfortable "ahhhh" while transitioning into a gentle hum by closing the lips.
- Ask the patient to produce comfortable repetitions of "ma-ma-ma" or "na-na-na," followed by prolongation of the /m/ or /n/ sound after a few repetitions.
- Ask the patient to produce bilabial raspberries, and transition those into a gentle hum.
- Ask the patient to gently produce a /z/ or /v/ sound while monitoring the physical sense of vibration at the point of articulation. Shape this into a gentle hum.
- Ask the patient to mimic agreement with something by producing "Umm Hmm" slowly and repetitively with an upward pitch inflection on the "hmm."

Mastery of stage 1 necessitates the patient being able to consistently produce the treatment targets accurately in the context of the isolated gesture(s). The clinician can choose the appropriate level of mastery (e.g., 80%, 90%, or higher) prior to advancement based on the individual needs of the patient. Once the established level of mastery is achieved, the patient moves on to the next stage.

- Stage 2: Voice expansion
  - Gentle humming will be expanded into **hum + vowel**. While most vowel sounds can be used, the authors typically choose to utilize the /a/ vowel as the initial target. The patient is asked to support voice with an easy, efficient inhalation and then produce a hum for a few seconds followed by a vowel. The vowel should transition immediately from the hum (e.g., there should not be a voicing silence between them), such as "mmmmmmmmmahhhhhhhhhh." Depending on patient response in the prior stage, different facilitative gestures can be used for the onset stimulus (e.g., UmmmHmmmahhhhh; leaning over while humming; rounding the lips; etc.).
  - When the level of mastery for the vowel is achieved, the patient is next asked to expand gentle humming into **hum + numbers**. These productions are generated as "hmmm … one; hmmm … two; hmmm … three, etc.. The number should transition immediately from the hum. It may help the patient with perceptual focus of the targets (perceptions of effort, tension, and voice quality) if they first generate these productions with **chanting** (a steady pitch and loudness). When successful at chanting, they can then transition into productions with a descending intonation on the number. An alternative to numbers is to utilize single-syllable words that begin with a nasal sound (e.g., "hmmm … man"; "hmmmm … no," etc.).

○ When the level of mastery for the numbers or nasal words is achieved, the patient is next asked to produce a gentle **hum + nonnasal word**. This step is similar to the steps mentioned earlier, with the exception that single-syllable word stimuli are chosen which reflect variable consonant and vowel structures. As mentioned earlier, it can benefit the patient to initially produce these stimuli with chanting, and then transition to typical speech intonation. The clinician should prepare each treatment session with copious word stimuli to ensure practice quantity and variability.

○ When the level of mastery for nonnasal single-syllable words is achieved, the patient is next asked to produce the **same stimuli without the preceding hum** (i.e., the hum is shaped away). It is important at this step to remind the patient of efficient respiratory support and the focus on effort, sites of tension, and voice quality. The previously identified regions of vibrotactile energy should be monitored by the patient to facilitate resonant productions. The single words produced without hum should be low loudness and generated with adequate airflow at the onset of phonation. The clinician should monitor these factors and bring to the patient's attention if poor technique resurfaces.

○ When the level of mastery for words without the humming cue is achieved, the patient is next asked to produce **sentences**. As with previous stimuli, each production is generated with focus on vibrotactile sensations, sense of effort, and voice quality. It can sometimes benefit the patient to first produce stimuli while chanting, and then move to more typical speech intonation once the targets are mastered using the chant context. Sentence stimuli should be varied and numerous to provide the patient with adequate practice opportunities.

• Stage 3: Generalization

○ Once the patient reaches mastery of the previous stage, they then move to producing the target voice with frontal resonance while **reading paragraphs** (e.g., from a book, magazine, or preselected **passages**). As with the previous stages, the patient is encouraged to consciously monitor frontal resonance, perceived effort levels, sites of tension, and voice quality during productions.

○ Once the appropriate level of mastery is achieved, the patient moves on to produce the target frontal resonance voice while engaging the clinician in **conversation**.

○ To facilitate carryover, the final step is for the clinician to monitor the patient while they engage in **conversation with others**. This can include conversations on the phone, in person with familiar individuals, and in person with those unfamiliar to the patient. Digital devices have also been developed to facilitate acquisition and maintenance of frontal resonant voice production.[37]

8.8.3 Vocal Function Exercises

Voice disorders that result in or from obligatory weakness and subsequent deconditioning (e.g., vocal fold paresis and vocal fold atrophy),[17,38] as well as functional voice disorders that demonstrate inefficient neuromuscular control and/or primary or compensatory muscular imbalance in the subsystems supporting voice production may have the potential for responding to exercises that facilitate **neuromuscular adaptation**. As with any other skeletal muscle, the laryngeal muscles should respond to the stress of physical rehabilitation by adapting to improve functional capacities. To increase muscular strength, tone, coordination, and/or endurance, a muscle must be exposed to repeated stress (e.g., a load or fatiguing task). In turn, the muscle and its neuromotor pathways will adapt to this stress through a process of physiological change. A classic example is weightlifting, where specific muscle groups are exposed to repeated stress in the form of exercise(s) presenting an overload (heavy weight). With repeated exposure to this overload, the targeted muscles adapt through a process of hypertrophy, where muscle cells gain volume and a greater number of neuromotor pathways and motor units are recruited during contraction. This adaptation makes the muscle increase in both size and ability to generate greater contraction strength. Muscle adaptation can also be responsive to long duration, repetitive motion. For example, progressive exposure to increased contraction durations is needed to allow muscular adaptions that will permit a runner to complete extended distance runs versus the reduced endurance requirements of leg muscles for sprinting.[39] Similar adaptations have been demonstrated in both dysphonic and nondysphonic speakers participating in vocal function exercise (VFE) programs.[40,41,42,43,44,45,46,47]

VFEs comprise a voice treatment program developed by Joseph Stemple which rehabilitates or enhances vocal function through repeated stress applied to the respiratory and laryngeal musculature. The program consists of a four-exercise set which is repeated four times daily, typically two repetitions of the set in the morning and two repetitions in the afternoon. The role of the SLP in administering this treatment includes skilled instruction and regular monitoring of exercise technique and progressive performance outcome. These elements are critical if VFEs are to challenge the target muscle groups in a manner that is specific to phonation for communication purposes. VFEs have been applied successfully to populations with both vocal hyperfunction and vocal hypofunction.

The exercises comprising the VFE program are illustrated in ▶ Fig. 8.4 and have been thoroughly described in previous publications.[1,10] The application of VFE is demonstrated in **Video 8.2**. Each exercise is designed to target adaptation in laryngeal muscles specific to voice demands during communication and/or vocal performance. VFE include exercises requiring sustained, controlled contraction of the vocal fold adductor muscles (warm-up), dynamic and controlled contraction of the vocal fold tensor muscles to elongate the vocal folds (stretch), dynamic and controlled contraction of the vocal fold tensor and relaxer muscles to shorten the vocal folds (contract), and coordination of all adductor and tensor muscles during sustained phonation at different fundamental frequencies (power). Instructions for the four exercises are briefly described as follows:

• **Exercise 1: Warm-up**: The clinician explains, models, and then elicits a sustained /i/ vowel for as long as possible at a target pitch equal to the musical note F above middle C (**~ 350 Hz**) for females or F below middle C (**~ 175 Hz**) for males.

○ Instruction should also emphasize appropriate respiratory support and coordination of airflow with vocal fold adduction (e.g., easy onsets).

○ The patient is prompted to produce vowels at reduced vocal loudness (below conversational loudness) but with "engaged" vocal folds—that is, without breathiness (if possible—for instance, when the physiological impairment is not glottal incompetency).

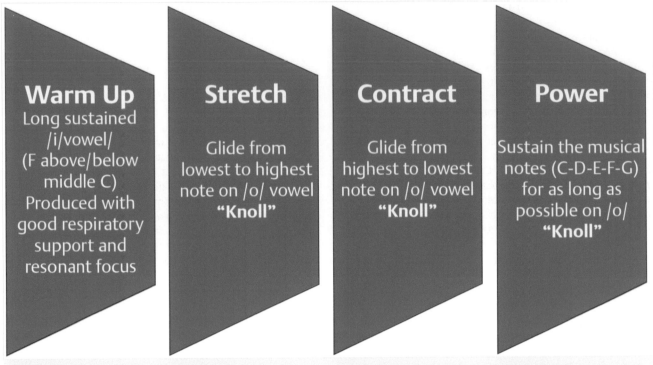

Warm Up
Long sustained
/i/vowel/
(F above/below
middle C)
Produced with
good respiratory
support and
resonant focus

Stretch

Glide from
lowest to highest
note on /o/ vowel
"Knoll"

Contract

Glide from
highest to lowest
note on /o/ vowel
"Knoll"

Power

Sustain the musical
notes (C-D-E-F-G)
for as long as
possible on /o/
"Knoll"

Fig. 8.4 Vocal function exercises.

- The patient is also instructed to utilize **resonant focus** when producing the vowel. Prompts to produce the /i/ sound with exaggerated nasal resonance can facilitate this.
- The goal is a maximum duration of phonation free of any voice breaks (see below for determining objective goals for this exercise).
- Numerous pitch pipes and tone generators are available via mobile applications and can be used as an auditory model for the target pitch.
- Trained vocalists are often very good at approximating the target pitch. For nonvocalists or patients with significant dysphonia, the clinician may need to set the target pitch somewhat higher or lower depending on patient characteristics.
- In some cases, it might be appropriate to simply have the patient produce this exercise at a comfortable pitch, with a subsequent goal to increase pitch as muscles adapt to the exercise demands.
- **Exercise 2: Stretch.** The clinician explains, models, and then elicits a slow, controlled pitch glide from the lowest possible frequency to the highest possible frequency, on the vowel /o/ as in the word "knoll."
  - Respiratory support, coordination, resonant focus, and soft intensity are also emphasized when instructing the patient.
  - Perceptual goals include an absence of pitch breaks throughout the range and the widest range possible. The presence or location of breaks and the extent of the frequency range can be measured objectively using acoustic software.
  - Some patients have difficulty producing the target /o/ vowel in "knoll." As alternatives, the stimulus can be modified by eliciting the /u/ vowel by slowly gliding upward on the word "whoop," or even using lip trills with a slow, upward gliding pitch.

- **Exercise 3: Contract.** The clinician explains, models, and then elicits a slow, controlled pitch glide from the highest possible frequency to the lowest possible frequency, on the vowel /o/ as in the word "knoll."
  - Respiratory support, coordination, resonant focus, and soft intensity are also emphasized when instructing the patient.
  - Goals are the same as for Exercise 2.
  - Similar modifications as suggested in Exercise 2 can be utilized.
- **Exercise 4: Power.** The clinician explains, models, and then elicits a sustained /o/ vowel as in the word "knoll" for as long as possible at five different target pitches. This results in five separate maximum prolongation productions.
  - Female (and preadolescent males) target pitches are the notes middle C-D-E-F-G (corresponding to approximate frequencies of **262**, **294**, **330**, **350**, and **392 Hz**, respectively).
  - Adult male target pitches are notes C-D-E-F-G below middle C (corresponding to frequencies of **131**, **147**, **165**, **175**, and **196 Hz**, respectively).
  - Respiratory support, coordination, resonant focus, and soft reduced loudness are also emphasized when instructing the patient.
  - Duration goals are the same for Exercise 1, for all five productions (see next section for calculation of goals).
  - Similar modifications for the vowel as suggested in Exercise 2 can be utilized. Additionally, some patients initially lack vocal control precise enough to closely approximate the target frequencies. In these cases, modifications can include producing an initial vowel close to the habitual pitch (e.g., "comfortable pitch") and then subsequent vowels at increasingly higher frequencies.

For exercises 1 (warm-up) and 4 (power), it is possible to set patient-specific goals relative to the individual speaker's physiological capacities. The patient's best vowel duration measurement (e.g., MPT obtained during the voice evaluation, or baseline measurements taken during the first treatment session) can be used as the initial baseline. If the clinician has access to a spirometer, obtaining a measurement of vital capacity (VC) will allow for the calculation of an estimate for expected maximum phonation time. Healthy nondysphonic speakers typically produce vowels with transglottal airflow rates between 100 and 200 mL/s, depending on vocal intensity. While it has been suggested that the lower end of this range may be used to estimate a target sustained vowel duration in both exercises 1 and 4 (e.g., VC/100),[1] this low airflow estimate can lead to inordinately long MPT expectations. We suggest that VC/150 (i.e., use an expected airflow value in the middle of the typically expected airflow range) will result in a more reasonable and attainable MPT for your patient. For example, if a patient's VC is measured at 3,000 mL, dividing this by 150 would derive a target sustained vowel of 20 seconds. This can be used as a benchmark toward which the patient attempts to progress. For exercises 2 (stretch) and 3 (contract), it is also possible to objectively measure frequency production using one of the many available mobile device applications that measure frequency/pitch. Healthy nondysphonic speakers should be able to produce controlled phonation across a wide pitch and frequency range. Extending the number and range of frequencies used in the VFE power exercise can also be both challenging and beneficial for the patient.

In addition to patients manifesting vocal hyperfunction, VFE and modifications of the program have been successfully administered to patients with hypofunction due to glottal incompetence associated with etiologies ranging from unilateral paralysis, atrophy, and presbylaryngis.[17,38,48,49,50] Patients with glottal incompetence often have difficulty engaging the vocal folds at reduced loudness levels. VFE can be modified in these cases by asking the patient to produce vowels at increased loudness.[1] This modification adds an additional stress to the respiratory and laryngeal muscles which potentially facilitates neuromotor adaptation in the form of increased motor unit recruitment during contraction to improve glottal closure.

Daily practice is a foundational element of VFE and patients should measure and log their performance with a tracking schedule each day (e.g., document the duration of Exercises 1 and 4, as well as the frequency of Exercises 2 and 3). This should be reviewed by the clinician with the patient during weekly or biweekly treatment sessions, depending on the treatment schedule (see Appendix 8.1 for a VFE exercise log example). Once a patient meets treatment goals, a tapering program can be established that terminates with Exercise 4 performed with one repetition once per day.[1] Production of Exercise 4 each day after treatment dismissal is thought to facilitate maintenance of the neuromuscular adaptions resulting from treatment.

Patient compliance (adherence) to treatment programs is a significant issue in voice rehabilitation and is one of the leading causes of treatment failure. Issues such as motivation, resistance, and personality characteristics are suspected to influence poor treatment compliance.[10] This can be mitigated by providing external models (e.g., video or audio recordings) of the exercises for home practice, which have been found to improve treatment adherence, self-efficacy beliefs, and outcomes.[9]

Commercial recordings of VFE are available for purchase, or the clinician can utilize custom video or audio recordings which can be stored on the patient's mobile device or computer.

8.8.4 Semioccluded Vocal Tract Exercises

Semioccluded vocal tract (SOVT) exercise programs utilize different techniques to narrow ("semiocclude") and elongate the anterior vocal tract to facilitate physiological changes in vocal fold vibratory characteristics and laryngeal muscle activation. At different fundamental frequencies, the supraglottal pressures generated by narrowing the anterior vocal tract while widening the supraglottal regions act as a force called **inertive reactance**, which influences glottal vibratory cycles and acoustic properties of sound. Inertive reactance acts as a backward directed pressure onto the surface of the of vocal folds, which interacts with (1) air pressure directed from the lungs through the glottis and (2) the stationary column of air in the laryngeal vestibule that is present immediately after the top edge of the vocal fold closes (the closed phase of vibration). The back pressure acts to facilitate separation of the vocal folds (the opening phase) by creating elevated supraglottal and intraglottal pressures. This is also thought to reduce vocal fold impact stress during the subsequent closing phase of vibration.[51,52] Semioccluded vocal tract configurations have the effect of **matching the impedance** to airflow exerted by the sound source (glottis) and sound filter (supraglottal regions), effectively boosting sound intensity in an efficient and economical manner.[53] By augmenting phonation in this way, it is thought that semioccluded vocal tract postures result in phonation with reduced effort and reduce excessive contraction of laryngeal muscles during voice production.

Many of the vocal tract configurations used in voice treatment programs are types of semiocclusions made through lip rounding, which narrows (i.e., semioccludes) the vocal tract to produce an inertive reactance force during the exercise. Lip trills and nasal humming can also be considered examples of SOVT postures. Various techniques have been employed to encourage and achieve voice with semiocclusion of the vocal tract, including phonating through straws and tubes, with the latter also being used while placed in different depths of water.[54,55] Andrade et al studied the effects of various SOVT techniques and suggested that those introducing a secondary vibratory source into the vocal tract via lip trills, tongue trills, or use of LaxVox tubes (35-cm silicone tubes with approximate inner diameter of 10 mm) placed into water (with the bubbling water acting as the secondary source of vibration) resulted in improved physiological and acoustic results.[56]

It has also been demonstrated that smaller diameter straws result in greater back pressures (due to increased inertive reactance) than larger diameter straws. The degree of back pressure when tubes are submerged into water (as with LaxVox tubes) is *influenced by the submerged depth of the straw*, with greater depths resulting in greater back pressures.[56] SOVT techniques are used most frequently to target primary vocal hyperfunction or compensatory hyperfunction (e.g., compensatory strain and effort) secondary to glottal incompetence such as vocal fold paresis.

Titze proposed a program of therapy which incorporates semiocclusive exercises that introduce the greatest degree of inertive reactance first within less natural voicing contexts followed by progression to contexts that offer less inertive reactance but are more naturalistic.[53] Suggestions for progression are as follows, and specific criteria for mastery (e.g., % accurate productions) can be individualized for the patients as they move through the hierarchy:

a) Highly resistant (small diameter) stirring straw (greatest inertive reactance).
b) Less resistant (larger diameter) drinking straw.
c) Bilabial or labiodental fricative.
d) Lip or tongue trill.
e) Nasal consonants.
f) /u/ and /i/ vowels (less inertive reactance).

Specific techniques for implementing this hierarchy include initial stimuli composed of non-speech pitch glides, followed by vocalizations through the straws/tubes with exaggerated intonation patterns as in singing or conversation. As the patient becomes familiar with sensations of less vocal effort and strong frontal resonance, the exercises can then be shaped from SOVT to speech production.[53]

Kapsner-Smith et al recently published results from a randomized-controlled trial demonstrating positive clinical effects of SOVT exercises in speakers with dysphonia.[57] Speakers received treatment once a week for 6 weeks, with treatment technique consisting of voicing tasks through a 14.1-cm-long stirring straw with a 0.4-cm diameter. In each treatment session, patients were asked to complete the following tasks:

• 10 pitch glides (up and back down).
• 10 accent repetitions—exaggerating prosody by creating pitch and loudness "hills" that progressively increase in frequency and intensity (think of a police siren that gets louder and higher in pitch with each sound pulse).
• 10 repetitions of familiar song melodies vocalized through the straw.
• 5 repetitions of reading five-to-ten sentence paragraphs, vocalized through the straw.

The treatment program included home practice where speakers produced each exercise for 1 minute, four different times during the day. Results indicated significant improvement in Voice Handicap Index (VHI) scores and CAPE-V ratings compared to pretreatment measurements, and equivalent clinical outcomes compared to VFE treatment.

Findings from Andrade et al[56] and Kapsner-Smith et al,[57] along with the theory-driven recommendations of Titze, can be used to develop an evidence-based method for administering SOVT exercises as part of a vocal rehabilitation program such as that illustrated in ▶ Fig. 8.5.[53] This program utilizes the four exercises from Kapsner-Smith et al[57] combined with the SOVT hierarchy suggested by Titze.[53] At each semiocclusion level (y-axis in ▶ Fig. 8.5), the patient completes the four exercise sets (x-axis) at a determined level of mastery. Percent correct to determine mastery would be judged by clinician and patient perceptions of production accuracy either during the straw phonation or on voice production immediately after the SOVT exercise. When a patient masters exercises at a specific level of semiocclusion, he or she then moves on to the next level (up the y-axis). As with all voice rehabilitation programs, homework programs would be included to facilitate

mastery and carryover of functional gains. An example of a homework tracking log that a patient can use is provided in Appendix 8.2.

8.9 Manual (Tactile) Circumlaryngeal Therapy

Hands-on manipulation of the larynx has been demonstrated to be an effective treatment for patients with functional voice disorders related to excessive musculoskeletal tension, as is typical in cases of MTD (a form of hyperfunction). Many patients with MTD present with the hyoid and larynx in a habitually elevated position during voice production. This elevated laryngeal positon is thought to negatively influence phonation flexibility by limiting the speaker's ability to manipulate vocal fold length and tension, as well as adversely influence vocal fold vibratory dynamics. Aronson and Bless noted that, if laryngeal muscle "cramping" is a cause of dysphonia, gentle massage can relax and lower the larynx, as well as reduce associated pain or discomfort.[5] They further described a manual approach for assessing laryngeal musculoskeletal tension by palpating the laryngeal region and unloading excessive muscle activity through massage and manipulation of the larynx. This method of tactile laryngeal manipulation has also been referred to as one form of **digital manipulation**, and a video example is provided in **Video 8.3**.[2]

Manual circumlaryngeal therapy (MCT) is a laryngeal musculoskeletal treatment which has been developed beyond Aronson's original techniques by Roy et al as a treatment program for patients with MTD.[58,59,60] The administration of MCT typically follows positive confirmation of excessive laryngeal tension through palpation during the voice evaluation. Roy has described three techniques, sometimes referred to as **laryngeal reposturing** that can be used alone or in conjunction with circumlaryngeal massage.[59] Each technique is applied while the patient produces sustained vowels (e.g., /u/), with the goal of briefly altering habitual muscular hyperfunction and establishing an improved voice quality which can then be shaped into new, effective motor patterns for voice production. A description of each is as follows:

• **Laryngeal pushback**: The clinician can support the patient's head with one hand placed on the base of the skull. With the free hand, the clinician locates the hyoid bone, placing the thumb on one greater cornu and the index and/or middle finger on the other greater cornu. As the patient sustains a vowel (they can be prompted with "comfortable pitch and loudness"), the clinician applies inward (medial) pressure at a slightly downward angle. The region of influence should include the hyoid bone, base of tongue (which is connected to the hyoid), and the thyrohyoid space (located immediately below the hyoid).

  ○ The degree of pressure applied might vary from patient to patient depending on their comfort level and the degree of muscular tension present. A useful starting guide is to exert enough pressure so that tip of the thumbnail blanches.[60] To effect change, there must be enough pressure applied to influence muscular activity. Therefore, the clinician must avoid being timid when administering this technique.

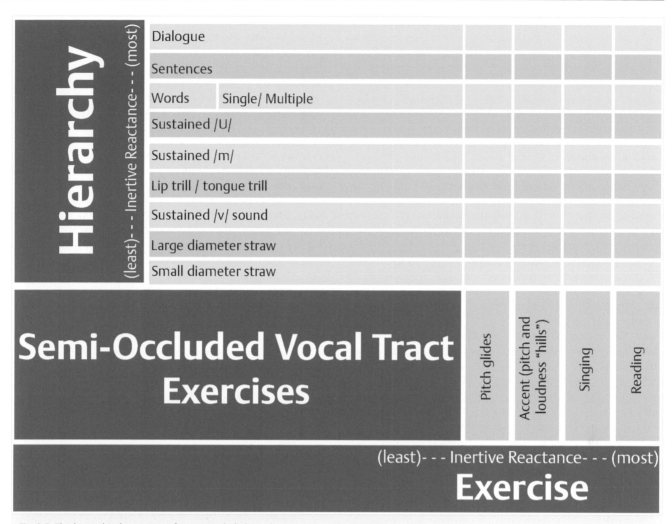

Fig. 8.5 The hierarchical structure of a semioccluded vocal tract treatment program.

○ The patient should be prompted to take breaths and repeat sustained vocalizations for four or five seconds consecutively. The clinician will release the manual pressure and then continue repeating the laryngeal pushback, experimenting with different degrees and angles of pressure. The clinician listens to the patient's voice quality throughout this process, and when a positive change occurs, the clinician notes the pressure and angle at which they are eliciting the improvement. The patient is also made aware of the change and the pushback is repeated multiple times.

○ As the improved voice quality becomes more consistent, the clinician should begin to release pressure as the patient vocalizes, with the goal of maintaining the improved voice without pressure. At this point, the clinician may want to introduce negative practice so that the patient can begin to differentiate improved vs. hyperfunctional modes of laryngeal motor control. As the improved voice stabilizes, the clinician elicits different vowels and words, progressing to **phrases**, sentences, and conversation. Throughout this process, if improved voice quality does not stabilize or if the patient is unable to release the excessive laryngeal tension, other reposturing techniques should be attempted and can be alternated with the laryngeal pushback.

• **Hyoid pulldown**: Supporting the patient's head in the same manner as above, the clinician places his or her free hand so that the thumb and fingers are positioned over the superior border of the hyoid bone. The clinician then exerts downward pressure onto the larynx as the patient sustains vowels. This traction should have the effect of manually lowering the larynx. This typically results in a lowering of pitch which can be brought to the patient's attention. As the patient continues to vocalize, the clinician releases and then re-exerts pressure, following a similar progression as described earlier in laryngeal pushback.

• **Combination (pushback + pulldown):** This technique combines the laryngeal pushback and hyoid pulldown. With the patient's head supported, the clinician applies inward pressure along with downward traction to the superior border of the thyroid cartilage. This has the effect of displacing the thyroid posteriorly while moving it inferiorly. Roy has suggested that the combination technique can be effective for patients with glottal incompetence related to hyperfunction.[59]

It can be useful to combine **circumlaryngeal massage** with laryngeal reposturing techniques to maximize the potential for releasing excessive laryngeal musculoskeletal tension. The goal of laryngeal massage is the same as reposturing, in that the clinician applies pressure and manipulates the laryngeal tissue in order to "unload" hyperfunctional muscle activity and elicit a more normal and efficient voice. Aronson and Bless described a technique for laryngeal massage which can be utilized diagnostically or as a treatment technique.[5] Procedural aspects of the technique are as follows (and demonstrated in **Video 8.3**):

- The clinician first *locates the hyoid bone*. A useful strategy is to first palpate the thyroid cartilage centrally and find the thyroid notch. The notch is readily sensed in most patients with exception to those who have excessive neck tissue or fibrosis from scar or radiation. Once the notch is located, the clinician can place a finger immediately above, which will locate the thyrohyoid space. The body of the hyoid bone will be palpated by rotating a finger off the thyroid cartilage to a location above the thyrohyoid space.
- With the hyoid body located the clinician places a thumb and finger(s) on either side so that they encircle the greater cornu, near their tips.
- The clinician begins to apply light pressure in a circular motion. The patient is asked to report any discomfort or pain, and their facial and body reactions to the massage should be monitored. The patient can be prompted to take comfortable breaths and sustain a low intensity vowel, such as /u/. The clinician and patient listen to the quality of this sound to determine if any improvements occur.
- The clinician lowers his or her fingers into the thyrohyoid space, continuing to apply pressure in a circular motion. The tissue should be manipulated centrally beginning at the thyroid notch and moving laterally toward the undersurface of the greater cornu of the thyroid. The clinician should continue to knead this space and attempt to facilitate a greater distance between the thyroid cartilage and hyoid bone. The patient is asked to report discomfort or pain throughout the procedure, and prompted to continue vocalizing during the manipulation.
- The clinician moves his or her fingers to the lateral plates of the thyroid cartilage near the sternocleidomastoid muscles and continues to apply pressure in a circular motion, asking the patient to report pain or discomfort while they continue to vocalize.
- While applying circular pressure, the clinician can begin to apply downward traction to displace the larynx inferiorly. This displacement can be palpated by moving a finger into the thyrohyoid space to check for expansion. With the fingers remaining on the lateral margins of the thyroid cartilage, the clinician can gently attempt to move the larynx laterally, from side to side. Resistance to this passive manipulation is a sign of laryngeal tension, and a goal of continued massage is to release this tension to increase flexibility of laryngeal movement. The patient is prompted to continue vocalizing as the manipulation progresses.

The process of laryngeal reposturing and/or circumlaryngeal massage can take time to effect change in neuromuscular hyperfunction. When a positive response is realized in the form of improved voice quality and reports of reduced vocal effort from the patient, the improved voice should be shaped from vowels to words with subsequent removal of the manual pressure. Following this the clinician should prompt **phrases**, sentences, and conversation from the patient using the new motor behaviors. Clinicians should not be surprised if positive responses to the treatment take upward of 30 minutes (or more) in some patients. While persistence is required, the clinician should also be able to adapt to patient responses and, if improvement in voice quality is unlikely with circumlaryngeal treatment, they should move on to a different approach (see any of the techniques described earlier).

Mathieson et al have described in detail a version of manual treatment called **laryngeal manual therapy** (LMT).[61] The technique of LMT focuses initially on the sternocleidomastoid and submandibular region as opposed to the thyrohyoid space and thyroid cartilage. MCT is usually applied with the clinician positioned to the side or in front of the patient, while LMT is applied with the clinician standing behind the patient.[61] LMT also differs from MCT in other ways, such as the use of both hands to manipulate the laryngeal region, and no prompts for vocalization while the manipulation is taking place.[62] Mathieson et al demonstrated significant effects of the LMT technique on acoustic measures and patient perceptions of discomfort in 10 speakers diagnosed with MTD, who each received one 45-minute treatment session.[61] The substantial improvement in vocal abilities and perceptions of vocal effort noted by Mathieson et al after only 45 minutes of treatment demonstrate the utility of laryngeal manual manipulation in patients with MTD.

8.10 Direct Interventions: Comprehensive Voice Treatment Programs for Vocal Hypofunction

Vocal hypofunction refers to a state of vocal fold muscular hypokinesia manifested by glottal incompetence. The most salient perceptual effects of glottal incompetence are a **breathy voice quality** and **reduced vocal loudness**. However, the clinician should note that many patients with vocal hypofunction develop a secondary hyperfunctional component to compensate for the underlying primary impairment. They do this by recruiting any or all residual motor units of the intrinsic and extrinsic laryngeal muscles. Strain, roughness, hoarseness, and fatigue are the common results, and many of the voice treatment programs noted in the previous section dealing with hyperfunctional voice can be adapted to address both compensatory hyperfunction as well as the underlying hypofunction.

Some voice treatments have been developed specifically for hypofunction caused by muscular weakness, deconditioning, atrophy, or reduced movement. These physiological impairments are most often associated with conditions such as vocal fold paresis/paralysis, presbylaryngis, and the hypokinetic dysarthria of Parkinson's disease. Voice treatment programs targeting hypofunction share a set of focused exercise training principles, most notably *specificity* and *overload*. These programs are specific to phonation by requiring varied vocal utterances as part of the treatment program, and they can provide an overload in the form of maximum effort to the point of muscular **fatigue** or in the form of **resistance** (e.g., see subsequent discussion on expiratory muscle strength training). Treatments applied specifically to vocal hypofunction will be described later. This is not an exhaustive list, and we have attempted to organize these based on those treatments with at least minimal well-designed research evidence to support their effectiveness.

8.10.1 LSVT-LOUD: The Lee Silverman Voice Treatment

LSVT LOUD is an intensive voice treatment program originally developed for vocal hypofunction associated with Parkinson's disease (Lee Silverman is the name of a former patient who first received the treatment). The technique associated with LSVT LOUD utilizes exercises requiring increased vocal intensity by prompting the patient to produce loud phonation with conscious awareness of effort in various speaking contexts.[63] LSVT LOUD is a commercial product requiring training and certification before a clinician can provide the technique using the LSVT brand.

The classic hierarchy of the LSVT protocol includes three exercises: (1) maximum duration of sustained phonation, produced with loud phonation; (2) fundamental frequency range exercises, produced with loud phonation; and (3) speech loudness exercises (**phrases**/sentences), produced with loud phonation. Over the course of the treatment program, speech stimuli progress from single words and **phrases** to sentences, paragraphs, and finally conversational speech. Multiple repetitions of each exercise are completed during a treatment session, and exercises are repeated during treatment and nontreatment days. The full LSVT LOUD program requires 16 treatment sessions spread out over 4 consecutive weeks of therapy. Since the original program was developed, several modifications have been implemented with positive clinical outcomes.[64,65]

LSVT LOUD is structured, intensive, and supported by a strong base of research evidence.[19,63,66,67] The protocol is grounded in essential concepts, including (**1**) a conscious focus on "thinking loud" during voice production, (**2**) high motor effort levels, (**3**) an intensive treatment regime, (**4**) targeted calibration of sensory and motor systems, and (**5**) quantification of performance and progress. Quantification is achieved by measurement of vowel duration, frequency range, and/or speech intensity for each repetition of the different exercises. The clinical outcomes achieved with LSVT may be related to the effect of the treatment on impairments that occur in addition to muscular rigidity. These beneficial effects include improvements in amplitude scaling of vocal effort, internal cueing of movement performance, movement planning and programming, and sensory processing.[63] An example of the application of LSVT is demonstrated in **Video 8.4**.

8.10.2 Phonation Resistance Training Exercises

A number of treatment programs have been adapted from the structure and techniques of LSVT, which include **Phonation Resistance Training Exercises** (PhoRTE—pronounced "four-tay" as in the Italian word *forte*, meaning strong). Preliminary efficacy of PhoRTE was demonstrated by Ziegler et al in a case series of five speakers diagnosed with presbyphonia.[68] The PhoRTE treatment program consists of exercise sets similar to LSVT, as follows:

- Loud maximum sustained phonation on /a/.
- Loud ascending and descending pitch glides over the entire pitch range on /a/.
- Participant-specific functional **phrases** using a loud and high pitch voice.
- **Phrases** from Exercise 3 in a loud and low pitch voice.

In the study of Ziegler et al, participants received once-weekly treatment sessions over 4 weeks and completed two repetitions of each exercise as daily homework. Posttreatment outcomes included significant improvements in perceived voice-related quality of life and vocal effort.[68] This study also compared PhoRTE to VFE in a similar group of speakers with presbylaryngis and found comparable results. Both treatment groups demonstrated improved voice outcomes compared to a nontreatment control group.

The authors of PhoRTE noted differences in the program compared to the LSVT protocol. These included fewer treatment sessions, requirements for pitch alterations during functional **phrases** (repetitions of loud with high pitch and loud with low pitch), and fewer repetitions of exercises during home practice.[68] Another substantial difference is that PhoRTE is not a commercial product requiring certification or annual maintenance training. Otherwise the structure and progression of the treatment program is very similar to LSVT, and conceptually the PhoRTE exercises are likely influencing similar motor and sensory pathways that research has demonstrated LSVT effects in many patients receiving the treatment.

8.10.3 SPEAK OUT!

Another voice treatment program based on the LSVT model is SPEAK OUT!. This program targets high-intensity phonation with patient cues to speak with "intent." The concept of "intent" is explained as a cognitive focus on the sounds and words being produced, so that attention is allocated to the actual words and **phrases**.[2] It shares a similar structure to LSVT in that it is intensive by requiring multiple sessions each week, and each treatment session is structured in the same way. Implementation of SPEAK OUT! also requires certification through workshop training. The program requires daily exercises targeting increased vocal loudness with a focus on speaking with intent during the following tasks: (**1**) high-intensity warm-up vocalizations, (**2**) high-intensity sustained vowel production, (**3**) high-intensity pitch glides, (**4**) high-intensity counting, (**5**) high-intensity reading, and (**6**) high-intensity cognitive exercises requiring patients to complete carrier **phrases** with novel sentences and conversational speech.

Each treatment session of SPEAK OUT! includes approximately 45 minutes of exercises, and patients will complete homework exercises each day using a guidebook. Unlike the original LSVT protocol, patients are not required to complete 16 sessions (they may be dismissed from therapy upon meeting goals earlier). One preliminary study demonstrated positive clinical effects of SPEAK OUT! characterized by increased vocal intensity in a case series of six speakers with Parkinson's disease.[69] Another retrospective report found similar clinical effects in a group of 72 PD speakers.[70]

8.11 Special Issues in Voice Treatment

8.11.1 Treatment for Paradoxical Vocal Fold Motion and Chronic Cough

Paradoxical vocal fold motion (PVFM), also known as vocal cord dysfunction (VCD), is manifested by vocal fold adduction during inspiration, effectively narrowing the airway and making it difficult to breathe. As described in Chapter 2, the underlying cause of the disorder is idiopathic, although it is most likely a multifactorial etiology and has been associated with laryngeal sensory dysfunction.[71] It has been categorized as a spectrum disorder within a larger category of impairments called **episodic laryngeal breathing disorders**.[72] Diagnosis necessitates a thorough case history which should include inquiry about possible onset triggers of PVFM episodes. Although difficult to establish in most patients, exposure to PVFM triggers while viewing the larynx during endoscopy can provide visual confirmation of the suspected impairment. Triggers become a central focus of treatment where goals center on awareness of physical reactions and conscious neuromotor control over respiratory and laryngeal subsystems in response to the inciting factors.

While PVFM triggers are specific to individuals (e.g., they can include physiological exertion, psychological reactions, reflux, allergies, postnasal drip, exposure to certain odors, and coughing episodes), a core treatment technique can be effective for a wide range of patients. While variations in treatment techniques for PVFM have been published and/or implemented clinically, many treatments center on at least three major goals (1) education and identification of triggers, (2) awareness of the specific physiological reactions to triggers, and (3) control of breathing cycles immediately before and/or during a PVFM episode. An example of these goals applied in a clinical setting is provided in **Video 8.5**.

- **Education and identification** includes teaching the patient, using language he or she can understand, the physiology of breathing and voice production. Following this, the patient is educated regarding the physiological impairments underlying PVFM episodes—that is, what occurs in the larynx. The clinician and patient then go through a process of discovery specific to triggers that the patient is able to associate with PVFM episodes. The process should include a focus on those that are more commonly reported, including:
  - Physical stress (e.g., exercise).
  - Psychological stress/anxiety.
  - Reflux (the laryngopharyngeal kind).
  - Postnasal drip (e.g., allergies. colds).
  - Environmental triggers (e.g., odors, dust, allergens, smoke).
- **Awareness of physiological reactions** specific to neuromuscular and cognitive reactions to stimuli which elicit PVFM episodes and the initial stages of reaction to the triggers. The following reactions are often reported by those experiencing PVFM, and should be explored with the patient along with other possible physiological and cognitive responses:
  - Tightening of respiratory (rib cage and diaphragm) muscles for breathing.
  - Tightening of larynx.
  - Tightening of neck muscles.
  - Tightness in the shoulders.
  - Wheezing (stridor).
  - Shortness of breath.
  - Coughing.
  - Tightness in the throat.
  - Hoarseness.
  - A feeling not being able to breathe.
- **Control of breathing cycles** involves rehabilitating the patient's ability to control respiratory and laryngeal muscles during respiration. There are many different techniques for achieving this goal, and the following is one example of an effective process.
  - **Progressive relaxation**—a process that teaches the patient how to control tension in skeletal muscles, which can assist in preventing or minimizing PVFM episodes.
    - The clinician prompts the patient to purposely increase muscle tension in an isolated muscle or muscle group, such as the hand or forearm.
    - The clinician prompts the patient take a deep, easy breath in and tense the muscle as much as possible (e.g., squeeze) for about 4 or 5 seconds (e.g., if focusing on the hand, the patient can make a fist as tightly as possible). The clinician monitors for tension in other muscle groups and works with the patient to isolate tension to the target muscle only.
    - It can be helpful to ask the patient to hold his/her breath while he/she is tensing the muscle.
    - The patient is asked to focus on the perception of tension in that muscle during the contraction.
    - After 4 or 5 seconds, the patient is asked to exhale and quickly relax the target muscle.
    - The clinician prompts the patient to focus on the perception of relaxation in the target muscle.
    - The clinician then prompts the patient to describe their perceptions of tension and contrast that with relaxation.
    - The process is repeated in the same muscle.
    - The process then moves to a different muscle group, and should continue so that multiple muscles in different parts of the body are included. Among these should include the neck muscles and chest wall muscles.
    - The goal is for the patient to be able to (**1**) purposely increase and decrease tension in selected muscles and (**2**) describe the perception of elevated tension and appropriate relaxation in those muscles. Attainment of these goals translates to the patient manifesting neuromotor control over skeletal muscle tension and cognitive awareness of tension levels in different muscle groups.
  - **Open throat (relaxed throat) breathing** is a respiratory strategy that facilitates breathing cycles (inspiration/expiration) completed with relaxed oral and laryngeal muscles. This breathing method can be effective for controlling respiratory and laryngeal muscles at the onset or during PVFM episodes.
    - The clinician prompts the patient to inhale slowly through the nose for 3 or 4 seconds, with a relaxed throat. Prompts for a relaxed throat can (1) allow the tongue to lie on the floor of the mouth, (2) gently close the lips, (3) allow the jaw to relax, and (4) when inhaling think as if they were yawning.

– The clinician then prompts the patient to exhale slowly through pursed lips or while prolonging an unvoiced fricative such as /s/, /sh/ or /f/.

– The clinician monitors the patient to ensure he or she is not breath holding prior to exhalation.

– The patient repeats this process multiple times until they demonstrate mastery.

The patient should be given homework exercises to establish carryover of mastery. An example could include 10 to 20 open throat breath repetitions, completed five different times per day (e.g., five sets spread out across a day). The patient is instructed that focused relaxation and open throat breathing are the strategies to utilize at the first sign of a PVFM episode.

An additional strategy to mitigate the duration of severity of a PVFM is to sniff briskly, and then exhale through pursed lips (or unvoiced /s/, /f/), and repeat. The sniff is generally accompanied by rapid and wide abduction during inspiration. Teaching the patient to slow down their breathing rate can be another effective strategy for preventing or minimizing PVFM episodes. For exercise-induced PVFM, the onset of an episode might necessitate stopping the exercise until the symptoms resolve. However, if the clinician can work with the patient during exercise performance, it is possible to learn similar neuromuscular control techniques during performance so that the patient can continue competition.

Chronic cough can occur alone or with PVFM and, in some patients, serves as a trigger for PVFM episodes.[73] Cough is also a phonotraumatic behavior that can cause chronic dysphonia and mid-membranous lesions.[74] As described in Chapter 2, chronic cough is defined as consistent cough present for more than 8 weeks. Vertigan and Gibson have published recommendations for a program of cough control intervention administered by SLPs. The approach is detailed in Appendix 8.3 and is further described in the study of Vertigan et al.[71] It consists of four components:

1. Education.
2. Cough control technique.
3. Vocal hygiene training.
4. Psychoeducational counseling.

Positive clinical outcomes for this program have been reported in a randomized clinical trial. Vertigan et al reported findings from experimental and control cohorts, noting that patients treated with the cough control intervention manifested improvements in breathing, cough, voice, and upper airway symptom scores in addition to acoustic measures of dysphonic severity compared to a control group.[75] Positive clinical outcomes have also been reported in additional studies which have utilized a similar technique focusing on respiratory training and cough control.[76,77]

8.11.2 Professional Voice Users

Professional voice users comprise individuals whose **professional career and livelihood are *dependent* on voice production**. Included within this category are vocal performers who utilize their voice for artistic expression and/or entertainment (this would include singers, actors, vocal percussionists, etc.), teachers, clergy, lawyers, auctioneers, and telemarketers, to name a few. Teachers and singers comprise the bulk of professional voice users who seek treatment for voice impairments.[78] The voice treatment techniques described earlier are usually appropriate when habilitating or rehabilitating the professional voice user. However, career requirements usually necessitate modifications to vocal hygiene recommendations and home practice schedules because these individuals usually have to continue speaking and/or singing on a regular basis to earn income.

It should be noted that while voice therapists with a background in professional voice training (singing pedagogy) may work with singers on their performance or artistic technique, **a background as a trained singer *is not a requirement* to provide services as a voice therapist/vocologist to singers or other professional voice users**. A strong foundation of knowledge and skills specific to anatomy and physiology, voice impairment, diagnostic processes, and rehabilitation options along with clinical experience will enable SLPs to focus their clinical practice on voice-impaired populations, including different types of vocal performers. When working with singers, **those without a trained singing background will need to collaborate with the singing teacher when technique and/or performance issues are thought to contribute to the existing problem**. Many singers, for example, develop voice impairments due to behaviors unrelated to singing performance. Most of the comprehensive voice treatment approaches discussed earlier in this chapter are appropriate for singers and other professional voice users when addressing impairments related to the speaking voice. In many cases, the reduction in physiological impairment and disability from these treatments indirectly carryover into the singing voice. ASHA has provided guidance on the curriculum recommendations that provide important foundational knowledge and skills for working with voice-impaired populations, including vocal performers.[79]

Professional and amateur singers are often more aware of the sound and feel of their voice than other clinical populations. Because of this, they may report symptoms which are difficult for the clinician to perceive through auditory-perceptual analyses without additional vocally demanding tasks or observation of performance examples. These are cases where acoustic and/or aerodynamic analyses can contribute to the diagnostic process in a very meaningful way, as these measures will often reveal subtle and/or intermittent changes in vocal function that the ear might miss during initial perceptual judgements.[80] At the same time, singers can be skilled at compensating for impairment in such a way that they are unaware of an existing physical injury to the vocal folds, and only seek treatment when the injury begins to affect performance.[81]

Common signs and symptoms reported by amateur and professional singers include (**1**) vocal fatigue, (**2**) loss of pitch range—usually in the high notes, (**3**) excessive air or breathiness in the voice—usually in the higher notes, and (**4**) vocal strain or excessive effort during performance. It is also important to understand that many singers have a strong emotional attachment to their voice, and vocal impairments can affect their psyche in ways that are different from nonsingers. The professional singer, as with other professional voice users, is dependent on his or her singing voice for earning income but is also connected to his or her voice as an instrument of emotional and artistic expression. These various physical and psychological issues are usually reflected in the elevated scores obtained from self-perceived handicap assessments, and the interrelationship of these factors should be taken into consideration when evaluating and treating the professional or amateur singer.[82]

Unique tools have been developed for evaluation purposes specific to the singing voice, including the **Singing Voice Handicap Index** and the **Modern Singing Handicap Index**.[82,83] Additional history information is also recommended when evaluating singers so that treatment can address all potential factors related to the voice disorder. This information can include specifics on (**1**) singing styles (e.g., genre), (**2**) current or past vocal training, (**3**) practice schedules, (**4**) performance schedules, and (**5**) performance environment. Most vocal impairments experienced by singers and other professional voice users are related to hyperfunction, phonotrauma, and poor vocal hygiene, which can be addressed with many of the previously described voice treatment techniques.

A useful tool for voice therapists working with singers is a keyboard or other device (e.g., tone producing computer program or handheld pitch pipe) which can be used to model different musical notes. The clinician should note specific regions of the pitch range that may present difficulty for a speaker or singer (e.g., pitches that are close to the transition between modal and falsetto register are often regions of poor vocal control and possible hyperfunction for the untrained singer). ▶ Fig. 8.6 illustrates how musical notes are organized on a typical piano keyboard, with corresponding frequencies associated with the different semitones (i.e., musical note equivalents). An example of a voice treatment session with a singer provided by a singing voice specialist is demonstrated in **Video 8.6**.

8.11.3 Transgender Voice Issues

The word "transgender" is an umbrella term referring to any of the following individuals: **trans men** (born female but identifies as male), **trans women** (born male but identifies as female), or **transsexual** (trans man or trans woman who seek to permanently transition to the gender they identify with). Although the labeling of transgender individuals with a psychiatric condition is a controversial issue, the aforementioned categories are currently classified under the term "gender dysphoria," a psychiatric diagnosis in the Diagnostic and Statistical Manual of Mental Disorders (DSM-V). Some argue that labeling all trans people as manifesting a mental illness is not only wrong and uninformed but also potentially detrimental to the individual.[84] Those supporting this inclusion in the DSM note the necessity for health insurance coverage and legal protection from discrimination.

Transgender people often seek treatment to habilitate voice quality and/or vocal function and better approximate the gender to which they identify. Unfortunately, many academic programs do not provide adequate training opportunities with these individuals, as evidenced by reports that many practicing clinicians do not feel they have adequate knowledge and skills to provide clinical services to transgender people.[84] Even though transgender people represent a low incidence subset of treatment-seeking populations, SLPs can provide services which facilitate the functional voice goals of these individuals.

The most common transgender groups seeking voice treatment are trans women and male-to-female transsexuals (MFTs).

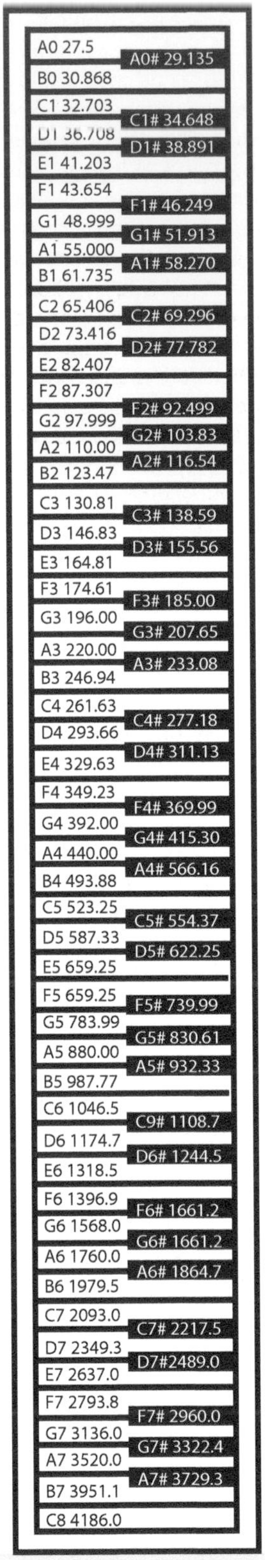

Note	Freq	Sharp	Freq
A0	27.5	A0#	29.135
B0	30.868		
C1	32.703	C1#	34.648
D1	36.708	D1#	38.891
E1	41.203		
F1	43.654	F1#	46.249
G1	48.999	G1#	51.913
A1	55.000	A1#	58.270
B1	61.735		
C2	65.406	C2#	69.296
D2	73.416	D2#	77.782
E2	82.407		
F2	87.307	F2#	92.499
G2	97.999	G2#	103.83
A2	110.00	A2#	116.54
B2	123.47		
C3	130.81	C3#	138.59
D3	146.83	D3#	155.56
E3	164.81		
F3	174.61	F3#	185.00
G3	196.00	G3#	207.65
A3	220.00	A3#	233.08
B3	246.94		
C4	261.63	C4#	277.18
D4	293.66	D4#	311.13
E4	329.63		
F4	349.23	F4#	369.99
G4	392.00	G4#	415.30
A4	440.00	A4#	566.16
B4	493.88		
C5	523.25	C5#	554.37
D5	587.33	D5#	622.25
E5	659.25		
F5	659.25	F5#	739.99
G5	783.99	G5#	830.61
A5	880.00	A5#	932.33
B5	987.77		
C6	1046.5	C9#	1108.7
D6	1174.7	D6#	1244.5
E6	1318.5		
F6	1396.9	F6#	1661.2
G6	1568.0	G6#	1661.2
A6	1760.0	A6#	1864.7
B6	1979.5		
C7	2093.0	C7#	2217.5
D7	2349.3	D7#2489.0	
E7	2637.0		
F7	2793.8	F7#	2960.0
G7	3136.0	G7#	3322.4
A7	3520.0	A7#	3729.3
B7	3951.1		
C8	4186.0		

Fig. 8.6 Notes on a typical piano/synthesizer keyboard. Each octave along the keyboard corresponds to whole notes C–D–E–F–G–A–B, with half notes (sharps/flats) located between C–D, D–E, F–G, G–A, and A–B. This results in 12 different notes, or semitones, within any octave. It is useful to identify (and mark) middle C on the keyboard, which corresponds to the C note in the fourth octave and a frequency of 261 Hz. A number of vocal exercises, including VFE, use this note as a reference.

An overarching goal for these individuals is to pass (i.e., be perceived by others) as female, not only visually but also via auditory-perception. A number of speech and voice characteristics can influence the perception of female voice and are valid treatment targets, including the modification of **vocal pitch and F$_0$** (higher), **voice quality** (i.e., subtle breathiness), **prosody, articulation** (resonance via lip spreading and forward tongue position), and **vocabulary**, among others.[85,86,87,88] For visual cues of femininity, nonverbal targets can include (**1**) greater maintenance of eye contact during conversation, (**2**) more fluid hand gestures, (**3**) greater variation of facial expressions, and (**4**) feminine posture.[88] Among voice characteristics, the greatest concern for MFT is often vocal pitch/F$_0$. While transgender female-to-male vocal F$_0$ can be altered through hormone supplementation, the voice of MFT transsexuals does not substantially change secondary to treatment with feminizing hormones which facilitate development of other female characteristics.[89,90]

Treatment targets specific to vocal pitch/ F$_0$ and voice quality for MFT include consistent production of connected speech with an average F$_0$ at or above 180 Hz in the context of a subtle breathy voice quality.[87] Speakers can also influence resonance so that formant frequencies approximate those of biological females by shaping the oral cavity through lip spreading and forward tongue position.[88] When voice treatment is not effective for habilitating vocal pitch/F$_0$ to the needs of the individual, there are surgical alternatives which have been shown to permanently increase vocal pitch and frequency. Specifically, laryngeal framework surgery in the form of cricothyroid approximation has been successful for increasing vocal F$_0$ toward expected biological female ranges.[91,92]

8.11.4 Childhood Voice Issues

Voice disorders in children are common, with estimates of dysphonia prevalence in school-age children ranging from 6 to 9%.[93,94] Children with vocal impairments often experience midmembranous lesions, which may be related to the immature development of the vocal fold layers. Vocal nodules are the most frequent vocal pathology, diagnosed in 25 to 82% of children who seek treatment for voice problems.[95,96,97]

Vocal nodules result from phonotrauma, which in children is often associated with inappropriate vocal behaviors such as shouting, loud talking, vocal noises, and excessive throat clearing.[1] As with all cases of vocal nodules, initial treatment should always be conservative. There are reasons for this which are similar for children and adults, including (**1**) the prognosis for elimination of vocal nodules is favorable, especially if they are not long-standing, and (**2**) the underlying etiology of the impairment (vocal behaviors) can be directly targeted. Another reason why treatment for nodules in children should be conservative is that some children, even without voice therapy, will change vocal behaviors after puberty such that nodules gradually reside. This natural resolution has been found in 35 to 45% of children assessed prior to and after the onset of puberty.[98,99] For the remaining children, however, nodules remain a problem and can continue to affect communication, social interactions, and academic participation.[23]

Vocal nodules occur more frequently in boys than in girls, although at postpuberty nodules are more likely to remain chronic in females.[97,99,100] SLPs treating children with voice disorders need to consider their unique personality characteristics. For example, Roy et al found that children with vocal nodules tended to be rated more frequently as extroverts compared to their peers without vocal nodules.[101] The personality traits of children with vocal nodules are associated with excessive vocal use, but it is also important to realize that children with voice disorders experience negative social and emotional consequences and can be concerned about their problems, especially older children.[102] In addition, Hersan and Behlau noted the following special considerations when administering voice treatment to children[103]:

- Young children are not always aware of the nature of their problem and some children do not identify their voice as "abnormal."
- Although an adult may be able to project that an improvement in voice production may lead to increased satisfaction in personal or occupational life, a child may not make the same connection.
- It is not always easy to persuade a child to remember proper ways of voice production.
- Cause–effect relationships should be explicitly applied to situations that are concrete and meaningful to the child.
- Children of different ages manifest different maturity levels.
- Many children need extra motivation for carrying-over lessons learned in therapy—practice activities outside of the therapy room should be fun and involve others.
- Parental/caregiver involvement is important to facilitate success.

Children are different from adults, both physiologically and psychologically. As a result, several treatment approaches specific to children have been developed. While older children who demonstrate motivation and treatment compliance can be effectively treated with any of the techniques previously described in this chapter, some techniques and programs have considered the preferences and learning styles of younger children. One example is the **Boone Voice Program for Children**. This program consists of assessment, education, and treatment materials developed to engage younger children in the rehabilitation process. Among the treatment techniques include frontal focus, changing loudness, and utilization of the chewing method. These techniques are employed in games or play-based contexts to facilitate the child's interest and motivation.

Voice treatments utilized for disorders in adults can also be applied or adapted to children. Stone and Casteel reported on the application of SnF for functional dysphonia in children and further described its administration in a detailed case study.[1,26] Stemple et al also reported on the application of VFEs to a child with vocal hyperfunction.[1] Wilson described a rule-based intervention program which considers the learning styles of younger males and females.[94] This 10-stage approach is centered on the development of "rules" to eliminate or reduce phonotraumatic behaviors and/or inappropriate vocal behaviors (e.g., in children common behaviors include inappropriate respiratory support, hard glottal attacks, excessive muscle tension, and speaking too loud). For each target behavior, rules are established with the child and then addressed in a hierarchical structure, using various methods to teach appropriate use of the rules, including different facilitative techniques. The hierarchy is as follows:

1. Explain the voice rule (e.g., "use a soft vocal loudness").
2. Make child aware of inappropriate use of the rule in others.
3. Make child aware of appropriate use of the rule in others.

4. Make child aware of inappropriate use in the child.
5. Make child aware of appropriate use in the child.
6. Make child aware of where child uses voice inappropriately.
7. Make child aware of where child uses voice appropriately.
8. Work with children so that they are able to follow the rule some of the time (e.g., one or two situational contexts).
9. Work with children so that they are able to follow the rule most of the time (e.g., a majority of situational contexts).
10. Work with children so that they are able to follow the rule always.

There are several strategies that clinicians can employ when utilizing this hierarchical approach, including video modeling and role playing to demonstrate appropriate and inappropriate adherence to the different voice rules (i.e., for stages 2–5). Later stages in the hierarchy also require the child to intentionally focus on how and when they violate the rule, which can engage the child in the process. At stage 8 of this hierarchy, one or two situations where inappropriate use of a rule occurs are selected as targets, and the focus is on changing behavior during those situations. Self-assessed observations in the form of tallying violations/adherence to voice rules are another strategy that can establish child engagement with the rehabilitation process. Older children can tally their own violations of the different rules, but for younger children the clinician may need to employ the assistance of teachers and parents. When possible, the SLP can also observe a child in these situations and tally behaviors. As the child eliminates the inappropriate behavior, the next stage in the hierarchy is addressed by adding more situational contexts and making criteria for success more stringent (e.g., stages 8–10 require adherence to the rule some of the time, most of the time, and then all of the time).[94]

8.12 Development of Voice Treatment Goals

Regardless of voice treatment orientation, the process of intervention will be guided by the selection of specific approach(s) which address the underlying physiological impairment causing the voice problem. The chosen treatment approach(es) will further inform the treatment goals set for the desired outcomes. Not all treatments are designed to achieve the same outcome, and the clinician must decide which approaches will restore or enhance function while meeting the needs of the patient. Some voice treatments, administered to the right patient with a specific disorder, can be effective in one session. This is not typical, however. In most cases, vocal rehabilitation takes weeks to months before the patient achieves a level of function that meets his or her expectations. Because of this, it is typically appropriate to set long-term and short-term goals that will guide the rehabilitation process.

Long-term and short-term treatment goals are individualized to the specific patient, and are developed to address the specific physiological impairment, activity limitations (handicap), and patient's needs. Long-term goals specify the desired final, functional outcome and are typically broader than short-term goals. Long-term goals also take time—usually over the course of several months—to attain. A common clinical phenomenon is that many patients share similar physiological impairments, among which

include a physiological imbalance in the neuromuscular control of the vocal subsystems.[1] This means that some specific treatment goals are appropriate for a wide range of individuals, including those with hyperfunctional and hypofunctional voice disorders.

The following are examples of long-term treatment goals that have applied to a wide range of clinical populations, and which can be used as a template upon which to build goals more specific to an individual patient. The individual characteristics of the patient will determine the timeframe and specific criteria of the long-term goals.

8.12.1 Long-Term Goals*

- Within 8 weeks, the patient will acquire vocalization skills to meet personal and professional needs while maintaining the health of the true vocal folds.
  - For example, this goal might be appropriate for a professional voice user experiencing MTD.
- Within 8 weeks, the patient will manifest a reduction or elimination of the underlying pathology while improving overall health of the true vocal folds.
  - For example, a patient with a mid-membranous lesion who is a professional voice user but does not want surgical intervention as a primary approach.
- Within 8 weeks, the patient will maximize efficiency of the vocal mechanism through improved neuromuscular control of the vocal subsystems.
  - For example, the patient will be able to produce effective voice without fatigue to meet production and/or performance needs.
- Within 8 weeks, the patient will achieve improved/normal voice quality validated with perceptual and/or acoustic measures.
  - For example, a patient with moderate to severe dysphonia, regardless of diagnosis and etiology.
- Within 8 weeks, the patient will return to vocal activities of daily living with reduction and/or elimination of complaints regarding vocal production.
  - For example, a patient whose physiological impairments result in a vocal handicap characterized by fatigue and/or pain.
- Within 8 weeks, the patient will acquire skills to reduce, avoid exacerbations, and/or eliminate speech breathing difficulties and/or coughing episodes.
  - For example, patients with PVFM or chronic cough.
- Within 8 weeks, the patient will demonstrate generalization of goals in varied speaking contexts during their vocal activities of daily living, as reported by the patient.
  - This goal would be appropriate to target functional carryover of improved vocal function outside of the treatment room. The goal can be made more stringent by requiring reports of generalization accuracy from family members and/or caregivers.

8.12.2 Short-Term Goals*

Short-term goals specify the measurable steps through which successful progression will facilitate achievement of the long-term goals. Short-term goals contain greater specificity than long-term goals, and are modified as the patient meets criteria. A useful model to follow when writing short-term goals is the

SMART framework, which stands for: **s**pecific, **m**easurable, **a**ttainable, **r**ealistic, and **t**imely.[104] The following are examples of short-term treatment goals that have applied to a wide range of clinical populations. Notice that each of these goals contains three essential elements: the **expected behavior**, the **context** in which the behavior will be displayed, and the **criteria** for success. Depending on the prognosis, the stated duration of each short-term goal will be specific to the patient. These goals were developed based on the framework of Kimberly Coker, MS, CCC-SLP.

- Within 2 weeks, the patient will demonstrate an understanding of voice production physiology (the BEHAVIOR) by describing the interaction of the vocal subsystems during phonation (the CONTEXT) with 100% accuracy (the CRITERION).
  - This short-term goal is an example that might be used as part of a rehabilitation plan that includes patient **education**. This goal might be one of the first short-term goals applied as an initial step toward attainment of many of the long-term goals listed above.
- Within 2 weeks, the patient will demonstrate the ability to identify modifications of vocal demands by listing at least three alternatives and/or adjustments to current vocal requirements in 100% of situational contexts (work, home, and social).
  - This is an example of a short-term goal related to the larger goal of establishing **vocal hygiene**.
- Within 3 weeks, the patient will demonstrate implementation of a hydration regimen throughout a full day with 80% compliance across three consecutive sessions/weeks, as self-reported by the patient.
  - This is another example of a short-term goal which might apply to a larger goal of establishing vocal hygiene.
- Within 2 weeks, the patient will eliminate or reduce phonotraumatic behaviors through modification of voice production (replace "voice production" with a specific vocal characteristic, such as loudness, strain, and pitch) demonstrated in the treatment room with 80% success.
  - This is an example of a short-term goal which might apply to numerous treatments designed to reduce or **eliminate phonotraumatic behaviors**.
- Within 4 weeks, the patient will establish volitional control of respiration as evidenced by utilization of diaphragmatic breathing with 80% accuracy during structured speaking tasks.
  - This is an example of a goal related to the larger objective of **rebalancing the physiological subsystems** of voice. Addressing efficient respiratory patterns increases body awareness, reduces tension throughout voice producing mechanism, and produces efficient respiratory support needed for speaking.
- Within 4 weeks, the patient will demonstrate improved voice quality through enhanced coordination of the vocal subsystems in hierarchical speech tasks with 80% accuracy at each level of the hierarchy.
  - This is an example of a goal that might apply to numerous treatments for vocal hyperfunction or hypofunction which are organized around a hierarchical framework (e.g., see sections (Stretch-and-Flow" and Resonant Focus") and seek to achieve **physiological balance**. The goal does not necessitate complete elimination of an impairment (e.g., a polyp or paresis), only improved vocal output as perceived by listeners.

- Within 3 weeks, the patient will exhibit decreased upper body tension during conversation or performance, as evidenced by a reduction in reported symptoms *and* observable signs of hyperkinetic muscular behaviors in 3 consecutive weeks/sessions.
  - This is another example of a goal that might relate to achieving a physiological balance, specifically in the context of hyperfunctional behaviors.
- Within 2 weeks, the patient will utilize open throat breathing and relaxation techniques in the context of physical exertion with 70% accuracy.
  - This is an example of a short-term goal which might apply to a patient with PVFM. The wording "*in the context of physical exertion…*" can be changed to reflect a specific trigger that elicits onsets of paradoxical episodes. As the patient masters the behaviors, the criterion level can be increased.

8.13 Conclusion

The purpose of this chapter has been to provide the voice therapist with an overview of the philosophies and frequently used methods of indirect and direct behavioral voice treatment. It is clear that adequate voice treatment must be based on the necessary prerequisite of a detailed and strong diagnostic hypothesis regarding the underlying physiological problem(s) that have led to the presenting voice disorder. Once the diagnostic hypothesis has been determined, the treatment methods described in this chapter (either by themselves or in conjunction with the pharmaceutical and/or surgical medical treatments previously described) can provide the pathway to improved voice function for our patients.

Case Study

Part 1

Mrs. Lopez is a 34-year-old woman referred for voice therapy subsequent to a diagnosis of primary MTD. She is an elementary school teacher, which means that she is a professional voice user dependent on her voice for income. She has experienced chronic dysphonia for the past 5 months, which began shortly after an upper respiratory infection at the beginning of the school year. She complains of excessive effort and strain when speaking, and vocal fatigue near the end of each work day. In the evaluation report, she did report a history of frequent voice difficulties during the teaching year but, she had made it through each year without needing to see a health professional about her voice. She indicated that the current problem is the longest period of time that dysphonia had remained present. Her goal for voice therapy is to improve her voice quality and stamina, such that she can make it throughout a working day without becoming hoarse and her voice wearing out.

Questions

1. Does the diagnosis of primary muscle tension dysphonia versus secondary muscle tension dysphonia influence the voice treatment choice? Explain your answer.
2. At a physiological level, what would explain a patient's report of vocal strain and vocal fatigue?

3. What relevance does the patient's report of upper respiratory infection have in the context of the current problem?

Part 2

Read the following article:

Roy N, Gray SD, Simon M, Dove H, Corbin-Lewis K, Stemple JC. An evaluation of the effects of two treatment approaches for teachers with voice disorders: a prospective randomized clinical trial. J Speech Lang Hear Res 2001;44(2):286–296.

Questions

1. Based on the evidence from this article, which voice treatment program would you select for Mrs. Lopez? Explain your answer.
2. Describe the framework of vocal function exercises, and the specific exercises which constitute the program.

8.14 Review Questions

1. Which of the following terms refers to the science and practice of voice habilitation?
   a) Speech–language pathology.
   b) Vocology.
   c) Stroboscopy.
   d) Logopedics.
   e) None of the above.
2. Which kinetic motor pattern is associated with muscle tension dysphonia (MTD)?
   a) Hyperkinesia.
   b) Hypokinesia.
   c) Dyskinesia.
   d) Diadochokinesia.
   e) None of the above.
3. Which of the following best defines direct interventions?
   a) Treatments that modify the cognitive, behavioral, psychological, and physical environment in which voicing occurs.
   b) Treatments that modify the specific impairment related to the environmental cause of a disorder.
   c) Treatments that modify vocal behavior through one or more physiological domains.
   d) Treatments aimed at educating patients, parents, or caregivers regarding vocal health and hygiene.
   e) None of the above.
4. Which of the following best defines indirect interventions?
   a) Treatments that modify the cognitive, behavioral, psychological, and physical environment in which voicing occurs.
   b) Treatments that modify the specific impairment related to the environmental cause of a disorder.
   c) Treatments that modify vocal behavior through one or more physiological domains.
   d) Treatments aimed at educating patients, parents, or caregivers regarding vocal health and hygiene.
   e) None of the above.

5. The domains of a vocal hygiene program could include
   a) Rest, ice, elevation, heat.
   b) Heat, hydration, rest, voice practice.
   c) Voice practice, vocal habits, hydration, counseling.
   d) Hydration, respiratory health, vocal habits, antireflux precautions.
   e) All of the above.
6. An organized group of treatments, typically structured in sequence with each other, and administered using one or more delivery methods defines what?
   a) Voice treatment program.
   b) Voice tool.
   c) Voice therapy.
   d) Vocology.
7. Level I of stretch-and-flow voice treatment elicits what behavior from the patient?
   a) A steady flow of unvoiced air without effort through rounded lips, as in a slow, comfortable exhalation.
   b) Voiceless airflow along with slow (stretched out) movements of the articulators, using minimal effort.
   c) Voiced airflow along with slow (stretched out) movements of the articulators.
   d) A normal voice quality with an appropriate rate of speech.
   e) All of the above.
8. Which voice treatment utilizes the conscious perception of vibrotactile sensations in the oral and nasal cavities to reduce excessive laryngeal motor activation during sound production?
   a) Stretch-and-flow.
   b) Resonant therapy.
   c) LSVT LOUD.
   d) Confidential voice.
   e) All of the above.
9. In what way is laryngeal manual therapy (LMT) different from manual circumlaryngeal therapy (MCT)?
   a) Circumlaryngeal massage manipulates the muscles of the laryngeal region.
   b) LMT utilizes the laryngeal pushback.
   c) LMT initially focuses on the sternocleidomastoid and submandibular region.
   d) LMT utilizes the hyoid pulldown.
   e) None of the above.
10. Which of the following voice disorders would Phonation Resistance Training Exercises (PhoRTE) be most appropriate for?
    a) Muscle tension dysphonia.
    b) Mutational falsetto.
    c) Presbylaryngis.
    d) Vocal nodules.
    e) All of the above.
11. Vocal function exercises (VFEs) consist of how many types of exercises in each set?
    a) 3.
    b) 4.
    c) 6.
    d) 10.
    e) 20.

12. What is inertive reactance in relation to voice production?
    a) The aerodynamic force which helps adduct the lower edges of the vocal folds during phonation.
    b) The reinforcement of vibratory amplitude which occurs with increased medial compression.
    c) The reaction of acoustic energy and aerodynamic energy in the subglottal regions.
    d) A backward-directed pressure onto the surface of the vocal folds which occurs when the anterior oral cavity is semioccluded.
    e) None of the above.

13. When performing circumlaryngeal massage, what is the first step?
    a) Knead the lateral margins of the larynx in the vicinity of the sternocleidomastoid.
    b) Locate the hyoid bone.
    c) Apply pressure to the thyrohyoid space.
    d) Apply a downward traction on the thyroid cartilage.
    e) None of the above.

14. On which factors to SLP base treatment selection when working with voice-impaired patients?
    a) The patient's needs and preferences.
    b) The underlying impaired physiology.
    c) The research evidence that supports a specific treatment.
    d) The competency (knowledge and skill) of the clinician.
    e) All of the above.

15. Which domain of direct intervention would the treatments of push/pull exercises, maximum phonation time (MPT), and flow phonation fall under?
    a) Somatosensory.
    b) Vocal function.
    c) Musculoskeletal.
    d) Respiratory.
    e) All of the above.

16. Which domain of direct interventions is circumlaryngeal massage treatment associated with?
    a) Somatosensory.
    b) Vocal function.
    c) Musculoskeletal.
    d) Respiratory.
    e) All of the above.

17. Relative to cough control intervention, which of the following is a specific cough control technique?
    a) Open throat breathing.
    b) Steam inhalation.
    c) Education.
    d) Adequate water intake.
    e) All of the above.

18. What is the approximate prevalence of dysphonia in school-aged children?
    a) 3 to 5%.
    b) 6 to 9%.
    c) 10 to 15%.
    d) 20 to 25%.
    e) 50%.

19. What is another commonly used name for paradoxical vocal fold motion (PVFM)?
    a) Puberphonia.
    b) Muscle tension dysphonia.
    c) Vocal cord dysfunction.
    d) Carcinoma.
    e) None of the above.

20. The second exercise of vocal function exercises (VFE) is called "stretch." What tasks does it require the patient to perform?
    a) Sustain sound for as long as possible at five vocal frequencies (pitches).
    b) Glide from the lowest to the highest vocal frequency.
    c) Glide from the highest to the lowest vocal frequency.
    d) Sustain one vowel for as long as possible at a target pitch.
    e) None of the above.

21. Which voice treatment program was originally developed structured around four weekly sessions for 4 consecutive weeks?
    a) VFE.
    b) RVT.
    c) LSVT.
    d) SOVT.

22. Which of the following voice treatment programs would be appropriate to use as a primary approach for glottal insufficiency?
    a) RVT and frontal focus.
    b) SOVT and PhoRTE.
    c) Chewing and LSVT.
    d) PhoRTE and LSVT.
    e) None of the above.

23. A frequent voice treatment goal established for trans women and male-to-female transsexuals (MFT) is to
    a) Pass as a male based on auditory-perception of their speaking voice.
    b) Pass as a female based on auditory-perception of their speaking voice.
    c) Produce a larger physiological frequency range.
    d) Produce a smaller physiological frequency range.
    e) None of the above.

24. Which of the following would be an appropriate treatment approach for paradoxical vocal fold motion (PVFM)?
    a) RVT.
    b) LSVT.
    c) Open throat breathing.
    d) Digital manipulation.

25. The laryngeal pushback and hyoid pulldown are part of what treatment program?
    a) Vocal function exercises.
    b) Manual circumlaryngeal therapy.
    c) Resonant voice therapy.
    d) Semioccluded vocal tract exercises.
    e) None of the above.

26. A treatment protocol for chronic cough might include:
    a) Education.
    b) Cough control technique.
    c) Vocal hygiene training.
    d) Psychoeducational counseling.
    e) All of the above.

8.15 Answers and Explanations

1. Correct: Vocology (**b**).
   (**b**) Vocology is a term used to denote the science and practice of voice habilitation. Speech–language pathologists who diagnose and treat patients with voice disorders on a regular basis, and some teachers of singing, refer to themselves as "vocologists." (**a**) Speech–language pathology is a profession with the disciple of communication sciences and disorders. (**c**) Stroboscopy is a term used to denote laryngeal imaging via an endoscope paired with a stroboscopic light. (**d**) Logopedics is a term referring to the diagnosis and treatment of speech disorders—it is synonymous with speech–language pathology.

2. Correct: Hyperkinesia (**a**).
   (**a**) Kinetics is the study of movement. Hyperkinesia is a form of excessive laryngeal motor activation and is often referred to as vocal hyperfunction. Vocal hyperfunction is exemplified by MTD, where the impaired physiological balance in the vocal subsystems usually includes excessive activation of intrinsic and extrinsic laryngeal, supralaryngeal, and respiratory muscles. (**b**) Hypokinesia refers to a condition of reduced kinetic activation of muscles, often associated with paresis, paralysis, and presbylaryngis. (**c**) Dyskinesia is a term typically used for voluntary motor activation, as tremors or chorea. (**d**) Diadochokinesis is a term referring to measures of movement speed.

3. Correct: Treatments that modify vocal behavior through one or more physiological domains (**c**).
   (**c**) Direct interventions include treatments that modify vocal behavior through one or more physiological domains including musculoskeletal, respiratory, vocal function, auditory, and somatosensory modification. (**a**) Treatments that modify the cognitive, behavioral, psychological, and physical environment in which voicing occurs are referred to as indirect interventions. (**b**) Treatments focusing on manipulation of environmental causes relate to indirect forms of intervention. (**d**) Treatments aimed at educating patients, parents, or caregivers regarding vocal health and hygiene would fall into the realm of indirect interventions using pedagogy and/or counseling.

4. Correct: Treatments that modify the cognitive, behavioral, psychological, and physical environment in which voicing occurs (**a**).
   (**a**) Indirect interventions are those treatments that modify the cognitive, behavioral, psychological, and physical environment in which voicing occurs. (**b**) Treatments focusing on manipulation of environmental causes relate to direct forms of intervention. (**c**) Indirect interventions are those treatments that modify the cognitive, behavioral, psychological, and physical environment in which voicing occurs. (**d**) Treatments aimed at educating patients, parents, or caregivers regarding vocal health and hygiene would fall into the realm of direct interventions using pedagogy and/or counseling.

5. Correct: Hydration, respiratory health, vocal habits, antireflux precautions (**d**).
   (**d**) Hydration, respiratory health, vocal habits, and antireflux precautions are four domains of a vocal hygiene program which can be administered to most patients with vocal impairments. Although vocal hygiene alone is not sufficient for rehabilitating most vocal impairments, its combination with direct and indirect interventions can reinforce their clinical effects. (**a, b, c**) While many of the terms listed in choices (**a, b, c**) are incorporated into rehabilitation programs, their combination is not typically implemented in clinical voice practice.

6. Correct: Vocology (**d**).
   (**d**) A voice treatment program is an organized group of treatments, typically structured in sequence with each other, and administered using one or more delivery methods. Traditionally, these have been referred to as "eclectic voice therapy." (**b**) A voice tool is a term synonymous with voice treatment, meaning a singular technique, not a comprehensive program. (**c**) Voice therapy is a term synonymous with voice rehabilitation, meaning the process of enhancing or restoring vocal abilities to a desirable (habilitation) or previous (rehabilitation) level of function. (**d**) Vocology refers to the science and practice of voice habilitation.

7. Correct: A steady flow of unvoiced air without effort through rounded lips, as a slow, comfortable exhalation (**a**).
   (**a**) Stretch-and-flow (SnF) is structured as a hierarchy of progressively challenging vocal tasks which initially focus on the respiratory domains, where level I requires voiceless airflow control techniques. Once the patient masters control of unvoiced air flow without any speech articulation, he/she can move on to the next step of the hierarchy. (**a, b, c**) After level I of SnF is mastered, the patient progresses through a hierarchy of increasing skills which progressively increase the degree of vocal fold adduction onto the stream of airflow, including voiceless airflow with slow articulation moving to a breathy voice, and then to a more engaged glottal contact pattern. The program culminates with mastery of coordinated neuromuscular control characterized by phonation in connected speech produced with equilibrium between respiration, phonation, and resonance.

8. Correct: Resonant therapy (**b**).
   (**b**) The perceptual target of RVT is the conscious awareness of focused, oral vibratory sensations in the context of easy phonation. Although the perceptual focus of RVT is on resonance, the physiological requirements for accurate resonant productions require coordination of respiratory, laryngeal, and supralaryngeal muscle. (**a, c, d**) Stretch-and-flow is initially structured with a focus on the respiratory domains with voiceless airflow control techniques. The technique associated with LSVT LOUD utilizes exercises requiring increased vocal intensity by prompting the patient to produce loud phonation with conscious awareness of effort in various

speaking contexts. Confidential voice is a facilitative approach which utilizes low intensity or low impact phonation to minimize phonotrauma.

9. Correct: LMT initially focuses on the sternocleidomastoid and submandibular region (**c**).

(**c**) The technique of LMT focuses initially on the sternocleidomastoid and submandibular region as opposed to the thyrohyoid space and thyroid cartilage. MCT is usually applied with the clinician positioned to the side or in front of the patient, while LMT is applied with the clinician standing behind the patient. LMT also differs from MCT in other ways, such as the use of both hands to manipulate the laryngeal region, and no prompts for vocalization while the manipulation is taking place. (**a, b, d**) Both LMT and MCT manipulate the muscles in the laryngeal region. MCT utilizes the laryngeal pushback and hyoid pulldown, not LMT.

10. Correct: Presbylaryngis (**c**).

(**c**) PhoRTE targets vocal hypofunction, a kinetic category to which presbylaryngis falls. The PhoRTE treatment program consists of exercise sets similar to LSVT. One aim of PhoRTE is increase laryngeal muscle activation to achieve improved glottal closure. (**a, b, d**) Muscle tension dysphonia, mutational falsetto, and vocal nodules fall into the category of vocal hyperfunction. PhoRTE targets increased laryngeal muscle activation, which would be contraindicated in those disorders.

11. Correct: 4 (**b**).

(**b**) The VFE program consists of a four-exercise set which is repeated four times daily, typically two repetitions of the set in the morning and two repetitions in the afternoon. The four different exercises are referred to as warm-up, stretch, contract, and power. (**a, c, d**) The VFE program consists of a four-exercise set. The patient repeats the four different exercises two times each, twice per day, so that a total of four sets are completed per day, two in the morning and two in the afternoon/evening.

12. Correct: A backward-directed pressure onto the surface of the of vocal folds which occurs when the anterior oral cavity is semioccluded (**d**).

(**d**) Inertive reactance acts as a backward-directed pressure onto the surface of the of vocal folds, which interacts with (**a**) air pressure being directed from the lungs through the glottis and (**b**) the stationary column of air in the laryngeal vestibule that is present immediately after the top edge of the vocal fold closes (the closed phase of vibration). The back pressure acts to facilitate separation of the vocal folds (the opening phase) by creating elevated supraglottal and intraglottal pressures. (**a**) Elasticity and differential pressures with the glottis are the phenomena which help close the lower edges of the vocal folds during phonation. (**b**) Increased medial compression can influence vibratory dynamics including vibratory amplitude, but this is not inertive reactance. (**c**) Acoustic energy and aerodynamic energy within the subglottal region is not referred to as inertive reactance. The nature of these interactions remains unclear.

13. Correct: Locate the hyoid bone (**b**).

(**b**) The first step in the application of circumlaryngeal massage is to locate the hyoid bone. A useful strategy is to first palpate the thyroid cartilage centrally and find the thyroid notch. (**a, c, d**) Encircling and kneading the lateral margins of the larynx, applying pressure to and increasing the thyrohyoid space, and applying downward pressure are later steps in the process of circumlaryngeal massage.

14. Correct: All of the above (**e**).

(**e**) Treatment decisions should be chosen while taking into account all of the listed factors. (**a, b, c, d**) While individual factors are important and need to be accounted for when choosing treatments, clinicians should take into account multiple factors which will lead to the selection of the most effective and efficient treatments to meet the needs of the patient.

15. Correct: Vocal function (**b**).

(**b**) The vocal function domain involves direct modification of phonation. Treatment techniques fall within the categories of glottal contact, pitch modification, and vegetative vocalization. Push/pull exercises, MPT, and flow phonation are associated with glottal contact treatments. (**a**) The somatosensory domain of direct interventions is associated with modification of somatic and visual put. (**c**) The musculoskeletal domain is associated with modification of muscular, skeletal, and connective tissue. (**d**) The respiratory domain is associated with modification of respiratory function.

16. Correct: Musculoskeletal (**c**).

(**c**) The musculoskeletal domain is associated with modification of muscular, skeletal, and connective tissue. When you apply pressure to the muscles and connective tissues of the laryngeal region with your hand and fingers, it is referred to as "digital manipulation," which falls under neck modification treatments with the musculoskeletal domain. (**a**) The somatosensory domain of direct interventions is associated with modification of somatic and visual put. (**b**) The vocal function domain is associated with modification of phonation. (**d**) The respiratory domain is associated with modification of respiratory function.

17. Correct: Open throat breathing (**a**).

(**a**) Open throat breathing is a technique used to gain volitional control over respiratory and laryngeal physiology and also to inhibit cough. To facilitate control, the patient is asked to inhale through the nose slowly while relaxing the oro/pharyngeal/laryngeal muscles by resting the tongue on the floor of the mouth, closing the lips gently, and allowing the jaw muscles to relax as if beginning to yawn. The patient is then asked to exhale slowly through pursed lips or on a sustained /s/ sound for approximately 5 to 10 seconds. This process is then repeated. (**b, d**) Steam inhalation and adequate water intake are part of vocal hygiene, which is included in cough control intervention but not as a cough control technique. (**C**) Education is a separate domain with cough control intervention.

18. Correct: 6 to 9% (**b**).

(**b**) The approximate prevalence of dysphonia in school-age children, based on research reports, is between 6 and 9%. Among the disorders causing dysphonia in school-age children, vocal nodules are the most frequent vocal pathology, diagnosed in 25 to 82% of children who seek treatment. (**a**) 3 to

5% underestimates the true number of school-age children who experience dysphonia. (**c, d, e**) Prevalence rates significantly higher than 10% likely overestimate the number of school-age children who experience dysphonia, based on current research evidence.

19. Correct: Vocal cord dysfunction (**c**).

(**c**) PVFM is also referred to as vocal cord dysfunction (VCD)—to date no universally accepted term has been accepted and no other names for this disorder also exist. (**a**) Puberphonia is a term used synonymously with mutational falsetto. (**b**) Muscle tension dysphonia is a functional voice disorder while PVFM falls into the category of idiopathic. (**d**) Sarcoma refers to a type of cancer, which does not include PVFM.

20. Correct: Glide from the lowest to the highest vocal frequency (**b**).

(**b**) The stretch exercise of VFE requires the patient to produce a slow, controlled pitch glide from the lowest possible frequency to the highest possible frequency, on the vowel /ɔ/ as the word "knoll." (**a**) Sustaining five different vocal frequencies describes the power exercise of VFE. (**C**) Gliding from the highest to the lowest describes the relax exercise of VFE. (**D**) Sustaining a vowel at one target pitch describes the warm-up exercise of VFE.

21. Correct: LSVT (**c**).

(**c**) The full LSVT LOUD program requires 16 treatment sessions spread out over 4 consecutive weeks of therapy. Since the original program was developed, a number of modifications have been implemented with positive clinical outcomes. (**a, b, d**) RVT (resonant voice therapy), VFE (vocal function exercises), and SOVT (semioccluded vocal tract exercises) can vary the duration of their administration, dependent on patient's progress.

22. Correct: PhoRTE and LSVT (**d**).

(**d**) PhoRTE and LSVT are related voice treatment programs used to target glottal sufficiency resulting in hypoadduction. (**a**) RVT and frontal focus are primarily used to treat vocal hyperfunction. (**b**) SOVT is used to treat vocal hyperfunction. (**c**) Chewing is used to treat vocal hyperfunction.

23. Correct: Pass as a female based on auditory-perception of their speaking voice (**b**).

(**b**) The most common transgender groups seeking voice treatment are trans women and male-to-female transsexuals (MFTs). An overarching goal for these individuals is to pass (i.e., be perceived by others) as female, not only visually but also via auditory-perception. (**a, c, d**) A number of speech and voice characteristics can influence the perception of female voice and are valid treatment targets, including the modification of vocal pitch and F_0 (higher), voice quality (i.e., subtle breathiness), prosody, articulation (resonance via lip spreading and forward tongue position), and vocabulary, among others. MFTs typically do not want to produce an F_0 in the range of a male and do not require increases or decreases in their physiological frequency range.

24. Correct: Open throat breathing (**c**).

(**c**) Open throat breathing is a respiratory strategy that facilitates breathing cycles (inspiration/expiration) completed with relaxed oral and laryngeal muscles. This breathing method can be effective for controlling respiratory and laryngeal muscles at the onset or during PVFM episodes. (**a**) RVT is used to treat vocal hyperfunction, most commonly associated with primary or secondary muscle tension dysphonia. (**b**) LSVT is used to treat hypofunction—for example, patients with glottal sufficiency due to Parkinson's disease or vocal fold paralysis. (**d**) Digital manipulation is used to treat hypofunction or hyperfunction through manual palpation and manipulation of the larynx. It is not commonly used to target PVFM.

25. Correct: Manual circumlaryngeal therapy (**b**).

(**b**) Manual circumlaryngeal therapy includes sequential application of the laryngeal pushback, hyoid pulldown, and combination of both (pushback + pulldown) to alter hyperfunctional laryngeal contraction patterns. (**a**) Vocal function exercises consist of four different exercises completed two times each, twice a day. (**c**) Resonant voice therapy targets vibrotactile sensations perceived during frontal resonance to alter hyperfunctional laryngeal contractions. (**d**) Semioccluded vocal tract exercises do not require placing the hands on the anterior neck.

26. Correct: All of the above (**e**).

(**e**) Education, cough control techniques, vocal hygiene, and psychoeducational counseling comprise the elements of a comprehensive behavioral treatment for chronic cough. Medical treatment may also be required. (**a, b, c, d**) Chronic cough requires multiple targets in the domains of knowledge (via education), behavioral changes (cough control techniques), vocal health (via vocal hygiene), and psychoeducational counseling.

Videos

Video 8.1 Resonant voice therapy. (From Aronson A, Bless D. Clinical Voice Disorders. 4th ed. New York: Thieme Publishers; 2009.)

Video 8.2 Vocal function exercises. (From Aronson A, Bless D. Clinical Voice Disorders. 4th ed. New York: Thieme Publishers; 2009.)

Video 8.3 The manual laryngeal muscle tension reduction technique. (From Aronson A, Bless D. Clinical Voice Disorders. 4th ed. New York: Thieme Publishers; 2009.)

Video 8.4 Lee Silverman voice treatment. (From Aronson A, Bless D. Clinical Voice Disorders. 4th ed. New York: Thieme Publishers; 2009.)

Video 8.5 Vocal cord dysfunction. (From Aronson A, Bless D. Clinical Voice Disorders. 4th ed. New York: Thieme Publishers; 2009.)

Video 8.6 Singing. (From Aronson A, Bless D. Clinical Voice Disorders. 4th ed. New York: Thieme Publishers; 2009.)

Appendix 8.1 Example of vocal function exercise tracking log

Week of:	Day						
	Monday	Tuesday	Wednesday	Thursday	Friday	Saturday	Sunday
Warm-up 1							
Warm-up 2							
Stretch 1							
Stretch 2							
Contract 1							
Contract 2							
Power 1a							
Power 1b							
Power 1c							
Power 1d							
Power 1e							
Power 2a							
Power 2b							
Power 2c							
Power 2d							
Power 2e							

Notes:
Each exercises two times, twice per day (morning, afternoon).
For warm-up 1 and 2, record time.
For stretch and contract 1 and 2, record highest/lowest frequency, respectively.
For power 1 and 2, record times.

Appendix 8.2 Example of semioccluded vocal tract exercise tracking log

Week of:	Day						
	Monday	Tuesday	Wednesday	Thursday	Friday	Saturday	Sunday
Pitch glides 1							
Pitch glides 2							
Pitch glides 3							
Pitch glides 4							
Accents 1							

(Continued)

continued									
Week of:	**Day**								
Accents 2									
Accents 3									
Accents 4									
Melody 1									
Melody 2									
Melody 3									
Melody 4									
Reading 1									
Reading 2									
Reading 3									
Reading 4									

Notes:
Each exercises for 1 minute, four times each day.
Place checkmark (√) in box when completing each exercise.

Appendix 8.3 Cough control intervention

Cough control intervention	
Goal	**Education/Training concepts**
Education	A cough can be triggered by irritation to the throat or lungs
	A cough protects the body by clearing the lungs and airway of material that irritates the body and secretions such as phlegm and mucous
	Cough is not always necessary. Cough can occur in response to irritation rather than because something needs to be cleared from the lungs
	In contrast with acute coughing, there may be no benefit to coughing once medical causes for cough have been excluded
	Coughing is both automatic and under conscious control
	The cause for cough cannot be found in approximately 10% of patients
	Medical treatment for chronic cough is effective in 80% of patients
	Speech pathology treatment is effective for patients with cough that does not respond to medical treatment
	The aim of speech pathology treatment for cough is to increase conscious control over the cough and to reduce the irritation that triggers coughing
Cough control techniques	Identify precipitating sensations
	Distraction techniques • Sip of water • Suck on ice or candy • Chew gum
	Cough suppression swallow • Dry swallow • Effortful swallow

(Continued)

continued

Cough control intervention	
	Open throat breathing
	Exhale through pursed lips
	Repeat /p/ sound with delayed burst release (creates inertive reactance)
	Focus relaxation (centering on larynx)
	Panting
Vocal hygiene training	Reduce laryngeal irritation • Avoid smoking or second-hand smoke • Breathe through nose • Avoid dehydrating substances • Avoid phonotraumatic vocal behaviors • Lifestyle strategies for reflux Improve hydration • Steam inhalation • Adequate water intake • Nonmedicated cough lozenges
Psychoeducational counseling	Validate patient's concern about cough
	Acknowledge they are not malingering
	Reinforce that cough is a physical response to an irritating stimulus—they can learn to control the response
	Cough may not be totally eliminated—but can be controlled
	Learning to control cough takes commitment to strategies, but can be successful

Source: Adapted from Vertigan et al[71] and Vertigan et al.[105]

References

[1] Stemple JC, Glaze L, Klaben B. The Voice and Voice Therapy. 4th ed. San Diego, CA: Plural Publishing; 2010

[2] Boone DR, McFarlane SC, Von Berg SL, Zraick RI. The Voice and Voice Therapy. 9th ed. Boston, MA: Pearson; 2014

[3] Dagli M, Sati I, Acar A, Stone RE, Jr, Dursun G, Eryilmaz A. Mutational falsetto: intervention outcomes in 45 patients. J Laryngol Otol. 2008; 122(3):277–281

[4] Borrett DS. Heidegger, Gestell and rehabilitation of the biomedical model. J Eval Clin Pract. 2013; 19(3):497–500

[5] Aronson AE, Bless DM. Clinical Voice Disorders. New York, NY: Thieme Medical Publishers; 2009

[6] Ruddy BH, Sapienza CM. Treating voice disorders in the school-based setting: working within the framework of IDEA. Lang Speech Hear Serv Sch. 2004; 35(4):327–332

[7] Dorland's Illustrated Medical Dictionary. Philadelphia, PA: W.B. Saunders; 1974

[8] Van Stan JH, Roy N, Awan S, Stemple J, Hillman RE. A taxonomy of voice therapy. Am J Speech Lang Pathol. 2015; 24(2):101–125

[9] van Leer E, Connor NP. Predicting and influencing voice therapy adherence using social-cognitive factors and mobile video. Am J Speech Lang Pathol. 2015; 24(2):164–176

[10] Stemple J, van Lear E. Successful voice therapy. In: Stemple J, Fry LT, ed. Voice Therapy: Clinical Case Studies. San Diego, CA: Plural Publishing; 2010

[11] Verdolini K, Druker DG, Palmer PM, Samawi H. Laryngeal adduction in resonant voice. J Voice. 1998; 12(3):315–327

[12] Fröschels E. Chewing method as therapy: a discussion with some philosophical conclusions. AMA Arch Otolaryngol. 1952; 56(4):427–434

[13] Brodnitz FS. Keep Your Voice Healthy: A Guide to the Intelligent Use and Care of the Speaking and Singing Voice. New York, NY: Harper Brothers; 1975

[14] Froeschels E, Kastein S, Weiss DA. A method of therapy for paralytic conditions of the mechanisms of phonation, respiration and glutination. J Speech Hear Disord. 1955; 20(4):365–370

[15] Cantarella G, Viglione S, Forti S, Pignataro L. Voice therapy for laryngeal hemiplegia: the role of timing of initiation of therapy. J Rehabil Med. 2010; 42(5):442–446

[16] El-Banna M, Youssef G. Early voice therapy in patients with unilateral vocal fold paralysis. Folia Phoniatr Logop. 2014; 66(6):237–243

[17] Mattioli F, Menichetti M, Bergamini G, et al. Results of early versus intermediate or delayed voice therapy in patients with unilateral vocal fold paralysis: our experience in 171 patients. J Voice. 2015; 29(4):455–458

[18] Yamaguchi H, Yotsukura Y, Sata H, et al. Pushing exercise program to correct glottal incompetence. J Voice. 1993; 7(3):250–256

[19] Ramig LO, Sapir S, Fox C, Countryman S. Changes in vocal loudness following intensive voice treatment (LSVT) in individuals with Parkinson's disease: a comparison with untreated patients and normal age-matched controls. Mov Disord. 2001; 16(1):79–83

[20] Logemann JA, ed. Management of the patient with oropharyngeal swallowing disorders. In: Evaluation and Treatment of Swallowing Disorders. Austin, TX: Pro-Ed; 1998

[21] D'Alatri L, Galla S, Rigante M, Antonelli O, Buldrini S, Marchese MR. Role of early voice therapy in patients affected by unilateral vocal fold paralysis. J Laryngol Otol. 2008; 122(9):936–941

[22] McFarlane SC, Holt-Romeo TL, Lavorato AS, Warner L. Unilateral vocal fold paralysis: perceived vocal quality following three methods of treatment. Am J Speech Lang Pathol. 1991; 1:45–48

[23] Sapienza C, Hoffman Ruddy B. Voice Disorders. 2nd ed. San Diego, CA: Plural Publishing; 2013

[24] Watts CR, Diviney SS, Hamilton A, Toles L, Childs L, Mau T. The effect of stretch-and-flow voice therapy on measures of vocal function and handicap. J Voice. 2015a; 29(2):191–199

[25] Gartner-Schmidt J. Flow phonation. In: Voice Therapy – Clinical Case Studies. San Diego, CA: Plural Publishing; 2010

[26] Stone RE, Casteel R. Restoration of voice in nonorganically based dysphonia. In: Filter M, ed. Phonatory Voice Disorders in Children. Springfield, IL: C.C. Thomas; 1982

[27] Watts CR, Hamilton A, Toles L, Childs L, Mau T. A randomized controlled trial of stretch-and-flow voice therapy for muscle tension dysphonia. Laryngoscope. 2015b; 125(6):1420–1425

[28] Fröschels E, Jellinek A. Practice of Voice and Speech Therapy. Boston, MA: Expression Company Publishers; 1941

[29] Chen FC, Ma EP, Yiu EM. Facial bone vibration in resonant voice production. J Voice. 2014; 28(5):596–602

[30] Verdolini-Marston K, Burke MK, Lessac A, Glaze L, Caldwell E. Preliminary study of two methods of treatment for laryngeal nodules. J Voice. 1995; 9(1):74–85

[31] Nanjundeswaran C, Li NY, Chan KM, Wong RK, Yiu EM, Verdolini-Abbott K. Preliminary data on prevention and treatment of voice problems in student teachers. J Voice. 2012; 26(6):816.e1–816.e12

[32] Roy N, Weinrich B, Gray SD, Tanner K, Stemple JC, Sapienza CM. Three treatments for teachers with voice disorders: a randomized clinical trial. J Speech Lang Hear Res. 2003; 46(3):670–688

[33] Behrman A, Haskell J. Exercises for Voice Therapy. San Diego, CA: Singular; 2008

[34] Chen SH, Huang JL, Chang WS. The efficacy of resonance method to hyperfunctional dysphonia from physiological, acoustic and aerodynamic aspects: the preliminary study. Asia Pac J Speech Lang Hear. 2003; 8(3):200–203

[35] Chen SH, Hsiao TY, Hsiao LC, Chung YM, Chiang SC. Outcome of resonant voice therapy for female teachers with voice disorders: perceptual, physiological, acoustic, aerodynamic, and functional measurements. J Voice. 2007; 21(4):415–425

[36] Coker K. Resonant Voice Therapy. Oral presentation at the Texas Voice Symposium, January 21, 2017, Fort Worth, TX

[37] van Leer E, Pfister RC, Zhou X. An iOS-based cepstral peak prominence application: feasibility for patient practice of resonant voice. J Voice. 2017; 31 (1):131.e9–131.e16

[38] Radhakrishnan N, Scheidt T. Modified vocal function exercises: a case report. Logoped Phoniatr Vocol. 2012; 37(3):123–126

[39] Rainoldi A, Gazzoni M, Melchiorri G. Differences in myoelectric manifestations of fatigue in sprinters and long distance runners. Physiol Meas. 2008; 29(3):331–340

[40] Gillivan-Murphy P, Drinnan MJ, O'Dwyer TP, Ridha H, Carding P. The effectiveness of a voice treatment approach for teachers with self-reported voice problems. J Voice. 2006; 20(3):423–431

[41] Nguyen DD, Kenny DT. Randomized controlled trial of vocal function exercises on muscle tension dysphonia in Vietnamese female teachers. J Otolaryngol Head Neck Surg. 2009; 38(2):261–278

[42] Pasa G, Oates J, Dacakis G. The relative effectiveness of vocal hygiene training and vocal function exercises in preventing voice disorders in primary school teachers. Logoped Phoniatr Vocol. 2007; 32(3):128–140

[43] Roy N, Gray SD, Simon M, Dove H, Corbin-Lewis K, Stemple JC. An evaluation of the effects of two treatment approaches for teachers with voice disorders: a prospective randomized clinical trial. J Speech Lang Hear Res. 2001; 44 (2):286–296

[44] Sabol JW, Lee L, Stemple JC. The value of vocal function exercises in the practice regimen of singers. J Voice. 1995; 9(1):27–36

[45] Stemple JC, Lee L, D'Amico B, Pickup B. Efficacy of vocal function exercises as a method of improving voice production. J Voice. 1994; 8(3):271–278

[46] Tay EY, Phyland DJ, Oates J. The effect of vocal function exercises on the voices of aging community choral singers. J Voice. 2012; 26(5):672.e19–672.e27

[47] Tsai YC, Huang S, Che WC, Huang YC, Liou TH, Kuo YC. The effects of expiratory muscle strength training on voice and associated factors in medical professionals with voice disorders. J Voice. 2016; 30(6):759.e21–759.e27

[48] Gorman S, Weinrich B, Lee L, Stemple JC. Aerodynamic changes as a result of vocal function exercises in elderly men. Laryngoscope. 2008; 118 (10):1900–1903

[49] Gorman S. 2010

[50] Sauder C, Roy N, Tanner K, Houtz DR, Smith ME. Vocal function exercises for presbylaryngis: a multidimensional assessment of treatment outcomes. Ann Otol Rhinol Laryngol. 2010; 119(7):460–467

[51] Laukkanen AM, Titze IR, Hoffman H, Finnegan E. Effects of a semioccluded vocal tract on laryngeal muscle activity and glottal adduction in a single female subject. Folia Phoniatr Logop. 2008; 60(6):298–311

[52] Titze IR. The human instrument. Sci Am. 2008; 298(1):94–101

[53] Titze IR. Voice training and therapy with a semi-occluded vocal tract: rationale and scientific underpinnings. J Speech Lang Hear Res. 2006; 49 (2):448–459

[54] Guzman M, Castro C, Testart A, Muñoz D, Gerhard J. Laryngeal and pharyngeal activity during semioccluded vocal tract postures in subjects diagnosed with hyperfunctional dysphonia. J Voice. 2013; 27(6):709–716

[55] Paes SM, Zambon F, Yamasaki R, Simberg S, Behlau M. Immediate effects of the Finnish resonance tube method on behavioral dysphonia. J Voice. 2013; 27(6):717–722

[56] Andrade PA, Wood G, Ratcliffe P, Epstein R, Pijper A, Svec JG. Electroglottographic study of seven semi-occluded exercises: LaxVox, straw, lip-trill, tongue-trill, humming, hand-over-mouth, and tongue-trill combined with hand-over-mouth. J Voice. 2014; 28(5):589–595

[57] Kapsner-Smith MR, Hunter EJ, Kirkham K, Cox K, Titze IR. A randomized controlled trial of two semi-occluded vocal tract voice therapy protocols. J Speech Lang Hear Res. 2015; 58(3):535–549

[58] Roy N, Leeper HA. Effects of the manual laryngeal musculoskeletal tension reduction technique as a treatment for functional voice disorders: perceptual and acoustic measures. J Voice. 1993; 7(3):242–249

[59] Roy N. Assessment and treatment of musculoskeletal tension in hyperfunctional voice disorders. Int J Speech-Language Pathol. 2008; 10(4):195–209

[60] Roy N, Nissen SL, Dromey C, Sapir S. Articulatory changes in muscle tension dysphonia: evidence of vowel space expansion following manual circumlaryngeal therapy. J Commun Disord. 2009; 42(2):124–135

[61] Mathieson L, Hirani SP, Epstein R, Baken RJ, Wood G, Rubin JS. Laryngeal manual therapy: a preliminary study to examine its treatment effects in the management of muscle tension dysphonia. J Voice. 2009; 23(3):353–366

[62] Van Lierde KM, De Bodt M, Dhaeseleer E, Wuyts F, Claeys S. The treatment of muscle tension dysphonia: a comparison of two treatment techniques by means of an objective multiparameter approach. J Voice. 2010; 24 (3):294–301

[63] Sapir S. Multiple factors are involved in the dysarthria associated with Parkinson's disease: a review with implications for clinical practice and research. J Speech Lang Hear Res. 2014; 57(4):1330–1343

[64] Halpern AE, Ramig LO, Matos CE, et al. Innovative technology for the assisted delivery of intensive voice treatment (LSVT®LOUD) for Parkinson disease. Am J Speech Lang Pathol. 2012; 21(4):354–367

[65] Spielman J, Ramig LO, Mahler L, Halpern A, Gavin WJ. Effects of LSVT Extended (LSVT-X) on voice and speech in Parkinson disease. Am J Speech Lang Path. 2007; 16:95–107

[66] Huber J, Stathopoulos E, Ramig L, Lancaster S. Respiratory function and variability in individuals with Parkinson disease: pre and post Lee Silverman Voice Treatment (LSVT®). J Med Speech-Lang Pathol. 2003; 11(4):185–201

[67] Sapir S, Ramig LO, Fox CM. Intensive voice treatment in Parkinson's disease: Lee Silverman voice treatment. Expert Rev Neurother. 2011; 11 (6):815–830

[68] Ziegler A, Verdolini Abbott K, Johns M, Klein A, Hapner ER. Preliminary data on two voice therapy interventions in the treatment of presbyphonia. Laryngoscope. 2014; 124(8):1869–1876

[69] Levitt JS. Case study: the effects of the "SPEAK OUT! ®" Voice Program for Parkinson's disease. Int J Appl Sci Technol. 2014; 4(2):20–28

[70] Watts CR. A retrospective study of long-term treatment outcomes for reduced vocal intensity in hypokinetic dysarthria. BMC Ear Nose Throat Disord. 2016; 16:2

[71] Vertigan AE, Bone SL, Gibson PG. Laryngeal sensory dysfunction in laryngeal hypersensitivity syndrome. Respirology. 2013; 18(6):948–956

[72] Shembel AC, Sandage MJ, Verdolini Abbott K. Episodic laryngeal breathing disorders: literature review and proposal of preliminary theoretical framework. J Voice. 2017; 31(1):125.e7–125.e16

[73] Ryan NM, Gibson PG. Characterization of laryngeal dysfunction in chronic persistent cough. Laryngoscope. 2009; 119(4):640–645

[74] Vertigan AE, Theodoros DG, Gibson PG, Winkworth AL. Voice and upper airway symptoms in people with chronic cough and paradoxical vocal fold movement. J Voice. 2007; 21(3):361–383

[75] Vertigan AE, Theodoros DG, Gibson PG, Winkworth AL. Efficacy of speech pathology management for chronic cough: a randomised placebo controlled trial of treatment efficacy. Thorax. 2006; 61(12):1065–1069

[76] Murry T, Tabaee A, Aviv JE. Respiratory retraining of refractory cough and laryngopharyngeal reflux in patients with paradoxical vocal fold movement disorder. Laryngoscope. 2004; 114(8):1341–1345

[77] Ryan NM, Vertigan AE, Bone S, Gibson PG. Cough reflex sensitivity improves with speech language pathology management of refractory chronic cough. Cough. 2010; 6:5

[78] Martins RH, do Amaral HA, Tavares EL, Martins MG, Gonçalves TM, Dias NH. Voice Disorders: Etiology and Diagnosis. J Voice. 2016; 30(6):761.e1–761.e9

[79] American Speech-Language-Hearing Association. Graduate curriculum on voice and voice disorders. 2003. Available at: http://www.asha.org. Accessed December 8, 2017

[80] Gaskill CS, Awan JA, Watts CR, Awan SN. Acoustic and perceptual classification of within-sample normal, intermittently dysphonic, and continuously dysphonic voice types. J Voice. 2017 Mar; 31(2):218–228

[81] Castelblanco L, Habib M, Stein DJ, de Quadros A, Cohen SM, Noordzij JP. Singing voice handicap and videostroboblaryngoscopy in healthy professional singers. J Voice. 2014; 28(5):608–613

[82] Paoliello K, Oliveira G, Behlau M. Singing voice handicap mapped by different self-assessment instruments. Codas. 2013; 25(5):463–468

[83] Cohen SM, Jacobson BH, Garrett CG, et al. Creation and validation of the Singing Voice Handicap Index. Ann Otol Rhinol Laryngol. 2007; 116 (6):402–406

[84] Hancock A, Haskin G. Speech-language pathologists' knowledge and attitudes regarding lesbian, gay, bisexual, transgender, and queer (LGBTQ) populations. Am J Speech Lang Pathol. 2015; 24(2):206–221

[85] Carew L, Dacakis G, Oates J. The effectiveness of oral resonance therapy on the perception of femininity of voice in male-to-female transsexuals. J Voice. 2007; 21(5):591–603

[86] Dacakis G, Oates J, Douglas J. Beyond voice: perceptions of gender in male-to-female transsexuals. Curr Opin Otolaryngol Head Neck Surg. 2012; 20 (3):165–170

[87] Gorham-Rowan M, Morris R. Aerodynamic analysis of male-to-female transgender voice. J Voice. 2006; 20(2):251–262

[88] Hancock AB, Garabedian LM. Transgender voice and communication treatment: a retrospective chart review of 25 cases. Int J Lang Commun Disord. 2013; 48(1):54–65

[89] Cosyns M, Van Borsel J, Wierckx K, et al. Voice in female-to-male transsexual persons after long-term androgen therapy. Laryngoscope. 2014; 124(6):1409–1414

[90] Gelfer MP, Schofield KJ. Comparison of acoustic and perceptual measures of voice in male-to-female transsexuals perceived as female versus those perceived as male. J Voice. 2000; 14(1):22–33

[91] Van Borsel J, Van Eynde E, De Cuypere G, Bonte K. Feminine after cricothyroid approximation? J Voice. 2008; 22(3):379–384

[92] Brown M, Perry A, Cheesman AD, Pring T. Pitch change in male-to-female transsexuals: has phonosurgery a role to play? Int J Lang Commun Disord. 2000; 35(1):129–136

[93] Carding PN, Roulstone S, Northstone K, ALSPAC Study Team. The prevalence of childhood dysphonia: a cross-sectional study. J Voice. 2006; 20(4):623–630

[94] Wilson DK. Voice Problems in Children. 3rd ed. Baltimore, MD: Williams & Wilkins; 1987

[95] Block BB, Brodsky L. Hoarseness in children: the role of laryngopharyngeal reflux. Int J Pediatr Otorhinolaryngol. 2007; 71(9):1361–1369

[96] Connelly A, Clement WA, Kubba H. Management of dysphonia in children. J Laryngol Otol. 2009; 123(6):642–647

[97] Van Houtte E, Van Lierde K, D'Haeseleer E, Claeys S. The prevalence of laryngeal pathology in a treatment-seeking population with dysphonia. Laryngoscope. 2010; 120(2):306–312

[98] Mori K. Vocal fold nodules in children: preferable therapy. Int J Pediatr Otorhinolaryngol. 1999; 49 Suppl 1:S303–S306

[99] De Bodt MS, Ketelslagers K, Peeters T, et al. Evolution of vocal fold nodules from childhood to adolescence. J Voice. 2007; 21(2):151–156

[100] Shah RK, Woodnorth GH, Glynn A, Nuss RC. Pediatric vocal nodules: correlation with perceptual voice analysis. Int J Pediatr Otorhinolaryngol. 2005; 69 (7):903–909

[101] Roy N, Holt KI, Redmond S, Muntz H. Behavioral characteristics of children with vocal fold nodules. J Voice. 2007; 21(2):157–168

[102] Connor NP, Cohen SB, Theis SM, Thibeault SL, Heatley DG, Bless DM. Attitudes of children with dysphonia. J Voice. 2008; 22(2):197–209

[103] Hersan R, Behlau M. Behavioral management of pediatric dysphonia. Otolaryngol Clin North Am. 2000; 33(5):1097–1110

[104] Doran GT. There's a S.M.A.R.T. way to write management's goals and objectives. Management Review. 1981; 70(11):35–36

[105] Vertigan AE, Theodoros DG, Winkworth AL, Gibson PG. Chronic cough: a tutorial for speech-language pathologists. J Med Speech-Lang Pathol. 2007; 15 (3):189–206

Suggested Readings

[1] Boone DR, McFarlane SC, Von Berg SL, Zraick RI. The Voice and Voice Therapy. 9th ed. Boston, MA: Pearson; 2014

[2] Brodnitz FS. Keep Your Voice Healthy: A Guide to the Intelligent Use and Care of the Speaking and Singing Voice. New York, NY: Harper Brothers; 1975

[3] Gartner-Schmidt J. Flow phonation. In: Voice Therapy – Clinical Case Studies. San Diego, CA: Plural Publishing; 2010

[4] Mattioli F, Menichetti M, Bergamini G, et al. Results of early versus intermediate or delayed voice therapy in patients with unilateral vocal fold paralysis: our experience in 171 patients. J Voice. 2015; 29(4):455–458

[5] Stemple JC, Lee L, D'Amico B, Pickup B. Efficacy of vocal function exercises as a method of improving voice production. J Voice. 1994; 8(3):271–278

[6] Stemple J, van Lear E. Successful voice therapy. In: Stemple J, Fry LT, eds. Voice Therapy: Clinical Case Studies. San Diego, CA: Plural Publishing; 2010

[7] Stone RE, Casteel R. Restoration of voice in nonorganically based dysphonia. In: Filter M, ed. Phonatory Voice Disorders in Children. Springfield, IL: C.C. Thomas; 1982

[8] Vertigan A, Theodoros D, Winkworth A, Gibson P. Chronic cough: a tutorial for speech-language pathologists. J Med Speech-Lang Pathol. 2007; 15(3):189–206

[9] Wilson DK. Voice Problems in Children. 3rd ed. Baltimore, MD: Williams & Wilkins; 1987

9 Voice Rehabilitation after Laryngeal Cancer

Summary

This chapter describes the consequences of medical treatments for laryngeal cancer and the rehabilitation options which can restore voice production abilities for individuals with significant vocal impairments secondary to those treatments. Historical and contemporary evidence-based approaches will be presented along with treatment frameworks to guide learning and inform clinical practice. A specific focus of this chapter will be on voice restoration secondary to laryngectomy. Although there has been a downward trend in this surgical procedure over the last few decades, the specialized knowledge and skill required of the speech–language pathologists for treating this population necessitates a dedicated chapter of this book.

Keywords: laryngectomy, voice prosthesis, artificial larynx, tracheoesophageal speech

9.1 Learning Objectives

At the end of this chapter, learners will be able to

- Describe the medical treatment options and current trends for the management of laryngeal cancer.
- Identify the physiological changes which occur secondary to chemoradiation applied to the laryngeal region.
- Compare and contrast the benefits and challenges of esophageal speech and use of an electronic larynx.
- Identify patient characteristics supporting the use of tracheoesophageal speech.
- Compare and contrast indwelling and non-indwelling voice prostheses produced by different commercial vendors.
- Describe the process of pulmonary rehabilitation for the laryngectomee.
- Identify solutions for clinical issues arising during the use of voice prostheses.

9.2 Introduction

Cancer is a disease resulting from irregular development and spread of abnormal cells in one or more parts of the body.[1] Laryngeal cancer (▶ Fig. 9.1) is a subtype of head/neck cancer, which also includes oropharyngeal cancers, nasopharyngeal cancers, sinus cancers, and salivary gland cancers. Among all cancers, laryngeal cancer is considered rare with an estimated number of new cases for the United States in 2016 approximating 13,500.[1] Laryngeal cancer occurs more frequently in males, with the male-to-female ratio approximately 3.5:1.[1,2]

The most significant risk factor for the development of laryngeal cancer is tobacco use (e.g., smoking cigarettes and/or inhaling cigar smoke) and the risk increases dramatically when smoking occurs in conjunction with the regular and heavy use of alcohol. However, individuals who do not smoke or consume alcohol can also develop laryngeal cancer. There is a growing awareness that some laryngeal cancers are associated with human papillomavirus (HPV) infection, with reports suggesting that approximately 25% of laryngeal squamous cell carcinomas are associated with HPV, especially type 16.[3] The impact of laryngeal cancer and the subsequent medical treatment on the physiology of phonation can be substantial. A description of the clinical characteristics associated with laryngeal cancer was provided in Chapter 2. The focus of this chapter will be the specialized knowledge that is needed regarding the voice evaluation and treatment which occurs after oncology management.

9.3 Medical Management for Laryngeal Cancer

Once laryngeal cancer has been confirmed, the approach to medical management will depend on factors such as (**1**) the patient's preferences, (**2**) the surgeon's or oncologist's recommendations, (**3**) knowledge and skills, (**4**) the site of cancer, and (**5**) the stage of cancer. Key considerations in the approach to treatment include the likelihood of eliminating the disease (cure) and the posttreatment quality of life for the patient. The approach to management for laryngeal cancer falls into three main categories: (**1**) surgery, (**2**) radiation therapy, and (**3**) chemotherapy. These treatments can be administered alone or in combination (e.g., surgery + radiation, or chemoradiation).

The stages of laryngeal cancer are identified in **Box 9.1**, and along with the site of the cancer within the larynx (subglottis, glottis, or supraglottis), the stage will greatly influence the choice of treatment. These stages relate to the TNM cancer staging system of the American Joint Committee on Cancer,[4] where

- T = Tumor characteristics (e.g., size, growth into surrounding tissues).
- N = Lymph node involvement.
- M = Metastasis (spread of cancer cells to sites distant to the origin).

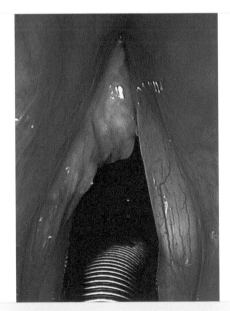

Fig. 9.1 Example of a T1 glottic cancer extending to the anterior commissure. (From Fried M, Tan M. Clinical Laryngology. 1st ed. New York: Thieme Publishers, 2014.)

Box 9.1 Stages of laryngeal cancer (from the National Cancer Institute. Retrieved from www.cancer.gov on 8/10/16).

Stage 0 (Carcinoma in situ [CIS])

In stage 0, abnormal cells (dysplasia) are found in the lining of the larynx. These abnormal cells may become cancer and spread into nearby normal tissue. Stage 0 is also called "carcinoma in situ."

Stage I

In stage I, cancer has formed. Stage I laryngeal cancer depends on where cancer began in the larynx:

○ **Supraglottis**: Cancer is in one area of the supraglottis only and the vocal cords can move normally.
○ **Glottis**: Cancer is in one or both vocal cords and the vocal cords can move normally.
○ **Subglottis**: Cancer is in the subglottis only.

Stage II

In stage II, cancer is in the larynx only. Stage II laryngeal cancer depends on where cancer began in the larynx:

○ **Supraglottis**: Cancer is in more than one area of the supraglottis or surrounding tissues.
○ **Glottis**: Cancer has spread to the supraglottis and/or the subglottis and/or the vocal cords cannot move normally.
○ **Subglottis**: Cancer has spread to one or both vocal cords, which may not move normally.

Stage III

Stage III laryngeal cancer depends on whether cancer has spread from the supraglottis, glottis, or subglottis.

Stage III cancer of the **supraglottis**:

○ Cancer is in the larynx only and the vocal cords cannot move, and/or cancer is in tissues next to the larynx. Cancer may have spread to one lymph node on the same side of the neck as the original tumor and the lymph node is 3 cm or smaller; or
○ Cancer is in one area of the supraglottis and in one lymph node on the same side of the neck as the original tumor; the lymph node is 3 cm or smaller and the vocal cords can move normally; or
○ Cancer is in more than one area of the supraglottis or surrounding tissues and in one lymph node on the same side of the neck as the original tumor; the lymph node is 3 cm or smaller.

Stage III cancer of the **glottis**:

○ Cancer is in the larynx only and the vocal cords cannot move, and/or cancer is in tissues next to the larynx; cancer may have spread to one lymph node on the same side of the neck as the original tumor and the lymph node is 3 cm or smaller; or
○ Cancer is in one or both vocal cords and in one lymph node on the same side of the neck as the original tumor; the lymph node is 3 cm or smaller and the vocal cords can move normally; or
○ Cancer has spread to the supraglottis and/or the subglottis and/or the vocal cords cannot move normally. Cancer has also spread to one lymph node on the same side of the neck as the original tumor and the lymph node is 3 cm or smaller.

Stage III cancer of the **subglottis**:

○ Cancer is in the larynx and the vocal cords cannot move; cancer may have spread to one lymph node on the same side of the neck as the original tumor and the lymph node is 3 cm or smaller; or
○ Cancer is in the subglottis and in one lymph node on the same side of the neck as the original tumor; the lymph node is 3 cm or smaller; or
○ Cancer has spread to one or both vocal cords, which may not move normally. Cancer has also spread to one lymph node on the same side of the neck as the original tumor and the lymph node is 3 cm or smaller.

Stage IV

Stage IV is divided into stage IVA, stage IVB, and stage IVC. Each substage is the same for cancer in the supraglottis, glottis, or subglottis.

Stage **IVA**:

○ Cancer has spread through the thyroid cartilage and/or has spread to tissues beyond the larynx such as the neck, trachea, thyroid, or esophagus. Cancer may have spread to one lymph node on the same side of the neck as the original tumor and the lymph node is 3 cm or smaller; or
○ Cancer has spread to one lymph node on the same side of the neck as the original tumor and the lymph node is larger than 3 cm but not larger than 6 cm, or has spread to more than one lymph node anywhere in the neck with none larger than 6 cm. Cancer may have spread to tissues beyond the larynx, such as the neck, trachea, thyroid, or esophagus. The vocal cords may not move normally.

Stage **IVB**:

○ Cancer has spread to the space in front of the spinal column, surrounds the carotid artery, or has spread to parts of the chest. Cancer may have spread to one or more lymph nodes anywhere in the neck and the lymph nodes may be any size; or
○ Cancer has spread to a lymph node that is larger than 6 cm and may have spread as far as the space in front of the spinal column, around the carotid artery, or to parts of the chest. The vocal cords may not move normally.

Stage **IVC**:

○ Cancer has spread to other parts of the body, such as the lungs, liver, or bone.

Staging details for laryngeal cancer TNM domains are shown in ▶ Table 9.1. The greater the number associated with T (T0–T4), N (N0–N3), and M (M0 or M1) in combination will be associated with a more advanced stage of cancer. Smaller lesions at less advanced stages (e.g., state I or II) are often managed with a single modality treatment, while larger lesions at higher stages (e.g., stage II or IV) are managed with combined modalities.

While the approach to laryngeal cancer management will be specific to each individual case, current trends in North America reveal that early-stage cancers (CIS, stages I and II) are treated most commonly with radiation therapy or surgery alone, or in combination.[5,6,7] Some larger (e.g., T2–T4) stage II cancers may include a combination of surgery plus radiation. Initial treatment with radiation or surgery results in similar

Table 9.1 TNM staging for laryngeal cancer based on the American Joint Committee on Cancer (based on Edge et al[4])

Domain	Characteristics
Primary tumor (T)	
Tx	Tumor cannot be assessed
T0	No evidence of primary tumor
Tis	Carcinoma in situ
• Supraglottis	
T1	Tumor limited to one subsite of supraglottic with normal vocal fold mobility
T2	Tumor invades more than one subsite of the supraglottic or glottis, without normal vocal fold mobility
T3	Tumor limited to the larynx with vocal fold fixation and/or invades the postcricoid area, medial wall of the piriform sinus, or preepiglottic tissues
T4	Tumor invades through the thyroid cartilage and/or extends to other tissues beyond the larynx
• Glottis	
T1 (a and b)	Tumor limited to one vocal fold (T1a) or both vocal folds (T1b) with normal mobility—may involve anterior or posterior commissure
T2	Tumor extends to the supraglottis and/or subglottis, and/or with impaired vocal fold mobility
T3	Tumor limited to the larynx with vocal fold fixation
T4	Tumor invades through the thyroid cartilage and/or extends to other tissues beyond the larynx
• Subglottis	
T1	Tumor limited to the subglottis
T2	Tumor extends to the vocal fold(s) with normal or impaired mobility
T3	Tumor limited to the larynx with vocal fold fixation
T4	Tumor invades through the cricoid or thyroid cartilage and/or extends to other tissues beyond the larynx
Regional lymph nodes	
Nx	Regional lymph nodes cannot be accessed
N0	No regional lymph node metastasis
N1	Metastasis in a single ipsilateral lymph node, 3 cm or less in dimension
N2 (a, b, and c)	Metastasis in a single ipsilateral lymph node, less than 6 cm (N2a); or metastasis in multiple ipsilateral lymph nodes, less than 6 cm (N2b); or metastasis in bilateral or contralateral lymph nodes, less than 6 cm (N2c)
N3	Metastasis in a lymph node more than 6 cm in dimension
Metastasis	
Mx	Presence of distant metastasis cannot be assessed

Table 9.1 continued

Domain	Characteristics
M0	No distant metastasis
M1	Distant metastasis

survival rates, although there is recent evidence to suggest that initial surgery results in better long-term larynx perseveration (e.g., function) than initial radiation for the earliest stage cancers when they are located at the level of the glottis.[7,8]

Surgical approaches for laryngeal cancers are described in ▶ Table 9.2. Stage I or II lesions typically include endoscopic-guided **transoral laser excision** or open **partial laryngectomies**, which can include **cordectomy** for glottic cancer, **supraglottic laryngectomy** for supraglottic cancer, or a **supracricoid laryngectomy** for more advanced lesions. Early-stage cancer which does not respond to initial radiation or surgery may require a **supracricoid laryngectomy** or a **total laryngectomy** to eliminate the recurring lesions (in this context, they are referred to as "salvage" procedures).

Research in the early 1990s demonstrated that survival rates are comparable when administering chemoradiation versus total laryngectomy for late-stage laryngeal cancers.[13] The standard treatment for later stage (III or IV) laryngeal cancer in North America is currently chemoradiation or radiation alone since these procedures "preserve" laryngeal structure.[14] Chemotherapy may be administered prior to radiation (referred to as "induction chemotherapy") or concomitant with radiation. However, because survival rates for advanced subglottic laryngeal cancers are substantially lower than those for glottic and supraglottic lesions, later stage subglottic cancers will usually be treated initially with surgery plus radiation (with the surgical procedure administered first).

While the increased utilization of chemoradiation as the frontline treatment for late-stage cancer does preserve laryngeal structure, clinical experience and published reports suggest that acute and late radiation effects can substantially impair laryngeal function.[14,15,16] Effects of radiation can result in voice and/or swallowing impairments due to the following effects:

• Acute effects:
  ◦ Inflammation and ulceration (mucositis).
  ◦ Swelling (edema).
  ◦ Dry mouth (xerostomia).
  ◦ Altered taste (dysgeusia).
  ◦ Hoarseness.
  ◦ Pain (odynophagia).
• Late effects:
  ◦ Fibrosis in dermis, muscles, nerves.
  ◦ Cranial nerve neuropathies.
  ◦ Muscular atrophy.

When used in combination, chemotherapy will typically exacerbate the adverse effects of radiation. In addition, the systemic administration of cancer-fighting chemicals can cause anemia, bruising or bleeding, hair loss, fatigue, and an increased susceptibility to infection during the course of treatment.

The lymphatic system of the head and neck drains a large part of the laryngeal tissues, especially the supraglottic and subglottic regions (on the other hand, the glottis contains relatively sparse lymphatic drainage). The consequence of this is

Table 9.2 Surgical options for laryngeal cancers

Procedure	Description
Transoral laser surgery	Applied using CO_2 laser with endoscopic visualization, and referred to as transoral laser microsurgery (TLM). Lesions are de-bulked and/or removed in pieces from the vocal fold tissue. Used most often for early-stage lesions, although some have used CO_2 laser for larger and/or more advanced lesions.[9] TLM is utilized to perform a partial laryngectomy when removing margins of tissue surrounding the lesion, and is currently the most common surgical modality for removing cancerous tumors[10]
Partial laryngectomy	Can be performed using cold steel instruments or CO_2 laser. Partial laryngectomy procedures leave a portion of the laryngeal structure intact, with the aim of removing all cancer while persevering function
• Cordectomy	A portion of the vocal fold tissue or all of the vocal fold is removed. This surgery may include one or more vocal fold layers, from the cover through the vocal ligament and body, and may extend from the vocal process to the anterior commissure[11]
• Supraglottic laryngectomy	Structures of the larynx superior to the vocal folds are removed. This may include the epiglottis, false vocal folds, thyroid cartilage, and aryepiglottic folds among other structures. Typically utilized for early-stage supraglottic lesions
• Supracricoid laryngectomy	Surgical excision of the true vocal folds, false vocal folds, ventricular spaces, and thyroid cartilage. For supraglottic lesions, it can include removal of the arytenoid cartilage and/or portions of the epiglottis.[12] Surgeons will reconstruct the larynx to preserve airway protection and voice by performing a cricohyoidopexy (hyoid bone attached to cricoid cartilage) or cricohyoidoepiglottopexy (hyoid *and* epiglottis are attached to cricoid). Used for larger (e.g., T2–T3) lesions and to avoid total laryngectomy
• Vertical laryngectomy	Removal of one true vocal fold, the corresponding vocal process of the arytenoid, and a portion of the ipsilateral thyroid cartilage and false vocal fold. The nature of this technique requires tracheostomy for a short duration postsurgery. Reconstruction can include tissue flaps to recreate the excised vocal fold
Total laryngectomy	Surgical removal of the entire laryngeal framework. Because the upper respiratory tract is separated from the lower tract, a permanent tracheal stoma will be required

that supraglottic cancers and subglottic cancers are prone to metastasize into the deep lymph nodes located in the neck (cervical lymph nodes), which can then result in the spread of cancerous cells to distant organs (▶ Fig. 9.2). While early-stage glottic cancers rarely spread into the lymph system, more advanced glottic tumors have a greater chance of spread.[17] Lymph node metastasis can occur on the ipsilateral side of lesion origin or in the contralateral nodes. When biopsy confirms cancer cells in the cervical lymph nodes, it necessitates their treatment

via radiation or surgical removal via a procedure known as a **neck dissection**. This may or may not be combined with post-surgical radiation treatment. This has implications for post-treatment voice rehabilitation, since the combination of substantial resections (which remove greater amounts of tissue) and radiation treatment can lead to fibrosis and possible limitations on certain alaryngeal speech options if a subsequent total laryngectomy is performed.

When late-stage laryngeal cancers do not respond to chemoradiation or when lesions present an imminent threat and/or substantial impairment, total laryngectomy (TL) may be needed as a "salvage" operation or alternative choice. Although currently the number of annual TL procedures has drastically reduced, prior to the 1990s, TL was the primary treatment for late-stage and aggressive laryngeal cancer.[18] As illustrated in ▶ Fig. 9.3, TL involves removal of the entire laryngeal framework and tissues, sealing off the pharyngeal cavity from the trachea (the two no longer communicate with each other, although the upper esophageal sphincter (UES) remains intact so that the pharynx remains connected to the esophagus for swallowing), and the creation of a tracheal stoma through which air will be inspired and expired for respiration. Individuals who have received TL are often referred to as a "**laryngectomee**" (the affix "-ee" marks a person affected by an action, in this case, the act of performing a laryngectomy).

Individuals undergoing laryngectomy might also be treated with an additional procedure at the time of surgery, called a **tracheoesophageal puncture** (TEP). A TEP creates a fistula (an opening) in the wall of tissue separating the trachea from the esophagus (the **tracheoesophageal (TE) wall**, as shown in ▶ Fig. 9.4. This puncture is created to facilitate placement of a speaking valve which will allow for respiratory airflow to be directed from the trachea into the esophagus for oral communication postsurgery.

9.4 Anatomical and Physiological Consequences of Laryngectomy

Removal of the larynx along with separation of the upper from lower respiratory tract will result in a number of permanent physiological changes to which an individual must adapt. Those scheduled to undergo a laryngectomy should be made aware of these changes prior to surgery so that they have time to consider and prepare for their presence. Suggestions for information provided to the patient by the speech–language pathologist (SLP) in the presurgical period are listed in ▶ Table 9.3. Unfortunately, presurgical consultation is not always feasible for many reasons, including (1) imminent requirement for surgery, (2) scheduling conflicts which arise between patient and/or various professionals, and/or (3) a lack of availability of interprofessional collaborative teams. A number of different health professionals might consult with the patient prior to surgery, including the otolaryngologist, radiologist, oncologist, and SLP. When the otolaryngologist plans to perform a primary TEP along with the laryngectomy procedure, it is important that both the physician and SLP counsel the patient in the preoperative period regarding the details of TE speech.

The information included in ▶ Table 9.3 relates to (1) the surgical alteration of laryngeal anatomy and function, (2) the

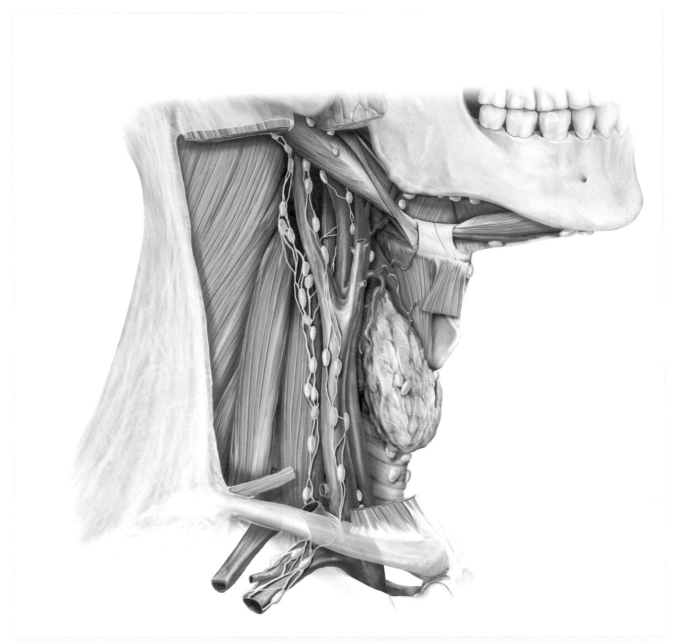

Fig. 9.2 The deep lymph nodes located in the neck serve as sites for regional metastasis of laryngeal cancer, and may necessitate treatment via radiation or surgical removal via neck dissection. (From Baker E. Anatomy for Dental Medicine, 2nd ed. New York: Thieme Medical Publishers, 2016.)

postsurgical changes in breathing and phonation, (3) potential lifestyle changes, and (4) the choices for postlaryngectomy voice restoration. When consulting with the patient, the SLP must consider that many will experience psychological stress and anxiety due to their diagnosis and pending surgery. This can influence their ability to process information provided to them. The same is true for the immediate postsurgical period. The SLP should take time to provide rational explanations, rather than simple brute facts, regarding the changes the patient will experience. Additional explanations for the information shown in ▶ Table 9.3 can include the following:

- The vocal folds have been removed so that the natural sound generator for speech is no longer available. However, individuals will be able to speak again, and multiple options will be available.

- Because air no longer moves through the nose, oral cavity, pharynx, and larynx, there is an absence of filtering, warming, and moistening of air by cilia and mucosa of the upper respiratory tract. This can result in irritation to the mucosal lining of the trachea and lungs, with subsequent coughing and increased production and buildup of mucous secretions.
- The lack of air movement through the nose can cause changes in the sensitivity to smell, taste, and changes in the ability to whistle, sniff, sip, and spit.
- Individuals will still cough, although the burst of air resulting from cough will travel through the stoma, not the mouth (they must learn to cover the stoma, not the mouth, when coughing).
- The disconnection between lower and upper respiratory tracts prevents direction of pulmonary air through the nose,

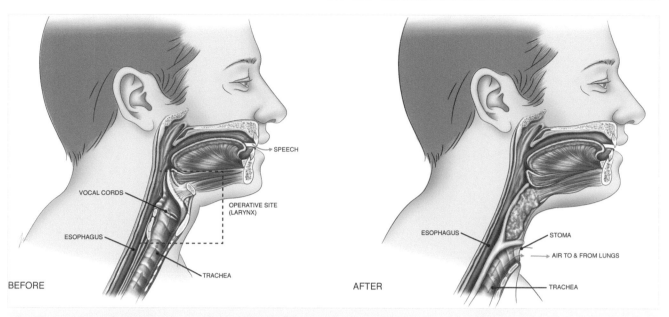

Fig. 9.3 Surgical site of total laryngectomy. The entire laryngeal framework is removed, disconnecting the upper and lower airways from each other. The communication between the pharynx and esophagus remains intact for swallowing.

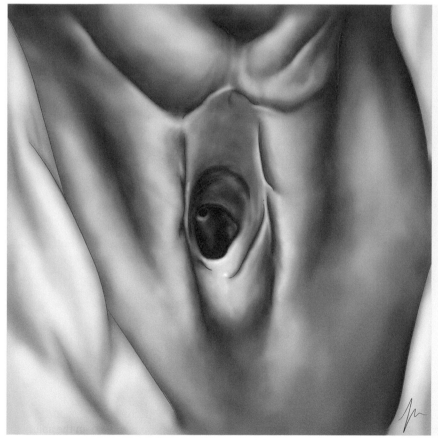

Fig. 9.4 A permanent tracheal stoma (tracheostoma) is created at the base of the neck during the laryngectomy procedure which connects the lower respiratory tract (trachea, bronchi, and lungs) directly to the outside environment. A tracheoesophageal puncture (TEP—visible as the opening within the stoma) can also be created at the time of laryngectomy (primary TEP) or as a secondary procedure after laryngectomy (secondary TEP) to facilitate oral communication using a speaking valve.

making it difficult to clear the nostrils by "blowing" the nose. Individuals will still experience nasal secretions (e.g., runny nose), and may need to wipe their nose with a tissue more frequently.
- Due to the presence of an open stoma leading directly to the trachea and lungs, individuals must be extra careful around water (e.g., bathing).

- Some individuals may have trouble lifting very heavy objects due to the impairments caused by loss of the glottal effort closure reflex and an inability to fixate the thorax by impounding air below the vocal folds—air instead can leak out of the stoma.
- Some patients may require a tracheostoma tube or vent (a.k.a., laryngectomy tube) to prevent stenosis (i.e., narrowing) of the

Table 9.3 Topics discussed with laryngectomees in the presurgical and postsurgical periods

Presurgery	
Anatomical and physiological changes	Surgery will remove the larynx—the sound source for voice will no longer be available
	A permanent stoma will be created—inspiration and expiration of air occurs through that
	If primary tracheoesophageal puncture will be performed, an opening will be created in the wall of tissue separating trachea and esophagus
	Absence of air filtering, warming, and moistening by upper respiratory tract
	Potential changes in the ability to smell, taste, sniff, sip
	Coughing through stoma instead of mouth
Special concerns	Difficulty blowing the nose
	May have difficulty being understood on telephone
	Must be extra careful around water
	Potential changes in ability to lift heavy objects
	May need tracheostoma tube temporarily
	Reinforce that they will speak again—in fact, they have multiple options
	Immediately postsurgery, writing or messaging via digital devices will be available
Communication options	Artificial electronic larynges—describe and show
	Esophageal speech—describe and provide video examples if possible
	Tracheoesophageal speech—describe and provide video examples if possible
Postsurgery	
Stoma and pulmonary care	Recommend covering stoma to minimize inhalation of particles which irritate trachea and lungs
	Describe and demonstrate heat and moisture exchangers
	Describe and demonstrate baseplates and adhesives
	Describe strategies for protecting stoma around water
	Describe maintenance of stoma and airway hygiene—regular inspection, removal of buildup, hydration of tissues
	Explain components and demonstrate operative techniques of artificial electronic larynges
Communication options	Describe and demonstrate (if possible—or show videos) esophageal speech
	Describe and demonstrate (via products and videos) tracheoesophageal speech
	Discuss patient's preferences regarding communication

Table 9.4 Alaryngeal communication options, along with the pros and cons of each

Method	Pros	Cons
Artificial larynx	○ Low cost and reimbursable ○ Easy to learn ○ Skilled users are highly intelligible	○ Poor voice quality—can be perceived as "robotic" ○ Most devices require use of hand ○ Depending on extent of surgical procedures, can cause discomfort with certain placements ○ Fibrotic tissue can inhibit sound transmission to oral cavity
Esophageal speech	○ Lowest cost option ○ Does not require use of hands ○ No surgery or equipment needed	○ Difficult to learn for many speakers ○ Potential for poor voice quality and vocal intensity ○ Limited utterance length and reduced speech intonation ○ UES spasms can inhibit speech production
Tracheoesophageal speech	○ Best voice quality ○ Hands-free options available ○ Uses speaker's own pulmonary air—improves utterance length and vocal intensity ○ Speech is more natural than with artificial larynx	○ Requires additional surgical procedure ○ Highest cost alternative ○ Requires frequent cleaning and maintenance ○ Without hands-free valve, will require use of hand ○ UES spasms can inhibit speech production

Abbreviation: UES, upper esophageal sphincter.

stoma. These need to be cleaned frequently to avoid mucus buildup and/or blockage. Tracheostoma tubes or vents may be removed once the threat of stenosis has passed.

One of the most substantial physiological changes postlaryngectomy is the creation of a permanent tracheal stoma at the base of the neck (▶ Fig. 9.4), through which the individual will now inspire and expire air when breathing. Prior to surgery, the upper respiratory tract protected the trachea and lungs by preventing undesired substances from reaching the lower airway and also warming, humidifying, and filtering inspired air. The point at which inspired air reaches tracheal and lung tissue is much closer to the outside environment after laryngectomy, which necessitates conscious awareness and intentional precautions. These precautions can include covering the stoma with various materials (e.g., a water shield when taking a shower, a cloth when leaving the home), or wearing special filters over the stoma which will compensate for the lost upper respiratory tract functions. More detail is provided in section "Pulmonary Rehabilitation for the Laryngectomee."

The vast majority of laryngectomees will be able to develop oral communication postsurgery, and most will have multiple communication options from which to choose. These options, along with pros and cons of each, are listed in ▶ Table 9.4. It is important to emphasize this fact during presurgical and immediate postsurgical consultations, as communication method will potentially be a major impact on quality of life for the laryngectomee.[19] In the immediate postsurgical period, while the patient is still healing, simple options are available including digital devices, writing, or simple communication boards. Patients who have undergone a primary TEP will be able to work on TE speech in the weeks after surgery. Two additional communication options include the use of an electronic artificial larynx and use of esophageal speech (ES).

9.5 Artificial Larynges

Humans communicate with one another using language and, for the vast majority of individuals, speech is the modality through which language is conveyed. It is obvious then that the loss of speech after laryngectomy can have consequences not only on the ability of one individual to communicate with another, but this disruption with communication may also affect routines for daily activities, and the overall psychological and emotional well-being of the patient. For many laryngectomees, use of an artificial larynx (AL) can provide relatively rapid postsurgical access to speech. ALs comprise one of the communication options which should be discussed during the presurgical consultation (▶ Table 9.3), and will require

education and instruction during the postsurgical period to develop mastery of use for effective and efficient communication.

ALs are external communication aids which allow a laryngectomee to produce speech. ALs can be powered pneumatically (e.g., using the speaker's own pulmonary energy) or using batteries, with battery-powered ALs sometimes referred to as an electronic AL (EAL) or "electrolarynx." Pneumatic devices, as illustrated in ▶ Fig. 9.5, are typically designed with a coupler that covers the stoma, an internal vibratory source in the form of a thin rubber membrane powered by pulmonary air, and tubing which can be placed into the mouth to direct the acoustic energy for articulation. Pneumatic ALs have some unique advantages over electronic ALs including lower cost and the use of the speaker's own air supply for power instead of batteries, which also reduces maintenance costs. However, there are hygiene issues that a patient must consider due to the need for cleaning the stoma coupler and tube that will be placed in the mouth to deliver sound energy. In addition, the position of the tube within the mouth may also influence the ability to articulate some sounds precisely.

Treatment that incorporates a pneumatic AL can include goals centered on (**1**) operational procedure, (**2**) articulation, and (**3**) maintenance.[20] Speakers must learn how to adequately join the coupler to the stoma and time its placement with expiratory airflow and the initiation of speech. Exploration and practice with placement of the mouth tube is also needed to facilitate the most effective transmission of sound energy into the oral cavity with minimum interference on articulation. Low maintenance of pneumatic ALs is one of their advantages, although speakers will need to be educated regarding cleaning

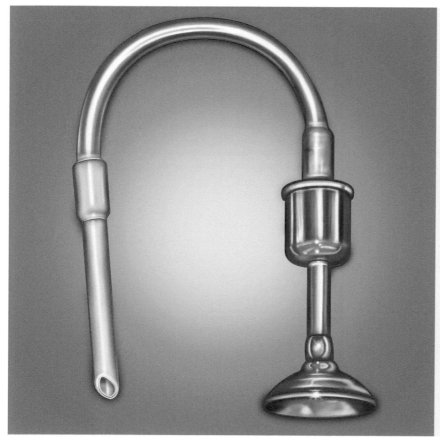

Fig. 9.5 Example of a pneumatic artificial larynx (Tokyo Artificial Larynx, Limco Solutions, LLC; www.limcosolutions.com). The rubber membrane serving as the vibratory source is housed in the chamber immediately in front of the stoma coupler.

of mucous from the stoma coupler in addition to clearing saliva that may occlude the mouth tube. When user skills are adequate for effective and efficient operation, pneumatic AL voice quality can be perceptually preferred over other forms of alaryngeal speech, including EALs.[21,22]

The choice of a pneumatic AL over an EAL may be a function of cost, accessibility, ease of use, personal preference, and culture among other factors. Liao suggested that English-speaking communities utilize EALs more than pneumatic ALs, which aligns with the authors' experiences that a majority of laryngectomees in the United States choose electronic devices.[23] EALs are battery-powered handheld devices which produce acoustic energy through a piston striking an internal membrane to sustain a vibratory tone. Recent models incorporate digital processing that allows for greater control of the frequencies and intensities produced by the device. As illustrated in ▶ Fig. 9.6, sound production from EALs is initiated by depressing a button located on the device frame, and then coupling the device head to the speaker's neck to transmit acoustic energy into the oral cavity for articulation.

EALs have *advantages* over pneumatic devices and other forms of alaryngeal speech production, which include the following:
- Can be a logical choice in advanced age due to ease of use.
- Intraoral adaptors can be used when sound transmission through neck or cheek is difficult.
- Hygiene issues are a minimal concern for neck/cheek placement.
- Ease of use suggests EALs are a good choice for those with poor physical or mental health.
- Maybe a good alternative if one fails at esophageal speech (ES).

- Useful as a backup device for those who primarily depend on ES or TE speech.
- Easily learned.
- If vibration is easily radiated into the oral cavity, intelligibility can be excellent.

There are *disadvantages* also, including the following:
- Produces an unnatural, somewhat "robotic" sound.
- Some elements of speech are difficult to produce using the EAL (/h/ sounds, cognates).
- Calls attention to the speaker.
- Requires the use of one hand.
- Maintenance (batteries, replacement devices) can be expensive.
- If it breaks, the patient is unable to communicate orally.

The treatment hierarchy for EALs is illustrated in ▶ Table 9.5, and moves from the development of simple operational skills to more advanced skills that will facilitate efficient use. In the acute postsurgical period, the tissue of the neck may be edematous and sensitive such that placement of an EAL on the neck may be too uncomfortable for the patient. Intraoral adaptors are also available when sound transmission through the neck is impaired. Some patients, due to significant postsurgical or postradiation scarring, may experience discomfort when pressing the EAL against the neck or may be unable to find a supple position on the neck where they can place the head of the EAL for sound transmission. These patients may require permanent use of an intraoral adaptor.

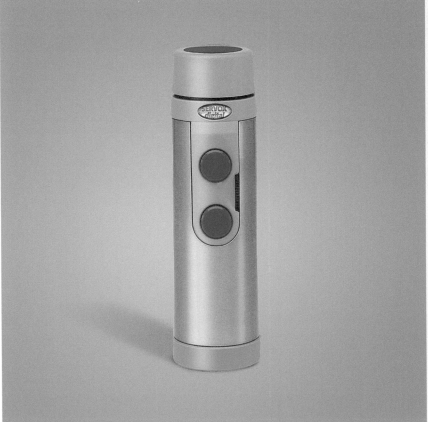

Fig. 9.6 An example of an electronic artificial larynx (InHealth Technologies). This particular product has two buttons to activate sound and a sliding knob to control loudness.

Table 9.5 Treatment hierarchy for electronic artificial larynges (EAL)

Target knowledge/ skill	Key concepts
Education and orientation	When specific unit is chosen, describe components of device including pitch controls, volume controls, battery compartments, and/or charging instructions
	Educate patient on routine care and maintenance of device
	Demonstrate and assess ability to exhibit basic operational procedures, including orientation of device in a preferred hand, initiating sound with preferred finger(s), arm/hand movements with device in hand, and coupling of intraoral adaptor if needed
Placement	Locate the placement on neck which promotes most effective sound transmission to vocal tract—the goal is for sound to resonate in the oral cavity for speech articulation. Soft tissue will transmit sound well, while stiff tissue will reflect sound. Radiation treatment can cause stiff scar tissue on neck, so experiment with placement by seeking areas allowing for greater sound transmission into vocal trace
	When neck transmission is poor, try different locations on tissue under the mandible, on the cheek, and/or the oral adapter
On-Off timing	Instruct the patient on the application of the EAL head against the skin of the neck or cheek with the device on—practice varied coupling pressures with the goal of finding the most effective resonant sound quality. If the intraoral adaptor is needed, find the mouth placement which facilitates maximum transmission of sound with minimum interference with articulation
	Instruct the patient to synchronize the tone onset (pressing tone button) with speech articulation. Initiating the tone early or late introduces a perceptually distracting buzz which can interfere with speech intelligibility. Appropriate timing also approaches more natural speech phrasing (e.g., we do not constantly produce phonation in-between **phrases** when speaking)
Articulation	Build articulation skills by moving through a hierarchy of open sounds (those characterized by resonance and which are easier to produce with EAL—e.g., vowels, glides, nasals) to more closed sounds
	/h/, fricatives, affricates, and distinctions between plosive cognates are typically the most difficult to produce
	Help patient develop strategies to differentiate production of cognates (voiced/voiceless distinctions), which are the most difficult. Shortening articulation time of voiceless and lengthening voiced cognates is one strategy. Attempting to generate oral/pharyngeal pressures to create frication noise for voiceless cognates is another

Table 9.5 continued

Target knowledge/ skill	Key concepts
Rate and phrasing	If stoma noise is present when producing stop consonants, work on reducing muscle tension during articulation
	As articulation skills develop, work on developing a faster rate of speech with appropriate pausing to facilitate intelligibility
	A natural speech rate with intelligible articulation should be the goal
Pitch and loudness adjustment	Instruct patient to modify intonation using strategies to adjust pitch and loudness. Most EALs have a loudness control knob which may be needed in noisy situations. Some devices have multiple buttons for differential pitch control
	Loosening the EAL head (slightly unscrew it) can influence loudness (reduces overall amplitude of tone)
	Pitch can also be varied by altering the amount of coupling pressure against the skin, moving the EAL head above or below the most resonant placement area (e.g., to a region with stiffer tissue), or extending/flexing the neck

Source: Adapted from Blom.[24]

9.6 Esophageal Speech

Esophageal speech is a method of sound production requiring a speaker to "load" air into the esophagus from above and then expel that air back through the **UES**. The UES can serve as a pseudoglottis (replacement for the vocal folds) that oscillates to create sound energy. Many readers of this book might have produced sound with the UES when belching. In fact, the early learning stages of ES can take advantage of this familiarity. As ES skill develops, the perceptual features will often transition to a low pitched, rough vocal quality which can serve as the primary method of communication. Although ES can be difficult to acquire for many speakers, those who master it can communicate efficiently and effectively for most communicative needs.[25]

The UES has also been referred to as the **pharyngo-esophageal segment** (PES), which distinguishes it as an anatomical region rather than an isolated muscular structure.[26] While PES and UES are often used synonymously, the PES is an anatomical region versus a specific sphincteric muscle in the case of the UES. The UES is composed of the distal fibers of the inferior pharyngeal constrictor (the cricopharyngeus muscle) and the circular muscle fibers that are part of the proximal esophagus (▶ Fig. 9.7). At rest, the UES is in a tonically active contracted state. This tight sphincter-like closure forms a high-pressure barrier between the esophagus and the pharynx which prevents air from passing into the esophagus during inhalation.

The UES will intermittently relax and dilate (open) to allow passage of contents during various physiologic events including belching, swallowing, and vomiting. During swallowing, the degree of UES dilation is a function of three physiological

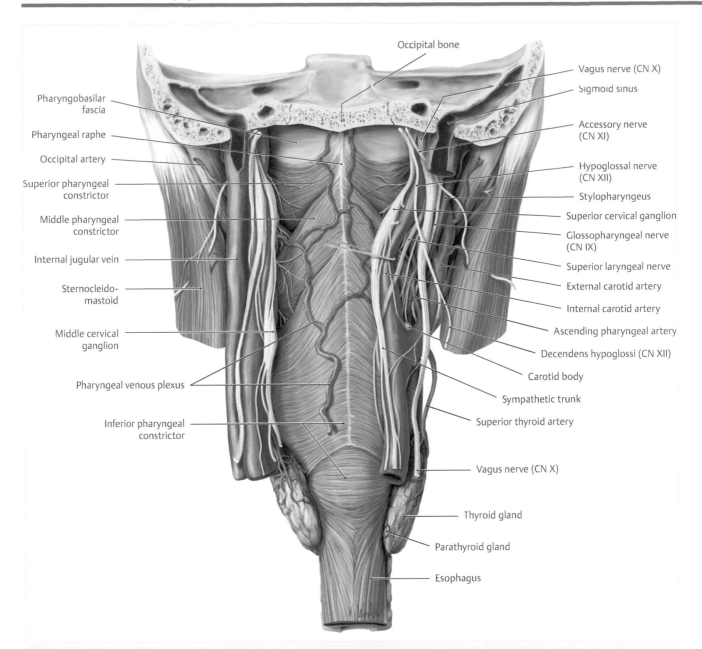

Fig. 9.7 Muscles of the pharynx (inferior pharyngeal constrictor) and esophagus forming the upper esophageal sphincter (UES), also known as the pharyngo-esophageal segment (PES). (From Baker EW et al. Anatomy for Dental Medicine. 1st ed. New York: Thieme Publishers, 2015.)

mechanisms: (1) central nervous system–mediated relaxation, (2) hyolaryngeal excursion, and (3) pressure from the bolus.[27] Muscles of the pharynx and tongue can also volitionally contract to create high pressure in the lower pharynx which can overcome the UES resting tone and load air into the esophagus from above, as when someone intentionally burps (e.g., a dry burp—without first drinking or consuming food).

The effective and efficient volitional loading of air into the esophagus is a key step in the ability to utilize ES. It has been estimated that as many as 25 to 75% of speakers attempting to learn ES fail to attain this goal.[26,28,29] Reasons for the high failure rate are likely multifactorial and have been attributed to factors such as the surgical method for laryngectomy, premorbid anatomical variability, esophageal motility and UES

pressure adaptations after surgery, adverse effects from radiation, the speaker's physiological status (health), and psychosocial factors.[26,30] Some individuals can also present with a spasmodic UES segment postsurgery or scar secondary to iatrogenic injury which can also complicate the attainment of ES.

Achievement of skilled ES use requires frequent and intensive practice regimens and can be likened to the process of mastering a new motor skill. The foundational skill for ES is the ability to load air into the upper esophagus and then expel that air in a manner which oscillates the UES. During the early treatment sessions, the clinician can assess this ability by simply asking the patient if they are able to make any type of burping sound—and if so, instructing the patient to demonstrate. If they are unable to spontaneously produce sound, it can be helpful for the clinician to provide a model and elicit replication from the patient. A useful target to model and elicit from the patient during this period of training is the open vowel /a/—for example, asking the patient to load air into the esophagus and produce an /a/ sound. As the patient demonstrates skill in this ability, the clinician should determine the patient's ability to sustain this sound (e.g., maximum prolongation). The clinician should continue to explore different vowels (requiring different tongue positions and consequent variable vocal tract pressures) with the patient to seek out facilitative contexts. The ability to create sound with the UES in these early stages can be a positive predictor for future success.

When observing the patient producing a basic esophageal sound, the clinician should observe the natural physiological strategy used to accomplish the task. Ideally, the patient will learn to utilize an efficient method of esophageal air loading which can then facilitate progression through the stages of ES mastery. Four loading strategies have been described and can be used as physiological treatment goals: (**1**) consonant injection, (**2**) glossopharyngeal press, (**3**) inhalation, and (**4**) the swallowing method.[31] It is important to realize that patients can learn to develop efficient and effective ES using one or more loading methods consecutively, or adapt a method to fit their physiological abilities. The primary clinical goal is to establish a method of injection that facilitates communication which meets the patient's needs, and it is often wise to follow the patient's lead when exploring what method or adaptation works for them. There are various techniques for teaching ES (see the study of Doyle for a review of different instruction strategies[26]), and the following steps and stimuli for progressing through a treatment hierarchy are only one example of many that might be utilized.

Consonant injection takes advantage of the increased vocal tract pressure that is an obligatory consequence of stop (plosive) production. The patient can utilize stop consonant phonemes and their associated pressures to load air into the esophagus both within a phrase and at phrase boundaries (e.g., pauses) when plosives occur in the sound structure of words, making this loading technique one of the more efficient strategies.[26,31] As with any method for teaching ES, initial training begins with the exploration of sound generation (see the preceding paragraphs). The patient can then be asked to produce plosive sounds by placing their tongue in the articulatory position for a /p/, /t/, and then /k/ while repeating each sound multiple times. With strong, quick movements of the articulators, they should perceive the increased vocal tract pressure. They are then asked to repeat with an esophageal sound, loading air into esophagus prior to releasing articulatory position for the lips (for the bilabial plosive) or tongue (for the lingual plosives). It will be important to encourage the patient during this early stage, as early success with ES sound generation can be difficult for many patients. Persistence will be a key.

The clinician should develop treatment stimuli and home practice stimuli containing targets at the various stages of the treatment hierarchy (CV, CVC, multisyllabic, etc.). These lists will need to be extensive because learning ES requires frequent and intensive practice distributed over periods of time throughout the day. Initial stimuli should include consonants /p/, /t/, and /k/ in CV structures (e.g., /pa/, /ta/, /ka/), as some patients may find it easier to load the esophagus using one sound over another due to the different physiological requirements for their production.[26] Close attention may reveal greater success using a particular plosive, which can be used to facilitate progression through the subsequent stages of treatment. Instruction in consonant injection and other loading methods will move through single-syllable stimuli in (**1**) CV and then (**2**) CVC structures, followed by progression to (**3**) multisyllabic and (**4**) multiword stimuli, (**5**) **phrases**, (**6**) sentences, and then (**7**) connected speech.[32]

As the patient develops skills meeting treatment goal requirements of producing sound with different vowels at the CV stage, the subsequent goal should require the patient to increase the duration of the vowel sound. As the patient increases his or her effectiveness at producing variable CV structures and prolonging sound for more than a few seconds, CVC stimuli should be introduced. It can be useful to first include CVC stimuli with the same initial and final plosive (e.g., "pop" and "tot"), as this context can be the foundation for which the patient will learn to produce multisyllabic stimuli (e.g., "popper" and "totter") and later utilize consonant injection within **phrases** during connected speech.

The **glossopharyngeal press** method requires the patient to obstruct the anterior oral regions using the tongue tip with the anterior dorsum raised to the hard palate, while using the posterior tongue (e.g., posterior dorsum and tongue base) to compress a volume of air into the pharynx. The patient will begin a loading gesture with an open mouth, and then close it quickly to capture air. As the posterior tongue compression pushes the air into a smaller pharyngeal space, the pressure builds until it is enough to overcome the resistance of the UES.[25,26,31] Because posterior movement of the tongue is not an articulatory movement for English speech sounds, utilization of the glossopharyngeal press must occur at pauses during connected speech. This creates less efficiency than use of consonant injection, although skilled ES speakers who use this method can learn to load air rapidly such that pauses between injections do not substantially detract from the communication process. Skill development can follow similar stimuli and structures as those described in the preceding paragraphs.

The **inhalation method** of air injection requires patients to inhale quickly through their stoma to create a pressure differential between the distal esophagus and pharyngeal region above the UES.[26] Lauder also suggested the accompaniment of a rapid "sniffing" gesture to facilitate this pressure differential.[25] The method requires the lips to be parted and the tongue to be flat or in a neutral position—there will be no active tongue contraction during the inhalation gesture. As air quickly enters the trachea, it will cause the pressure differential on either side of the UES to increase (pressure decreases in the esophagus relative to the pharyngeal space, so that the differential between the two spaces is greater), such that air will move through it and into the esophagus.[26]

The **swallowing method** of air injection is considered the least efficient due to the non-speech gesture (swallowing) that is needed to facilitate loading of air, and the amount of time required for each loading cycle. The patient is instructed to capture air in the oral cavity by closing the mouth from an open position, and then to swallow the air using a typical swallow gesture. Lauder suggested that patients having difficulty with initial learning of the swallow method can use sips of water to facilitate a swallow and subsequent belch, although this strategy should not be used frequently and should be eliminated as soon as loading skills become consistent.[25]

9.7 Tracheoesophageal Speech

In the absence of skilled ES ability, TE speech is considered the most efficient method of alaryngeal voice production and is the method of communication used by a majority of laryngectomees today.[33] ▶ Fig. 9.3 illustrated the postlaryngectomy anatomy showing the trachea sutured to the anterior neck creating a stoma. In order for a patient to use TE speech, a tracheoesophageal puncture (TEP) must be performed. The puncture is created so that it is immediately accessible through the opening of the stoma (▶ Fig. 9.4).

The TEP can be performed as a primary procedure at the time of laryngectomy (referred to as **primary TEP**), or as a secondary procedure on a later date after laryngectomy (**secondary TEP**). A majority of patients undergoing laryngectomy will receive a primary TEP.[33,34,35] Once the puncture is created, a voice prosthesis can be placed inside to stent the puncture and facilitate air injection into the esophagus which will subsequently vibrate the UES, as illustrated in ▶ Fig. 9.8.

A patient receiving a primary TEP may have the voice prosthesis placed at the time of surgery or in the weeks postsurgery. When placed during primary surgery, the tracheoesophageal wall length is measured and the prosthesis is placed by the surgeon. The surgeon may instead place a catheter into the puncture and refer to the SLP *7 to 14 days* later for prosthesis placement. This allows time for the tissue to heal and the patient to recover from surgery. The catheter can also serve as a feeding port for nutrition intake during the immediate postlaryngectomy period. When a patient receives a secondary TEP, a catheter is placed into the puncture and the voice prosthesis will be placed by the SLP approximately *3 to 5* days postsurgery. In many patients, the initial prosthesis length will be in the range of 8 to 10 mm. However, the length of the puncture can change over time, especially in the months after surgery. Eventually this length can range from 4 to 22 mm or more.

A minority of patients may require placement of a **laryngectomy tube** postsurgery. As illustrated in ▶ Fig. 9.9, these tubes are curved to fit inside the trachea and maintain stenting of the stoma. Laryngectomy tubes are utilized for patients experiencing or at risk for stenosis of the stoma. Some patients scheduled for postsurgical radiation might also require a laryngectomy tube.[36] Laryngectomy tubes are typically used until the risk of stenosis is minimal or the process of wound healing is complete. In rare instances, patients may not be able to utilize stoma housings (see below) and will utilize a laryngectomy tube that can accommodate filters and speaking valves.

Initial treatment provided by the SLP will consist of (**1**) counseling and education regarding TE speech, (**2**) measurement of the puncture length, (**3**) selection of the appropriate prosthesis, (**4**) placement of the prosthesis, and then (**5**) training in use of

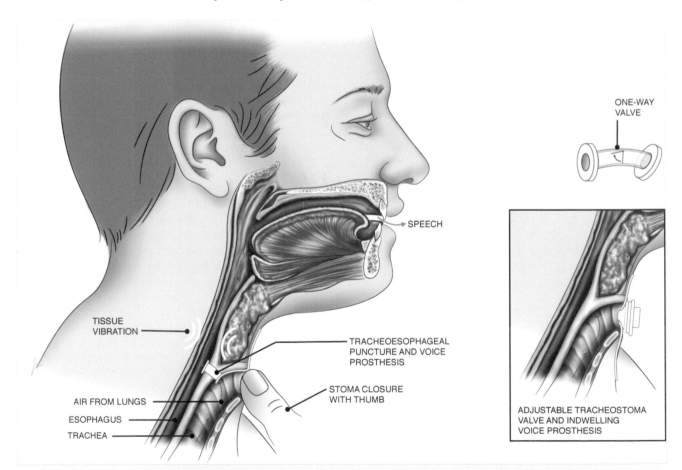

Fig. 9.8 A voice prosthesis is placed into the tracheoesophageal puncture. This occludes the puncture and maintains patency. When a speaker inhales, seals their stoma, and then exhales, the open channel running through the center of the prosthesis will allow air to flow from the trachea, through the prosthesis, and into the esophagus. A one-way valve inside the prosthesis opens into the esophagus, but will prevent food or liquid from flowing into the trachea. (From Probst R et al. Basic Otorhinolaryngology. 1st ed. New York: Thieme Publishers, 2015.)

the prosthesis followed by (**6**) training in care and maintenance procedures specific to the type of prosthesis. Counseling and education are critical in this early stage of treatment to both reassure the patient and facilitate knowledge and skill development which will promote subsequent learning. Topics to include during this stage of treatment include

- The anatomy of the TE puncture—what it is connecting.
- The importance of maintaining puncture dilation (something must be in the puncture at all times to prevent resealing through natural wound healing).
- Care and maintenance of the stoma and tracheal side of the puncture.
- The construction and function of a voice prosthesis.
- The different types (non-indwelling, indwelling) and commercial brands of voice prostheses—it is beneficial to have product examples with you.
- Care and maintenance of the voice prosthesis.
- The process of coordinating inhalation, stoma occlusion, and exhalation for TE speech.

- The mechanics of digitally occluding the stoma (using different fingers).
- Stoma housings.
- Filters, heat/moisture exchangers, and hands-free speaking valves.
- Troubleshooting and actions to take when leakage and/or difficult voicing is present.

If a patient is scheduled to receive or is considering a secondary TEP, some clinicians chose to conduct an **insufflation test** to assess the vibratory function of the UES. This test may have also been performed prior to the laryngectomy to determine if any UES spasm or constriction is present. Insufflation testing requires a commercially available test kit. The clinician will route a flexible catheter containing an internal lumen through the nasal cavity, pharynx, and into the distal esophagus. The other end of the catheter is connected to a coupler which fits over the stoma. Once in place, the clinician asks the patient to inhale, the clinician (or patient) then occludes the stoma coupler with a finger, and asks the patient to exhale while attempting to produce "ahhh." Air will be routed through the internal lumen of the catheter and into the esophagus. Typically, voicing is immediate and this will support a positive prognosis for future TE speech abilities. If the catheter has been properly placed into the esophagus and the stoma coupler adequately covered, a lack of voicing could be due to a number of different factors. These include (1) excessive muscular tension on the part of the patient (multiple trials asking them to attempt more relaxed productions can test this assumption), (2) a hypertonic UES, or (3) a spasmodic UES among others. However, clinicians should keep in mind research which has demonstrated that failure for voicing during insufflation testing *is not necessarily a good predictor* of later acquisition of TE speech.[37]

9.8 Tracheoesophageal Voice Prostheses

Voice prostheses are devices which fit into the TEP and incorporate a one-way valve that allows air to flow from the trachea to the esophagus while protecting the lower airway from tracheal aspiration.[38] Two basic types of voice prostheses are available for TE speech: indwelling and non-indwelling (▶ Fig. 9.10). An **indwelling** prosthesis will remain in the puncture until it needs to be changed, with routine daily maintenance being performed

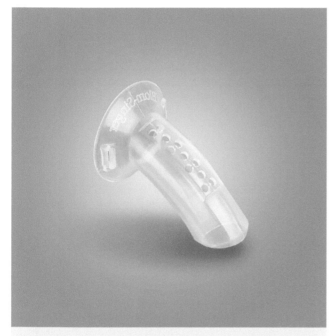

Fig. 9.9 Example of a laryngectomy tube for maintenance of stoma patency. (Used with permission from InHealth.)

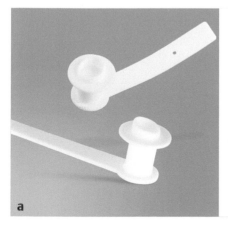
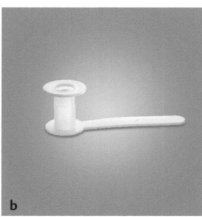

Fig. 9.10 Examples of non-indwelling (**a**) and indwelling (**b**) voice prostheses. (Used with permission from InHealth.)

by the patient or a caregiver *with the prosthesis in place*. Only an SLP removes and replaces an indwelling prosthesis. Depending on the manufacturer, indwelling prostheses come in diameters ranging from 16 to 22.5 French (**French** is a scale used to measure the diameter of catheters, and is often represented by "Fr": 1 Fr = 1/3 mm), and are constructed of more dense material with subtle design modifications which differentiate them from non-indwelling prostheses. A **non-indwelling** prosthesis *can be removed, cleaned, and reinserted daily by the patient*. Depending on the manufacturer, non-indwelling prostheses come in diameters ranging from 16 to 20 Fr. In the United States, the majority of prostheses prescribed for and utilized by laryngectomees are produced by InHealth Technologies or Atos Medical, although products from other manufacturers are also available. InHealth and Atos products are slightly different in their thickness, materials, design elements, and insertion methods. The following information will center on the design and function of these products.

Regardless of prosthesis type or brand, the voice prostheses consist of six basic parts, as illustrated in ▶ Fig. 9.11:
- Tracheal flange.
- Exterior shaft.
- Internal lumen (channel).
- Internal valve(s).
- Esophageal flange.
- Safety strap.

The tracheal and esophageal flanges are wider than the shaft and act in concert to seal the prosthesis against the tracheoesophageal wall. The shaft acts as a stent to maintain patency of the puncture. A prosthesis may consist of one or two internal valves. These valves are constructed so that they only open in one direction—toward the esophagus. This allows air from the trachea to flow through the channel, open the valve, and stream into the esophagus, but prevents material from the esophagus being aspirated into the trachea.

The choice of prostheses, including indwelling versus non-indwelling and specific brand, will be based on multiple factors. Patients who have good manual dexterity in at least one arm and hand, adequate eyesight, appropriate cognitive abilities, are motivated to maintain the prosthesis, and are concerned about costs may prefer to start with a non-indwelling prosthesis. In the authors' experience, a non-indwelling prosthesis as the initial choice is logical for patients receiving a secondary TEP because

most puncture tracts will change in length between the first and second placements. Starting with a non-indwelling can also help control costs. Patients who prefer not to remove a prosthesis frequently, desire a longer device life, or who have physical/cognitive limitations may prefer an indwelling prosthesis. Brand choice will be influenced by patient and clinician preferences, and informed by the research evidence which has studied device life over time. The selection of special prostheses (e.g., see Blom-Singer Advantage and Provox Acti-Valve below) is often dictated by the patient's experience with standard prosthesis device life over time—these are typically not the initial prostheses utilized.

9.8.1 InHealth Prostheses

InHealth Technologies produce the **Blom-Singer** brand of voice prostheses. This line of devices are named after the innovators of tracheoesophageal voice restoration, Dr. Eric Blom and Dr. Marc Singer.[39] The Blom-Singer voice prosthesis was the first commercially produced option available for laryngectomees in the United States, being introduced in the early 1980s. Blom-Singer currently manufactures five prosthesis options: two non-indwelling and three indwelling, and all Blom-Singer prostheses use an anterograde placement (i.e., placement from the front by inserting the prosthesis through the TEP at the tracheal side):
- **Non-indwelling low pressure** (▶ Fig. 9.12): The low-pressure Blom-Singer prosthesis is so named because the pressure generated as air moves through the prosthesis and into the esophagus is lower than the duckbill prosthesis (see below). As a non-indwelling prosthesis, the low pressure prosthesis can be inserted, removed, and maintained by the patient. A safety strap is designed to remain attached to the prosthesis, and is secured to the neck via tape or some other material. If the patient has physical or cognitive impairment, it is also possible for a caregiver or clinician to perform those functions. The low pressure prosthesis is currently priced at a

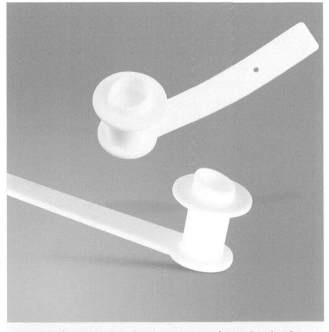

Fig. 9.12 Blom-Singer Low Pressure voice prosthesis. (Used with permission from InHealth.)

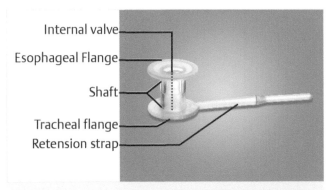

Internal valve
Esophageal Flange
Shaft
Tracheal flange
Retension strap

Fig. 9.11 Elements of a voice prosthesis. (Used with permission from InHealth.)

low-to-mid cost range (e.g., under $100), making it an economic choice for some patients. It comes in 16 and 20 Fr options, and can use a gel-cap insertion method for initial or re-insertion. This method of insertion utilizes a small, hollow gel cap which covers the esophageal flange of the prosthesis and eases the placement into the TEP. The gel cap will dissolve after insertion and allow the esophageal flange to unfold against the esophageal wall to hold the prosthesis firmly in place. Multiple lengths of the low-pressure prosthesis are available to accommodate the patient's specific anatomy.

- **Non-indwelling duckbill** (▶ Fig. 9.13): The Duckbill prosthesis is also inserted, maintained, and replaced by the patient, caregiver, or clinician. It generates higher air pressures which, for some patients, promotes more efficient and effective UES vibration. Like the low-pressure prosthesis, the Duckbill prosthesis includes a retention strap that is designed to remain on the prosthesis. One drawback of the Duckbill is that the high air pressure in the esophagus during voice production can cause "gastric filling," where some air moves inferiorly (rather than superiorly) past the lower esophageal sphincter into the stomach resulting in possible discomfort for the patient. The Duckbill is the lowest cost prosthesis produced by InHealth, and is available only in 16 Fr versions. As with the low-pressure prosthesis, multiple lengths are available. Because of the rounded end on the esophageal side of the shaft, the Duckbill does not need a gel cap for insertion.

- **Indwelling classic** (▶ Fig. 9.14): The Blom-Singer classic indwelling prosthesis comes in sterile (for surgical placement) and nonsterile (for postsurgical placement) versions. It is inserted, removed, and replaced only by a clinician. The classic indwelling comes in 16 and 20 Fr options and is available in multiple lengths. A gel cap insertion method is used to place

this prosthesis into the TEP. The esophageal flange of this prosthesis is radiopaque, allowing clinical verification of fit via X-ray. This prosthesis is thicker than the alternative indwelling options and has other design differences such as larger flanges. These promote a more secure adherence to the tracheal and esophageal sides of the tracheoesophageal wall, preventing its dislodgement. While the safety strap can remain attached to the Classic Indwelling, the prosthesis is designed so that this strap can be removed (via cutting with scissors) once secure placement is confirmed. Because of the design differences and added cost of manufacture, the Classic Indwelling is a more expensive option than non-indwelling prostheses.

- **Indwelling Advantage** (▶ Fig. 9.15): The Advantage indwelling prosthesis has a unique design element characterized by the incorporation of silver oxide into the internal valve. In theory, this extends device life through preservation of valve function because the silver oxide helps prevent the formation of biofilm on and around the valve (as described further below, biofilm is the primary cause of internal valve failure). The Advantage comes in 16 and 20 Fr options, is available in multiple lengths, and utilizes the gel cap insertion method. It is also available in two valve options: hard or soft. The hard valve has a reinforced titanium ring in the shaft and is only available in 20 Fr diameters. The Advantage is costlier than the Classic Indwelling, although one study noted that the use of an Advantage prosthesis resulted in a longer device life than use of the Classic Indwelling which, along with discontinuation of medications to prevent biofilm and reduction in the number of clinical visits, resulted in an overall lowering of healthcare costs.[40]

- **Indwelling Dual Valve** (▶ Fig. 9.16): The Dual Valve indwelling is designed with two internal valves: a primary valve

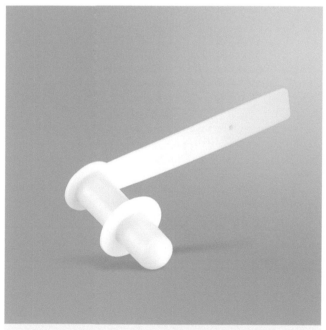

Fig. 9.13 Blom-Singer Duckbill (high pressure) voice prosthesis. (Used with permission from InHealth.)

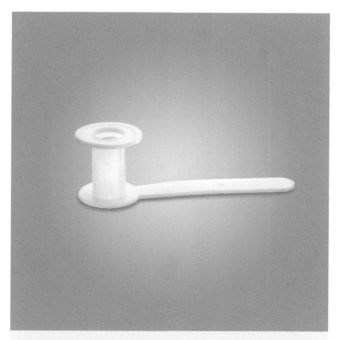

Fig. 9.14 Blom-Singer Classic Indwelling voice prosthesis. (Used with permission from InHealth.)

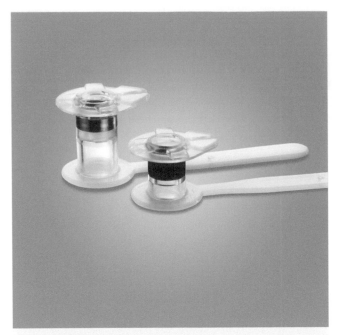

Fig. 9.15 Blom-Singer Advantage indwelling voice prosthesis. (Used with permission from InHealth.)

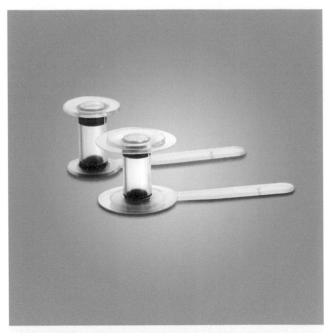

Fig. 9.16 Blom-Singer Dual Valve indwelling voice prosthesis. (Used with permission from InHealth.)

near the esophageal end of the shaft and a secondary valve near the tracheal end. This design can add life to the prosthesis and protect the patient from tracheal aspiration when the primary valve fails. The Dual Valve is available only in a 20 Fr option but comes in multiple lengths. As with all Blom-Singer prostheses other than the Duckbill, it is inserted using the gel cap method. Like the Advantage prosthesis, the Dual Valve also contains silver oxide embedded in the valves. It also shares the higher cost of the Advantage.

InHealth also provides modified prostheses to accommodate individual patient needs. These modifications include larger flanges to better prevent dislodgement, stronger valves, and varied (nonstandard) shaft lengths.

9.8.2 Atos Medical Voice Prostheses

Atos Medical produces the Provox brand of voice prostheses. These products were first made available to patients in the early 1990s and have evolved over time into four different options:

- **NID**: The Provox NID (stands for "non-indwelling") is Atos' low-pressure non-indwelling prosthesis option. The NID can be inserted and maintained by the patient (or caregiver/clinician if needed). It is available in 17 and 20 Fr options along with multiple lengths. Among the differences between this and the Blom-Singer Low Pressure prosthesis is the material and density used in valve construction. It comes with a special inserter that allows for anterograde placement. It also has a unique safety medallion designed to prevent the prosthesis from falling into the trachea. Like the Blom-Singer Low Pressure prosthesis, the NID is priced at a low to mid-range cost. Lewin et al reported

significantly longer device life of the NID compared to other non-indwelling prostheses.[41]

- **Provox 2**: The Provox 2 is the second-generation indwelling prosthesis version produced by Atos. It replaced the original Provox 1, which required a retrograde insertion method (placement through the oral cavity, into the esophagus, and then through the puncture from the esophageal side). The Provox 2 can be inserted anterograde using a special insertion tool that comes with the prosthesis. As with any indwelling prosthesis, it is inserted, removed, and replaced only by the clinician. The Provox 2 is designed as a 22.5-Fr prosthesis that is available in multiple lengths to fit the individual characteristics of the patient. In general, it is higher cost than the Blom-Singer Classic Indwelling.

- **Vega**: The Vega is the newest generation Provox indwelling prosthesis, meant to replace the Provox 2. Anterograde insertion of the Vega utilizes a unique insertion tool which comes with the prosthesis (the product comes as a kit). It is available in 17, 20, and 22.5 Fr diameter options along with multiple length choices. The internal valve is made of special material which in theory reduces biofilm development. It is higher in cost than the Provox 2, although a recent study found significantly greater device life of the Vega compared to the Provox 2 and Blom-Singer Classic Indwelling.[42]

- **Acti-Valve**: The Acti-Valve is a 22.5-Fr indwelling option designed for patients who have experienced decreased prosthesis device life due to valve failure or negative esophageal pressures which cause the valve to open during breathing and swallowing. It consists of a unique valve design incorporating magnets which prevent the valve from opening inadvertently. The magnets come in three different strengths which can be selected based on the needs of the patient. The valve mechanism needs to be lubricated on a regular basis using a proprietary lubricant provided by Atos Medical. The Acti-Valve is inserted by the clinician using an anterograde approach and comes in different lengths. It is one of the most expensive prostheses on the market. However, recent studies have demonstrated that patients utilizing the Acti-Valve experienced longer device life compared to those using other indwelling and non-indwelling prostheses.[42,43]

9.9 Assessment, Measurement, and Insertion of Voice Prostheses

The clinical process of voice prosthesis assessment, measurement, and insertion requires development of a protocol that will account for the multidimensional factors that can potentially influence patient success. ▶ Table 9.6 shows an example of the domains of inquiry and specific questions to which answers are sought during the initial stages of this process. The information obtained will help guide the patient's and clinician's decision-making processes with regard to the specific prostheses that might best meet the patient's needs.

Before seeing a patient, the clinician will need to have ready materials which will allow safe and effective prosthesis measurement and/or insertion. A recommended material setup includes the following:
- Gloves.
- Face shield.
- Disposable gown.
- Tissues and gauze.
- Hemostat.
- Straight and angled scissors (medical grade).
- Headlamp.
- Angle tip and straight forceps.
- 14-Fr catheters.
- Puncture dilator (▶ Fig. 9.17).
- Tape (which can adhere to skin).
- Puncture measurement device (▶ Fig. 9.18).

The process of measurement for the initial prosthesis generally follows the following schedule:
1. Premeasurement counseling, education, and assessment questions (▶ Table 9.6).
2. Remove catheter from puncture tract (do not discard).
3. Ask patient to produce voice with an open puncture to assess function (inhale, occlude stoma, and exhale while attempting to say "ahhhh").
4. Place measuring device into puncture to acquire length.
5. Place dilator/replace catheter into puncture.

Once the correct puncture tract length is known, the appropriate prosthesis can be selected. Some clinics maintain supplies of different prosthesis types and lengths. In these cases, the prosthesis can be inserted and tested right away. When this is not the case, the clinician must submit a prescription and order the prosthesis on behalf of the patient. The prosthesis can then be mailed (overnight if needed) to either the clinician or patient

Table 9.6 Domains and questions which can be used to guide the initial process of assessment for prosthesis placement after puncture has been created

Domain of assessment	Questions to be answered
Medical history	What preexisting conditions exists? Can these influence the patient's motor and/or cognitive abilities needed to learn TE speech?
	What operational procedures were performed? Was this a primary or secondary puncture?
	Were there any postoperative complications? Was the patient irradiated at any time?
	Any preexisting condition/comorbidity that can affect learning new tasks?
	What is the patient's current diet level?
	Does the patient require a laryngectomy tube?
Tracheostoma status	Is the skin surrounding the stoma healthy or does it appear inflamed/irregular?
	Will the topography of the stoma support peristomal housings? Is there an adequate stomal lip to support intrastromal housings?
	Is the diameter of the stoma adequate for occlusion with one of the patient's fingers?
	Is the tracheal airway clear or is it blocked with mucus and/or other debris?
	Are any abnormal tracheoesophageal fistulas, other than the puncture, visible?
TE puncture status	Is a catheter in place or was a prosthesis placed during primary TEP surgery?
	Does the orientation of the puncture allow for direct anterograde access, or has the puncture migrated to a more difficult position?
	Is there any granulation tissue or other abnormal tissue surrounding the puncture?
Current communication status	What is the current primary means of communication?
	Is the patient able to read and write?
	How legible is their handwriting?
	Do they have any visual, auditory, or fine motor hand–eye coordination deficits that may affect ability to perform tasks?
	Does the patient have an artificial electronic larynx? If so, are they skilled in its use?

Abbreviations: TE, tracheoesophageal; TEP, tracheoesophageal puncture.

(if it is not the initial prosthesis and only if it is a non-indwelling type). Prosthesis insertion generally follows the following schedule:
1. The prosthesis is prepared based on the manufacturer's instructions (e.g., gel cap system for Blom-Singer or with loading tool for Provox).

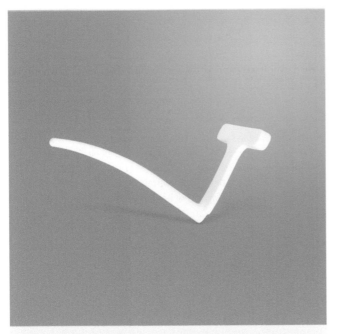

Fig. 9.17 Example of a dilator used to dilate/occlude the tracheoeso-phageal puncture during removal and replacement of a voice prosthesis. (Used with permission from InHealth.)

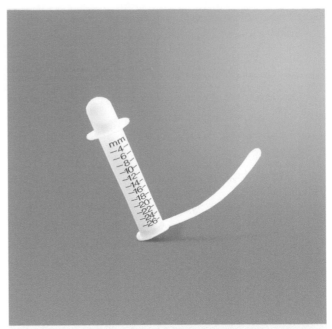

Fig. 9.18 Example of a measurement device used to measure the length of the tracheoesophageal puncture track for initial fitting and/or replacement of a voice prosthesis. (Used with permission from InHealth.)

2. The catheter or old prosthesis is removed from the puncture tract.
3. A dilator is inserted into the puncture tract (typically the tract will be dilated 2 Fr above the diameter of the prosthesis to be inserted. For example, a 22-Fr dilator would be used to prepare insertion of a 20-Fr prosthesis).
4. The dilator is removed and the prosthesis is inserted into the puncture tract based on the manufacturer's instructions.
5. Clinical checks are performed to assess whether the prosthesis is adequately seated within the puncture tract. These checks include (1) rotating the prosthesis 360 degrees—it should rotate freely within the puncture tract, and the retention flange should not kink or get stuck while the prosthesis is rotating; (2) gently tugging on the prosthesis—the clinician should feel resistance which confirms that the esophageal flange has fully extended; and (3) leak test—ask patient to swallow a small amount of green-dyed water while the clinician uses a headlamp to assess whether or not any liquid moves through the prosthesis channel or around the prosthesis on the tracheal side.
6. The clinician asks the patient to produce voice by inhaling, occluding the stoma, and exhaling while attempting to say "ahhh."

In most patients, initial voicing attempts will be successful and subsequent training to improve skills can be planned. However, some patients are unable to achieve adequate voicing during the initial prosthesis placement. The reasons for this can be multifactorial and clinical investigation will be needed to determine the actual cause(s). The following are some of the reasons for voicing difficulty at the time of initial insertion, and additional causes of voicing difficulty are provided in ▶ Table 9.7:
• Functional tension (muscular hyperfunction).
• Hypertonic UES.

• Spasmodic UES.
• Esophageal stricture.
• Posterior flange not fully seated.
• Prosthesis is too short.
• Prosthesis is too long.

9.10 Troubleshooting Tracheoesophageal Voice Prostheses

Patient factors and device characteristics (e.g., indwelling versus non-indwelling) can influence the lifespan of a voice prosthesis.[43] At some point, all voice prostheses will fail and need to be replaced. The most common cause of voice prosthesis failure is malfunction of the internal one-way valve. The most common cause of valve malfunction is the colonization of **biofilm** on and/or around the valve which interferes with how it seals the internal channel. Biofilm consists of fungal and bacterial microbes (e.g., *Candida albicans*) which migrate onto the prosthesis from oral, pharyngeal, esophageal, and potentially tracheal sites of origin. In a majority of patients, both fungal and bacterial microbes are present in the biofilm material.[44] Broad spectrum antifungal and antibacterial treatments can help extend device life for some patients who experience prosthesis failure due to biofilm formation.

When the internal valve fails, the consequence will be leakage through the internal channel of the prosthesis. The patient will first notice this because they will either cough when drinking liquids, or notice material inside the prosthesis or surrounding the tracheal side of the puncture when performing daily maintenance. In addition to biofilm formation, there are other causes of valve malfunction and many

Table 9.7 Common causes of TE speech difficulty and potential solutions to be tested during the process of troubleshooting

Problem	Solution
Leakage through middle—at the time of insertion	
Prosthesis is too short—posterior flange not fully seated and/or valve compression in tract	Remeasure to fit correct length
Prosthesis is too long—contacts posterior esophageal wall	Remeasure to fit correct length
Excessive esophageal back pressure	Prosthesis with increased valve resistance
Leakage through middle—after successful insertion	
Valve failure—biofilm growth	Replace prosthesis Consider prostheses with biofilm resistance
Valve failure—old prosthesis	Replace prosthesis
Valve stuck—mucus/bolus material	Clean/flush prosthesis
Leakage around prosthesis—at the time of insertion	
Posterior flange not fully seated	Apply inward pressure while rotating Remove and reinsert Swallow saliva to dissolve gel cap (for Blom-Singer)
Prosthesis too short	Remeasure and fit correct length
Prosthesis too long	Remeasure and fit correct length
Irregular puncture shape	Consider customized prosthesis options
Puncture dilation due to insertion trauma	Allow time for puncture to contract before subsequent leak test Consider not dilating to size larger than prosthesis
Leakage around prosthesis—after successful insertion	
Prosthesis too long—pistons within tract	Remeasure and fit correct length
Structural changes to puncture	Consider custom prosthesis Consider medical referral for puncture management
Lack of UES vibration (no sound)—at the time of insertion	
UES spasm/hypertonicity	Consider insufflation test Consider Botox/lidocaine injections Myotomy should have already been performed
Prosthesis too long	Remeasure and fit correct length
Excessive thumb/finger pressure against stoma	Patient training/education
Lack of UES vibration (no sound)—after successful insertion	
Mucus/secretion plugging prosthesis	Clean prosthesis
Posterior narrowing/closure of puncture	Dilate puncture Refer for medical management if repuncture is necessary

Abbreviations: TE, tracheoesophageal; UES, upper esophageal sphincter.

other possible causes of TE speech difficulty. The more common causes of difficulty and potential solutions are illustrated in ▸ Table 9.7.

9.11 Pulmonary Rehabilitation for the Laryngectomee

Laryngectomy results in a disconnection between the upper and lower respiratory tracts. Prior to surgery, individuals inspired air through the mouth and/or nose. This routed air past warm, moist epithelial tissue containing cilia in addition to nasal hairs. The respiratory epithelium and nasal hairs served to (1) warm, (2) humidify, and (3) filter air making its way to the lungs. This function provided a barrier to harmful microbes and pathogens which could potentially irritate the lower respiratory tissues. After surgery, this function is lost as the individual will inhale air through the stoma and directly into the trachea. However, it will still be important to maintain health of the tissues in the trachea and lungs. To replace this lost function, SLPs can implement pulmonary rehabilitation strategies to help the patient restore, maintain, and/or improve the condition of tissues in the lower respiratory tract.

At a minimum, patients should be educated and instructed on methods for filtering air inhaled through the stoma. There are multiple options for this, ranging from simple cloth coverings to commercial heat and moisture exchangers (HMEs). Filters made from fabric or other materials can filter large particles but may not be sufficient for small or microscopic particles drawn into the trachea during inspiration. In addition, these filters do not replace the humidifying and warming effects on inspired air formerly provided by the upper respiratory tract. Lower respiratory tract health is often maximized when utilizing HMEs, which act as a substitute for the loss of natural warming, humidifying, and filtering abilities and restore the cellular function of tracheal epithelium.[45,46,47] Thus, HMEs provide multidimensional benefits to the patient, which include the following:

- Increased temperature in lungs.
- Increased humidity in lungs.
- Increased respiratory resistance for improved pulmonary function.
- Reduced respiratory tract secretions and coughing.
- Improved stomal hygiene.
- Stomal HME attachments and designs can facilitate TE speech production.
- Some HME designs have side openings versus front/anterior opening for potential added protection.

▸ Fig. 9.19 illustrates an example of a commercially available HME. Some products contain treated material which inhibits the growth of microorganisms within the porous filter and improves the filtration capabilities of the HME. These products are typically replaced daily and require a stoma housing to fix the device over the stoma. Stoma housings, as illustrated in ▸ Fig. 9.20, are available in various shape and material designs. They are adhered to the skin surface surrounding the stoma. Stoma housings can also be used to connect **hands-free speaking valves** over the stoma. These valves open and close based on respiratory pressures (e.g., open during passive breathing; closed during speech production) and can incorporate HMEs into the design. When the speaking

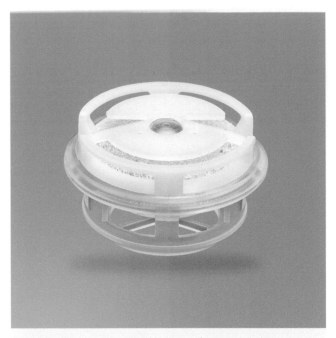

Fig. 9.19 Example of an InHealth Heat and Moisture Exchanger cartridge. A treated foam filter is located inside the housing. (Used with permission from InHealth.)

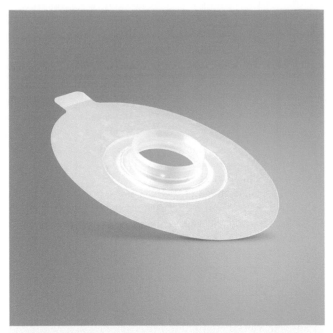

Fig. 9.20 Example of an InHealth stoma housing. (Used with permission from InHealth.)

valves close, they force air into the voice prosthesis without the need to manually occlude the stoma, freeing the hands to perform other functions while communicating.

9.12 Conclusion

The voice therapist must be prepared to address the treatment needs of those patients who have unfortunately developed laryngeal cancer. This chapter has reviewed information dealing with the nature of laryngeal cancer (common causes, sites, stages), various forms of medical treatment (e.g., chemotherapy, radiation therapy, surgical options), and the various options currently available for those who undergo complete laryngectomy to reacquire speech production. The voice therapist should be prepared to discuss the relative pros and cons of treatment options such as esophageal speech, artificial larynges, and tracheoesophageal speech with patients and their care givers so that effective and efficient communication may be achieved.

Clinical Case Study

Part 1

Mr. Spiccoli is a 58-year-old man with a history of laryngeal cancer and status-post laryngectomy approximately 12 days prior to visiting you for evaluation and placement of a voice prosthesis. He received a primary TEP, but a prosthesis was not placed at that time. He presents in the office with a 14-Fr red rubber catheter inserted through the puncture tract to maintain patency. You proceed to educate and council Mr. Spiccoli regarding the various prostheses options and their basic

function, and he decides to move forward with a Blom-Singer Low Pressure non-indwelling prosthesis.
1. Assuming your facility has this prosthesis in stock, *what materials or tools* will you need to evaluate and then fit the prosthesis?
2. List the steps you will take to appropriately measure the puncture tract length.
3. Once an accurate length has been established, what are the steps to be taken to appropriately place the prosthesis and then verify that it is seated correctly?

Part 2

Mrs. Spiccoli is able to use the Low Pressure indwelling with no apparent difficulty, and after further education is able to demonstrate understanding of appropriate care and maintenance. He leaves with a 16-Fr 10-mm prosthesis in place. Approximately 1 month later, he is back in your office complaining of leakage around the outside of the prosthesis and through the center of the prosthesis, whenever he drinks liquids.

Read the following article:

Lewin JS, Baumgart LM, Barrow MP, Hutcheson KA. Device life of the tracheoesophageal voice prosthesis revisited. JAMA Otolaryngol Head Neck Surg 2017;143(1):65–71.
1. What is the most likely cause of leakage through the middle of the prosthesis?
2. What are the possible causes of leakage around the outside of the prosthesis?
3. As this is Mr. Spiccoli's first prosthesis, are you surprised that there is leakage around the outside? Explain your answer.

9.13 Review Questions

1. Recent estimates of the number of new cases for laryngeal cancer in the United States each year is approximately
   a) 25,000.
   b) 10,200.
   c) 13,500.
   d) 108,000.
   e) None of the above.

2. In the TNM cancer staging system, what does the acronym stand for?
   a) Treatment, number, medicine.
   b) Time, name, modulus.
   c) Treatment, name, metastasis.
   d) Tumor, node, metastasis.
   e) All of the above.

3. Which treatment approach is currently more common for early-stage laryngeal cancers?
   a) Radiation.
   b) Surgery.
   c) Chemotherapy.
   d) Both a and b.
   e) None of the above.

4. Which of the following are late effects of radiation treatment?
   a) Fibrosis.
   b) Cranial nerve neuropathy.
   c) Muscle atrophy.
   d) All of the above.
   e) None of the above.

5. Which of the following sites of laryngeal cancer is less prone to spread via the lymphatic system?
   a) Glottic.
   b) Supraglottic.
   c) Subglottic.
   d) All of the above.
   e) None of the above.

6. When laryngeal cancers do not respond to initial treatment via chemoradiation or when lesions present an imminent threat and/or substantial impairment, total laryngectomy may be needed. This type of total laryngectomy is called a _____ procedure.
   a) Surgical.
   b) Salvage.
   c) Secondary.
   d) Primary.
   e) None of the above.

7. Which of the following could potentially prevent presurgical counseling when a patient is scheduled for a laryngectomy?
   a) Lack of available oncologist.
   b) Surgical need is imminent.
   c) SLP lacks knowledge.
   d) None of the above.
   e) All of the above.

8. Which of the following is a physiological change that might occur postlaryngectomy?
   a) Loss of visual acuity.
   b) Loss of sense of touch in facial region.
   c) Loss of sense of smell.
   d) Loss of auditory acuity.
   e) None of the above.

9. Why, after laryngectomy, can a patient no longer inspire air through the mouth and nose?
   a) The inspiratory muscles are weakened secondary to the surgery.
   b) The surgical swelling inhibits the flow of air through the pharyngeal region.
   c) The patient is required to be on a respirator for at least 2 weeks postsurgery.
   d) The surgery creates a separation between the upper and lower respiratory tract.
   e) None of the above.

10. Which of the following is an advantage of an electronic artificial larynx over a pneumatic artificial larynx?
    a) Hygiene issues are a minimal concern for neck/check placement.
    b) Calls attention to the speaker.
    c) Maintenance can be expensive.
    d) Requires the use of one hand.
    e) All of the above.

11. Individuals who use esophageal speech for communication vibrate which structure as a replacement for the vocal folds?
    a) Pharyngeal walls.
    b) Tongue base.
    c) Upper esophageal segment (UES).
    d) Lower esophagus.
    e) None of the above.

12. Which of the following is the least efficient method of loading air for esophageal speech production?
    a) Consonant injection.
    b) Glossopharyngeal press.
    c) Swallowing.
    d) Gulping.
    e) All of the above.

13. Mr. Jones underwent a total laryngectomy. During the surgery, the surgeon also created a fistula (hole) in the tissue separating the trachea from the esophagus. This procedure is known as what?
    a) Tracheal puncture.
    b) Esophageal fistula.
    c) Primary tracheoesophageal puncture.
    d) Secondary tracheoesophageal puncture.
    e) None of the above.

14. Which of the following is a true statement:
    a) Tracheoesophageal voice production is the least efficient form of communication postlaryngectomy.
    b) A tracheoesophageal puncture can be left open overnight to promote esophageal and tracheal hygiene.
    c) Most patients who attempt tracheoesophageal speech fail and will eventually utilize an artificial larynx or esophageal speech.
    d) All of the above.
    e) None of the above.

15. Which of the following would be an appropriate reason for patients to choose an indwelling prosthesis rather than a non-indwelling prosthesis?
    a) They have limited financial resources.
    b) Their upper limb dexterity and vision are limited.
    c) They live very close to their clinician.
    d) All of the above.
    e) None of the above.

9.14 Answers and Explanations

1. Correct: 13,500 (**c**).

   (**c**) Among all cancers laryngeal cancer is considered rare, with the estimated number of new cases in the United States in 2016 approximating 13,500. (**a, b, d**) While prevalence and incident rates related to cancers change over time due to multifactorial reasons, current estimates of laryngeal cancers are more than 10,000 new cases per year but less than 20,000 new cases.

2. Correct: Tumor, node, metastasis (**d**).

   (**d**) In the TNM system, T stands for tumor characteristics (e.g., size, growth into surrounding tissues), N stands for lymph node involvement, and M stands for metastasis (spread of cancer cells to sites distant to the origin). (**a, b, c**) In the TNM system, T stands for Tumor characteristics (e.g., size, growth into surrounding tissues), N stands for lymph node involvement, and M stands for metastasis (spread of cancer cells to sites distant to the origin).

3. Correct: Both a and b (**d**).

   (**d**) While the approach to laryngeal cancer management will be specific to the individual, current trends in the North America reveal that early-stage cancers (CIS, stages I and II) are treated most commonly with radiation therapy or surgery alone, or in combination. (**a, b, c**) Because chemotherapy and radiation therapy "preserve" laryngeal structure, the standard treatment for later stage (III or IV) laryngeal cancer is currently chemoradiation or radiation alone.

4. Correct: All of the above (**d**).

   (**d**) Acute and late radiation effects can substantially impair laryngeal function and cause voice and/or swallowing impairments due to acute and late effects. Late effects include tissue fibrosis, cranial nerve neuropathy, and muscle atrophy. (**a, b, c**) Late effects of radiation treatment include tissue fibrosis, cranial nerve neuropathy, and muscle atrophy.

5. Correct: Glottic (**a**).

   (**a**) The tissue in the region of the glottis contains relatively sparse lymphatic drainage. (**b, c, d**) The lymphatic system of the head and neck drains a large part of the laryngeal tissues, especially the supraglottic and subglottic regions (on the other hand, the glottis contains relatively sparse lymphatic drainage).

6. Correct: Salvage (**b**).

   (**b**) When late-stage laryngeal cancers do not respond to chemoradiation or when lesions present an imminent threat and/or substantial impairment, total laryngectomy (TL) may be needed as a "salvage" operation or alternative choice. (**a, c, d**) Prior to 1990, many laryngeal cancers were treated with surgery. Currently, many late-stage cancers are treated with chemoradiation as the initial management option. When this fails, "salvage" surgeries may be needed.

7. Correct: Surgical need is imminent (**b**).

   (**b**) Presurgical consultation is not always feasible for many reasons, including (1) imminent surgery is required, (2) scheduling conflicts which arise between patient and various professionals, and/or (3) unavailability of interprofessional collaborative teams. (**a, c, d**) Cancer patients will work with an oncologist to decide the course of management. SLPs who are licensed and certified, and who work with cancer patients, should demonstrate the appropriate knowledge and skills to treat this population if they are working under the professional code of ethics.

8. Correct: Loss of sense of smell (**c**).

   (**c**) The lack of air movement through the nose can cause changes in the sensitivity to smell, taste, and changes in the ability to whistle, sniff, sip, and spit. (**a, b, d**) Patients undergoing laryngectomy should not experience changes in vision, touch, or hearing compared to their presurgical status.

9. Correct: The surgery creates a separation between the upper and lower respiratory tracts (**d**).

   (**d**) Laryngectomy separates the upper from lower respiratory tract, affecting the process of negative pressure breathing. Air will flow into the lungs through the stoma, not the mouth and nose. (**A**) Muscles of inspiration are typically not affected by laryngectomy. (**b**) Although significant swelling occurs around the site of surgery and can influence postsurgical swallowing function, patients will inhale through the stoma not the mouth and nose. (**c**) Unless major surgical complications arise, patients undergoing laryngectomy do not require a respirator postsurgery.

10. Correct: Hygiene issues are a minimal concern for neck/check placement (**a**).

    (**a**) Many users of electronic artificial larynges can use a neck placement to transmit sound into the oral cavity. Pneumatic devices always require insertion of a mouthpiece. (**b, c, d**) There are disadvantages of electronic artificial larynges (EALs), which include the following: EALs produce an unnatural sound, some elements of speech are difficult to produce using the EAL (/h/ sounds, cognates), EALs call attention to the speaker, EALs require the use of one hand, maintenance can be expensive, and if it breaks, the patient is unable to communicate orally.

11. Correct: Upper esophageal segment (UES) (**c**).

    (**c**) The UES serves as a pseudoglottis during esophageal speech. Air loaded into the esophagus causes pressure below the UES which will result in oscillation. (**a, b, d**) The pharyngeal walls, tongue base, and lower esophagus do not vibrate during esophageal speech.

12. Correct: Swallowing (**c**).

    (**c**) The swallowing method of air injection is considered the least efficient due to the non-speech gesture (swallowing) that is needed to facilitate loading of air, and the amount of time required for each loading cycle. (**a, b**) Conant injection and glossopharyngeal press are two of the most efficient methods for loading air into the esophagus. (**c**) There is no loading method called "gulping."

13. Correct: Primary tracheoesophageal puncture (**c**).

    (**c**) Primary tracheoesophageal punctures are performed at the same time as the laryngectomy surgery. (**a**) Tracheal punctures are not part of the surgical procedure for creating a tracheoesophageal puncture. (**b**) An esophageal fistula would be a negative consequence of surgery. (**d**) Secondary tracheoesophageal punctures are performed at a later date than the laryngectomy.

14. Correct: None of the above (**e**).

    (**e**) No choices accurately reflect use of tracheoesophageal speech. It is the most efficient form of communication postlaryngectomy, the puncture tract must always have something inside to maintain patency, and a majority of patients who attempt tracheoesophageal speech are successful.

    (**a**) Tracheoesophageal speech is the most efficient form of communication postlaryngectomy. (**b**) A tracheoesophageal puncture must always have something inside to maintain patency—it can close up in a matter of hours. (**c**) A majority of patients who attempt tracheoesophageal speech are successful.

15. Correct: Their upper limb dexterity and vision are limited (**b**). (**b**) Daily removal and cleaning of non-indwelling prostheses requires adequate dexterity in the upper limbs in addition to adequate vision. (**a**) In general, the cost of non-indwelling prostheses is less than indwelling options. (**c**) Patients who live close to their clinical professionals typically do not have to worry about access to help in an emergency, whether they are using a non-indwelling or an indwelling prosthesis.

References

[1] American Cancer Society. Cancer Facts & Figures 2016. Atlanta: American Cancer Society; 2016

[2] Jemal A, Siegel R, Xu J, Ward E. Cancer statistics, 2010. CA Cancer J Clin. 2010; 60(5):277–300

[3] Torrente MC, Rodrigo JP, Haigentz M, Jr, et al. Human papillomavirus infections in laryngeal cancer. Head Neck. 2011; 33(4):581–586

[4] Edge S, Byrd DR, Compton CC, Fritz AG, Greene FL, Trotti A, eds. AJCC Cancer Staging Manual. New York:Springer-Verlag; 2010

[5] De Santis RJ, Poon I, Lee J, Karam I, Enepekides DJ, Higgins KM. Comparison of survival between radiation therapy and trans-oral laser microsurgery for early glottic cancer patients; a retrospective cohort study. J Otolaryngol Head Neck Surg. 2016; 45(1):42

[6] Khaja SF, Hoffman HT, Pagedar NA. Treatment and survival trends in glottic carcinoma in situ and Stage I cancer from 1988 to 2012. Ann Otol Rhinol Laryngol. 2016; 125(4):311–316

[7] Brady JS, Marchiano E, Kam D, Baredes S, Eloy JA, Park RC. Survival impact of initial therapy in patients with T1-T2 glottic squamous cell carcinoma. Otolaryngol Head Neck Surg. 2016; 155(2):257–264

[8] Kujath M, Kerr P, Myers C, et al. Functional outcomes and laryngectomy-free survival after transoral CO2 laser microsurgery for stage 1 and 2 glottic carcinoma. J Otolaryngol Head Neck Surg. 2011; 40 Suppl 1:S49–S58

[9] Sandulache VC, Kupferman ME. Transoral laser surgery for laryngeal cancer. Rambam Maimonides Med J. 2014; 5(2):e0012

[10] Fried MP, Tan M. Clinical Laryngology: The Essentials. New York: Thieme; 2015

[11] Remacle M, Van Haverbeke C, Eckel H, et al. Proposal for revision of the European Laryngological Society classification of endoscopic cordectomies. Eur Arch Otorhinolaryngol. 2007; 264(5):499–504

[12] Sperry SM, Rassekh CH, Laccourreye O, Weinstein GS. Supracricoid partial laryngectomy for primary and recurrent laryngeal cancer. JAMA Otolaryngol Head Neck Surg. 2013; 139(11):1226–1235

[13] Wolf GT, Fisher SG, Hong WK, et al. Department of Veterans Affairs Laryngeal Cancer Study Group. Induction chemotherapy plus radiation compared with surgery plus radiation in patients with advanced laryngeal cancer. N Engl J Med. 1991; 324(24):1685–1690

[14] Lefebvre JL, Rolland F, Tesselaar M, et al. EORTC Head and Neck Cancer Cooperative Group, EORTC Radiation Oncology Group. Phase 3 randomized trial on larynx preservation comparing sequential vs alternating chemotherapy and radiotherapy. J Natl Cancer Inst. 2009; 101(3):142–152

[15] Johns MM, Kolachala V, Berg E, Muller S, Creighton FX, Branski RC. Radiation fibrosis of the vocal fold: from man to mouse. Laryngoscope. 2012; 122 Suppl 5:S107–S125

[16] Wall LR, Ward EC, Cartmill B, Hill AJ. Physiological changes to the swallowing mechanism following (chemo)radiotherapy for head and neck cancer: a systematic review. Dysphagia. 2013; 28(4):481–493

[17] Birkeland AC, Rosko AJ, Issa MR, et al. Occult nodal disease prevalence and distribution in recurrent laryngeal cancer requiring salvage laryngectomy. Otolaryngol Head Neck Surg. 2016; 154(3):473–479

[18] Hoffman HT, Porter K, Karnell LH, et al. Laryngeal cancer in the United States: changes in demographics, patterns of care, and survival. Laryngoscope. 2006; 116(9, Pt 2) Suppl 111:1–13

[19] Robertson SM, Yeo JC, Dunnet C, Young D, Mackenzie K. Voice, swallowing, and quality of life after total laryngectomy: results of the west of Scotland laryngectomy audit. Head Neck. 2012; 34(1):59–65

[20] Salmon SJ, Goldstein LP. The Artificial Larynx Handbook. New York: Grune & Stratton; 1978

[21] Green G, Hults M. Preferences for three types of alaryngeal speech. J Speech Hear Disord. 1982; 47(2):141–145

[22] Ng ML, Kwok CL, Chow SF. Speech performance of adult Cantonese-speaking laryngectomees using different types of alaryngeal phonation. J Voice. 1997; 11(3):338–344

[23] Liao JS. An acoustic study of vowels produced by alaryngeal speakers in Taiwan. Am J Speech Lang Pathol. 2016; 25(4):481–492

[24] Blom ED. Approaches to treatment. In: Salmon SJ, Goldstein LP, eds. The Artificial Larynx Handbook. New York: Grune & Stratton; 1978

[25] Lauder E. Self-Help for the Laryngectomee. San Antonio, TX: Lauder Publisher; 1991

[26] Doyle PC. Foundations of Voice and Speech Rehabilitation Following Laryngeal Cancer. San Diego, CA: Singular Publishing; 1994

[27] Logemann JA. Evaluation and Treatment of Swallowing Disorders. Austin, TX: PRO-ED; 1997

[28] Gates GA, Ryan W, Cantu E, Hearne E. Current status of laryngectomee rehabilitation: II. Causes of failure. Am J Otolaryngol. 1982; 3(1):8–14

[29] Schaefer SD, Johns DF. Attaining functional esophageal speech. Arch Otolaryngol. 1982; 108(10):647–649

[30] Dantas RO, Aguiar-Ricz LN, Oliveira EC, Mello-Filho FV, Mamede RC. Influence of esophageal motility on esophageal speech of laryngectomized patients. Dysphagia. 2002; 17(2):121–125

[31] Deem JF, Miller L. Manual of Voice Therapy. Austin, TX: PRO-ED; 2000

[32] Waldrop WF, Gould MA. Your New Voice. Chicago, IL: American Cancer Society; 1956

[33] Moon S, Raffa F, Ojo R, et al. Changing trends of speech outcomes after total laryngectomy in the 21st century: a single-center study. Laryngoscope. 2014; 124(11):2508–2512

[34] Boscolo-Rizzo P, Zanetti F, Carpené S, Da Mosto MC. Long-term results with tracheoesophageal voice prosthesis: primary versus secondary TEP. Eur Arch Otorhinolaryngol. 2008; 265(1):73–77

[35] Gitomer SA, Hutcheson KA, Christianson BL, et al. Influence of timing, radiation, and reconstruction on complications and speech outcomes with tracheoesophageal puncture. Head Neck. 2016; 38(12):1765–1771

[36] Jensen KM. The Modern Laryngectomee. Malmo, Sweden: Practical SLP; 2013

[37] Callaway E, Truelson JM, Wolf GT, Thomas-Kincaid L, Cannon S. Predictive value of objective esophageal insufflation testing for acquisition of tracheoesophageal speech. Laryngoscope. 1992; 102(6):704–708

[38] Blom ED, Singer MI. Tracheoesophageal puncture prostheses. Arch Otolaryngol. 1985; 111(3):208–209

[39] Singer MI, Blom ED. An endoscopic technique for restoration of voice after laryngectomy. Ann Otol Rhinol Laryngol. 1980; 89(6, Pt 1):529–533

[40] Leder SB, Acton LM, Kmiecik J, Ganz C, Blom ED. Voice restoration with the advantage tracheoesophageal voice prosthesis. Otolaryngol Head Neck Surg. 2005; 133(5):681–684

[41] Lewin JS, Portwood MA, Wang Y, Hutcheson KA. Clinical application of the Provox NiD voice prosthesis: a longitudinal study. Laryngoscope. 2014; 124(7):1585–1591

[42] Kress P, Schäfer P, Schwerdtfeger FP, Rösler S. Are modern voice prostheses better? A lifetime comparison of 749 voice prostheses. Eur Arch Otorhinolaryngol. 2014; 271(1):133–140

[43] Lewin JS, Baumgart LM, Barrow MP, Hutcheson KA. Device life of the tracheoesophageal voice prosthesis revisited. JAMA Otolaryngol Head Neck Surg. 2017; 143(1):65–71

[44] Somogyi-Ganss E, Chambers MS, Lewin JS, Tarrand JJ, Hutcheson KA. Biofilm on the tracheoesophageal voice prosthesis: considerations for oral decontamination. Eur Arch Otorhinolaryngol. 2017; 274(1):405–413

[45] Foreman A, De Santis RJ, Sultanov F, Enepekides DJ, Higgins KM. Heat and moisture exchanger use reduces in-hospital complications following total laryngectomy: a case-control study. J Otolaryngol Head Neck Surg. 2016; 45(1):40

[46] Hilgers FJ, Aaronson NK, Ackerstaff AH, Schouwenburg PF, van Zandwikj N. The influence of a heat and moisture exchanger (HME) on the respiratory symptoms after total laryngectomy. Clin Otolaryngol Allied Sci. 1991; 16(2):152–156

[47] van den Boer C, Muller SH, van der Noort V, et al. Effects of heat and moisture exchangers on tracheal mucociliary clearance in laryngectomized patients: a multi-center case-control study. Eur Arch Otorhinolaryngol. 2015; 272(11):3439–3450

Suggested Readings

[1] Jensen KM. The Modern Laryngectomee. Malmo, Sweden: Practical SLP; 2013

[2] Kress P, Schäfer P, Schwerdtfeger FP, Rösler S. Are modern voice prostheses better? A lifetime comparison of 749 voice prostheses. Eur Arch Otorhinolaryngol. 2014; 271(1):133–140

[3] Lauder E. Self-Help for the Laryngectomee. San Antonio, TX: Lauder Publisher; 1991

[4] Lewin JS, Baumgart LM, Barrow MP, Hutcheson KA. Device life of the tracheoesophageal voice prosthesis revisited. JAMA Otolaryngol Head Neck Surg. 2017; 143(1):65–71

Index

Note: Page numbers set in **bold** or *italic* indicate headings or figures, respectively.

A

accessory nerve *17*
acoustic analysis
– amplitude 138
– autocorrelation 100
– case study *152*
– cepstral 138, *139*, 141
– cepstral, methodological considerations **140**
– condenser microphone 97, *98*
– continuous/running speech 138, 140, 142, *143*, 144, *144–145*
– decibels, averaging of **154**
– digital recording basics, *see* digital recording basics
– dominant harmonic 138
– dynamic range measurement **122**
– frequency measures **100**
– frequency weighting 119
– fundamental frequency, *see* fundamental frequency (F0)
– headset microphone calibration 120, *120*
– high-quality recordings requirements **96**
– limitations of **137**
– low/high spectral ratio **146**
– mean fundamental frequency 100
– measurements used in **99**
– microphone 97, *97*, *98*
– microphone XLR plug 97
– minimum vocal sound level/intensity 122
– modal intensity measurement **119**, 121
– mouth to microphone distance **118**
– multivariate forms of **144**
– overview 95
– period 100, *101*
– perturbation measures, *see* perturbation measures
– phantom power 97
– phonation threshold pressure (PTP) 122
– preamplifier *97*, **97**
– quality, *see* quality
– quefrency 138
– rationale **95**
– recording environment **119**
– sound level meters 118, *119*
– spectral-based 139
– vocal sound level (intensity), *see* intensity
– voice analysis software 96, *96*, *98*
– waveform matching 100
– zero-crossing 100
Acoustic Voice Quality Index (AVQI)
– CSID vs. 147
– overview 138
– principles **147**, *148*
ADSV
– cepstral analysis **140**, *143–145*
– cepstral analysis instructions **155**
aerodynamic analyses
– acoustic power 173

– aerodynamic efficiency 173
– aerodynamic power 173
– case study **179**
– equipment manufacturers **183**
– glottal efficiency 173, 175
– glottal insufficiency 162, 166
– laryngeal efficiency 173
– lung capacity 162, **162**, *163*
– MPT 174–175, **178**
– overview 161–162
– phonation and **161**
– phonation efficiency, *see* phonation efficiency
– resistance measurements 174
– s/z ratio 174, 176–177, **179**
– subglottal pressure, *see* subglottal pressure
– transglottal airflow, *see* transglottal airflow
– vital capacity, *see* vital capacity
airflow *170*, 174, 178, **179**
Aithal, V. U. 106
allergist/Immunologist 213
alpha motor neurons 2
amplitude 204
amyloidosis 46
anatomy of phonation
– alpha motor neurons 2
– arytenoid cartilages 6, *7*, 8
– connective tissues 7, *9*
– corniculate cartilages 7, *7*, 8
– cough, production of 2
– cricoid cartilage 5, *6*, 8
– cuneiform cartilages 7, *7*, 8
– diaphragm 2, *3*
– epiglottis 6, *6*, 8, *8*
– extrinsic laryngeal muscles 10, *11*, 18
– glottis 1
– hyoid bone *4*, 6
– intercostal muscles innervation 2, *4*
– intrinsic laryngeal muscles **11**, *12–13*, 18
– laryngeal adductor reflex 1, *2*
– laryngeal cartilages 8, *8*
– laryngeal framework *4*, *5–6*
– laryngeal membranes, ligaments 10
– laryngeal muscles 10, *11*, 18
– larynx evolution, roles **1**
– nasal cavity *198*
– nucleus ambiguus 2
– overview 1
– phrenic nerve 2
– pneumotaxic center 3
– pyramidal (voluntary) pathways 2
– respiration, nervous system regulation of **2**, *5*
– respiration, rates of 3
– respiratory function **2**, *3–4*
– reticular formation 3, *5*
– solitary tract nucleus 2, *2*
– thyroid cartilage *4*, 6, 8
– vagus nerve 1, *2*
anchoring bias 72
Andrade, P. A. 240
anterior commissure 5, 216
anterior gap closure pattern 205
antibiotics 220
antihistamine 220
antireflux agents 220

antitussive agents 220
arthritis 46
artificial larynx 266, *267*, **267**, *268*, 269
aryepiglottic folds 7, *9*, 10
aryepiglottic muscle 12–13, *13*, 18
arytenoid
– adduction 215
– cartilages 6, *7*, 8
– overrotation 201
– prolapse *49*, 201
– repositioning 215
arytenopexy 215
asymmetry 204
Atos Medical prostheses **276**
auditory modification 228, *228*
automatic voicing **231**
availability bias 72
Awan, S. N. 102, 106, 113, 115, 121, 127, 129, 131, 141–142, 146–147, 151, 163, 167, 172, 176–177
axonal sprouting 51

B

Backman, H. 164
bacterial/fungal infections 46
Baltopoulos, G. 164
Banh, J. 127, 129, 131
Barsties, B. 141, 164
basement membrane zone, of vocal folds 8, *10*, 37, *38*
Beckett, R. L. 171, 174, 178
Bennett, S. 102
billing, reimbursement issues 205, **205**
Blom-Singer prostheses *274*, **274**, *275–276*, *280*
Boltezar, I. H. 127, 129
Boone Voice Program for Children 247
Boone, D. R. 174, 177
botulinum toxin 50, 218
breathing
– clavicular *84*, **84**
– cycles control 244
– diaphragmatic-abdominal **83**
– thoracic **83**
Brown, W. S., Jr. 121

C

calcium hydroxylapatite 218
cancer (laryngeal), *see* carcinoma
– artificial larynx 266, *267*, **267**, *268*, 269
– Atos Medical prostheses **276**
– case study **280**
– chemoradiation 262
– chemotherapy 262
– cordectomy 263
– esophageal speech 266, **269**, *270*
– InHealth prostheses *274*, **274**, *275–276*, *280*
– laryngectomy, consequences of **263**, 266
– medical management for **260**
– metastases 262, *264*
– neck dissection 262
– overview 260, *260*
– partial laryngectomy 263
– radiation therapy 261

– risk factors 260
– stages of **261**
– supracricoid laryngectomy 263
– supraglottic laryngectomy 263
– surgical approaches 262–263
– TNM staging 261–262
– total laryngectomy 263, *265*
– tracheoesophageal puncture 263, *265*, 272, *272*, 273, *273*
– tracheoesophageal speech *265*, 266, 272, **272**, *273*
– tracheoesophageal voice prostheses *273*, **273**, *274*
– transoral laser surgery 263
– vertical laryngectomy 263
candidiasis 57
Cantarella, G. 167, 172
carcinoma, *see* cancer (laryngeal)
– clinical characteristics 46, 53, *54*, **54**
– described **54**
– supraglottic, subglottic 54
– treatment **55**
carcinoma in situ 53
Carroll, L. M. 178
Carson, C. 141
central nervous system 14, **14**
cepstral analysis
– methodological considerations **140**
– peak prominence 139, *139*, 141–142
– peak prominence, standard deviation **145**
– principles of **138**, *139*, 141
cepstral/spectral index of dysphonia
– applications of **145**
– AVQI vs. 147
– CAPE-V sentences **146**
– examples of *144–145*, **146**
– interpretation of 146
– listener-perceived severity ratings 147
– low/high spectral ratio **146**
– low/high spectral ratio standard deviation **146**
– mathematical formulas 147
– Rainbow Passage **146**
– sustained vowels **146**
– validation of 141, 147
checking action 83
chewing **231**
childhood voice issues **247**
cholinesterase inhibitors 220
chronic cough
– acute 61
– clinical characteristics **60**
– described **60**
– etiology 61
– medications causing **221**
– production of 2
– refractory 61
– subacute 61
– treatment *61*, **61**
– voice therapy 244, 245, **256**
circumlaryngeal massage 241–242
clavicular breathing *84*, **84**
closure duration 205
closure patterns caused by mass lesions 204–205
collagen 218
combination (pushback + pull-down) 241

complete closure pattern 205
compressive phase, of cough 2
confirmation bias 72
Consensus Auditory-Perceptual Evaluation of Voice (CAPE-V) scale 76, 77, 78
consonant injection 271
continuous/running speech 138, 140, 142, *143*, 144, *144–145*
conus elasticus 7, *9*, 10
cordectomy 263
corniculate cartilages 7, **7**, 8
corticosteroids, inhaled 57
cough, *see* chronic cough
counseling 228, *228*, **230**, **256**
Cox, V. O. 102
CPP, *see* cepstral peak prominence
cranial nerves 14, *14*, 15, *17*
cricoarytenoid ligament 10
cricoid cartilage 5, *6*, 8
cricothyroid
– joint 5, *6*
– ligament 7, *9*, 10
– muscles 12–13, *13*, 18
– repositioning 216, *218*
– subluxation 216, *218*
cricotracheal ligament 5, *6*, 10
CSID, *see* cepstral/spectral index of dysphonia
cuneiform cartilages 7, **7**, 8
cysts, *see* vocal fold cysts

D

Dastolfo, C. 167, 172
De Virgilio, A. 178
deafness/hearing impairment
– evaluation/diagnosis **81**, **86**
– fundamental frequency (F0) 117, **117**
– intensity **123**, 124
– perturbation 137
– voice evaluation/diagnosis **83**
decibels, averaging of **154**
decongestants 220
Deem, J. F. 127, 129, 131
deep inspiration assessment 200
deep layer of lamina propria, of vocal folds 8, *10*
Denor, S. L. 102, 106
diagnosis, *see* voice evaluation/diagnosis
diagnosis momentum 72
diaphragm 2, *3*
diaphragmatic-abdominal breathing **83**
Diercks, G. R. 141
differential pressure pneumotach *165*, *170*, **170**
digastric muscle 11, *11*, 18
digital manipulation **233**
digital recording basics
– analog-to-digital conversion **97**
– audio format **99**
– bits of resolution 99
– clipping 99, *100*
– file compression 99
– quantization **99**
– sampling rate **98**, *98*, 99
– signal amplitude, recording quality and **99**
– signal-to-noise ratio 99, *100*
diplophonia 78, 85

distributed tissue changes
– cepstral peak prominence 142
– fundamental frequency (F0) 116, 117
– intensity **123**, 124
– voice evaluation/diagnostic 80, 82, **84**, **86**
Doherty, E. T. 102, 106, 127
duration
– control, normal vs. disordered individuals **84**
– evaluation/diagnosis **83**
Dwire, A. 127
dynamic range measurement **122**
dynamic voicing assessment 200
dysarthria
– clinical characteristics 46, 52
– described **51**
– evaluation of 80
– flaccid 53
– hypokinetic 52
– Lewy bodies, Lewy neurites 52
– spastic 52
– subtypes **52**
– treatment 52
dysphonia, *see* voice therapy
– adductor spasmodic 111, *111*, 135, *135*, 138
– case study **206**
– cepstral/spectral index of **145**
– characterization 74
– defined 1, 71
– disruption type, severity ratings **75**
– ICD-10 codes 190
– patient, effects on **74**
– physiology **227**
– reversal **227**
– SOVT exercises 240
– spasmodic, surgical options 213
– treatment approach **227**
– vocal hyperfunction/hypofunction 227
Dysphonia Severity Index (DSI)
– evaluation of 151, **151**
– in nondysphonic, dysphonic voice 151
– principles of **151**
dysphonic physiology reversal (DPR) **227**, *229*
dysplasia 53
dyspnea 3
dystonic movements, assessment of 202

E

Eckel, F. C. 174, 177
edema, inflammation
– assessment **44**, 200
– clinical characteristics 31, **43**, *44*
– described **43**
– etiology **43**
– ICD-10 codes 190
– medications causing **221**
– polypoid changes 43
– treatment **44**
edematous polyp, *see* vocal fold pseudocysts
education, identification 244, 249, **256**
electrolarynx 267, **267**, *268*, 269
EMG testing 213
endocrinologist 213
endoscopy, *see* stroboscopy

– anesthetic **190**
– certification, licensure 188, **189**
– competencies **189**, **209**
– endoscopes 186, *186*, **190**, 192, **192**, *193*
– light source **194**
– medical diagnoses **189**, 190
– overview 186
– rationale for **191**
– scope of practice **187**, 190
– vibratory dynamics **202**
epiglottis 6, *6*, 8
episodic laryngeal breathing disorders 244
erythema 43
erythema/hypervascularity assessment 200, *200–201*
erythroleukoplakia 53, *54*
erythroplakia 53, *53*
esophageal speech 266, **269**, *270*
essential voice tremor
– assessment of 202
– BTX injections 219
– clinical characteristics 46, **51**
– described **51**
– etiology **51**
– evaluation of 81
– physiologic 51
– treatment **51**
estimated mean flow rate (eMFR) 171
eupnea 3
evaluation, *see* voice evaluation/diagnostic
expectorants 220
expulsive phase, of cough 2
extrinsic laryngeal muscles **10**, *11*, 18

F

facial nerve 15, *17*
false vocal folds 7, *9*
fat injection 218
Fendel, D. M. 127, 129, 131
Fendler, M. 177
Finger, L. S. 127, 129, 131
Fisher, H. B. 106, 127
Fitch, J. L. 102
flow phonation **233**, *234*
French scale 273
Frenkel, M. L. 131
frequency 77
– *See also* fundamental frequency (F0)
– acoustic measures **100**
– highest phonational frequency 112–113
– mean fundamental frequency 100
– musical note/frequency equivalents 112
frontal resonance treatment
– characteristics of **235**
– generalization 237
– principles of **235**
– vibrotactile energy location 236
– voice expansion 236
Fu, S. 167, 172
functional aphonia/dysphonia, *see* psychogenic dysphonia/aphonia
functional dysphonia, *see* muscle tension dysphonia
fundamental frequency (F0), *see* specific disorders
– adulthood, senescence 101, 105, *115*, **115**

– blurred images 204
– coefficient of variation **101**, 106
– coefficient of variation, in Praat **105**, *108–110*
– control physiology 19, *20*
– deafness/hearing impairment 117, **117**
– detection of 194
– distributed tissue change **116**, 117
– gender differences 115, *115*
– highest phonational frequency 112–113
– in voice-disordered persons **116**
– infancy, childhood 101, 105, **114**
– intonation capability 101
– mass lesions **116**, 117
– mean speaking **101**, 102
– mean speaking, in Praat **105**, *108–110*
– measures of 100, **100**, *101*
– measures, limitations of **118**
– mucosal wave 204
– musical note/frequency equivalents 112
– neurological disorders **116**, 117
– normalization of 104
– pitch sigma **101**, 106
– pitch stability 101
– psychological disorders 117, **117**
– puberty **114**
– race, possible effect of **116**
– standard deviation **101**, 106
– standard deviation, in Praat **105**, *108–110*
– sustained vowels 104–105, *105*, 110, *110*, 111, *111*
– total phonational frequency range **111**, 113
– total phonational frequency range, in Praat **113**, *114*
– vocal training effects on **116**
fundoplication 57
fungal infections, *see* bacterial/fungal infections

G

gastroenterology 212
Gelfer, M. P. 102, 106, 127, 129, 131
Gelfoam 218
geniohyoid muscle 11, *11*, 18
Gilbert, H. R. 102
Gillespie, A. I. 167, 172
glossopharyngeal nerve *17*
glossopharyngeal press 271
glottal adduction exercises **232**
glottal attack exercises 233
glycerine 218
Golden Rule of voice therapy 191, 211
Goy, H. 102, 121, 127, 129, 131, 151, 176
Gramuglia, A. C. 176
granulomas, *see* vocal process granulomas
GRBASI scale 76

H

habilitation 225
habitual loudness 82
habitual pitch **77**, *78*, 80
Hakkesteegt, M. M. 151

half-swallow boom 233
Hallin, A. E. 113, 121
hands-free speaking valves 279
harmonics-to-noise ratio 125, **128**, 131, 137, **137**
Hartl, D. M. 167, 172
Hema, N. 106
Heman-Ackah, Y. D. 141
highest phonational frequency 112–113
Hirano, M. 171, 178
Holbrook, A. 102
Hollien, H. 102, 106, 113
Holmberg, E. B. 167, 172
Honjo, I. 102
Horii, Y. 102, 106, 127, 129
hourglass closure pattern 205
Hudson, A. I. 102
humming 230
hyaluronic acid 218
hydration 229–230
hyoepiglottic ligament 6, 8, 10
hyoid bone **4**, 6
hyoid pulldown 241
hyperfunctional voice
– cepstral peak prominence 142
– evaluation of **80**, 83, **83**, **86**
– facilitative approaches **230**
– fundamental frequency (F0) 117, **117**
– intensity **123**, 124
– perturbation 137
hypoglossal nerve 15, 17

I

ICD-10 codes 190
immobility of vocal folds, see vocal fold paralysis/paresis
impedance matching 239
incomplete closure pattern 205
indwelling advantage prostheses 275, 276
indwelling classic prostheses 275, 275
indwelling dual valve prostheses 275, 276
indwelling prosthesis 273, 273
inertive reactance 239
inflammation, see edema, inflammation
inhalation method 271
InHealth prostheses **274**, **274**, 275–276, 280
injection augmentation 217–219
inspiratory phase, of cough 2
insufflation test 273
insurance 206
intensity, see loudness
– adults/senescent adults, values 121, **122**
– aging effects **122**
– control, physiology 20, **20**
– deafness/hearing impairment **123**, 124
– distributed tissue changes **123**, 124
– frequency weighting 119
– gender differences 122
– in voice-disordered subjects **123**
– infancy/children, values 121, **122**
– mass lesions **123**, 124
– measurement, considerations in **118**
– measures in normal subjects **122**

– modal intensity measurement **119**, 121
– modal, measurement of **119**, 121
– mouth to microphone distance **118**
– neurological disorders **123**, 124
– psychological disorders **123**, 124
– puberty, values **122**
– race effects on **123**
– recording environment **119**
– sound intensity level 118
– sound level meters **118**, 119
– sound pressure level 118
– vocal training effects **123**
interarytenoid muscle 12–13, 18
intermediate layer of lamina propria, of vocal folds 8, 10
intrinsic laryngeal muscles 18
inverse square law 118
irregular closure pattern 205
Isshiki, N. 102
Iwata, S. 178
Izadi, F. 102

J

Jackson, B. 102, 106, 113
jitter 125, **126**, 127, 136–137, **137**
jitter factor 126
jitter ratio 126
Joshi, A. 178

K

Kapsner-Smith, M. R. 240
Karnell, M. P. 127
Kent, R. D. 102, 127, 129, 131
knowledge enhancement 229

L

lamina densa, of vocal folds 37, 38
lamina lucida, of vocal folds 37, 38
Larson, G. W. 177
laryngeal adductor reflex 1, 2
laryngeal cancer, see carcinoma
laryngeal diadochokinesis assessment 200
laryngeal dystonia, see spasmodic dysphonia
laryngeal framework surgery 215
laryngeal manual therapy 242
laryngeal papillomatosis
– clinical characteristics 46, 56, **56**
– described **56**
– treatment **56**
laryngeal pushback 240–241
laryngeal reposturing 240
laryngeal stenosis 46
laryngeal trauma 73
laryngeal ventricle 8, 9
laryngeal vestibule 7, 9
laryngeal web
– acquired 58
– clinical characteristics 46, 58, **58**
– congenital 58, 58
– described **58**
– pediatric 58
– treatment **58**
laryngectomy
– communication options, postsurgery 266–267
– consequences of **263**, 266

– partial 263
– pulmonary rehabilitation **279**, 280
– supracricoid 263
– supraglottic 263
– total 263, 265
– tracheal stoma creation 265, 266
– tubes 272, 273
– vertical 263
laryngitis
– clinical characteristics 46, **57**
– described **57**
– etiology **57**, 73
– ICD-10 codes 190
– infections 57, 58
– medications 57
– treatment **57**
laryngocele 46, **58**
laryngologists 211
laryngomalacia **22**, 46, **58**, 59
laryngopharyngeal reflux 57, 74
laryngoplasty 215, **216–217**
laryngoscopes 192, 212
laryngoscopy 186, 191, 212
– See also endoscopy, stroboscopy
laryngoscopy, procedural technique **194**
larynx
– anteroposterior compression assessment 202
– artificial 266, 267, **267**, 268, 269
– cartilages 8, 8
– discolored plaques assessment 54, 201
– evolution, roles **1**
– excessive mucous assessment 40, 200
– extrinsic muscles **10**, **11**, 18
– framework **4**, 5–6
– intrinsic muscles **11**, 12–13, 18
– membranes, ligaments 10
– muscle innervation 18
– muscles **10**, **11**, 18
– tissue color assessment 200, 200
laser resection 215
lateral cricoarytenoid muscle 12–13, 13, 18
lateral cricothyroid ligament 7, 9, 10
lateral thyrohyoid ligament 5, 10
Lee Silverman Voice Treatment (LSVT-LOUD) 52, 123, **243**
Leino, T. 176, 178
Lessac-Madsen Resonant Voice Therapy (LMRVT) 235
leukoplakia 53, 53
Liang, F. Y. 167, 172
lingWaves 96, 96
Linville, S. E. 106, 113, 121, 127
loudness, see intensity
– evaluation/diagnosis **81**
– habitual loudness 81, **81**, 82
– instability 81
– normal vs. disordered individuals **82**
– range **82**
– variability **81**, 82
Lowell, S. Y. 141
Ludlow, C. L. 127, 129
Lundy, D. S. 176, 178
lung capacity 162, **162**, 163
Lycke, H. 113, 121

M

Ma, E. P. 113, 122, 167, 172

manual circumlaryngeal therapy **240**
Martin, D. 127, 129
Maslan, J. 176
mass lesions
– closure patterns caused by 205
– exophytic 201, 203
– fundamental frequency (F0) **116**, 117
– intensity **123**, 124
– irregular medial edge 201, 203
– resection, cold instruments 213
– subglottal pressure and 166
– voice evaluation/diagnostic **80**, **82**, **84**, **86**
Mathieson, L. 242
McCauley, R. 127
McGlone, J. 102
McGlone, R. E. 102
McMullan, P. M. 178
mean fundamental frequency 100
medialization thyroplasty 215–216, 216–217
median cricothyroid ligament 7, 9, 10
median thyrohyoid ligament 5, 10
Mendes Tavares, E. L. 177
microflap dissection 213
microlaryngoscopy 213, 214
modal intensity measurement **119**, 121
Modern Singing Handicap Index 246
modified voice rest 219
Mohseni, R. 176
Moran, M. J. 102
Morris, R. J. 102, 106, 113, 121
movement observations 201
MPT 174–175, **178**
mucosa-drying medications **220**
mucosal wave 204
Mueller, P. B. 102, 106, 177
Multi-Speech 96, 96
Murry, T. 102, 106, 127
muscle tension dysphonia
– case study **249**
– cepstral peak prominence 142
– clinical characteristics 31, **34**, **34**
– described **30**
– etiology **30**
– evaluation of **80**, 83, **83**, **86**
– fundamental frequency (F0) 117, **117**
– hard glottal attacks 34
– intensity **123**, 124
– manual circumlaryngeal therapy **240**
– perturbation 137–138
– primary vs. secondary 30
– psychological processes and **35**
– Trait Theory 35
– treatment **35**
– vegetative voicing **231**
– ventricular phonation 34
muscular process, of arytenoid cartilages 6
muscularis muscle 12–13, 18
musculoskeletal modification 228, 228
mutational falsetto
– cepstral peak prominence 142
– clinical characteristics 31, **37**
– described **36**
– etiology **36**
– evaluation of **80**
– fundamental frequency (F0) 117, **117**

– treatment **37**
mylohyoid muscle 11, *11*, 18

N

nasal cavity anatomy *198*
nasoendoscopes, *see* under endoscopy
Nawka, T. 176
Nemr, K. 176
neurological disorders
– cepstral peak prominence 142
– evaluation/diagnosis **80**
– fundamental frequency (F0) **116**
– intensity **123**
neurologist 213
neurology of phonation
– central nervous system 14, **14**
– corticobulbar tract 14, *14*
– corticospinal tract 14, *14*
– cranial nerves 14, *14*, 15, *17*
– extrapyramidal pathway 14
– laryngeal muscles innervation 18
– motor plans, programs 14, *16*
– peripheral nervous system **15**, *17*
– pyramidal pathway 14
– upper motor neurons 14
– voicing 14, *16*
nodules, *see* vocal fold nodules
non-indwelling duckbill prostheses 275, *275*
non-indwelling low pressure prostheses 274, *274*
non-indwelling prosthesis 273, *273*
nonkeratinized stratified squamous epithelium, of vocal folds 8, *10*
normal vs. disordered individuals **85**
NSAIDs 220
nucleus ambiguus 2
Nyquist Theorem 98

O

oculomotor nerve *17*
office-based phonosurgery 216
olfactory nerve *17*
omohyoid muscle 11, *11*, 18
Omori, K. 127, 129
oncologist 212
open (relaxed) throat breathing 244–
   245
optic nerve *17*
Orlikoff, R. F. 106, 127, 129, 131
otolaryngology office examination
– debriefing **212**
– diagnosis **212**
– imaging 212
– laryngeal visualization **212**
– patient history **211**
– patient questionnaires **211**
– physical examination **212**
– referral **212**

P

pachydermia 57
papilloma, *see* laryngeal papillomatosis
paradoxical vocal fold movement
– clinical characteristics **60**
– described **60**
– treatment **60**, 244
Parker, P. A. 177
partial laryngectomy 263

pedagogy 228, *228*, **229**
Pedersen, M. F. 102, 113
PENTAX Medical Phonatory Aerodynamic System *165*, **171**
period-doubling 133–134, *135*
period-tripling 134, *135*
periodicity 204
peripheral nervous system **15**, *17*
perturbation measures
– age effects **136**
– general expectations 137
– in aphonia 135, *136*
– in normal/typical subjects **136**
– in Praat **131**, *132–135*
– in severe dysphonia 135, *135*
– in voice-disordered persons **136**
– methodological considerations
   in 137
– principles of **124**
– race effects **136**
Petrović-Lazić, M. 106
pharmaceutical management 220, **220**
pharmaceutical management
   ADRs **220**
pharyngo-esophageal segment 269,
   270
phase relationships 204
phonation efficiency
– described 162
– intrinsic laryngeal muscles **11**, *12–
   13*
– laryngeal impairment sensitivity **175**
– measurement considerations **175**
– measurement methods **175**
– normal vs. dysphonic speakers 176,
   176, 177–178
phonation quotient **170**
phonation resistance training exercises
   (PhoRTE) **243**
phonation threshold pressure
   (PtP) 166
phonetogram, *see* Voice Range Profile
phonomicrosurgery 213, *214*
phonomicrosurgery, voice recovery 219, **219**
phonoscopy, phonoscopic examination 186
phonosurgery 213
phonosurgery, office-based 216
phonotrauma **37**, 226
phonotraumatic behaviors elimination 249
phrenic nerve 2
physiological balance 249
physiological reactions awareness 244
physiological subsystems rebalancing 249
physiology of phonation
– Bernoulli effect 19–20
– cover-body theory 15
– elastic recoil 20
– flow vortices 15, 20
– fundamental frequency control **19**,
   20
– inertive reactance 19
– intraglottal pressure gradient 15
– medial compression 15, 20
– musical timbre 21
– myoelastic-aerodynamic theory of
   phonation 19
– processes **15**, *19*, 20
– recoil force 19

– source-filter theory 21
– supraglottal resonance **20**, *21–22*
– sustained phonation 19
– tracheal pull 20
– transglottal airflow 15, *19*, 20
– vertical phase difference 15, *19*
– vocal intensity control 20, **20**
– voice quality **20**, *21–22*
piano/synthesizer keyboard notes *246*
Piccioni, P. 164
Pistelli, F. 164
pitch
– break 78
– evaluation/diagnosis **77**
– glide assessment 200
– habitual pitch **77**, *78*, 80
– instability 79
– normal vs. disordered patients **79**
– range 79
– sigma **101**, 106
– stability 101
– total pitch range **79**
– variability 78, *79*
pneumotach-based systems **171**
pneumotachograph masks 165, *165*,
   168, *169*
polypoid degeneration, corditis 43, *44*
polyps, *see* vocal fold polyps
posterior cricoarytenoid muscle 12–
   13, *13*, 18
posterior gap closure pattern 205
postnasal drip 74
Praat
– cepstral analysis **140**
– cepstral analysis instructions **155**
– mean F0, standard deviation, coefficient of variation *96*, *98*, **105**, *108–
   110*
– overview 96
– perturbation measures **131**, *132–
   135*
– total phonational frequency
   range *113*, *114*
premalignant lesions
– clinical characteristics 46, *53*, **53**, *54*
– described **53**
– treatment **54**
premature closure 72
presbylaryngis
– cepstral peak prominence 142
– clinical characteristics 46, **55**, *56*
– described **55**
– glottal incompetence 55, *56*
– treatment **55**
presbyphonia, *see* presbylaryngis
professional voice users 29, 74, **245**,
   246
progressive relaxation 244
prostheses
– assessment of 277, **277**
– Atos Medical **276**
– Blom-Singer 274, **274**, *275–276*, 280
– case study **280**
– insertion of **277**
– measurement of 277, *278*
– tracheoesophageal voice 273, **273**,
   274
– troubleshooting 278, **278**, 279
Provox prostheses **276**
pseudocysts, *see* vocal fold pseudocysts
pseudosupraglottic swallow 233
psychogenic dysphonia/aphonia
– clinical characteristics 31, **36**

– described **35**
– etiology **36**
– treatment **36**
puberphonia, *see* mutational falsetto
push/pull exercises 232

Q

quadrangular membrane 7, *9*, 10
quality
– acoustic analysis correlates *124*, **124**,
   125
– amplitude modulation 133
– breathiness 132, *133*, 136
– cycle-to-cycle variations 125
– evaluation/diagnosis **85**
– harmonics 124, *125*
– harmonics-to-noise ratio 125, **128**,
   131, 137, **137**
– interharmonic peaks 134, *134*
– jitter 125, **126**, 136–137, **137**
– shimmer 125, **126**, 129, *129*, 136–
   137, **137**
quick sniff through the nose followed
   by /i/ assessment 200
quiet breathing assessment 200

R

Radiesse voice gel 218
Ramig, L. A. 102, 113, 129
Rau, D. 171, 174, 178
recurrent laryngeal nerve 15
regularity 204
rehabilitation 225
Reinke's edema 40, 43, *44*, 110, *110*
Reinke's space, of vocal folds 8, *10*
relative amplitude perturbation jitter 126
relative average perturbation
   shimmer 126
resonant focus **230**
Resonant Voice Therapy (RVT) 235
respiration, regulation of *2*, *5*
respiratory epithelium 7, *9*
respiratory health 229–230
respiratory modification 228, *228*
Ringel, R. L. 102, 113, 129
Rosen, C. A. 167
Rosenthal, A. L. 141, 167, 172
roughness 134, *134*
Roy, N. 138, 240
Ryan, W. J. 121

S

s/z ratio 174, 176–177, **179**
Sandoughdar, N. 176
scar, *see* vocal fold scar
Scarpino, S. 106
Scherer, R. C. 127, 129, 131
selective laryngeal adductor denervation–reinnervation surgery 213
Selent, M. 102
semioccluded vocal tract therapy **239**,
   241, **255**
Shearer, W. M. 177
shimmer 125, **126**, 129, *129*, 136–137,
   137
Shipp, T. 102, 106
short-term instability 125
Silastic implant 215, *217*

silicone–polydimethylsiloxane 218
Singing Voice Handicap Index 246
singing voice specialists 225
Siupsinskiene, N. 113, 121
slow vital capacity 163
smoking 80, 110, *110*
Smolej Narancić, C. N. 164
solitary tract nucleus 2, *2*
somatosensory modification 228, *228*
Sorenson, D. N. 177
spasmodic dysphonia
– abductor **50**
– adductor **50**
– clinical characteristics 46, **50**
– described **50**
– etiology **50**
– treatment **50**
SPEAK OUT! 52, **243**
spectral tilt 146
SpeechTool 96, *96*
spindle (elliptical) gap closure pattern 205
spirometry **163**
Stemple, J. C. 127
sternohyoid muscle 11, *11*, 18
sternothyroid muscle 11, *11*, 18
steroids 220
stiffness 204
Stoicheff, M. L. 102, 106
strap muscles 10, *11*
stretch-and-flow (SnF) therapy **233**, *234*, 247
stroboscopy, *see* endoscopy
– adverse events 199
– anesthetic **190**
– certification, licensure 188, **189**
– clinician position **195**
– competencies **189**, **209**
– domains of observation *200*, **200**, *201–203*
– endoscope handling *196*, **196**, *197*
– endoscope insertion (flexible) *198*, **198**, *199*
– endoscope insertion (rigid) **197**
– evaluation protocol **199**
– FAQs **187**
– greeting, history **194**
– instrumentation *191*, **191**
– light source **194**
– medical diagnoses **189**, 190
– observations, interpretation of **199**
– overview 186
– patient position **195**, *196*
– positioning, endoscope technique **195**, *196*
– preevaluation **194**
– principles of **187**, *188–189*
– procedural technique **194**
– procedure explanation **195**
– rationale for **191**
– scope of practice **187**, 190
– vibratory dynamics **202**
– vocal tasks **199**
stylohyoid muscle 11, *11*, 18
subglottal pressure
– described 162, **164**, *165*
– laryngeal impairments sensitivity **166**, 167
– measurement considerations **166**
– measurement methods *168*, **168**, *169*
– normal vs. dysphonic speakers 167, **169**

sulcus, *see* vocal fold sulcus
superficial layer of lamina propria, of vocal folds 8, *10*, 37, *38*
superior laryngeal nerve 15
supracricoid laryngectomy 263
supraglottic laryngectomy 263
surgical injury, iatrogenic 73
sustained vowels 126, 132, *132*, 133, *133*, 200
swallowing method 271
symmetry 204

T

Tait, N. A. 177
Tan, W. C. 164
Teflon 218
thoracic breathing **83**
thyroarytenoid muscle 12, *12*
thyroepiglottic ligament 6, *8*, 10
thyroepiglottic muscle 12–13, *13*, 18
thyrohyoid membrane 5, 10
thyrohyoid muscle 11, *11*, 18
thyroid cartilage advancement 216
thyroid notch 5
thyroid prominence (Adam's Apple) 5, 20
thyroidectomy 48
thyroplasty 215–216, *216–217*
Titze, I. R. 239–240
tongue advancement **231**
total laryngectomy 263, *265*
total phonational frequency range **111**, 113
total phonational frequency range, in Praat **113**, *114*
total voice rest 219
tracheoesophageal puncture 263, *265*, *272*, **272**, *273*, *273*
tracheoesophageal speech *265*, 266, *272*, **272**, *273*
tracheoesophageal voice prostheses *273*, **273**, *274*
transgender voice issues **246**
transglottal airflow
– defined 162, **170**
– differential pressure pneumotach *165*, **170**, *170*
– estimated mean flow rate (eMFR) 171
– laryngeal impairments sensitivity **171**
– measurement considerations 162, **171**
– measurement methods **171**
– measurement of *165*, **170**
– normal vs. dysphonic speakers 172, **173**
– phonation quotient **170**, 174, 178, **179**
– pneumotach-based systems *170*, **171**
transoral laser surgery 263
trigeminal nerve 15, *17*
trochlear nerve *17*

U

U=P/R formula 170

V

vagus nerve 1, *2*, 3, 15, *17–18*
vascular injury
– capillary lakes 44
– clinical characteristics 31, **44**
– described 44, *45*
– ectasias 44, *45*
– etiology **44**
– hemorrhage 44, *45*
– spider telangiectasias 44
– treatment **45**
– varices 44, *45*
VC/MPT formula 170
vegetative vocalization 226
vegetative voicing **231**
ventricular (thyroventricularis) muscle 12–13, *13*
ventricular folds 7, *9*, 202
ventricular ligaments 7, *9*, 10
vertical laryngectomy 263
Vertigan, A. E. 245
vestibular folds 7, *9*
vestibular ligament 10
vibratory dynamics **202**
video endoscopes 192
vital capacity
– defined 162, *163*
– laryngeal impairments sensitivity **163**
– measuring **163**
– values in healthy populations *163*, 164
vocal cord dysfunction, *see* paradoxical vocal fold movement
vocal efficiency 162
vocal fold
– atrophy, bowing 201, *203*
– bowing 55, *56*
– closure patterns caused by mass lesions 205
– cover, anatomy 8, *10*
– edema 43, *44*
– hemorrhage 44, *45*
– histology **8**, *10*
– injections 217
– nonvibrating segments 205
– reduced elongation 201
– vertical level difference 205
– vibratory dynamics **202**
vocal fold cysts
– clinical characteristics 31, **41**, *42*, 46, **55**
– described 41, **55**
– epidermoid 41
– etiology **41**
– mucous retention 41
– treatment **42**
vocal fold nodules
– case study 90
– clinical characteristics 31, **39**
– described 37, *38–39*
– etiology **37**
– ICD-10 codes 190
– in children 247
– sustained vowels *111*
– treatment **39**
vocal fold paralysis/paresis
– abductor/adductor 45
– assessment of 201
– bilateral abductor/adductor **49**
– case study **62**, **221**
– clinical characteristics 46, **48**

– described **45**
– etiology 47, **48**
– ICD-10 codes 190
– SLN 45, **49**
– treatment **49**
– unilateral abductor/adductor 48, **48**, *49*
vocal fold polyps
– case study **90**, **152**
– clinical characteristics 31, **40**, *40*
– described 39
– edematous 40
– etiology **39**
– ICD-10 codes 190
– pedunculated 40
– sessile 40
– treatment **40**
vocal fold pseudocysts
– clinical characteristics 31, **41**
– described 40
– etiology **40**, *41*
– treatment **41**
vocal fold scars 46, **59**
vocal fold sulcus
– clinical characteristics 46, **59**
– physiological 59
– sulcus vergeture 59
– sulcus vocalis 59
– treatment **60**
vocal function exercises 52
– compliance (adherence) 239
– contract 238
– glottal incompetence 239
– goal setting 239
– low vocal intensity 237
– power 238
– principles of **237**, *238*
– resonant focus 238
– stretch 238
– tracking schedule 239
– warm-up 237
vocal function modification 228
vocal habits 229–230
vocal hygiene **229**, 230, 249, **256**
vocal impairment, *see* voice disorders
vocal irritants 230
vocal ligament, of vocal folds 8, 10, *10*
vocal process granulomas
– clinical characteristics 31, **42**, *43*, 46, **55**
– described **42**
– etiology **42**, 55
– ICD-10 codes 190
– treatment **43**
vocal process, of arytenoid cartilages 6
vocal sound level, *see* intensity
vocal tremor 78
vocalis muscle 8, *10*, 12–13, 18
vocologists, voice therapists 225
Vogel, A. P. 141
voice analysis software *96*, **96**, *98*
voice disorders, *see* specific disorders
– classifications **29**
– disability 29
– dysphonia 28
– etiology 29
– functional **29**, 74
– functional, clinical characteristics **30**, 31
– handicap 29
– hyperfunctional 29
– ICD-10 codes 190
– idiopathic **30**, **60**

– impairment 29
– mild 28
– moderate 28
– muscle misuse 29
– nonorganic 29
– organic 30, 45, **45**, 46
– organic, neurological subtypes **45**
– overview 28
– pharmaceutical management 220, **220**
– prevalence 29
– psychogenic 29
– psychological **80**, **83**
– severe 28
– surgical management **213**, *214*
– vocal abuse, misuse 37
– vocal hyperfunction 29
– voice care team 211
voice evaluation/diagnosis
– age-related changes 79
– assessment vs. evaluation vs. diagnosis **69**
– auditory-perceptual evaluation **75**, *86*
– breathiness **85**
– case history content **72**
– characteristics, terminology **77**
– clavicular breathing *84*, **84**
– considerations **71**
– deafness, hearing impairment **81**, **83**, **86**
– definitions 69
– development of problem **73**
– diaphragmatic-abdominal breathing 83
– disruption type, severity ratings **75**
– distributed tissue change **80**, **82**, **84**, **86**
– duration **83**
– duration control, normal vs. disordered individuals **84**
– equal-appearing interval scales 76, **76**, *78*, *79*

– error in 72
– etiologies, possible **75**
– expiratory/phonatory function coordination testing 83
– gender differences 79
– habitual loudness *81*, **81**, 82
– habitual pitch **77**, *78*, 80
– handicap, self-perception of **87**
– harshness **85**
– health status **75**
– hoarseness **85**
– instability **85**, *86*
– loudness **81**
– loudness instability 81
– loudness range **82**
– loudness variability **81**, *82*
– loudness, normal vs. disordered individuals **82**
– mass lesions **80**, **82**, **84**, **86**
– monoloudness 81
– monopitch 78
– nature of problem **72**
– neurological disturbance **80**, **82**, **84**, **86**
– organization of **69**, *70*
– patient, dysphonia effects on **74**
– perceptual, limitations of **87**
– phonation breaks 81
– pitch **77**
– pitch break 78
– pitch instability 79
– pitch range 79
– pitch variability 78, *79*
– pitch, normal vs. disordered patients **79**
– preevaluation information **71**
– prognosis 74
– protocol *70*, 71, **71**
– psychological disorders **80**, **83**
– quality **85**
– quality of life/handicap scales role **87**

– quality, normal vs. disordered individuals **85**
– reduced respiratory capacities **84**
– roughness **85**
– shakiness 78
– strain **85**
– thoracic breathing **83**
– total pitch range **79**
– usage description **74**
– variability vs. consistency **74**
– visual analog scales **76**, *77*, *78*
voice habilitation/rehabilitation 225
Voice Handicap Index (VHI) 87, *88–89*
Voice Range Profile
– elicitation procedures **149**, *150*
– evaluation of **150**, 151
– principles of **148**, *149*
– studies of 149
voice therapy, *see* specific modalities
– childhood voice issues **247**
– chronic cough **244**, 245, **256**
– digital manipulation **233**
– direct interventions (comprehensive) **233**, **242**
– direct interventions (facilitative) 228, **230**, **232**
– dysphonic physiology reversal **227**, *229*
– eclectic **227**
– etiologic **226**
– hygienic **226**
– indirect interventions 228, **229**
– method of delivery 228, *228*
– organizational framework for *228*, **228**, *229*
– orientations 226
– overview 225
– physiologic **226**
– psychogenic **226**
– rationale 226
– symptomatic **226**
– terminology 225–226
– transgender voice issues **246**

voice treatment programs
– comprehensive **233**
– eclectic 233
– frontal resonance treatment **235**
– goal setting **248**
– long-term goals **248**
– manual circumlaryngeal therapy **240**
– physiological 233
– semioccluded vocal tract **239**, *241*, **255**
– short-term goals **248**
– stretch-and-flow **233**, *234*, 247
– tracking log **255**
– vocal function exercises **237**, *238*
voice tremor, *see* essential voice tremor
voicing 14, *16*
von Leden, H. 178

W

Walton, J. H. 127, 129, 131
Wang, C. C. 178
Watts, C. R. 141, 178
Weinrich, B. 164, 167
whispering 220
Wolfe, V. 106, 127, 129, 131
Wuyts, F. L. 122, 151–152

Y

Yiu, E. M. 167, 172
Yumoto, E. 131

Z

Zheng, Y. Q. 167, 172
Zhuge, P. 176
Ziegler, A. 243
Zraick, R. I. 101, 164, 167, 172–173
Zwirner, P. 127, 129, 131